COMMON ABBREVIATIONS USED IN THE TEXT

2D	two-dimensional
3D	three-dimensional
4D	four-dimensional
A2C	apical two chamber
A4C	apical four chamber
AAR	area at risk
ABI	ankle-brachial index
ACC	American College of Cardiology
ACEI	angiotensin-converting enzyme inhibitor
ACR	American College of Radiology
ACS	acute coronary syndrome
ADP	adenosine diphosphate
AF	atrial fibrillation
AHA	American Heart Association
AMI	acute myocardial infarction
APMHR	age-predicted maximal heart rate
ARVC	arrhythmogenic right ventricular cardiomyopathy
AS	aortic stenosis
ASD	atrial septal defect
ASL	arterial spin labeling
ATP	adenosine triphosphate
AUC	appropriate use criteria; area under the curve
BMI	body mass index
BOLD	blood-oxygen-level–dependent
BP	blood pressure
BSA	body surface area
bSSFP	balanced steady-state free precession
C	carbon
CABG	coronary artery bypass graft
CAD	coronary artery disease
CAV	coronary allograft vasculopathy
CE	contrast enhanced
CFR	coronary flow reserve
CHD	congenital heart disease
CI	confidence interval
CIED	cardiac implantable electronic device
CK	creatine kinase
CKD	chronic kidney disease
CMR	cardiovascular magnetic resonance
CMRS	cardiovascular magnetic resonance spectroscopy
CNR	contrast-to-noise ratio
CoV	coefficient of variation
Cr	creatinine
CRT	cardiac resynchronization therapy
CS	compressed sensing
CSA	cross-sectional area
CSPAMM	complementary spatial modulation of magnetization
CT	computed tomography
CTO	chronic total occlusion
CVA	cerebrovascular attack
DBP	diastolic blood pressure
DCM	dilated cardiomyopathy
DCMR	dobutamine stress cardiovascular magnetic resonance
DENSE	displacement encoding with stimulated echoes
DIR	double inversion recovery
DSA	digital subtraction angiography
DSE	dobutamine stress echocardiography
DTI	diffusion tensor imaging
DTPA	diethylenetriamine pentaacetic acid
DUS	doppler ultrasound
DWI	diffusion weighted imaging
EAM	electroanatomic map
ECG	electrocardiogram
ECV	extracellular volume
ED	end diastole
EDV(I)	end-diastolic volume (index)
EF	ejection fraction
EGE	early gadolinium enhancement
eGFR	estimated glomerular filtration rate
EMB	endomyocardial biopsy
EPI	echo planar imaging
ESC	European Society of Cardiology
ESV(I)	end-systolic volume (index)
FDA	US Food and Drug Administration
FDG	fluorodeoxyglucose
FFR	fractional flow reserve
FHS	Framingham Heart Study
FID	free induction decay
FLASH	fast low angle shot
fMRI	functional magnetic resonance imaging
FOV	field of view
FPP	first-pass perfusion
FSE	fast spin echo
FT	feature tracking; Fourier transform
FWHM	full width at half maximum
GBCA	gadolinium-based contrast agent
Gd	gadolinium
GRAPPA	generalized autocalibrating partially parallel acquisition
GRE	gradient recalled echo
HARP	harmonic phase
HASTE	half-Fourier single-shot turbo spin echo
HCM	hypertrophic cardiomyopathy
HDL	high-density lipoprotein
HF	heart failure
HFpEF	heart failure with preserved ejection fraction
HFrEF	heart failure with reduced ejection fraction
HIP	high-intensity plaque
HLA	horizontal long axis
HOCM	hypertrophic obstructive cardiomyopathy
HR	heart rate
ICC	intraclass correlation coefficient
ICD	implantable cardioverter-defibrillator
ICM	ischemic cardiomyopathy
IHD	ischemic heart disease
IPH	intraplaque hemorrhage
IQR	interquartile range
IR	inversion recovery
IVUS	intravascular ultrasound
LA	left atrial; left atrium
LAD	left anterior descending (coronary artery)
LCX	left circumflex (coronary artery)
LDL	low-density lipoprotein
LGE	late gadolinium enhancement
LV	left ventricle; left ventricular

LVEDVP	left ventricular end-diastolic pressure		**Qs**	systemic flow
LVEF	left ventricular ejection fraction		**RA**	right atrial; right atrium
LVNC	left ventricular noncompaction		**RARE**	rapid acquisition with relaxation enhancement
LVOT	left ventricular outflow tract		**RCA**	right coronary artery
MACE	major adverse cardiac event		**RF**	radiofrequency
MAP	mean arterial pressure		**ROC**	receiver operator characteristic; receiver operator curve
MAPSE	mitral annular plane systolic excursion		**ROI**	region of interest
MBF	myocardial blood flow		**RPP**	rate pressure product
MBV	myocardial blood volume		**RV**	right ventricle; right ventricular
MDCT	multidetector computed tomography		**RVED(I)**	right ventricular end-diastolic volume (index)
MESA	Multiethnic Study of Atherosclerosis		**RVEF**	right ventricular ejection fraction
MI	myocardial infarction		**RVOT**	right ventricular outflow tract
MIP	maximal intensity projection		**RVSP**	right ventricular systolic pressure
MMP	metalloproteinases		**SAR**	specific absorption rate
Mn	manganese		**SAX**	short axis
MOCO	motion corrected		**SBP**	systolic blood pressure
MOLLI	modified Look-Locker inversion recovery		**SCMR**	Society for Cardiovascular Magnetic Resonance
MPO	myeloperoxidase		**SD**	standard deviation
MPR	multiplanar reconstruction/reformatting; myocardial perfusion reserve		**SEE**	standard error of the estimate
MR	magnetic resonance		**SENSE**	sensitivity encoding
MRA	magnetic resonance angiography		**ShMOLLI**	shortened modified Look-Locker inversion recovery
MRI	magnetic resonance imaging		**SI**	signal intensity
MRS	magnetic resonance spectroscopy		**SNR**	signal-to-noise ratio
MT	magnetization transfer		**SPAMM**	spatial modulation of magnetization
MTC	magnetization transfer contrast		**SPECT**	single-photon emission computed tomography
MVD	microvascular disease		**SSFP**	steady-state free precession
MVO	microvascular obstruction		**STEAM**	stimulated echo acquisition mode
MVO$_2$	myocardial oxygen consumption		**STEMI**	ST elevation myocardial infarction
MVP	mitral valve prolapse		**STIR**	short-inversion time inversion recovery
MVR	mass/volume ratio		**STS**	Surgical Thoracic Society
NHLBI	National Heart, Lung, and Blood Institute		**SVC**	superior vena cava
NSF	nephrogenic systemic fibrosis		**SV(I)**	stroke volume (index)
NSTEMI	non–ST elevation myocardial infarction		**SVR**	systemic vascular resistance
NYHA	New York Heart Association		**T**	Tesla
OR	odds ratio		**T1W**	T1 weighted
P	phosphorus		**T2W**	T2 weighted
PAD	peripheral arterial disease		**TD**	delay time
PCA	phase contrast angiography; principal component analysis		**TE**	echo time
PCI	percutaneous coronary intervention		**TEE**	transesophageal echocardiography
PCMR	phase contrast magnetic resonance		**TFE**	turbo field echo
PCr	phosphocreatine		**TGA**	transposition of the great arteries
PDA	patent ductus arteriosus; posterior descending artery		**TI**	inversion time
PDW	proton-density weighted		**TIA**	transient ischemic attack
PET	positron emission tomography		**TOF**	tetralogy of Fallot
PLAX	parasternal long axis		**TR**	repetition time
PMR	plaque:myocardial signal ratio		**TSE**	turbo spin echo
POC	point of care		**TTC**	triphenyltetrazolium chloride
PPM	permanent pacemaker		**TTE**	transthoracic echocardiography
PSAX	parasternal short axis		**USPIO**	ultrasmall superparamagnetic particles of iron oxide
PSIR	phase-sensitive inversion recovery		**VCAM**	vascular cell adhesion molecule
PWV	pulse wave velocity		**VENC**	velocity encoded
QALY	quality-adjusted life year		**VF**	ventricular fibrillation
QCA	quantitative coronary angiography		**VSD**	ventricular septal defect
Qp	pulmonary flow		**VT**	ventricular tachycardia
			XMR	combined x-ray cardiac magnetic resonance laboratories

CARDIOVASCULAR MAGNETIC RESONANCE

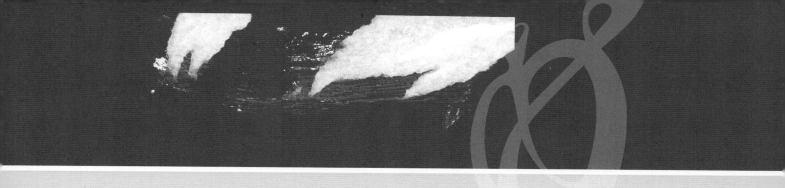

CARDIOVASCULAR MAGNETIC RESONANCE

A COMPANION TO **BRAUNWALD'S HEART DISEASE**

THIRD EDITION

WARREN J. MANNING, MD, FACC, FACP, FAHA, FISMRM, FSCMR
Professor of Medicine and Radiology
Harvard Medical School
Section Chief, Non-invasive Cardiac Imaging and Testing
Cardiovascular Division
Beth Israel Deaconess Medical Center
Boston, Massachusetts

DUDLEY J. PENNELL, MD, FRCP, FACC, FESC, FAHA, FRCR, FMedSci, FSCMR
Professor of Cardiology
National Heart and Lung Institute
Imperial College London;
Director, Cardiovascular Magnetic Resonance Unit
Royal Brompton Hospital
London, United Kingdom

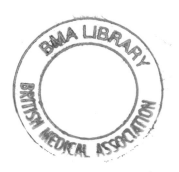
ELSEVIER

ELSEVIER

1600 John F. Kennedy Blvd.
Ste 1800
Philadelphia, PA 19103-2899

Notices

Knowledge and best practice in this field are constantly changing. As new research and experience broaden
our understanding, changes in research methods, professional practices, or medical treatment may become
necessary.

Practitioners and researchers must always rely on their own experience and knowledge in evaluating and
using any information, methods, compounds, or experiments described herein. In using such information
or methods they should be mindful of their own safety and the safety of others, including parties for
whom they have a professional responsibility.

With respect to any drug or pharmaceutical products identified, readers are advised to check the most
current information provided (i) on procedures featured or (ii) by the manufacturer of each product to be
administered, to verify the recommended dose or formula, the method and duration of administration,
and contraindications. It is the responsibility of practitioners, relying on their own experience and
knowledge of their patients, to make diagnoses, to determine dosages and the best treatment for each
individual patient, and to take all appropriate safety precautions.

To the fullest extent of the law, neither the Publisher nor the authors, contributors, or editors, assume
any liability for any injury and/or damage to persons or property as a matter of products liability,
negligence or otherwise, or from any use or operation of any methods, products, instructions, or ideas
contained in the material herein.

Previous editions copyrighted 2010 and 2002.

Library of Congress Cataloging-in-Publication Data

Names: Manning, Warren J., 1957- editor. | Pennell, Dudley J., 1958- editor.
Title: Cardiovascular magnetic resonance : a companion to Braunwald's heart disease / [edited by] Warren J.
    Manning, Dudley J. Pennell.
Other titles: Cardiovascular magnetic resonance (Manning) | Complemented by (expression): Braunwald's
    heart disease. 11th edition.
Description: Third edition. | Philadelphia, PA : Elsevier, [2019] | Complemented by: Braunwald's heart disease /
    edited by Douglas P. Zipes, Peter Libby, Robert O. Bonow, Douglas L. Mann, and Gordon F. Tomaselli. 11th
    ed. 2018. | Includes bibliographical references and index.
Identifiers: LCCN 2018006374 | ISBN 9780323415613 (hardcover : alk. paper)
Subjects: | MESH: Cardiovascular Diseases–diagnosis | Magnetic Resonance Imaging–methods | Diagnostic
    Techniques, Cardiovascular
Classification: LCC RC683.5.M35 | NLM WG 141.5.M2 | DDC 616.1/207548–dc23 LC record available at
    https://lccn.loc.gov/2018006374

Executive Content Strategist: Robin Carter
Senior Content Development Specialist: Jennifer Ehlers
Publishing Services Manager: Catherine Jackson
Book Production Specialist: Kristine Feeherty
Design Direction: Renee Duenow

Printed in China

Last digit is the print number: 9   8   7   6   5   4   3   2   1

Working together
to grow libraries in
developing countries

www.elsevier.com • www.bookaid.org

To the joys, inspirations, and blessings of my life—
mom and dad, Susan Gail, Anya and Elie, Sara
and Jeremy, Isaac, Raziel, and JJ.

—WJM

To the memory of my parents, Terence and Joan;
the love of my wife, Elisabeth;
and the joy of my daughter, Indigo.

—DJP

CONTRIBUTORS

Mehmet Akçakaya, PhD
Department of Electrical and Computer Engineering
Center for Magnetic Resonance Research
University of Minnesota
Minneapolis, Minnesota

Francisco Alpendurada, MD, PhD
Consultant
CMR Unit, Royal Brompton Hospital
London, United Kingdom

Evan Appelbaum, MD
Department of Medicine
Cardiovascular Division
Beth Israel Deaconess Medical Center
Harvard Medical School
Boston, Massachusetts

Andrew Arai, MD
Chief, Advanced Cardiovascular Imaging Laboratory
National Institutes of Health
National Heart, Lung, and Blood Institute
Bethesda, Maryland

Dominique Auger, MD, PhD
Adjunct Professor of Medicine
Cardiology
Centre Hospitalier de l'Université de Montréal;
Associate Professor of Medicine
McGill University Health Center
Montreal, Quebec, Canada

Robert S. Balaban, PhD
Scientific Director, NHLBI
Laboratory of Cardiac Energetics
National Heart, Lung, and Blood Institute
National Institutes of Health
Bethesda, Maryland

Jeroen J. Bax, MD, PhD
Professor of Cardiology
Department of Cardiology
Leiden University Medical Center
Leiden, The Netherlands

Nicholas G. Bellenger, MD
Consultant Cardiologist
Royal Devon and Exeter Hospital
Exeter, United Kingdom

David A. Bluemke, MD, PhD
Department of Radiology
School of Medicine and Public Health
University of Wisconsin-Madison
Madison, Wisconsin

René M. Botnar, PhD
Division of Imaging Sciences and Biomedical Engineering
King's College London
London, United Kingdom

Craig Ronald Butler, MD, MSc
Associate Professor of Medicine
Division of Cardiology
University of Alberta
Edmonton, Alberta, Canada

Peter Caravan, PhD
A.A. Martinos Center for Biomedical Imaging
Massachusetts General Hospital
Boston, Massachusetts

Csilla Celeng, MD, PhD
Department of Radiology
University Medical Center Utrecht
Utrecht, The Netherlands

Michael L. Chuang, MD, ScM
Cardiovascular Imaging Core Laboratory
Beth Israel Deaconess Medical Center
Boston, Massachusetts

Albert de Roos, MD, PhD
Professor of Radiology
Department of Radiology
Leiden University Medical Center
Leiden, The Netherlands

Victoria Delgado, MD, PhD
Consultant Cardiologist
Department of Cardiology
Leiden University Medical Center
Leiden, The Netherlands

Rohan Dharmakumar, PhD
Cedars-Sinai Medical Center
University of California
Los Angeles, California

Marc R. Dweck, MD, PhD
Translational and Molecular Imaging Institute
Zena and Michael A. Wiener Cardiovascular Institute
Icahn School of Medicine at Mount Sinai
New York, New York;
Centre for Cardiovascular Science
University of Edinburgh
Edinburgh, United Kingdom

Afshin Farzaneh-Far, MD, PhD
Section of Cardiology
Department of Medicine
University of Illinois at Chicago
Chicago, Illinois;
Department of Medicine
Division of Cardiology
Duke University
Durham, North Carolina

Zahi A. Fayad, PhD
Translational and Molecular Imaging Institute
Zena and Michael A. Wiener Cardiovascular Institute
Icahn School of Medicine at Mount Sinai
New York, New York

David Firmin, PhD
Director of Physics
CMR Unit
Royal Brompton Hospital
Professor of Biomedical Imaging
National Heart and Lung Institute
Imperial College London
London, United Kingdom

Mark A. Fogel, MD, FACC, FAHA, FAAP, FNASCI
Professor of Pediatrics (Cardiology) and Radiology
The Perelman School of Medicine at the University of Pennsylvania
Director of Cardiac Magnetic Resonance
The Children's Hospital of Philadelphia
Philadelphia, Pennsylvania

Herbert Frank, MD
Professor of Internal Medicine
Director, Department of Internal Medicine
University Hospital Tulln and Medical University of Vienna
Tulln, Austria

Matthias G. Friedrich, MD
Professor of Medicine and Diagnostic Radiology
McGill University;
Adjunct Professor of Radiology
Université de Montréal
Montreal, Quebec, Canada;
Professor of Medicine
Heidelberg University
Heidelberg, Germany;
Adjunct Professor
Cardiac Sciences and Radiology
University of Calgary
Calgary, Alberta, Canada

Eric M. Gale, PhD
Assistant Professor in Radiology
A.A. Martinos Center for Biomedical Imaging
Massachusetts General Hospital
Boston, Massachusetts

Tal Geva, MD
Cardiologist-in-Chief
Department of Cardiology
Boston Children's Hospital
Professor of Pediatrics
Harvard Medical School
Boston, Massachusetts

John D. Grizzard, MD
Department of Radiology
VCU Health Systems
Richmond, Virginia

Brian P. Halliday, MBChB (Hons), MRCP
BHF Clinical Research Fellow
National Heart and Lung Institute
Imperial College London;
Clinical Research Fellow
Cardiovascular Magnetic Resonance Unit and Cardiovascular
    Research Centre
Royal Brompton and Harefield NHS Trust
London, United Kingdom

Michael Hansen, PhD
Investigator
National Heart, Lung, and Blood Institute
National Institutes of Health
Bethesda, Maryland

Thomas H. Hauser, MD, MMSc
Director of Nuclear Cardiology
Beth Israel Deaconess Medical Center
Assistant Professor of Medicine
Harvard Medical School
Boston, Massachusetts

Susie N. Hong, MD, MSc
Assistant Professor
Department of Medicine
Division of Cardiovascular Medicine
Assistant Professor
Department of Diagnostic Radiology and Nuclear Medicine
University of Maryland Medical Center
Baltimore, Maryland

Till Huelnhagen, Dipl.-Ing.
Berlin Ultrahigh Field Facility (B.U.F.F.)
Max-Delbrueck Center for Molecular Medicine in the Helmholtz
    Association
Berlin, Germany

W. Gregory Hundley, MD
Department of Internal Medicine (Cardiology Section)
Department of Radiology
Wake Forest University School of Medicine
Winston-Salem, North Carolina

El-Sayed H. Ibrahim, PhD
Medical College of Wisconsin
Milwaukee, Wisconsin

Esra Gucuk Ipek, MD
Department of Medicine
Section for Cardiac Electrophysiology
Johns Hopkins University School of Medicine
Baltimore, Maryland

Michael Jerosch-Herold, PhD
Department of Radiology
Brigham and Women's Hospital and Harvard Medical School
Boston, Massachusetts

Robert M. Judd, PhD
Duke Cardiovascular Magnetic Resonance Center
Duke University Medical Center
Durham, North Carolina

Jennifer Keegan, PhD
Principal Physicist
Cardiovascular Research Centre
Royal Brompton Hospital
Adjunct Reader
National Heart and Lung Institute
Imperial College London
London, United Kingdom

Peter Kellman, PhD
Staff Scientist
National Heart, Lung, and Blood Institute
National Institutes of Health
Bethesda, Maryland

Muhammad Shahzeb Khan, MD
Department of Internal Medicine
John H. Stroger Jr. Hospital of Cook County
Chicago, Illinois

Faisal Khosa, MD, MBA, FFRRCSI, FRCPC, DABR
Assistant Professor
Department of Radiology
Vancouver General Hospital
Vancouver, British Columbia, Canada

Kiran Khurshid, MBBS, MD
Research Fellow
Department of Radiology
Vancouver General Hospital
Vancouver, British Columbia, Canada

Philip J. Kilner, MD
Consultant, CMR Unit
Royal Brompton Hospital
London, United Kingdom

Daniel H. Kim, MD
Professor of Medicine
Department of Medicine
Division of Cardiology
University of Alberta
Edmonton, Alberta, Canada

Raymond J. Kim, MD
Duke Cardiovascular Magnetic Resonance Center
Duke University Medical Center
Durham, North Carolina

W. Yong Kim, PhD
Department of Cardiology
Aarhus University Hospital
Aarhus, Denmark

Christopher M. Kramer, MD
Ruth C. Heede Professor of Cardiology
Professor of Radiology
University of Virginia Health System
Charlottesville, Virginia

Eric V. Krieger, MD
Associate Professor of Medicine
Department of Medicine
Division of Cardiology
University of Washington School of Medicine
University of Washington Medical Center
Seattle Children's Hospital
Seattle, Washington

Raymond Y. Kwong, MD, MPH
Department of Medicine
Cardiovascular Division
Brigham and Women's Hospital
Harvard Medical School
Boston, Massachusetts

Jay S. Leb, MD
Assistant Professor
Department of Radiology
Columbia University Medical Center
New York, New York

Robert Lederman, MD
Cardiovascular Branch
Division of Intramural Research
National Heart, Lung, and Blood Institute
National Institutes of Health
Bethesda, Maryland

Tim Leiner, MD, PhD, EBCR
Professor of Radiology
Department of Radiology
University Medical Center Utrecht
Utrecht, The Netherlands

Debiao Li, PhD
Cedars-Sinai Medical Center
University of California
Los Angeles, California

David Lopez, MD
Heart and Vascular Institute
Cleveland Clinic
Weston, Florida

Alicia M. Maceira, MD, PhD, FESC
Director, Cardiovascular Imaging Unit
ERESA Medical Center
Valencia, Spain

Heiko Mahrholdt, MD
Department of Cardiology
Robert-Bosch-Krankenhaus
Stuttgart, Germany

Marcus R. Makowski, MD
Department of Radiology
The Charité
Berlin, Germany

Warren J. Manning, MD, FACC, FACP, FAHA, FISMRM
Professor of Medicine and Radiology
Harvard Medical School
Section Chief, Non-invasive Cardiac Imaging and Testing
Cardiovascular Division
Beth Israel Deaconess Medical Center
Boston, Massachusetts

Constantin B. Marcu, MD
Associate Professor of Cardiology
Director of Advanced Cardiac Imaging and Imaging Education
Cardiovascular Sciences
Brody School of Medicine at East Carolina
Greenville, North Carolina

Martin S. Maron, MD
Hypertrophic Cardiomyopathy Center
Division of Cardiology
Tufts Medical Center
Boston, Massachusetts;
Chanin T. Mast Center for Hypertrophic Cardiomyopathy
Morristown Medical Center
Morristown, New Jersey

Raad H. Mohiaddin, MD
Professor of Cardiovascular Imaging
Royal Brompton Hospital and Harefield NHS Trust
National Heart and Lung Institute
Imperial College London
London, United Kingdom

James C. Moon, MD, MRCP
Professor
Institute of Cardiovascular Science
University College London
Advanced Cardiac Imaging
Barts Heart Centre
London, United Kingdom

Manish Motwani, MB, ChB, PhD
Consultant Cardiologist
Manchester Heart Centre
Manchester University NHS Foundation Trust
Manchester, United Kingdom

Shiro Nakamori, MD, PhD
Postdoctoral Research Fellow
Harvard Medical School
Department of Medicine
Cardiovascular Division
Beth Israel Deaconess Medical Center
Boston, Massachusetts

Saman Nazarian, MD, PhD
Associate Professor of Medicine
Cardiac Electrophysiology
University of Pennsylvania Perelman School of Medicine
Philadelphia, Pennsylvania

Felix Nensa, MD
Department of Diagnostic and Interventional Radiology and
    Neuroradiology
University Hospital Essen
Essen, Germany

Stefan Neubauer, MD, FRCP, FACC, FMedSci
Professor of Cardiovascular Medicine
Head, Division of Cardiovascular Medicine
Director, Oxford Centre for Clinical Magnetic Resonance Research
Division of Cardiovascular Medicine
Radcliffe Department of Medicine
University of Oxford
John Radcliffe Hospital
Oxford, United Kingdom

Reza Nezafat, PhD
Department of Medicine
Cardiovascular Division
Beth Israel Deaconess Medical Center
Harvard Medical School
Boston, Massachusetts

Christoph A. Nienaber, MD, PhD
Royal Brompton & Harefield Hospital NHS Foundation Trust/
    Imperial College
Cardiology and Aortic Centre
London, United Kingdom

Thoralf Niendorf, PhD
Berlin Ultrahigh Field Facility (B.U.F.F.)
Max Delbrueck Center for Molecular Medicine in the Helmholtz
    Association
DZHK (German Centre for Cardiovascular Research) Partner Site
MRI.TOOLS GmbH
Berlin, Germany

Sara L. Partington, MD
Assistant Professor of Clinical Medicine
Philadelphia Adult Congenital Heart Disease Center
The Hospital of the University of Pennsylvania and the Children's
    Hospital of Philadelphia
Perelman Center for Advanced Medicine
Philadelphia, Pennsylvania

Ian Paterson, MD
Department of Medicine
Division of Cardiology
University of Alberta
Edmonton, Alberta, Canada

Katharina Paul, PhD
Berlin Ultrahigh Field Facility (B.U.F.F.)
Max-Delbrueck Center for Molecular Medicine in the Helmholtz
    Association
Berlin, Germany

Dudley J. Pennell, MD, FRCP, FACC, FESC, FAHA, FRCR, FMedSci
Professor of Cardiology
National Heart and Lung Institute
Imperial College London;
Director, Cardiovascular Magnetic Resonance Unit
Royal Brompton Hospital
London, United Kingdom

Ronald M. Peshock, MD
Professor of Internal Medicine and Radiology
Vice Chair of Information Technology
University of Texas Southwestern Medical Center
Dallas, Texas

Dana C. Peters, PhD
Magnetic Resonance Research Center
Associate Professor of Radiology and Biomedical Imaging
Yale University
New Haven, Connecticut

R. Nils Planken, MD, PhD, EBCR
Department of Radiology and Nuclear Medicine
Academic Medical Center
Amsterdam, The Netherlands

Sven Plein, MD, PhD
Professor of Cardiology
British Heart Foundation Professor of Cardiovascular Imaging
Honorary Consultant Cardiologist
Division of Biomedical Imaging
Leeds Institute of Cardiovascular and Metabolic Medicine
    (LICAMM)
University of Leeds
Leeds, United Kingdom

Andrew J. Powell, MD
Chief, Cardiac Imaging Division
Department of Cardiology
Boston Children's Hospital
Associate Professor of Pediatrics
Harvard Medical School
Boston, Massachusetts

Sanjay Prasad, MD, FRCP, FESC
Consultant Cardiologist
CMR Unit
Royal Brompton Hospital
Honorary Senior Lecturer
Cardiovascular Biomedical Research Unit
Royal Brompton Hospital and Imperial College London
London, United Kingdom

Claudia Prieto, PhD
School of Biomedical Engineering and Imaging Sciences
King's College London
St Thomas' Hospital
London, United Kingdom

Kuberan Pushparajah, BMBS, BMedSci, MD(Res)
Consultant Paediatric Cardiologist
Paediatric Cardiology
Evelina London Children's Hospital;
Clinical Senior Lecturer
Division of Imaging Sciences and Biomedical Engineering
King's College London
London, United Kingdom

Imran Rashid, MBBS, PhD
School of Biomedical Engineering and Imaging Sciences
King's College London
St Thomas' Hospital
London, United Kingdom

Reza S. Razavi, MD
Professor, Paediatric Cardiovascular Science
School of Biomedical Engineering and Imaging Sciences
King's College London;
Consultant Paediatric Cardiologist
Evelina London Children's Hospital
London, United Kingdom

Wolfgang G. Rehwald, PhD
Duke Cardiovascular Magnetic Resonance Center
Siemens Healthineers
Durham, North Carolina

Philip M. Robson, PhD
Translational and Molecular Imaging Institute
Zena and Michael A. Wiener Cardiovascular Institute
Icahn School of Medicine at Mount Sinai
New York, New York

Christopher T. Rodgers, MChem, DPhil
Associate Professor of Biomedical Imaging
Division of Cardiovascular Medicine
Radcliffe Department of Medicine
University of Oxford
John Radcliffe Hospital
Oxford, United Kingdom

Toby Rogers, BM BCh, PhD
Cardiovascular Branch
Division of Intramural Research
National Heart, Lung, and Blood Institute
National Institutes of Health
Bethesda, Maryland

Ethan J. Rowin, MD
Hypertrophic Cardiomyopathy Center
Division of Cardiology
Tufts Medical Center
Boston, Massachusetts;
Chanin T. Mast Center for Hypertrophic Cardiomyopathy
Morristown Medical Center
Morristown, New Jersey

James H.F. Rudd, MD, PhD
Division of Cardiovascular Medicine
University of Cambridge
Cambridge, United Kingdom

Hajime Sakuma, MD, PhD
Professor and Chairman of Radiology
Mie University Hospital
Mie University Graduate School/Faculty of Medicine
Mie, Japan

Michael Salerno, MD, PhD
Associate Professor
Departments of Medicine and Radiology
University of Virginia Health System
Charlottesville, Virginia

Thomas Schlosser, MD
Professor
Institute of Diagnostic and Interventional Radiology and
    Neuroradiology
University Hospital Essen
Essen, Germany

Juerg Schwitter, MD
Professor
Cardiovascular Department
Division of Cardiology
Director, Cardiac MR Center of the CHUV
University Hospital Lausanne, CHUV
Lausanne, Switzerland

Udo P. Sechtem, MD
Chairman, Department of Cardiology
Robert-Bosch-Krankenhaus
Stuttgart, Germany;
Associate Professor of Medicine and Cardiology
University of Tubingen
Tubingen, Germany

R. Brandon Stacey, MD, MS
Department of Internal Medicine (Cardiology Section)
Wake Forest University School of Medicine
Winston-Salem, North Carolina

Matthias Stuber, PhD
University of Lausanne
Lausanne, Switzerland

Teresa Sykora, MD
Consultant
Department of Internal Medicine
University Hospital Tulln and Medical University of Vienna
Tulln, Austria

Upasana Tayal, BMBCh, MRCP
MRC Clinical Research Fellow
National Heart and Lung Institute
Imperial College London
London, United Kingdom

Anneline S.J.M. te Riele, MD, PhD
Department of Medicine
Division of Cardiology
University Medical Center Utrecht
Netherlands Heart Institute
Utrecht, The Netherlands

Thomas A. Treibel, PhD
Professor
Institute of Cardiovascular Science
University College London
Advanced Cardiac Imaging
Barts Heart Centre
London, United Kingdom

Sotirios A. Tsaftaris, PhD
University of Edinburgh
Edinburgh, United Kingdom

Anne Marie Valente, MD
Associate Professor, Pediatrics and Internal Medicine
Harvard Medical School;
Staff Cardiologist, Pediatric Cardiology
Children's Hospital Boston;
Staff Cardiologist, Internal Medicine
Division of Cardiology
Brigham and Women's Hospital
Boston, Massachusetts

Harrie van den Bosch, MD
Department of Radiology
Catharina Hospital
Eindhoven, The Netherlands

Pieter van der Bijl, MB, ChB, MMed
Research Fellow
Department of Cardiology
Leiden University Medical Center
Leiden, The Netherlands

Albert C. van Rossum, MD, PhD
Chair, Department of Cardiology
VU University Medical Center
Amsterdam, The Netherlands

David C. Wendell, PhD
Duke Cardiovascular Magnetic Resonance Center
Duke University Medical Center
Durham, North Carolina

Jos J.M. Westenberg, PhD
Associate Professor
Department of Radiology
Leiden University Medical Center
Leiden, The Netherlands

Mark A. Westwood, MA, MD, FRCP
Consultant Cardiologist
Department of Cardiology
Barts Heart Centre
London, United Kingdom

Norbert Wilke, MD
Department of Radiology
Krankenhaus St. Anna
Höchstadt an der Aisch, Germany

Lukas Winter, R.rer.nat, Dipl.-Ing
Berlin Ultrahigh Field Facility (B.U.F.F.)
Max-Delbrueck Center for Molecular Medicine in the Helmholtz
    Association
Berlin, Germany

Hsin-Jung Yang, PhD
Cedars-Sinai Medical Center
University of California
Los Angeles, California

In 1900 the first Nobel Prize in Physics was awarded to Dr. Wilhelm Roentgen. His monumental discovery provided, for the first time, images of the heart in intact patients. Roentgenology, named in honor of its discoverer, ranks high among the greatest advances of modern medicine. The two specialties of Imaging Sciences and Cardiology developed hand-in-hand during the first half of the twentieth century. Imaging progressed with a variety of technologies that included angiography, echocardiography, radionuclide imaging, computed tomography, positron emission tomography, and cardiovascular magnetic resonance (CMR).

Of these, CMR offers a veritable treasure trove of information about the heart and great vessels. It not only provides excellent three-dimensional displays of the structure and function of the cardiac chambers and valves, but it is also useful in the assessment of the normal and diseased aorta. The lumina, walls, and obstructive lesions in the major coronary arteries can be visualized, and myocardial perfusion assessed. Myocardial ischemia, necrosis, infiltration, and fibrosis can be detected and quantified. When combined with the ability to determine myocardial viability and to measure cardiac high-energy phosphate stores noninvasively by CMR spectroscopy, the assessment of patients with ischemic heart disease is greatly enhanced. This noninvasive technique, which does not require ionizing radiation, can reduce the need for coronary angiography, now performed on more than 1.5 million patients each year in the United States alone.

Just as it became necessary for the pioneer cardiologists of the early 20th century to become familiar with cardiac radiology, it is now equally important for their successors to do the same with CMR. Warren J. Manning and Dudley J. Pennell, two distinguished leaders of this important technology, and their talented contributors to *Cardiovascular Magnetic Resonance* have taken an important step toward enabling clinicians and clinical investigators to accomplish this. They deserve the appreciation of cardiovascular specialists, radiologists, and trainees for producing this detailed and authoritative yet eminently readable book. We are very pleased to welcome this third edition of *Cardiovascular Magnetic Resonance* into the family of companions to *Heart Disease: A Textbook of Cardiovascular Medicine*.

Eugene Braunwald, MD
Peter Libby, MD
Robert O. Bonow, MD, MS
Douglas L. Mann, MD
Gordon F. Tomaselli, MD

Cardiovascular magnetic resonance (CMR) is a medical imaging field that excites great interest because it combines superb image quality with new techniques for probing the cardiovascular system in novel ways. What surprises is the versatility of the technology: blood flow, angiography, assessment of atherosclerosis, myocardial perfusion, focal necrosis, tissue characterization, oxygen saturation, spectroscopy, technology, and chemical composition are among the measurements that are being refined for clinical use, in addition to the well-known "gold standard" capabilities of CMR in defining anatomy, fibrosis, ventricular function, and blood flow. Such potential comes at a price, however, as this technology is not quickly learned, and high-quality clinical practice needs experience. Professional didactic and clinical training is required for all newcomers to the field and to maintain cutting-edge competency.

In the third edition of this textbook, we are excited to have partnered with the exceptional Braunwald companion series. This brings *Cardiovascular Magnetic Resonance* to a larger audience and cements our growing field in mainstream cardiology. Our aim is to continue to provide instruction in the current clinical practice of CMR, while also highlighting areas of clinical potential, which are presently in varying stages of development. If we succeed in drawing new investigators and clinicians to enter the field or in illuminating new areas for those already involved, then we will have achieved our objective—the healthy growth of competent and motivated practitioners in CMR for the benefit of clinical science, patient care, and the advancement of the field.

The reader should be forewarned that CMR is constantly developing, and no printed text can include all of the most recent developments; however, the foundations provided in these pages will serve the reader for many years to come. The future of CMR remains very bright. Join us on the journey!

Warren J. Manning, MD
Dudley J. Pennell, MD

ACKNOWLEDGMENTS

It takes a village to create a book. Like any large endeavor, this text is a success because of the efforts of the many individuals to whom we owe great thanks. These include the outstanding contributions of our primary authors and their collaborators; Robin Carter, our editor at Elsevier; Kristine Feeherty, our project manager; our office assistants, Lillian Robles at the Beth Israel Deaconess Medical Center, Boston, and Fei Wang at the Royal Brompton Hospital, London; the multitude of CMR mentors, trainees, and colleagues who have stimulated and educated us over the past three decades; and most of all our families for allowing us the time to pursue this endeavor among the myriad other activities that occupy our daily lives. To all, we express our thanks and appreciation.

Warren J. Manning, MD
Dudley J. Pennell, MD

CONTENTS

BRAUNWALD'S HEART DISEASE
FAMILY OF BOOKS

BRAUNWALD'S HEART DISEASE COMPANIONS

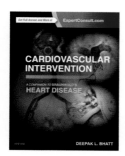

BHATT
Cardiovascular Intervention

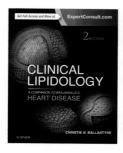

BALLANTYNE
Clinical Lipidology

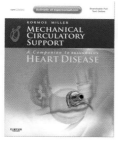

KORMOS AND MILLER
Mechanical Circulatory Support

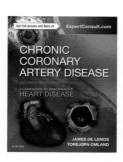

ANTMAN AND SABATINE
Cardiovascular Therapeutics

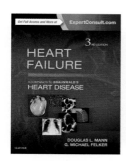

MCGUIRE AND MARX
Diabetes in Cardiovascular Disease

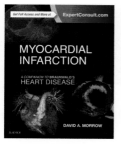

MORROW
Myocardial Infarction

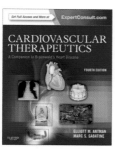

DE LEMOS AND OMLAND
Chronic Coronary Artery Disease

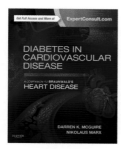

MANN AND FELKER
Heart Failure

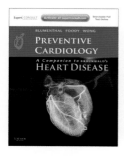

BLUMENTHAL, FOODY, AND WONG
Preventive Cardiology

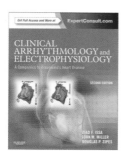

ISSA, MILLER, AND ZIPES
Clinical Arrhythmology and Electrophysiology

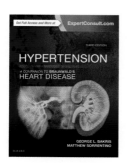

BAKRIS AND SORRENTINO
Hypertension

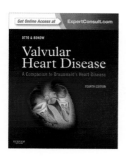

OTTO AND BONOW
Valvular Heart Disease

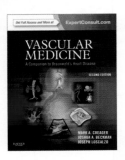

CREAGER, BECKMAN, AND LOSCALZO
Vascular Medicine

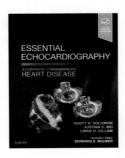

SOLOMON, WU, AND GILLAM
Essential Echocardiography

BRAUNWALD'S HEART DISEASE REVIEW AND ASSESSMENT

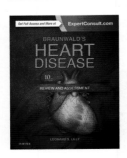

LILLY
Braunwald's Heart Disease Review and Assessment

BRAUNWALD'S HEART DISEASE IMAGING COMPANIONS

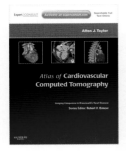

TAYLOR
Atlas of Cardiovascular Computer Tomography

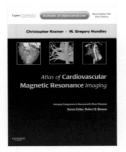

KRAMER AND HUNDLEY
Atlas of Cardiovascular Magnetic Resonance Imaging

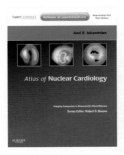

ISKANDRIAN AND GARCIA
Atlas of Nuclear Cardiology

1

Basic Principles of Cardiovascular Magnetic Resonance

Robert S. Balaban and Dana C. Peters

INTRODUCTION

This introduction to the basic principles of cardiovascular magnetic resonance (CMR) describes the concepts of magnetization, T1, T2, T2*, and image formation, and describes some common CMR pulse sequences and parameters. These basic ideas will require some time and rereading to fully appreciate, but each new concept will add to the understanding of CMR.

The human body is composed of mostly water, and a lot of fat. The water (H_2O) and fat contain many hydrogen atoms. Hydrogen atoms in turn are made up of a proton (^1H, the hydrogen nucleus) and an electron. Hydrogen protons are in very high concentration in the body, roughly ~100 molar.[a] These hydrogen protons within the body can be imaged through magnetic resonance imaging (MRI). MRI is possible because hydrogen protons have "spin" and all nuclei with spin interact with magnetic fields. Spin is called the "intrinsic angular momentum," and it is a fundamental property of protons. MRI physics is often called "spin physics" because it describes how the proton spins are used to image the body. In this chapter we will use the term *spin* to indicate the hydrogen proton's spin. MRI images these spins, and in this way it images the tissues in which they are embedded.

In the absence of a magnetic field, the spins are randomly oriented (Fig. 1.1A). But if placed in a large magnetic field (called B_0; i.e., the CMR scanner), the water spins partly align in the same orientation of this applied magnetic field much like iron filings (Fig. 1.1B), with larger magnetic fields causing greater alignment of the spins. In fact, the bulk magnetization, M_z, is proportional to the strength of the applied field. Unlike iron filings, however, the interaction of the spins with the B_0 field results in the spins rotating around the axis of the magnetic field (Fig. 1.1C). This is why the hydrogen nuclei in MRI are also referred to as spins: they spin (precess) around the B_0 field. The frequency of precession (v) is a very important

property of the spins in a magnetic field and is defined by the Larmor equation:

$$v = \frac{\gamma}{2\pi} B \qquad \text{Eq. 1.1}$$

where B is the magnetic field strength experienced by the spin, which is approximately B_0, but includes any variations as described below, v is the spin's precessional frequency in cycles/s or hertz (Hz), and γ (gamma) is the gyromagnetic ratio, which is a constant related to the mass and charge of the water proton, $\gamma/2\pi = 42.58 \times 10^6$ Hz Tesla for water protons. The precessional frequency for water protons at 1.5 Tesla (T; a common CMR field strength) is $v = 63.87 \times 10^6$ Hz, or roughly 64 MHz (about the frequency of an FM radio station and one of the reasons the CMR environment must be shielded from FM radio waves). Thus, at 3 T, the precessional frequency is twice this, $v = 127.74 \times 10^6$ Hz (Eq. 1.1).

The Larmor equation (see Eq. 1.1) looks simple, but it is the basis of CMR imaging. To determine the location of different magnetic spins, the magnetic field (B) is made to vary (linearly) with position using specialized coils of wire (called "gradient coils") inside the magnet. This results in a precessional frequency (v) that depends on a spin's location in the scanner. By measuring the number of spins precessing at each location (i.e., frequency), a magnetic resonance (MR) image is created[1] as will be discussed below.

DETECTION OF THE MRI SIGNAL

Alignment With the Main Magnetic Field

How can the MRI signal from water spins be detected in order to image the sample? Remember, when a sample (i.e., a patient) is placed in the main magnetic field (i.e., inside the bore of the magnet), the hydrogen spins align with that field (see Fig. 1.1B) and begin to precess at the Larmor frequency. We call the direction of the main magnetic field, B_0, the Z-axis direction or the longitudinal direction. Since the spins partially align with the B_0 field, they create a net magnetic field along the Z axis (oriented parallel with B_0). However, the spins precess or rotate around the Z axis in a random, incoherent fashion, resulting in no net magnetization in the X-Y plane (also called the transverse plane) (see Fig. 1.1C). Magnetization by the B_0 field (i.e., M_z) is *not* enough to generate an MR signal. The MR signal is measured as the

---

[a]The molarity of ^1H can be estimated as ~(2 moles hydrogen/mole H_2O) × (1 mole H_2O/18 g of tissue) × 1000 g/L (density of the body) ~ 100 mole/L.

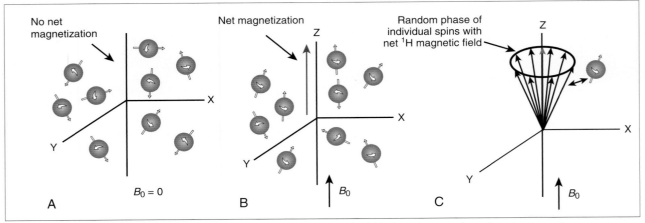

FIG. 1.1 Orientation of molecular spins. (A) With no magnetic field, the spins are oriented randomly, producing no net magnetization. (B) The spins orient with an applied magnetic field (B_0), producing a net magnetic field aligned along B_0. (C) The magnetized spins rotate around the B_0 field (the Z axis) in a random way, resulting in no net magnetization in the X-Y plane.

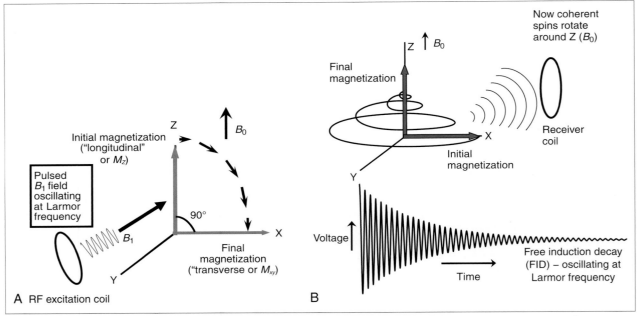

FIG. 1.2 Effects of a perpendicular B_1 magnetic field. (A) The B_1 field oscillating at the Larmor frequency of the spins is absorbed by the spins and causes a rotation around the B_1 field axis (Y axis). A 90-degree RF pulse is shown in which longitudinal magnetization (M_z) becomes transverse magnetization (M_{xy}). (B) Once the B_1 field is removed, the spins continue to rotate around the Z axis at the Larmor frequency, but the signal decays (in the X-Y plane) as equilibrium is reestablished. The result is a coherent oscillating magnetic field that is detected with the coil as the free induction decay *(FID)*. The FID is a decaying sinusoidal voltage signal with a frequency equal to the Larmor frequency of the spins. *RF,* Radiofrequency.

magnetization on the X-Y plane (called M_{xy}). The MR signal is detected by placing a receiver coil (loops of wire tuned to receive signals oscillating at the Larmor frequency) near the subject to detect any spin precession in the X-Y plane. A receiver coil, placed to detect the precession of spins in the X-Y plane, will not detect any signal if M_{xy} is zero (see Fig. 1.1C).

Radiofrequency Excitation

To create an MR signal, the water spins must be precessing in a coherent manner in the X-Y plane. To accomplish this task, another (less

powerful) magnetic field, with a strength that oscillates at the Larmor frequency is applied perpendicular to the main magnetic field (Fig. 1.2A). This process is called radiofrequency (RF) excitation, and the field is called an RF pulse or a B_1 field, since it uses a magnetic (B_1) field rotating at a high (radio wave) frequency. The frequency of this perpendicular B_1 field has to precisely match the Larmor frequency of the water to excite the spins in the presence of the stronger B_0 field. (This concept is analogous to exciting a piano string with a tuning fork. Only the string with the same resonant frequency as the tuning fork will efficiently absorb the energy from the fork and resonate. In fact, magnetic *resonance* imaging gets its name from the resonant frequency used for RF excitation.) The excitation field (B_1) has a strength of only a few gauss, compared to the B_0 field, which has a strength of 15,000 gauss at 1.5 T (1 T = 10,000 gauss). In addition, the B_1 field is only applied transiently (for milliseconds), long enough to temporarily deflect the spins into a plane perpendicular to B_0. This effect on the net magnetic field is illustrated in Fig. 1.2A, which shows a B_1 pulse that drives the magnetization completely into the transverse plane (X-Y plane). This is called a 90-degree pulse (or saturation pulse), referring to the angle through which the initial magnetization (M_z) moves relative to the Z axis. However, in practice, the B_1 pulse can be used to flip the magnetization by any angle from 0 to 180 degrees. A small B_1 pulse (<90 degrees) is called an alpha pulse, while a 180-degree pulse is called an inversion pulse. A 180-degree flip is achieved by applying the B_1 field for twice as long or with twice the strength as the 90-degree pulse. The RF pulse is usually directed along the X or Y axis and oscillates at the Larmor frequency, with an amplitude and shape that determine the true flip angle. Once the B_1 field is turned off, the only field affecting the magnetization is the B_0 field. Now the net magnetization of the water proton spin is in the transverse plane and can be detected as an oscillating signal in the receiver coil (Fig. 1.2B), precessing at the Larmor frequency. This is the signal measured in MRI.

After the RF excitation, the water spins will rotate around the B_0 field on the X-Y plane. Fig. 1.2B shows the signal detected by the receiver coil as the spins precess in the X-Y plane. The signal oscillates at the Larmor frequency and decays in amplitude with time; it is called a free induction decay (FID). The decay in net magnitude in the transverse plane is known as magnetic relaxation. The decay occurs because the spins, having absorbed energy from the transient B_1 field, which is now turned off, return to their original state in equilibrium with the B_0 field, with spins partially aligned along the Z axis (see Fig. 1.1C). This occurs via two extremely important processes called T1 and T2 relaxation. Nature abhors order and seeks to minimize the energy in the system by returning to equilibrium with the main magnetic field, B_0, through T1 and T2 relaxation. T1 and T2 relaxation are the foundations of MRI because they are responsible for MRI's excellent contrast.

T1 Relaxation

T1 relaxation, also known as spin-lattice relaxation, is the release of energy to the environment, or lattice, that results in the reestablishment of the magnetization along the Z axis. Thus T1 is the time constant by which the longitudinal (or Z) magnetization relaxes to its equilibrium value, M_0. After a 90-degree RF pulse, the Z magnetization, $M_z(t)$, is initially 0 but regrows with a relaxation time T1 to its equilibrium value (M_0).

$$M_z(t) = M_0(1 - e^{-t/T1}) \qquad \textbf{Eq. 1.2}$$

where t is the time after the 90-degree pulse. Each tissue type has a unique T1, which changes with field strength and in disease. Table 1.1 gives values for the normal T1 of many cardiac tissues, although reference values vary depending on the method of T1 quantification. Studies[2] using T1 mapping show that native T1 is longer than normal in acute

myocardial infarction and inflammatory diseases such as myocarditis. T1 is also longer in amyloid cardiomyopathy[3] and Anderson-Fabry disease. In siderotic disease (iron overload), native myocardial T1 is shorter.[4]

T2* and T2 Relaxation: The Effects of Spin Phase

The other form of relaxation, T2* (T2 star) relaxation, is that of the randomization of the phase of the spins. After RF excitation, all of the spins precess about the Z axis, with slight differences in the precessional rate, and this eventually results in "T2* decay." T2* decay comes from differences in the phase of each spin, so that the net X-Y magnetization, M_{xy}, decays to 0. The phase indicates the direction of the spin in the transverse plane. The phase (ϕ) of a spin in the transverse plane depends on its initial phase, ϕ_0, the precessional frequency of that spin, and the time, t, that it has spent in the transverse plane (assuming a constant frequency).

$$\phi = \phi_0 + 2\pi\nu t \qquad \textbf{Eq. 1.3}$$

Since this precessional frequency depends on the magnetic field (see Eq. 1.1), which changes slightly with location, time, and molecular environment, each spin on the transverse plane has a different frequency, and thus *phase*, and this phase difference generally increases with time (Eq. 1.3). Fig. 1.3A defines the phase (ϕ) of the spin magnetic field vector as the direction of the transverse magnetization relative to the X axis.

In Fig. 1.3B a phase diagram is used to show the changing phase relationships for three spins in a sample that are precessing at different frequencies. The magnetic field always varies because of imperfections in the main magnetic field and changes in the molecular environment. In this schematic, the three spins experience slightly different magnetic fields, one higher than B_0, one exactly B_0, and one lower. Therefore, after some time on the X-Y plane, each spin experiences phase accrual, until the net magnetization (the sum of all of the spins magnetization) decreases to 0.

Within a single pixel in a CMR image, there are a quintillion water spins, each with a slightly different frequency. Therefore, while all of the spins are precessing at about the Larmor frequency, at any time one spin might be precessing a little faster and another might be precessing a little slower.

T2* relaxation can be understood as the characteristic time in which the spins in the (X-Y) plane become so out of phase that the signal decays (dies out). The signal decays because the relative phase of the spins in a single voxel are different. After the initial excitation using a B_1 pulse, all of the spins on the transverse plane have identical phase but then begin to dephase quickly. This dephasing is described by a time constant T2*. The dephasing causes the bulk transverse magnetization, M_{xy}, to decay and approach 0, due to incoherent phase.

$$M_{xy}(t) = M_{xy_0}e^{-t/T2*} \qquad \textbf{Eq. 1.4}$$

Thus the CMR signal (M_{xy}) decays in a simple exponential way, with a time constant of T2*.

T2 Versus T2*

We need to further understand T2* and how it differs from T2. Both are related to dephasing due to variability in the main magnetic field. In general, two distinct processes contribute to the dephasing of spins in a voxel. The first mechanism is the true T2 decay that is unavoidable, irreversible, and dependent on the molecular interactions within the sample. T2 relaxation is also called spin-spin relaxation. It is called this because the mechanism of the relaxation process is through the interaction of spins in the sample with each other at or below the Larmor frequency, making this process dependent on the microscopic motions within the sample. The second process is T2* decay and includes T2

TABLE 1.1	**T1 and T2 Values**			
Field Strength		**1.5 T**		**3 T**
Tissue	T1 (ms)	T2 (ms)	T1 (ms)	T2 (ms)
Myocardium	950[71]	55[72]	1150[73]	40[74]
Arterial blood	1550[71]	250	1650[75]	200
Fat	260	110	320	70
Skeletal muscle	1000[76]	45[76]	1400[76]	50[76]

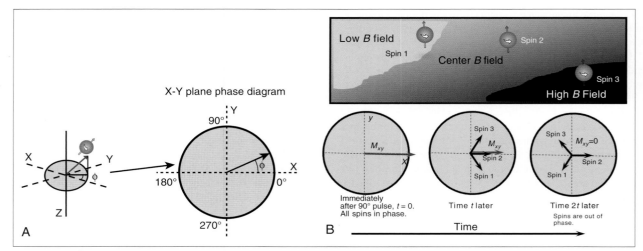

FIG. 1.3 The phase diagram. (A) A phase diagram is a view of the magnetization vectors projected into the X-Y plane. (B) The magnetic field of a sample varies as shown. Spins located in the lower field (spin 1), central field (spin 2), and higher field (spin 3) regions are followed in time after a 90-degree pulse using the phase diagram. The phase diagram presents the phases of the spins relative to spin 2, which is always shown with 0-degree phase. Note that spin 1 lags behind spin 2, while spin 3 is ahead, because it has a higher phase velocity. This difference is due to the higher frequency of the spins in the higher magnetic field. This process is called *dephasing*.

relaxation *and also* relaxation due to *static inhomogeneity* of the main magnetic field (B_0) within the sample. These B_0 field imperfections result from hardware imperfections and susceptibility-induced B_0 variations due to the influence of the body itself. In the heart, both the lung cavity and the deoxygenated blood in the right heart contribute to B_0 inhomogeneity. B_0 field imperfections also arise from any metallic objects (sternal wires, devices, etc.) near the heart. As illustrated in Fig. 1.3B, if the B_0 field is not homogeneous throughout the sample then the frequency of the spins in different regions will vary (see Eq. 1.1). These spins are called "off-resonance" spins. Both T2 and T2* processes result in a randomization of the spin phases as they precess at different frequencies, and a decrease in the net transverse magnetization. However, while T2 relaxation is irreversible, T2* relaxation can be partly reversed since some of it is due to static off-resonance: T2* includes the irreversible molecular spin-spin interactions (T2) and static off-resonance. Myocardial T2 relaxation rate is ~55 ms at 1.5 T (see Table 1.1),[5,6] while myocardial T2* is ~30 ms at 1.5 T.[7] *T2* is always less than T2 for all tissues*, because it includes effects of T2 relaxation, as well as off-resonance effects. Later we will describe how to obtain T2 contrast instead of T2* contrast.

These basic relaxation processes, T1, T2, and T2* are key in the generation of *image contrast* as well as determining the optimal image sequence for gathering information on cardiovascular anatomy, function, and physiology. What is important is that T1, T2, and T2* vary for different tissues, and in disease, thereby providing "contrast" in the CMR image (see Table 1.1). For example, the T1 and T2 values are prolonged with increasing water content, as with edema, which is present in different disease states.[8,9] Overall, myocardial remodeling, or myocyte replacement with connective tissue, also changes the water relaxation properties since the nature of the macromolecules in contact with water are critical for these relaxation processes. Finally, most exogenous, intravenously injected CMR contrast agents act by shortening T1[10–12] and T2/T2*[13,14] of the water spins. By appropriately modifying the imaging sequences, these changes in relaxation properties due to pathology or exogenous contrast agent can be highlighted or even mapped (measured on a pixel-by-pixel basis) in the heart. First,

the process of imaging—localizing the T1- or T2-weighted signal to a region—will be explained.

SPATIAL LOCALIZATION

To create a CMR image, the MR signal intensity from the sample (e.g., patient) must be determined in three dimensions (X, Y, and Z). Thus, for a single image, it is necessary to collect information on X, Y, and Z positions and signal amplitude. This signal amplitude can be T1, T2, or T2* weighted, as desired. This localization is performed using multiple measurements or repetition times (TRs). To localize signal to $Nx \times Ny$ voxels (e.g., a 128 × 128 matrix), approximately $Nx \cdot Ny$ signals (and Ny TRs) are needed. This is actually a limitation of CMR, resulting in a relatively slow image acquisition rate compared to many other modalities.

The simplest imaging experiment can be divided into four stages as shown in the block diagram in Fig. 1.4: (1) RF excitation with slice selection (localization in Z); (2) phase encoding (localization in Y); (3) gradient and RF rephasing/refocusing; and (4) frequency encoding (localization in X). Each stage is used to encode the MR data with information on the position and the amplitude of the water proton signal. By convention, the Z-position information is encoded with the slice-selection step, the X position is determined in the frequency-encoding/readout step, and the Y position is obtained with the phase-encoding step. In practice the frequency-encoding (X), phase-encoding (Y), and slice-selection (Z) directions can be rotated in any appropriate direction. MR is tomographic and can create an image of the body along any plane. Indeed, oblique imaging, slicing through a tissue at 45 degrees, or any other angle, is possible and common. In this way CMR differs from other modalities (e.g., computed tomography [CT] or two-dimensional [2D] echocardiography), because CMR can acquire images in any plane.

Magnetic Gradients

Spatial encoding in CMR is performed using magnetic field gradients applied to the main magnetic field: slice-select gradients, phase-encoding gradients, and frequency-encoding gradients. Gradient coils are special

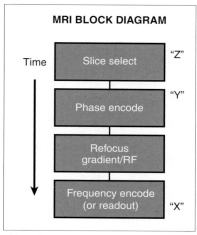

MRI BLOCK DIAGRAM

Time

Slice select — "Z"

Phase encode — "Y"

Refocus gradient/RF

Frequency encode (or readout) — "X"

FIG. 1.4 General imaging scheme for collecting a simple cardiovascular magnetic resonance image *(MRI)*. RF, Radiofrequency.

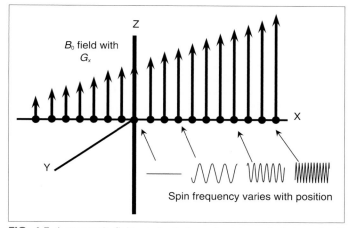

Z

B_0 field with G_x

Y

X

Spin frequency varies with position

FIG. 1.5 A magnetic field gradient. A gradient is applied along the X axis, causing the *B* field to vary from less than to greater than B_0 along X. This leads to a linear increase in spin frequency as a function of position along the X direction.

coils within the magnet that modify the main magnetic field *(B)*, causing its strength (but not direction) to change slightly in space.

$$B(x, y, z) = B_0 + G_x \cdot x + G_y \cdot y + G_z \cdot z \quad \text{Eq. 1.5}$$

where G_x, G_y, and G_z are called "gradient strengths," and x, y, and z are the spatial coordinates with $x = 0$, $y = 0$, $z = 0$ at the center of the magnet bore. Eq. (1.5) describes how the main magnetic field strength—which always is directed along the Z axis—varies spatially with x, y, and z. Fig. 1.5 demonstrates the variation of the *B* field in the presence of an x gradient. In the same way, gradients on the Y or Z axis vary the *B* field in y or z. Using gradients, the main magnetic field, with which spins align, and around which they precess, varies with spatial position inside the scanner. *Remember, this magnetic field points in the Z direction.* The gradients do not change this direction but slightly increase or decrease its strength spatially. These spatially varying magnetic fields are called gradients because they create a spatially varying magnetic field (a magnetic field gradient). Of course, since the magnetic field varies with position, the precessional frequency $v(x, y, z)$ and the phase

$\phi(x, y, z, t)$ of the spins also varies with position (see Eqs. 1.1 and 1.3, and Fig. 1.5).

$$v = \frac{\gamma}{2\pi} B(x, y, z) = \frac{\gamma}{2\pi}(B_0 + G_x \cdot x + G_y \cdot y + G_z \cdot z) \quad \text{Eq. 1.6}$$

The first term, $(\gamma/2\pi) \cdot B_0$, is just the Larmor frequency. In CMR, we usually describe M_{xy} magnetization in the "rotating frame." Therefore it is as if we are rotating with the spins at the Larmor frequency, and only *differences* between the spin's frequency and the Larmor frequency are important. In that frame, $v = \gamma/2\pi(G_x \cdot x + G_y \cdot y + G_z \cdot z)$. Also note that at any time, gradients on X, Y, and Z axes may be applied together or alone and the amplitudes can be slewed up and down or set to 0.

The phase $\phi(x, y, z, t)$ of the spins also varies with position. For a constant gradient, $\phi = \gamma B \cdot t = \gamma(G_x \cdot x + G_y \cdot y + G_z \cdot z) \cdot t$, and is related to the gradient strengths, the time *(t)* that the gradient is on, and the spin's location. Note that phase accumulation due to precession at the Larmor frequency $(\gamma \cdot B_0 \cdot t)$ is omitted, because the phase is described in the rotating frame. For nonconstant gradients (e.g., ramped gradients), the phase is proportional to the area of the gradient-time curve (gradient × time):

$$\phi(x, y, z, t) = \gamma[\text{area}(G_x, t) \cdot x + \text{area}(G_y, t) \cdot y + \text{area}(G_z, t) \cdot z] \quad \text{Eq. 1.7}$$

The idea of gradient "area" is very important. The gradient area is the product of the gradient amplitude, G, and the duration, t, of the gradient. The phase of a spin at any given time is proportional to the total gradient area and its location. Gradients cause the frequency and phase of the spins to depend on location, so that if frequency of a certain spin can be measured, its position is determined using slice selection, frequency encoding, and phase encoding.

Slice-Selective Excitation: Position in Z

During the slice-select stage, the RF excitation is performed to rotate the spins into the X-Y plane. During excitation, one of the spatial coordinates *(z)* is determined by only flipping (with the B_1) magnetization in a selected slice of the sample. The magnetization remains unchanged (i.e., aligned with B_0) *except* in that slice. The slice-selection process is illustrated in Fig. 1.6. A linear magnetic field gradient, G_z, is applied to the sample to vary the B_0 field along the slice direction (the Z axis). The magnetic field gradient causes the spins along this axis to have slightly different frequencies as defined by the Larmor equation:

$$v(z) = (G_z \cdot z) \cdot (\gamma/2\pi)$$

The B_1 field is used to excite the spins, but only within a range of precessional frequencies. If only a selected band of frequencies are excited (Δv), then a slice of spins with precessional frequencies in that range (Δz) is placed into the transverse plane, not affecting the rest of the sample. The "slice thickness" can be freely chosen by adjusting the Z gradient. Typical slices range from thin (e.g., 2 mm) slices to thick (e.g., 30 cm) slabs. The slice position can also be freely chosen. Furthermore, if no Z gradient is applied during the slice selection, this is equivalent to an infinite slab thickness, so that all of the spins in the body will be tipped into the transverse plane. This is called a "nonselective" (NS) RF pulse and is commonly used in CMR for preparation pulses.

How can the B_1 field, which oscillates at about the Larmor frequency, be used to excite only spins precessing within a range of frequencies? To excite a bandwidth of frequencies, the Z gradient is turned on, and the B_1 strength is modulated in time:

$$B_1(t) = B_{1_0} \cdot \sin(\pi \cdot t/T)/(\pi \cdot t/T) \quad \text{Eq. 1.8}$$

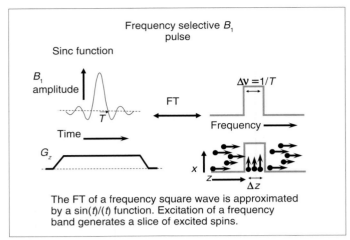

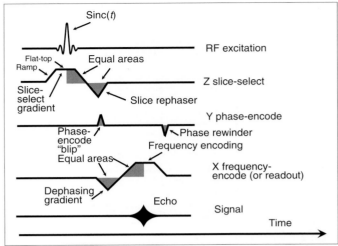

FIG. 1.6 The slice-selective B_1 pulse. The shape of the slice-selective B_1 pulse in time is $\sin(t)/t$. This is called a "sinc" function. It has the property that it excites a distinct band of frequencies. This is true because the Fourier transform *(FT)* of the sinc B_1 field is a square wave in frequency space. The excitation of a band of frequencies by the B_1, used in conjunction with the gradient G_z (similar to Fig. 1.5, but along the Z axis), causes a slice of spins to be placed on the transverse plane.

FIG. 1.7 Pulse sequence diagram. In a pulse sequence diagram a time line is shown for the B_1 pulse, the gradients on each axis, and the signal received. This convention is used in all pulse sequence diagrams. Here the slice-selection process is shown (see top portion of figure), in which a Z gradient is used with a sinc B_1 pulse. The frequency encoding is shown on the X axis. The frequency encoding shows a dephasing gradient, and then a flat top, during which time the signal is acquired, as indicated on the last line (signal). The phase-encoding gradient "blip" is often applied just prior to frequency encoding. Often after the frequency encoding, the phase-encoding gradient is rephased. During each repeated pulse sequence, only the phase-encoding strength changes. *RF*, Radiofrequency.

This B_1 shape, $\sin(t)/t$, is called a "sinc" function and is plotted in Fig. 1.6. This $B_1(t)$ excites a well-defined band of frequencies of width, $\Delta\nu = 1/T$, centered around the Larmor frequency. Here, a Fourier transform (FT) is used to show how the spins interpret the $\sin(t)/t$ pulse in terms of frequency. If a Z gradient is applied during the sinc RF excitation, then the band of frequencies excited is a "slice" of spins at a certain Z location, with a slice thickness Δz. Modifications to the sinc pulse are possible to optimize the performance and slice definition of this approach.[15,16]

The slice-selection process is summarized in the imaging "pulse sequence diagram" shown in Fig. 1.7. A pulse sequence diagram presents all of the gradients, the B_1 field excitation, and also marks the timing of data collection (i.e., when the receiver coil records the MR signal) on a time line. In Fig. 1.7 (boxed region), the slice-selection gradient is first increased to a constant level by a ramp. The gradient is maintained while the frequency selective (i.e., slice-selective) B_1 field is applied; note its sinc shape. Subsequently, the slice gradient is ramped down and the rephasing gradient is applied to remove the phase introduced by the slice-select gradient. After performing the slice-select excitation, only a slice of the sample has been placed in the transverse plane and all of the spins are in phase.

The rephasing Z gradient shown in Fig. 1.7 is performed so that all of the spins are "in phase" after the slice-selection process. During the 90-degree pulse the spins will dephase, depending on where they are in the slice (similar to that seen in Fig. 1.3B) since a magnetic field gradient is applied. Thus another magnetic field gradient of opposite magnitude must be applied to reverse the dephasing caused by the slice-selection process (shaded regions in Fig. 1.7). The gradient area to rephase the spins is half the slice-select area, since the spins reach the transverse plane exactly coincident with the peak of the RF sinc pulse. By applying the gradient in the opposite direction, the spins are forced back to the same phase as they had before application of the slice-select gradient. This small gradient is called a slice-rephasing gradient.

In summary, to selectively excite a slice, a linear magnetic field gradient G_z is placed along the axis to be sliced. A sinc B_1 field pulse is

applied, and only the predefined slice within the sample will be placed onto the transverse plane for further modification to create an image.

Frequency Encoding: Position in X

While the Z position is now known, X and Y positions remain unknown. If a gradient G_x is applied after the RF excitation in the X direction (called the "frequency-encoding direction" in MRI), recall that the frequency of the spins will reflect the locations of the spins in the X direction:

$$\nu(x) = (G_x \cdot x) \cdot (\gamma/2\pi)$$

(in the rotating frame). This is illustrated in Fig. 1.8 for three spins at different X locations. The spins are located along the X axis, and a magnetic field gradient in the X is turned on. One spin is located at $x = 0$, where the magnetic field remains B_0, but the others experience slightly higher fields. The signal received from each spin depends on its precessional frequency, as shown in Fig. 1.8, with each spin's signal oscillating at a different frequency. The combined signal from all three spins is measured (while G_x is "on") by the receiver coil as the MR signal. The location of each spin can then be determined using an FT, which converts time oscillating total signal into its frequency (i.e., location) components.

$$FT(\text{signal}) = \int \text{signal}(t) \cdot e^{-2\pi \cdot i\nu t} dt \qquad \textbf{Eq. 1.9}$$

where ν is related to the X location, as before. Using a frequency-encoding gradient, the MR signal provides a measure of the number of spins precessing at each frequency.

As shown in Fig. 1.7 (bottom two rows), the gradient is applied for a few milliseconds, during which the MR signal is measured. The

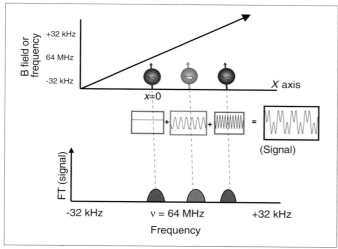

FIG. 1.8 Frequency encoding of position. A frequency-encoding (also called *readout*) gradient is applied on the X axis, causing the *B* field to vary from less than to greater than the main magnetic field. Three spins are shown at different X locations, with different precessional frequencies. The signal from the spins during the application of this gradient is acquired, and its frequency depends on location. The total signal is then Fourier transformed *(FT)* to provide a measurement of the number of spins precessing at each frequency, thereby indicating the X location of each spin.

gradient must remain on for a specific time during frequency encoding, in order to sufficiently record the oscillating signals with high fidelity.

Note that a dephasing gradient is applied with an area equal to half that of the readout gradient. The readout gradient is then ramped up and held constant for a period of time, and then the gradient is ramped back down to zero. This time (when G_x is constant) *is the time during which the signal is acquired—the data acquisition*. During this period the signal is continuously sampled, providing N_x time samples, where the spatial resolution (Δx) is related to N_x, by FOV/$N_x = \Delta x$. The field-of-view (FOV) is the size of the sample (the patient) in the imaging field. Remember that this signal is already localized in Z, and using slice-selective RF excitation, and is now localized in X using frequency encoding. The signal measured contains this X and Z information. However, it does not yet contain Y-position information.

Fig. 1.7 shows a pulse sequence called a gradient recalled echo (GRE) or gradient echo, since the readout gradient is used to refocus the dephasing gradient applied before it. A rephaser is sometimes applied also, which is similar to a dephaser but is applied after a gradient. A very thoughtful reader may wonder, why are the gradients always "ramped" up and down? The ramps reflect the reality that the magnetic field cannot be changed instantaneously, but rather the change is constrained by the scanner hardware. With current hardware, the gradient coils can be "slewed" to reach their maximum value (currently 4–8 gauss/cm) within about 100–200 ms. Slew rate is currently constrained by safety concerns related to peripheral nerve stimulation.

Phase Encoding: Position in Y

Y spatial information is determined through a process called *phase-encoding*. Just like frequency encoding, phase encoding occurs after the RF pulse. The spins can be phase encoded by transiently applying a magnetic field gradient (G_y) along the phase-encoding axis (Y axis by convention) as shown in Fig. 1.7 (labeled a "phase-encoding blip"). This transient gradient or blip imparts a phase to each spin proportional

to its area (gradient × time, Eq. 1.7), and to the spin's Y position. The phase-encoding gradient is applied prior to the frequency encoding. A rephaser is commonly applied after frequency encoding, to remove any phase accumulations in Y. However, many phase-encoding gradients of progressively increasing areas are required in order to localize a spin in the Y direction, depending on the object size (called an FOV), and the desired spatial resolution (Δy). The number of phase encodings (N_y) is given by the relationship FOV/$N_y = \Delta y$.

Recall that to determine the position of a spin within the sample, a gradient is applied, and the resulting frequency reports its position. Frequency is simply a measure of how fast the phase is changing in time (see Eq. 1.3). Phase encoding is a method for measuring the locations of the spins, by measuring their response to different strengths of Y gradient, and deducing their precessional frequency (and therefore location) from these measurements. Unlike frequency encoding, which provides the locations of spins in X with a single measurement, phase encoding is performed slowly, over N_y measurements. In successive measurements, the amplitude of the phase-encoding gradient is progressively increased, and the signal is measured. Each measurement is called a repetition, and the time to acquire a single measurement is called the repetition time (TR).

Fig. 1.9 describes the phase-encoding technique. Consider three spins, located at three Y positions, but at any position in X. The Y gradient is "blipped" on, increased for a time T, to a maximum value G_y, and then ramped down to 0. The area of the gradient ($G_y \cdot T$) and the spin's Y location determines the phase accumulation (see Eq. 1.7). With no G_y gradient on, all spins precess at the Larmor frequency and have the same phase. If the signal is measured from these spins, it is the bulk signal. The application of a gradient G_y for a short time T, results in a phase that depends on the spin's Y location. If a small gradient is used, the phase changes gradually with Y position. The sphere at $y = 0$ accumulates no phase, but the other spheres accumulate phase, depending on their Y location. A larger phase-encoding gradient causes even more phase accumulation at $y \neq 0$. Now two of the spins are completely out of phase. The signal measured during each phase-encoding blip is dependent on each spins' phase, which in turn is determined by each spins' Y location. With three phase encodings, it is not yet possible to locate the spins in Y, but after collecting the signal from multiple (32 to 512) phase-encoding steps, the signals can be used to determine Y locations, using the FT. It is important to realize that for each phase-encoding, *an entire frequency encoding must be collected*. When the readout signal is collected during phase encoding, each of the spins' phases is influenced by their position in Y and X. In this way, X and Y spatial information are encoded together. Thus this slow phase-encoding process provides the last piece of information, Y axis position, needed to create the MR image.

Raw *k*-Space Data and the Fast Fourier Transform

Fig. 1.7 shows all of the steps of spatial encoding. A separate echo is collected for each phase-encode step. The phase-encode step is most commonly applied immediately after the slice-select process, frequently at the same time as the dephasing gradient for readout occurs (as shown in Fig. 1.7). This is done to minimize the scan time. All of the frequency and phase-encoded raw data are combined to create *k-space* (Fig. 1.10). The *k*-space of Fig. 1.10 represents the raw data collected at each phase-encoding step. The phase- and frequency-encoding directions are labeled. MR imaging can be understood as acquiring *k*-space data. Each frequency encoding acquires a signal for a full line of *k*-space (k_x) at a single k_y value. Each phase-encoding step moves up along the phase-encoding axis (k_y) to acquire another frequency-encoding line. Once enough *k*-space signal is acquired, this *k*-space signal is converted into an image using a 2D FT. Ideally, the raw *k*-space data contains enough information,

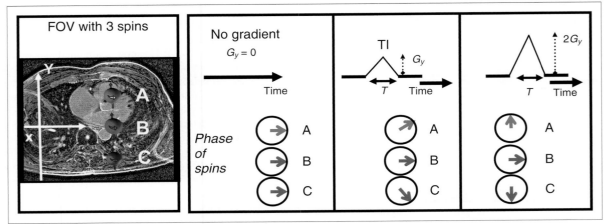

FIG. 1.9 Phase encoding. A Y gradient is transiently applied for a time T using larger and larger gradient strengths, G_y. Three spins, A, B, and C, located at three different Y locations, respond differently to the phase-encoding gradient. The gradient does not affect the spin at $y = 0$ (spin B) because it still precesses at the Larmor frequency. But the gradient causes spin A to precess more slowly and spin C to precess more quickly, resulting in phase differences proportional to the gradient strength (G_y) and the time t. These phase differences allow the locations of the spins to be determined. *FOV*, Field of view.

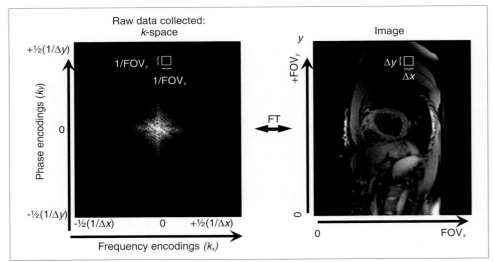

FIG. 1.10 The frequency-encoding data collected during each phase-encoding step is called the k-space signal. The k-space signal is collected on a grid. The k-space signal does not look like an image, but is transformed into an image using the Fourier transform. The spacing in k-space $(\Delta k_x, \Delta k_y)$ determines the field of view (FOV_x, FOV_y) of the image. The width of k-space is related to the pixel size of the image, as shown. Collecting "more" k-space reduces the pixel size.

so that after the 2D FT an image of infinite spatial resolution results. In reality, there are limits on the amount of data that can be collected. The Y resolution of the CMR image is directly related to the number of phase-encoded echoes that are collected ($\Delta y = FOV_y/N_y$), and therefore infinite spatial resolution would require infinite time to collect. The X resolution is related to the number of frequency-encoding data points acquired ($\Delta x = FOV_x/N_x$). It is easier to acquire very high resolution in the frequency-encoding direction, and often in CMR spatial resolution in the frequency-encoding direction is higher. In CMR, time is limited due to respiratory and cardiac motions, so the tradeoff between spatial resolution required to observe the structure of interest and scan time is critically important. Schemes to increase the efficiency of collecting k-space data (e.g., spiral, radial) will be discussed throughout this book.

PULSE SEQUENCES AND CONTRAST

Spin Echo Imaging

Among the very first pulse sequences used in CMR was the spin echo sequence and, even today, it is routinely used in its accelerated form (fast spin echo). As described earlier, in tissue, T2* causes rapid magnetic relaxation of water protons, compared with T2 relaxation. Thus the decay rate of the M_{xy} signal after an RF pulse excitation is actually a measure of T2*. Since T2* decay is a rapid process, it limits the time that we can detect the MR signal. As noted above, it's possible to circumvent and reverse some of the T2* dephasing, because some of it is caused by fixed B_0 field inhomogeneity. This reversal is accomplished using a classic and important MR method called spin echo imaging. This method uses

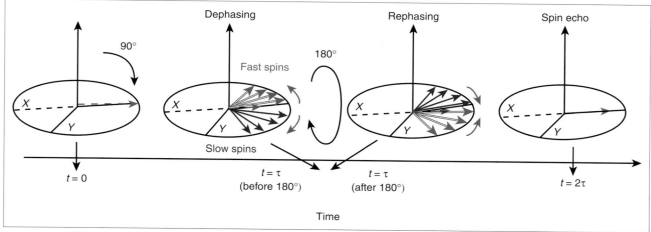

FIG. 1.11 Spin echo: effects of a 180-degree B_1 pulse after a 90-degree B_1 pulse. The spins are first excited by a 90-degree pulse, as in Fig. 1.2. After some time in which dephasing occurs (as in Fig. 1.3B), a 180-degree pulse is applied. The 180-degree pulse, by flipping the spins 180 degrees about the X axis, exchanges the phase position of the slower and faster spins, so that the faster spins are now lagging the slower spins. The faster spins begin to catch up, and after a time τ equal to the time of dephasing, the spins are all aligned in the same direction (have the same phase). This process is called "rephasing" or "refocusing" to form a spin echo.

two B_1 pulses to generate an "echo" (a signal), as outlined in Fig. 1.11. First, a 90-degree pulse is applied to create M_{xy} magnetization. Due to magnetic field imperfections, the magnetization begins to dephase. Next a 180-degree B_1 pulse is applied to flip the magnetization by 180 degrees around the X axis. This 180-degree flip is important, because now any slow spins (precessing slower than the Larmor frequency) are "ahead" of fast spins, so that the spins now drift back into phase (i.e., "rephase") taking the *same amount of time* to rephase that they were allowed to dephase. This is analogous to two people standing back to back in a field and then walking apart (90-degree pulse) at some fixed rate (but different rates for each person). At some time later, they reverse (180-degree pulse) their direction and now walk toward each other at their same "individual" pace. The time it takes them to reach each other will be the same amount of time as they walked apart. This is the nature of the echo that effectively recaptures all of the coherent transverse magnetization that had been destroyed by the B_0 field inhomogeneity in the sample. Note that the echo has both a rephasing as well as a dephasing period. The spins continue to dephase after reaching the coherent echo due to ongoing field inhomogeneity; just as in the field they would walk past each other and continue to "dephase." The signal at the time of the spin echo only decays by T2, not T2*.

The spin echo sequence is shown in Fig. 1.12. Note that it is almost identical to the GRE sequence (see Fig. 1.7), except for the 180-degree refocusing pulse. Even in this simple sequence, several factors of its design will change the contrast of the MR image, based on T1 and T2 relaxation. Since a 180-degree refocusing pulse is used in this sequence, the total time that the spins stay in the transverse plane, before the signal is measured, determines the amount of T2 relaxation that will occur (see Eq. 1.3). This time is called the *time to echo* or the *echo time (TE)* and is measured from the center of the slice-select sinc pulse to the center of the refocused echo during the readout or data acquisition (see Fig. 1.12). Generally, the longer the TE, the more T2 contrast or T2 weighting is generated in the image (see Eq. 1.4).

Another sequence timing parameter that influences the signal amplitude is based on T1 relaxation. The time between each slice excitation pulse is the critical factor in this sequence and is called the time to repetition or the TR (see Fig. 1.12). If a shorter TR is used between

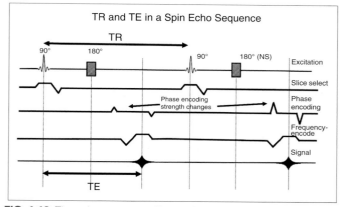

FIG. 1.12 The pulse sequence diagram for a spin echo pulse sequence. A 90-degree slice-selective excitation is followed by a 180-degree refocusing pulse, as described in Fig. 1.11. Then phase encoding on Y and frequency encoding on the X axis are performed. The repetition time *(TR)* and echo time *(TE)* are defined. The diagram shows two TRs. During each repeated TR, everything is the same, except that the phase-encoding strength changes, as shown.

slice-selective pulses, the spins' Z magnetization will not fully regrow between pulses, and this leads to a reduction in the MR signal. This reduction in signal is dependent on the TR and the T1 of the sample. Therefore **T1 weighting** *can be achieved using a short TR, combined with a short TE, so that T2 weighting is minimized.* **T2 weighting** *is achieved with a long TE and long TR.* "Proton density" weighting (i.e., how many spins are in each location) can be achieved with a short TE and a long TR.

As an example of the importance of TE, the MR water signals from normal (T2 ~55 ms) and acutely infarcted (T2 ~70 ms)[17] regions of the myocardium are shown in Fig. 1.13A. Note that the signal of both tissues decreases with increasing TE, but that the infarcted tissue signal decays more slowly, because of its longer T2. This results in a *contrast*, or increased difference, in signal between the normal and the infarcted

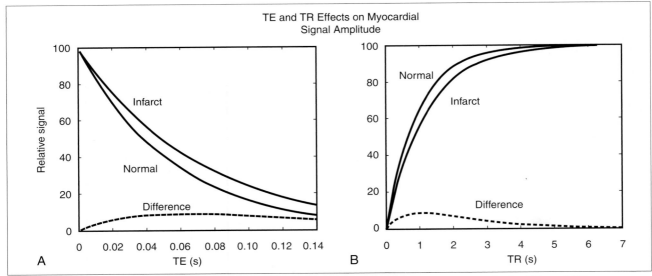

FIG. 1.13 Echo time *(TE)* and repetition time *(TR)* effects on myocardial signal amplitude. Effect of TE (A) and TR (B) on cardiovascular magnetic resonance signal amplitude, for normal and infarcted myocardium. Because the T1 and T2 of acutely infarcted myocardium differ from normal myocardium, contrast between these tissues can be created.

tissue at prolonged TEs. Inspecting the difference between the signal of the two tissue curves (dotted line), a TE of about 50 ms could be selected to optimize the contrast between these two tissue types. Thus, by simply adjusting the imaging parameters, fundamental information on the heart structure can be obtained. Conversely, pathology may be obscured if the imaging parameters are not ideal.

The impact of TR on signal amplitude is shown in Fig. 1.13B for a spin echo sequence. The effect of TR is illustrated for normal myocardium with a T1 of 950 ms and abnormal myocardium with a T1 of 1200 ms. Note that the shorter the T1 the more *rapidly* the pulses can be applied and still maintain the MR signal. Also apparent in Fig. 1.13B is that by varying the TR, the contrast or difference between tissues, can be altered. Thus the TR can be used to vary the image contrast based on T1. Note that a TR of 1 s would be optimal in generating the largest difference (or contrast; "dotted" line) between the normal and the infarcted tissue. Current CMR techniques perform T1 mapping or T1-weighted imaging using inversion recovery, as described below and in Chapter 2, to differentiate infarction and normal myocardium based on "native" T1.

Fast Spin Echo Imaging

The relatively long TRs required for full T1 relaxation is the major reason that the spin echo method is very rarely used: Scan time (TR · N_y) is too long. To circumvent this problem, one highly useful approach is to use multiple 180-degree refocusing pulses and to collect many echoes during each slice-selective excitation (see Fig. 1.13). This method, called fast spin echo (FSE) or turbo spin echo (TSE), is an important technique in CMR.[18] A phase-encoding gradient is applied between each 180-degree pulse, thereby providing multiple phase-encoded steps from a single 90-degree pulse. For CMR, typically 16 to 64 echoes are collected for each slice-selective pulse, thereby reducing the time to collect a spin echo image by 16 to 64 times, respectively. Since large blocks of time are required to collect all of these echoes, this method is usually restricted to relatively motion free phases of the cardiac cycle, such as diastole. The inherent high signal-to-noise ratio (SNR) of these FSE approaches supports very high spatial resolution images of the heart. In addition, true T2 contrast can be generated by acquiring the central phase-encoding data (which largely controls the image contrast) at a specific time within the echo train. This time is called the effective TE. The longer the time between the initial 90 degrees, and the acquisition of central *k*-space (i.e., the longer the effective TE), the more T2 weighting will occur. The FSE technique is very commonly used in CMR to visualize anatomy and measure sizes of cardiac chambers (Fig. 1.14 shows an FSE image). It is usually used with a black-blood preparation pulse described below. T2-weighted black-blood FSE has been advocated for identifying edematous tissue associated with acute infarct,[19] and for identifying the region at risk.[20] In Chapter 2, methods for quantifying myocardial T2 will be described, which are currently in greater use.

Gradient Echo Imaging

GRE imaging, like spin echo, is a fundamental CMR method and enjoys greater use than any other method. For imaging the beating heart, and other highly dynamic applications, gradient echo imaging (also known as GRE, FLASH, or TFE)[21] with very short TRs is one of the most commonly used methods in CMR. This sequence is shown (again) in Fig. 1.15, displaying multiple TRs. GRE imaging uses short TRs and lower flip angles. Furthermore, in GRE imaging the 180-degree refocusing pulse is eliminated. The signal on the transverse plane will then decay with T2* instead of T2, but this is acceptable if the TE is very short (TE < 3 ms). As the TR is shortened, the flip angle must be reduced to provide the optimal SNR per unit time. The flip angle provides maximum signal at steady state (i.e., after many slice-selective pulses) and is determined by a tradeoff. A larger flip angle provides more spins on the transverse plane (more signal), but less Z magnetization is preserved, and therefore the following echoes have less signal. A smaller flip angle provides less signal on the transverse plane, but more Z magnetization is preserved for subsequent echoes. The maximum signal at steady state is achieved using the Ernst angle for a given TR and T1:

$$\alpha = \cos^{-1}\left(e^{-TR/T1}\right) \qquad \text{Eq. 1.10}$$

This low flip angle RF pulse is also called an "alpha pulse" and is suitable for short TRs. Short TRs are needed for dynamic imaging. For example, the collection of 32 phase-encode lines in *k*-space, each with a 5-ms TR, requires 160 ms (5 ms × 32 phase-encode lines). This time

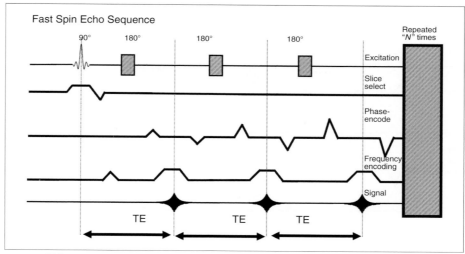

FIG. 1.14 Pulse sequence diagram for fast spin echo imaging. *TE,* Echo time.

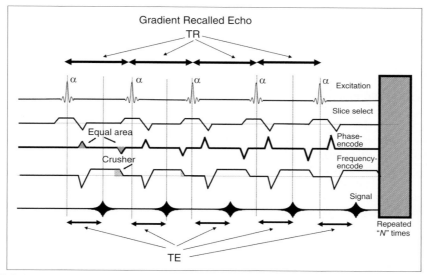

FIG. 1.15 Pulse sequence diagrams for gradient recalled echo imaging showing multiple repetition times *(TRs).* TRs and echo times *(TE)* are indicated.

is sufficiently short that 32 TRs can be acquired in the quiescent diastolic period. Thus data can be collected rather rapidly using a small excitation pulse rather than the 90-degree pulse. The GRE imaging method uses short TRs, low flip angles (alpha pulses), and no 180-degree refocusing pulse. Note that in GRE imaging (see Fig. 1.15), to keep the phase information intact, rewinding gradients are applied after each acquisition equal to and opposite to the phase-encoding gradient. Furthermore, the readout gradient is also rewound, so that on all axes, the spins are in phase after each TR. Usually an extra gradient is applied at the end of each TR on the X or Z axis, called a "crusher," "killer," or "spoiler" gradient (Fig. 1.16), which dephases any remaining transverse magnetization so that it does not contribute signal during the next phase-encode step (TR). These crushers are effective, but it is recognized that some residual magnetization remains during the approach to steady state, possibly affecting image contrast.[22] Although the fast GRE images have T2* dephasing, this does not usually reduce image quality, since very short TEs are achievable, unless a serious source of magnetic field inhomogeneity (e.g., a metallic implant) is present. Furthermore, the

GRE sequence can be used to quantify myocardial T2* (by imaging at multiple TE times) which may help detect diseases with myocardial iron deposition such as thalassemia[23-25] with good reproducibility.

Three-Dimensional Fast Gradient Echo: MR Angiography

The fast GRE pulse sequence is also used for contrast-enhanced MR angiography, which is the imaging of arteries and veins during the first pass of an exogenous contrast agent[26,27] or in steady state.[28] During the first pass of a gadolinium contrast agent, the blood T1 is reduced to ~30 ms. The Ernst angle equation (see Eq. 1.9) identifies an optimal angle of ~30 degrees for a TR of 5 ms. Because this method is three dimensional (3D), "phase-encoding" in Z (now called "slice encoding") is performed in the slice direction also. Therefore the scan time is $N_y \cdot N_z \cdot TR$, where N_z is the number of slice-encodings (slices). The acquisition of a 3D fast GRE volume provides high-quality images of vessels (see Chapters 43–46). However, without a contrast agent, the SNR of fast GRE imaging can be low, because the time between TRs, during

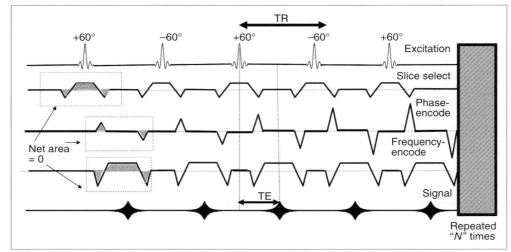

FIG. 1.16 Balanced steady-state free precession (SSFP) imaging. The sequence is identical to gradient recalled echo, except that the flip angle for SSFP is high and its sign is alternated in each repetition time *(TR)*. Also, the gradients in the SSFP sequence are fully rephased (see shaded areas), so that the net gradient area (summed over the TR) is zero, for each gradient axis. *TE*, Echo time.

which the longitudinal magnetization can regrow, is short. This limitation is partly overcome using balanced SSFP.

Balanced Steady-State Free Precession

Directly related to the GRE sequence is the balanced SSFP method (see Fig. 1.16). Today, almost all CMR imaging of ventricular function at 1.5 T employs this method, and it also is used for anatomical localization, valve visualization, and coronary artery imaging.[29] This very old technique[30] was later revived[31,32] because better scanner hardware allows for short TRs (e.g., 2–4 ms on 1.5 T) required for balanced SSFP. Balanced SSFP uses a pulse sequence identical to GRE (see Fig. 1.16), except for two distinctions. First, after each TR, the spins are rephased on each gradient axis (X, Y, and Z) to zero phase. No crushers, killers, or spoilers are used. This keeps the spins completely in phase (except for dephasing due to magnetic field inhomogeneities) so that the transverse magnetization can be reused in the next TR. For this reason the sequence is called "balanced." Second, a large flip angle (e.g., 60 degrees) is used, flipping spins around the positive and negative Y axis, in alternate TRs. This flip angle alternation scheme reuses the remaining transverse magnetization, and mixes it with longitudinal magnetization, for increased signal in each TR.

Balanced SSFP provides high SNR of blood and a unique T2/T1 weighting.[33] As stated above, balanced SSFP is highly sensitive to off-resonance, requires short TRs and large flip angles, and is challenging at 3 T, where off-resonance creates artifacts,[34] and RF heating concerns (specific absorption rate) limits the flip angle.

Echo Planar Imaging, Spiral and Radial

Analogous to reducing scan time, by replacing a spin echo acquisition by a fast spin echo acquisition, the GRE sequence can be accelerated by acquiring a train of gradient recalled echoes after a single RF pulse. This approach is called multiecho or echo planar imaging (EPI) and was among the first CMR imaging methods described.[35] For anatomy with long T2* tissues (e.g., the head), EPI can result in a complete image collection with a single slice-select pulse and a train of gradient echoes. EPI is the basis for the functional MRI (fMRI) technique widely used in brain mapping. Fig. 1.17 shows an EPI sequence, in which after a single RF excitation, frequency-encoding information at multiple

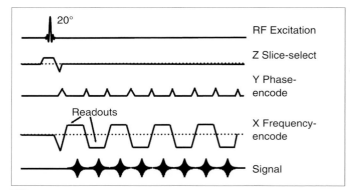

FIG. 1.17 Echo planar imaging (also called *multiecho imaging*), in which a portion of the frequency encodings are collected after each B_1 pulse. Here eight frequency encodings are collected after a single B_1 excitation pulse (here with a 20-degree flip angle). All of the CMR data can be acquired after a single excitation, or only a portion. The phase-encoding gradient is blipped with a constant area, which leads to increasing phase encoding, and readouts are acquired using both positive and negative lobes of the frequency-encoding gradient.

phase-encodings values are acquired. To reduce time between echoes, the readout gradient is rapidly reversed with every phase-encode step, so that MR signals are collected during both the positive and negative lobes of the readout gradient (arrows). This approach is challenging in the heart, where the T2* can be short[36] compared to the brain, but has found applications in cardiac perfusion[37] and the cardiac diffusion weighted imaging.[38] Because of the acquisition of many phase-encode steps after one RF excitation, the EPI method is fast, but results in poor SNR. EPI (along with spiral and radial described below) has *k*-space "trajectory" errors that need correction,[39–42] and image distortions due to off-resonance. However, these limitations can be overcome by only collecting a few (e.g., 3–9) phase-encode steps per slice-select RF excitation (instead all phase-encode steps) and repeating this process until all of the data have been collected.

Spiral imaging is similar to EPI, obtaining more image data after a single RF pulse, compared to conventional imaging, by continuously

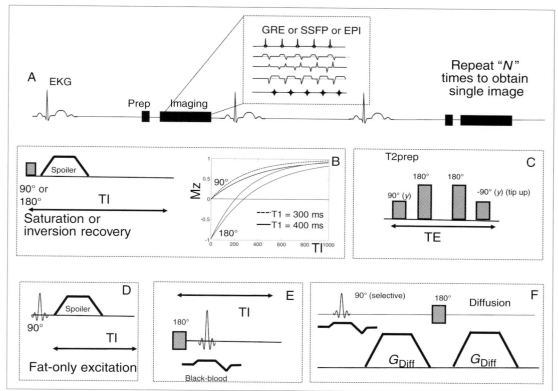

FIG. 1.18 Preparation pulses. (A) A preparation pulse precedes the acquisition of a segment of data (e.g., multiple repetition times [TR] with gradient recalled echo *[GRE]* or steady-state free precession *[SSFP]*), usually as part of an electrocardiogram *(ECG)*-gated acquisition. All preparations affect the longitudinal magnetization (M_z). (B) A nonselective 180-degree or 90-degree followed by an inversion time *(TI)* pulse generates T1 contrast, because M_z depends on the T1 and the TI time chosen. (C) T2prep uses the method of fast spin echo to refocus magnetization, which is then stored on the M_z axis. This results in Z magnetization, which depends on T2 of the imaged tissue. (D) Fat saturation is performed by exciting fat with a 90-degree pulse and then crushing the resulting fat M_{xy}. Using a short TI, the M_z of fat is 0 after the saturation pulse, and the fat signal is suppressed. (E) Black-blood preparation inverts all blood, and images at a TI when blood M_z magnetization is close to 0. The myocardial signal is unaffected, because a slice of interest is reinverted immediately after the 180 degrees. (F) Diffusion-encoding preparation. *EPI*, Echo planar imaging; *TE*, echo time.

sampling *k*-space in a spiral pattern,[43–45] and has found applications in flow imaging,[46] coronary imaging, and 3D late gadolinium enhancement,[47] where SNR is important. Radial imaging is another trajectory that acquires *k*-space data as radial spokes, analogous to CT. It has been applied to the heart, especially using undersampling of *k*-space for fast imaging.[48–51] Radial imaging was the first imaging method,[1] and its clinical utility has been facilitated by trajectory improvements and recent developments in reconstruction of undersampled MR data[52–55] using sparsity constraints. Spiral and radial also need trajectory correction. MR fingerprinting is a way of randomly sampling *k*-space with variable T1/T2 contrast.[56] In combination with advanced reconstruction methods, T1, T2, and proton density images can be generated.

Preparation Pulses

In CMR imaging, preparation pulses are often used to generate contrast, by generating M_z magnetization, which is T1 or T2 weighted. Fig. 1.18A shows how preparation pulses are used in CMR. First, a preparation pulse is applied, and then a segment (16–64 lines or more of *k*-space) of the MR data is acquired, at a certain time within the cardiac cycle. Then, either in the next cardiac cycle or after skipping one or more

cycles, another preparation pulse is applied and another segment of data is acquired. Fig. 1.18B–F shows a few important preparation pulses. Fig. 1.18B shows nonselective RF pulses, both a 90-degree "saturation recovery" pulse and a 180-degree "inversion recovery" pulse. These pulses generate T1 weighting, determined by the inversion time (TI) choice. A spoiler gradient destroys any M_{xy} magnetization, created by the RF pulse. These are commonly used for perfusion and late gadolinium enhancement.[57] They are nonselective, so that all spins experience these pulses. Adiabatic RF pulses are often used, which are less susceptible to B_0 inhomogeneity.[58] Eq. (1.2) describes the T1 weighting achieved for a 90-degree saturation pulse.

Fig. 1.18C shows a *T2prep* pulse.[59,60] This is also nonselective, affecting all of the spins in the magnetic field. A 90-degree excitation is followed by multiple 180-degree refocusing pulses. The signal decays by T2, just like fast spin echo imaging. However, the signal is tipped back to the Z axis with a 90-degree pulse, generating M_z magnetization that is weighted by the T2 of the tissue, with higher M_z for long T2 tissues. Thus this preparation pulse is called T2prep. Very importantly, Fig. 1.18D shows how fat saturation can be achieved using a 90-degree excitation of fat only, which is possible because the Larmor frequency of fat is different from that of water (~210 Hz difference at 1.5 T). After the saturation of fat, a spoiler kills the fat M_{xy}. Imaging then begins, with the fat signal suppressed. Fig. 1.18E shows a double inversion recovery (DIR) black-blood preparation.[61] This preparation consists of two inversion (180-degree) pulses, which immediately follow each other. The first inversion is a nonselective inversion pulse, which inverts all magnetization. The second inversion is a slice-selective inversion pulse, which reinverts a slice of interest, which is centered on the imaging slice but is slightly larger (by a factor of 1.5–2). This preparation is timed so that at the time of acquisition, all blood magnetization has regrown from $-M_z$ to 0 (i.e., is black). Any blood that was reinverted, because it was within the slice of interest, moves out of the imaging slice during systole. Any blood that has flowed into the slice will contribute no signal because it is nulled (see Fig. 1.10 for a black-blood image). Fig. 1.18F shows a "diffusion weighting" preparation. In this technique, the microstructure of the myocardium can be studied. The diffusion of water in the myocardium depends on the myocyte's orientation and therefore fiber structure. The diffusion is measured using preparation pulses: a 90-degree RF saturation pulse, to excite the spins, followed by the application of a maximal strength and rather long gradient (~10 ms, on any or multiple axes) to sensitize the signal to microscopic motions (diffusion). This is followed by a 180-degree refocusing pulse and an identical gradient that should rephrase any phase accumulation not due to spin motion. Cardiac diffusion imaging was proposed early on[62,63] but is only now gaining acceptance[38] due to lessening concerns about the influences of cardiac and respiratory motion. Many other preparation pulses, such as magnetization transfer (MT),[64] are available for generating contrast.

NEW HARDWARE ADVANCES

For CMR, a B_0 of 1.5 T is most commonly used; however, cardiac imaging at 3 T[65] provides equivalent or improved quality for coronary artery imaging,[66,67] late gadolinium enhancement, and perfusion,[68] and function,[34] and there is progress in CMR at 7 T.[69] The number of receiver coil channels has increased from a single surface coil or body coil to 16–32 channels routinely on new systems, up to 128 channels.[70] Higher gradient strengths of 80 mT/m are now available, which might hold promise for cardiac diffusion imaging.

REFERENCES

A full reference list is available online at ExpertConsult.com

2

Techniques for T1, T2, and Extracellular Volume Mapping

Peter Kellman and Michael Hansen

Many disease processes alter the local molecular environment of the myocardium, and consequently the longitudinal (T1) and transverse (T2) relaxation times can change. While such changes may be observed directly as changes in image contrast,[1–6] the tissue processes may be global and diffuse, hampering reliable detection of the disease. Quantitative methods for characterizing myocardial tissue based on parametric mapping of T1 and T2 have been proposed as an objective way of detecting and quantifying both focal and global changes in tissue. In combination with extracellular contrast agent injection, T1 mapping can also provide an estimate of the extracellular volume (ECV) fraction.

Native T1 mapping, as well as ECV mapping, is currently being explored as a diagnostic tool for a wide range of cardiomyopathies, and native T1 changes are detectable in both acute and chronic myocardial infarction (MI)[7,8] and may be used to characterize the edematous area at risk.[4,9,10] Elevated native T1 has also been reported in a number of diseases with cardiac involvement (e.g., myocarditis,[11] amyloidosis,[12] lupus,[13] and system capillary leakage syndrome[14]), and decreases in native T1 have been associated with Anderson-Fabry disease[15] and high iron content.[16,17] Native T2 mapping is used to detect edema in acute MI and myocarditis[18–20] and to identify the area at risk[4] in acute MI. Application of tissue characterization using parametric mapping for detection of disease is discussed elsewhere in this book.

This chapter describes state-of-the-art methods for measuring T1, T2, and ECV in the myocardium. Because the purpose of such techniques is a quantitative (objective) evaluation of biomarkers and disease, the discussion of the available techniques is framed in terms of accuracy, precision, and general reliability. In parametric mapping it is important to understand errors in quantification and other artifact mechanisms, which may be less familiar than conventional cardiovascular magnetic resonance (CMR) artifact mechanisms. Method imperfections may manifest themselves as subtle changes in measured tissue parameters, and artifactual changes may well be correlated with specific patient groups—that is, they are potential confounders. In particular, the estimated parameter values such as T1 may be affected by other variables such as myocardial wall thickness, T2, protocol settings, or scanner adjustments. Although this is not new to magnetic resonance imaging (MRI), where T1-weighted contrast may have some T2 contrast, these confounding effects may influence the interpretation of parametric maps. Normal values for parameters may depend on the field strength and the specific measurement technique or imaging protocol. Therefore well-controlled and optimized protocols are key to reproducibility, which is particularly important in applications aimed at the detection of subtle fibrosis and preclinical disease, and normal values need to be established for specific protocols. Limited spatial resolution will lead to errors caused by partial volume effects, particularly between myocardium and adjacent blood pool or fat tissue. Despite limitations, parametric mapping is a powerful tool in the assessment of diffuse myocardial disease.

T1 AND EXTRACELLULAR VOLUME MAPPING

Changes in both native T1 and T1 following the administration of gadolinium (Gd) contrast agents are considered important biomarkers, and multiple methods have been suggested for quantifying myocardial T1 in vivo.[21] In general, methods for measuring myocardial T1 consist of three components: (1) a perturbation of the longitudinal magnetization (i.e., an inversion or saturation), (2) an experiment to sample the relaxation curve as the longitudinal magnetization returns to its original level, and (3) a model used to fit the sampled curve and extract the myocardial T1. This chapter focuses on the technical aspects of key methods and imaging protocols and describes their limitations and the factors that influence their accuracy, precision, and overall reproducibility. The accuracy and precision of these measurements affect the detection and quantification of abnormal myocardial tissue.

Late gadolinium enhancement (LGE) is currently the primary tool for tissue characterization in CMR because it provides excellent depiction of MI and focal scar and has become an accepted standard for assessing myocardial viability.[22] LGE is also useful for detecting and characterizing fibrosis that is "patchy" in appearance, for example, as seen in nonischemic cardiomyopathies such as hypertrophic cardiomyopathy (HCM).[23] Diffuse myocardial fibrosis is, however, more difficult to distinguish using LGE, since the myocardial signal intensity may be nearly isointense and may be globally "nulled," thus appearing to be normal tissue.[24] Alternatively, quantitative measurement of myocardial T1 following the administration of an extracellular Gd contrast agent has been shown to be sensitive to increased ECV associated with diffuse myocardial fibrosis. However, a single postcontrast T1 measurement has limitations because of a variety of confounding factors such as Gd clearance rate, time of measurement, injected dose, body composition, and hematocrit.[25,26] These factors cause a significant variation in postcontrast T1, making it difficult to distinguish diseased and normal tissue based on absolute T1 values alone. Precontrast T1 varies with water content and may be elevated in cases of diffuse myocardial fibrosis. Precontrast T1 also varies significantly with field strength.[27] Direct measurement of ECV was initially developed for quantifying the myocardial extracellular fractional distribution volume[28] and has been proposed as a means for detection and quantification of diffuse myocardial fibrosis.[24,29–34] This approach is based on the change in T1 following administration of an extracellular contrast agent and circumvents the limitation of a single postcontrast T1 measurement in detecting a global change in T1. Myocardial ECV is measured as the percent of tissue composed of extracellular space, which is a physiologically intuitive unit of measurement and is independent of field strength.

ECV has been shown to correlate with collagen volume fraction in some diseases.[29,31]

Brief History of Methods for T1 Mapping in the Heart

Methods for measuring myocardial T1 were initially based on region of interest (ROI) analysis rather than pixelwise parametric maps. Inversion recovery (IR) images at different inversion times were acquired with multiple breath-holds[35] or IR cine protocols were used as a means of acquiring data in a single breath-hold.[36] These early methods were ROI-based schemes and were not suitable for pixelwise mapping. Pixelwise T1 mapping was introduced with the modified Look-Locker inversion recovery (MOLLI) imaging strategy,[37] which propelled the use of T1 mapping in CMR and inspired many new methods. MOLLI is widely used today with some protocol optimization and other adaptations. A shortened breath-hold adaptation with conditional curve fitting (ShMOLLI)[38] was proposed as a means of mitigating heart rate dependence as well as shortening the breath-hold. Further protocol optimization has been aimed at shortening the breath-hold and optimizing precision.[32,39] Motion correction was developed to mitigate respiratory motion for subjects with poor breath-holding,[40] and phase-sensitive IR reconstruction with motion correction further improved image quality.[41] A number of publications analyzed the accuracy of T1 measurements,[37,38,42–45] leading to a better understanding of the influence of various protocol parameters on T1 measurement errors. Saturation recovery (SR) methods developed initially for T1 measurements during first-pass contrast-enhanced perfusion (short acquisition period-T1 [SAP-T1])[46] have been recently adapted for T1 mapping using SR single-shot acquisition (SASHA),[47] with steady-state free precession (SSFP) readout as a means of mitigating the T1 underestimation in MOLLI and reducing the influence of confounding factors such as T2, magnetization transfer (MT), heart rate, and off-resonance. Even more recently, hybrid schemes have been proposed that incorporate both inversion and SR methods (saturation pulse prepared heart rate independent inversion-recovery [SAPPHIRE]).[48] ECV measurements were initially introduced using ROI-based measurement,[28–30] and pixelwise ECV mapping was later introduced.[33,39] Improvements to T1 and ECV mapping are continuously introduced, such as navigated methods for higher-resolution three-dimensional (3D)[49] or two-dimensional (2D) multislice.[50]

This chapter focuses on the basic concepts behind the widely used MOLLI and SASHA acquisition strategies for T1 mapping, followed by a review of factors influencing accuracy and precision. Discussion includes a description of other limitations and a summary of the pros and cons of various protocols.

T1-Mapping Methods

The currently used protocols for T1 mapping in the heart (Table 2.1) are based on IR or SR. Images are acquired at multiple time points on the recovery curve, and pixelwise curve fitting is performed to estimate the relaxation time parameter to produce a pixel map of T1. Images are generally acquired at the same cardiac phase and respiratory position to eliminate tissue motion. Although initial implementation involved multiple breath-holds, current methods generally use single breath-hold protocols with single-shot 2D imaging. To achieve higher spatial resolution and/or 3D imaging, segmentation may be required.

MOLLI, the original scheme, was proposed by Messroghli et al.[37] and is illustrated in Fig. 2.1. For each inversion, the MOLLI method samples the IR curve at multiple inversion times using single-shot imaging spaced at heartbeat intervals. Multiple inversions are used with different trigger delays to acquire measurements at different inversion times to sample the IR curve more finely. Recovery periods are needed between the inversions to ensure that samples from the different inversions are from the same recovery curve; that is, each inversion starts at

TABLE 2.1 Widely Used Inversion and Saturation Recovery Methods for T1 Mapping in the Heart

Inversion recovery (IR)	Multiple breath-hold FLASH[35]
	MOLLI[37]
	ShMOLLI[38]
	Modified MOLLI protocols[32,33,44,45]
Saturation recovery (SR)	SAP-T1[46]
	SASHA[47,51,52]
	SASHA VFA[53]
	SMART1[54]
Combined IR/SR	SAPPHIRE[48]

FLASH, Fast low angle shot; *MOLLI*, modified Look-Locker inversion; *SAP*, short acquisition period; *SASHA*, saturation recovery single-shot acquisition; *SAPPHIRE*, saturation pulse prepared heart rate independent inversion-recovery; *ShMOLLI*, shortened breath-hold modified Look-Locker inversion.

the same initial condition. The T1-map precision is related to the number and position of samples along the IR curve, and accuracy of the signal model is also affected by the sampling strategy due to the influence of the readout on the apparent recovery.

The MOLLI method uses an SSFP readout. The readout drives the IR to recover more quickly and reaches a steady state that is less than the equilibrium magnetization (M_0). The effect of the readout (Fig. 2.2) is an apparent recovery time referred to as T1*, which is less than the actual longitudinal recovery time, T1, which is the desired tissue parameter. As a result of the influence of the readout, the IR curve follows a three-parameter exponential signal model, $S(t) = A - B \exp(-t/T1^*)$, where t represents the inversion time and $T1^*$ is the apparent T1. The measured values may be fit to the three-parameter model to estimate A, B, and T1*, which may be used to approximate T1 ≈ T1* (B/A − 1). The derivation for the so-called Look-Locker correction factor (B/A − 1) is based on a continuous readout using fast low angle shot (FLASH).[55] Despite the fact that the MOLLI uses a gated SSFP readout, the signal model behaves as a three-parameter model where the Look-Locker correction is reasonably effective at low readout excitation flip angles (FAs).

The analytic relationship between T1* and T1 for SSFP has been derived for continuous SSFP under somewhat idealized conditions such as ideal slice profile.[56] Useful analytic derivations for gated SSFP with realistic slice profiles have not been developed due to complexity. Bloch simulations may be used to calculate the error inherent in this approximation[43] and to gain insight into the sensitivity of various protocol parameters and design variables. The influence of various parameters such as T2, heart rate, off-resonance, and actual FA are referred to as confounders and are discussed later.

A number of modifications (Table 2.2) to the original proposed MOLLI protocol have been proposed to shorten the acquisition duration or to improve the accuracy or precision.[32,38,39,44,45] A shorthand nomenclature is used to label these protocols. The notation captures how many inversions (or saturations) are included in the experiment, how many images are acquired after each inversion, and how long the waiting period is between inversions. For example, a 3(3)3(3)5 protocol would indicate that there are a total of three inversions; three images are acquired (over three RR intervals) after the first inversion; this is followed by a waiting period of three RR intervals, and then three images are acquired, followed by another three RR waiting period; finally, there is a third inversion, after which five images are acquired. In an extension of this nomenclature, an "s" can be added to the intervals to

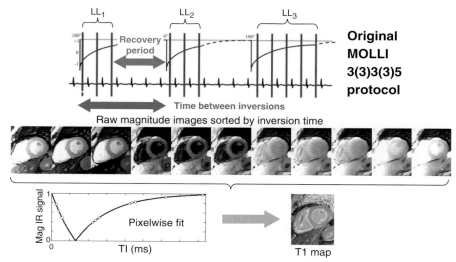

Raw magnitude images sorted by inversion time

FIG. 2.1 Modified Look-Locker inversion *(MOLLI)* recovery scheme for T1-mapping in the heart.[37] The original protocol employed 3 inversions with 3, 3, and 5 images acquired in the beats following inversions, and 3 heartbeat recovery periods between inversions, referred to here as 3(3)3(3)5. All images are acquired at the same delay from the R-wave trigger for mid-diastolic imaging. Curve fitting is performed on a pixelwise basis using the actual measured inversion times. *IR,* Inversion recovery. (From Kellman P, Hansen MS. T1-mapping in the heart: accuracy and precision. *J Cardiovasc Magn Reson.* 2014;16:2.)

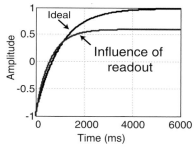

FIG. 2.2 The apparent inversion recovery (T1*) is influenced by the steady-state free precession readout. The effective inversion recovery is fit using a three-parameter model, and the T1 is estimated using the so-called Look-Locker correction. (From Kellman P, Hansen MS. T1-mapping in the heart: accuracy and precision. *J Cardiovasc Magn Reson.* 2014;16:2.)

TABLE 2.2   Reported Schemes for Modified Look-Locker Inversion Sampling

MOLLI	3(3)3(3)5	Messroghli et al.[37] (original publication)
	3(3)5	Ugander et al.[33] and Salerno et al.[44]
	5(3)3	Kellman et al.[39]
	4(1)3(1)2	Schelbert et al.[32]
	2(2)2(2)4	Salerno et al.[44]
	5(3s)3	Kellman et al.[57,58]
	4(1s)3(1s)2	Kellman et al.[57]
	5s(3s)3s	Kellman and Hansen[45]
	4s(1s)3s(1s)2s	Kellman and Hansen[45]
ShMOLLI	5(1)1(1)1(with conditional fitting)	Piechnik et al.[38]

MOLLI, Modified Look-Locker inversion; *ShMOLLI,* shortened breath-hold modified Look-Locker inversion.

indicate that images are acquired for a certain number of seconds and the waiting period is in seconds: that is, 5s(3s)3s would indicate two inversions with acquisition of images for at least 5 s, followed by a recovery of at least 3 s, and a second inversion with images acquired for at least 3 s. Because the number of electrocardiogram (ECG)-triggered images must be a whole number, the acquisition and recovery periods are rounded to the nearest multiple of the RR period to ensure an adequate duration. To avoid acquiring too few images for low heart rates (<60 beats per minute), the sequence never acquires fewer than the specified number of images: that is, 5 + 3 = 8 in this example. The recovery period is never less than the specified number of seconds. Acquiring and recovering with fixed minimum time periods helps gain independence of heart rate.

SR is an alternative to IR that has gained renewed attention. Despite having a reduced dynamic range, SR has potential for improved accuracy. SR methods that use a saturation preparation for each measurement have the benefit that each measurement becomes independent of the others. By starting the recovery from a saturated state, the prior history is erased. Recovery periods between successive measurements are not required unless longer SR times are needed for fitting. Shown in Fig. 2.3, the SASHA method[47] uses SSFP readout very similar to the earlier SAP-T1 method,[46] which used a spoiled gradient recalled echo (GRE) readout.

The SASHA method acquires multiple time points on the SR curve and does a pixelwise curve fit. To acquire a fully recovered image, an image is initially acquired before any saturation preparation: that is, starting from the equilibrium magnetization. Images are acquired on successive heartbeats using SR preparations with varying trigger delays. In the original proposed SASHA protocol, there are 10 images acquired at saturation delays uniformly spaced over the RR interval plus the initial fully recovered image, which serves as an important anchor point for the curve fit. The order in which the various delays are acquired is not significant for fitting, assuming ideal saturation. Importantly, the SR curve recovers as T1 and is not influenced by the readout so that it is not shortened to an apparent T1* < T1 as in the case of MOLLI.

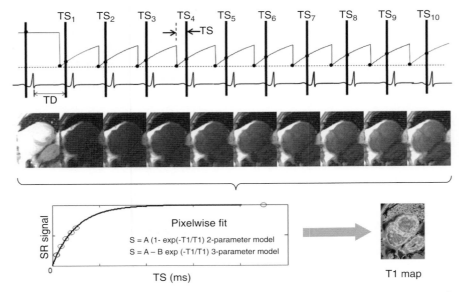

FIG. 2.3 Saturation recovery single-shot acquisition (SASHA) scheme for T1 mapping in the heart.[47] A single image is acquired without saturation and used as the fully recovered measurement followed by a series of saturation recovery images at different saturation recovery times (TSi). All images are acquired at the same delay from the R-wave trigger for mid-diastolic imaging. Curve fitting is performed on a pixelwise basis. (From Kellman P, Hansen MS. T1-mapping in the heart: accuracy and precision. *J Cardiovasc Magn Reson.* 2014;16:2.)

Therefore no correction is necessary, which eliminates the source of many inaccuracies of the IR-based MOLLI scheme. Because the readout does not lead to an apparent T1*, a higher FA readout is possible, which makes up for some of the lost dynamic range in using SR. The higher FA readout using SSFP with linear phase-encode ordering does slightly alter the shape of the recovery curve, causing an apparent bias: that is, the curve does not start at 0 for 0 delay. Thus the otherwise two-parameter signal model $S(t) = A(1 - \exp[-t/T1])$ for SR assuming ideal saturation becomes a three-parameter model $S(t) = A - B \exp(-t/T1)$. The three-parameter model also absorbs any imperfection in the saturation efficiency attributed to the RF saturation pulse. However, the cost of estimating the additional parameter is loss of precision. Therefore there is a tradeoff between accuracy and precision in considering whether to use two- or three-parameter fitting. Although a center-out phase-encode order in which the center of *k*-space is acquired first has the potential to completely remove the influence of the readout, the use of center-out ordering with SSFP is problematic because of artifacts, and the use of center-out FLASH is associated with a significant loss of signal-to-noise ratio (SNR). An improved version of SASHA[53] that uses variable flip angle (VFA) for SSFP readout minimizes the small bias attributed to a linear phase-encode order and therefore makes two-parameter fitting practical with negligible loss in accuracy. The SASHA VFA also has the benefit of improved transition to steady state, which greatly reduces ghost artifacts, particularly as a result of off-resonant fat, which was an issue with the original implementation.

The SASHA sampling scheme may be altered to acquire longer saturation delay measurements by allowing one or more heartbeat recovery periods between saturations. Measurements strategies that use recovery periods such as SMART1[54] may improve precision for specific ranges of T1 and heart rate but reduce the overall SNR efficiency somewhat. Optimized sampling strategies for SASHA are described for both two-[51] and three-parameter[52] fittings. Schemes that simply use a MOLLI strategy replaced with SR[59] incur the problems of an apparent T1* without

gaining the main benefits of SR. A combined IR/SR approach known as SAPPHIRE[48] gains many of the benefits of IR and SR but still retains some of the problems associated with IR. Each method has its strengths and weaknesses in terms of accuracy, precision, and overall reproducibility.

ECV Mapping Methods

The ECV in the myocardium may be estimated from the concentration of extracellular contrast agent in the myocardium relative to the blood in a dynamic steady state.[28,29,33] The ECV may be calculated as:

$$ECV = (1 - hct)\frac{\Delta R1_{myo}}{\Delta R1_{blood}} = (1 - hct)\frac{\left(\dfrac{1}{T1_{myo\ post}} - \dfrac{1}{T1_{myo\ pre}}\right)}{\left(\dfrac{1}{T1_{blood\ post}} - \dfrac{1}{T1_{blood\ pre}}\right)} \qquad \text{Eq. 2.1}$$

where hct is the hematocrit, and the change in relaxation rate $\Delta R1$ (where $R1 = 1/T1$) between precontrast and postcontrast is directly proportional to the Gd concentration, $\Delta R1 = \gamma[\text{Gd}]$ ($\gamma = 4.5$ L/mmol per second for Gd-DTPA). A dynamic steady state exists for tissues that have a contrast exchange rate with the blood, which is faster than the net clearance of contrast from the blood.[28] A dynamic steady state between the plasma and interstitium may be achieved by slow intravenous infusion[24,29] or by imaging 15 minutes following an intravenous bolus administration[32,33] for normally perfused myocardium, although 15 minutes may not be adequate for recently infarcted myocardium.[60] The bolus method is more generally used because it fits well with clinical workflow and permits conventional late enhancement imaging at the desired dose. The ECV formula (Eq. 2.1) implies that our myocardial ECV measurements include both the intravascular and extravascular space. The factor $(1 - hct)$, which varies between individuals, represents the blood volume of distribution (blood ECV) and converts the equation from a partition coefficient calculation to a myocardial ECV.

Precontrast and postcontrast image series are acquired in separate breath-holds, which are typically 15 to 30 minutes apart. Even small differences in respiratory position or changes in patient position attributed to movement will cause significant misregistration of the images. Care must be taken that the patient does not move, and coregistration of the precontrast and postcontrast images must be performed using a nonrigid image registration to mitigate in-plane motion.[40,41] The complete processing workflow may be fully automated[39] to include precontrast and postcontrast T1 mapping with respiratory motion correction and blood pool segmentation. A prototype ECV mapping tool has been integrated onto a clinical scanner.[61] Inline ECV mapping presumes that the hematocrit has been measured before the scan using point-of-care devices. For instances for which the hematocrit has not been measured, it is possible to estimate an approximate hematocrit from the value of blood T1 and use this derived *hct* for a synthetic ECV.[62] In this way, the ECV map may be available immediately following the completion of the postcontrast T1 map, regardless of whether or not *hct* was measured.

Although detecting global changes that are difficult to see in nonquantitative imaging has been a driver for quantitation, there is also potential value in cases of focal abnormalities in determination of whether remote tissue is in fact normal and in measurement of border zones. Given adequate precision, the strength of pixelwise mapping of T1 is the ability to detect small abnormalities and discriminate spatial structures. Fig. 2.4 illustrates T1 and ECV maps in cases ranging from focal scar to patchy to diffuse.

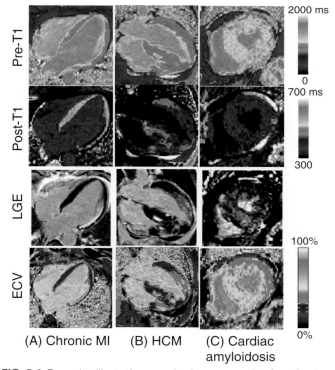

FIG. 2.4 Examples illustrating mapping in cases ranging from focal and patchy to diffuse disease. Native (precontrast) T1 maps (first row), postcontrast T1 maps (second row), late gadolinium enhancement *(LGE)* (third row), and extracellular volume fraction *(ECV)* maps (fourth row) for patients with (A) chronic myocardial infarction *(MI)*, (B) hypertrophic cardiomyopathy *(HCM)*, and (C) cardiac amyloidosis. (From Kellman P, Wilson JR, Xue H, Ugander M, Arai AE. Extracellular volume fraction mapping in the myocardium, part 1: evaluation of an automated method. *J Cardiovasc Magn Reson.* 2012;14:63.)

Reproducibility: Accuracy, Precision, and Confounding Factors

The sensitivity for detecting abnormal elevation of T1 and ECV derived from measurements of T1 is fundamentally limited by the reproducibility of T1 estimates. The reproducibility is affected by a number of factors that include measurement precision and accuracy as well as biological variability. It is important to establish normal baseline values and ranges[21] for the specific technique and protocol.

The precision refers to the effect of random noise on the measurement and is a function of the number and timing of measurements along the IR or SR curve, the SNR, the tissue T1, and the method of fitting. The precision of T1 methods has been well characterized,[45] and pixelwise maps of standard deviation (SD) attributed to thermal noise may be generated as a quality map.[57] Example T1 and corresponding SD maps are shown (Fig. 2.5) for a normal subject using four different mapping protocols. This example illustrates several points: (1) normal T1 values vary considerably by method and specific imaging protocol, (2) the SD varies across the heart as the SNR varies because of surface coil drop off with distance, and (3) different methods of T1 mapping have different precisions, leading to differing sensitivities.

Other factors contributing to measurement error that are not random further limit the reproducibility and are highly dependent on the technique and specific protocol. Some of these factors may depend on the scanner adjustments such as off-resonance errors[58] due to center frequency adjustment error, inability to shim the volume perfectly, or because of variation in the actual FA attributed to transmitter field inhomogeneity or FA adjustment error. Techniques must be designed to be robust in the presence of such variations because these variables are generally not well controlled. Variations may also relate to the actual tissue composition. For instance, IR methods using SSFP readout are dependent on the tissue T2[43,45,47] and MT resulting from the macromolecular content of proteins.[63] Still other variables relating to the patient such as heart rate, heart rate variability, and cardiac or respiratory motion may affect estimates of T1. The accuracy for a given technique may also be influenced by specific protocol parameters such as FA, matrix size, repetition rate (TR), and sampling strategy. The sensitivity of MOLLI (Fig. 2.6) and SASHA (Fig. 2.7) techniques has been calculated based on Bloch simulations for a common protocol with matrix size 256×144, partial Fourier factor 7/8, factor 2 acceleration, bandwidth 1085 Hz/pixel, TR = 2.8 ms, excitation FA (FA) 35 degrees, minimum TI 100 ms, and TI increment 80 ms. These calculations illustrate the dependencies on T2, HR, FA, and off-resonance leading to an underestimation of T1. The MOLLI-based methods have the largest sensitivity to adjustments and protocol parameters. For a 25% variation in transmit FA often seen in practice, the variation in apparent native T1 is 2%. For 100 Hz off-resonance, the variation in apparent native T1 can be as high as 4%. For heart variation from 60 to 120 beats per minute, there is a 2.5% variation in apparent native T1. Over the range of normal to highly edematous T2 (45 to 90 ms), the native T1 will vary approximately 4%. The SR-based method of SASHA is much less sensitive to these variables. However, the IR methods such as MOLLI achieve a higher precision.[45]

An example of how edematous myocardium may confound the measurement of native T1 (Fig. 2.8) is presented for a subject with acute MI. The edematous region of MI has an elevated value of T2 that is 15 ms greater than remote. The increase in T1 for this MI region is 227 ms above remote measured using MOLLI, and elevated 199 ms measured using SASHA. The difference in T1 elevation $227 - 199 = 28$ ms is explained in part due to the 15 ms elevation of T2 attributed to edema as seen in plot of MOLLI sensitivity to T2 (see Fig. 2.6) and

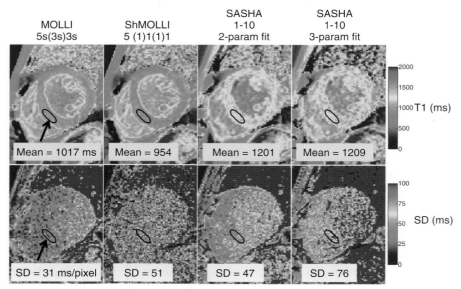

FIG. 2.5 Examples of in vivo T1 maps and corresponding pixelwise standard deviation *(SD)* maps acquired using modified Look-Locker inversion *(MOLLI)* 5s(3s)3s, shortened breath-hold MOLLI, and saturation recovery single-shot acquisition *(SASHA)* protocols with two- and three-parameter fitting. Variation in SD across the heart is apparent because of variation in signal-to-noise ratio from surface coil sensitivity roll-off. MOLLI has the best precision but underestimates T1 as a result of the approximate nature of the Look-Locker correction and because of magnetization transfer. Note that SASHA with two-parameter fitting has a small T1 underestimation; three-parameter fitting is more accurate but has significant loss of precision. (From Kellman P, Hansen MS. T1-mapping in the heart: accuracy and precision. *J Cardiovasc Magn Reson.* 2014;16:2.)

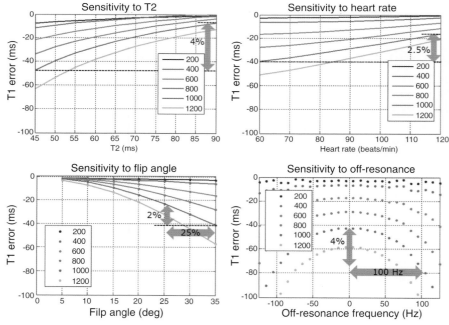

FIG. 2.6 Sensitivity of T1 estimates using the modified Look-Locker inversion method to T2, heart rate, flip angle, and off-resonance frequency using a 5s(3s)3s sampling scheme.[45]

because of the different degree of MT between the MI and remote region. The MT will be less in the edematous region because of increased water content; thus the T1 underestimation of MOLLI attributed to MT will be less, corresponding to an increased T1. The SASHA method is relatively insensitive to both T2 and MT.

Limitations and Potential Pitfalls

The use of T1 to characterize myocardial tissue is a simplification or first-order model. The myocardium consists of several compartments such as myocytes, interstitium, and capillaries, each with different constituent molecular makeup to include free water and macromolecules.

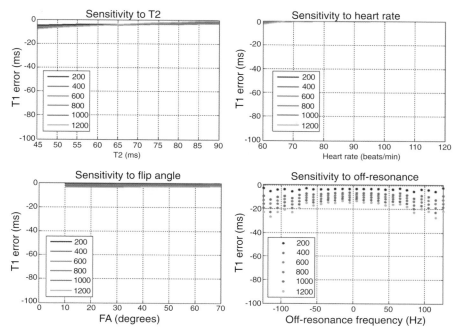

FIG. 2.7 Sensitivity of T1 estimates using the saturation recovery single-shot acquisition variable flip angle two-parameter method to T2, heart rate, flip angle, and off-resonance frequency using an NS + [(0)1][9] sampling scheme.[51]

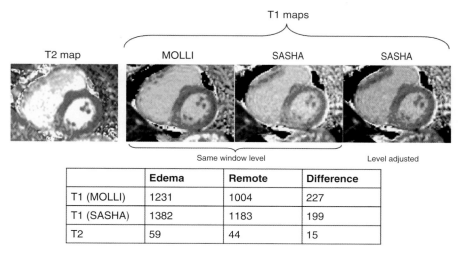

	Edema	Remote	Difference
T1 (MOLLI)	1231	1004	227
T1 (SASHA)	1382	1183	199
T2	59	44	15

FIG. 2.8 Example of T1 and T2 maps for subject with edematous acute myocardial infarction. The edematous region is elevated 15 ms above remote, and T1 is elevated 227 ms (using the modified Look-Locker inversion *[MOLLI]*) and 199 ms (using saturation recovery single-shot acquisition *[SASHA]*). The greater increase in apparent T1 for MOLLI edematous is because of the confounding effects of T2 and magnetization transfer. Note that the baseline values for SASHA are greater than for MOLLI.

The interactions between the proton spins contributing to the observed MRI signal are highly complex. Despite the fact that current T1 mapping largely ignores these complexities in measuring a single macroscopic T1, the T1 measurements have been demonstrated to have potential in clinical use.

The potential for quantification of myocardial tissue is to detect small changes as a result of disease processes or treatment. The desire to measure subtle changes places stringent requirements on reliability of the measurement. For this reason there is great emphasis on accuracy, precision, and general reproducibility. In addition to the confounding factors described earlier, wherein estimates of T1 may be affected by tissue T2, MT, patient heart rate, off-resonance (B_0), or actual FA (transmitted B_1), there are other artifact mechanism that may affect measurement. One of the most important limitations is the partial volume contamination of the myocardium by the adjacent blood pool signal, which is generally greater than the myocardium. The blood pool contamination is caused by both limited in-plane spatial resolution as well as through-plane. A voxel in a myocardial region may contain a mixture of myocardium and blood and thus be biased. The degree of bias as a result of this partial volume between myocardium and blood will depend

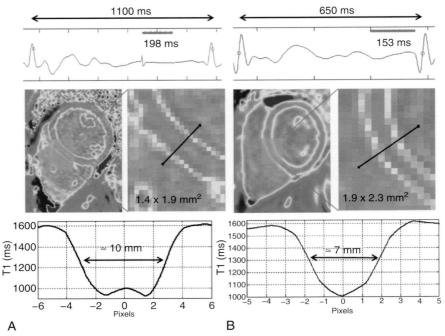

FIG. 2.9 Example of T1 maps in two subjects. (A) Subject with heart rate of 58 beats per minute acquired using a modified Look-Locker inversion protocol with 256 × 144 matrix. (B) Subject with heart rate of approximately 90 beats per minute using a 192 × 120 matrix. Although the interpolated maps are of good quality, the subject with higher heart rate and thinner wall has only about 3.5 pixels across the septum, leading to a degree of partial volume error in region of interest measurements. (From Kellman P, Hansen MS. T1-mapping in the heart: accuracy and precision. *J Cardiovasc Magn Reson.* 2014;16:2.)

on proximity to the blood pool as well as effective spatial resolution. With in-plane image resolution of 1.5 to 2 mm and thin myocardial walls (<1 cm), there may be only a few (2–5) pixel widths across the myocardial wall. Gibb's ringing can lead to fluctuations of ≥5% in T1 values even mid-wall, and errors can be much larger close to the blood myocardial boundary. For slices for which there is through plane angulation of the wall, particularly at the apex, there can be additional partial volume effects. Caution must be exercised in making and interpreting measurements for thin walls, particularly when comparing populations with different wall thickness.

Fig. 2.9 illustrates the effect of spatial resolution on native T1 maps for two subjects with different wall thickness and heart rates. Subject 1 (A) has a myocardial wall thickness of approximately 10 mm (approximately 6 pixels) in the septum and heart rate approximately 55 beats per minute. A profile plot of T1 across the septal wall shows a ringing of approximately 50 ms (5%) attributed to Gibb's effect and a smooth transition between the myocardium and adjacent blood pool of approximately 2 pixels. Subject 2 (B) has a thinner myocardial wall (approximately 7 mm) and a higher heart rate. At the higher heart rate (approximately 92 beats per minute), a slightly reduced matrix size was used to mitigate temporal motion blur, resulting in a myocardial wall thickness corresponding to 3 to 4 pixels. In this case, the measured T1 (see profile plot) is contaminated by adjacent blood for all but the mid-wall, thereby compromising the accuracy of measurements. Most clinical image viewers use interpolation to display images when zoomed, thus hiding the true resolution limits that would be apparent when displaying the pixelated image. Depending on the displayed range (window level), the zoomed and interpolated maps often appear to have distinct boundaries, even in situations with significant partial volume contamination.

In addition to limited spatial resolution, there may be additional blurring as a result of cardiac motion in cases of higher heart rates, variations in RR interval, or imaging during a period of cardiac cycle in which there is wall motion. The temporal duration of image acquisition can be reduced to mitigate blurring by using higher parallel imaging acceleration, although this may come at the expense of loss in SNR. The partial volume bias attributed to potential blurring at high heart rates is important to consider and is distinct from the previously described heart rate dependence of the MOLLI-type sequences. Finally, imperfect respiratory motion correction may lead to an additional source of blurring.

There are partial volume errors for voxels with a mixture of myocardium and fat.[64] This may occur at tissue boundaries or within the myocardium in the case of lipomatous metaplasia of replacement fibrosis, which is commonly seen in chronic MI or other scarring. The presence of fat leads to a bias in T1 measurement, which may be either a positive or negative bias depending on the specific protocol and off-resonance frequency. T1 biases will be additive or subtractive depending on whether the center frequency corresponds to the myocardium and fat is in-phase or out-of-phase, respectively. Lipomatous metaplasia is prevalent and often difficult to detect at low fat fractions. The influence on T1 at these low-fat fractions is significant and is readily misinterpreted. Although this may be mitigated to some extent by means of chemical shift fat suppression (i.e., fat saturation), the fat saturation may also influence the measurement of normal myocardial T1 if there is any significant off-resonance error caused by imperfect shim.

Quality maps such as goodness of fit or standard deviation maps[57] may be used for quality control as a means of detecting cases for which there is increased error because of cardiac or respiratory motion in cases where the motion is fairly extreme. However, quality maps do not account for all partial volume errors. Other potentially useful quality metrics are off-resonance field maps and FA maps. When ECV is elevated, it may not be clear whether this is because of fibrosis, edema, or both, which may be either diffuse or focal. In such instances, precontrast T1 or T2 maps, in addition to patient history and contextual imaging clues like signs of heart failure, may help to differentiate these mechanisms.

One of the attractive aspects of ECV measurement is that the value represents a quantitative measurement. However, biases in the measurement of precontrast and postcontrast T1 do not cancel out, and methods with different baseline normal values of T1 such as MOLLI and SASHA will yield different baseline normal values of ECV.

The ability to distinguish partial volume border pixels and correctly determine whether pixels are contaminated by partial volume effects, or are true pathophysiology such as subendocardial or subepicardial fibrosis, is a residual and important issue as it was shown in the T1 mapping example. This issue is not only important in terms of the visual readout but also may introduce biases into quantitative measurements, which become particularly significant in the context of more subtle diseases. One approach to reducing the bias in measurements is to restrict the measurement to the mid-wall region, although one must exercise caution for subjects with thin-walled myocardium or patients with thin rims of subendocardial fibrosis.

Summary

There are a number of methods and imaging protocols for T1 mapping in the heart, and new methods are emerging. A comparison of several of the widely used protocols is shown in Table 2.3. This assessment of pros and cons, albeit subjective, is meant to capture the key issues that relate to overall reproducibility and affect the ability to detect subtle changes in T1 from normal values. The inherent difficulty of tightly controlling the shim and uniformity of transmit FA in clinical scanners reduces the overall reproducibility of the MOLLI-based methods using IR and SSFP readout as compared with the SR approach. Limitations such as partial volume effects between myocardium and blood are common to all of these protocols. In this table, falsely elevated T1 due to partial volume with fat is considered an artifact.

ECV mapping appears promising to complement LGE imaging in cases of more homogenously diffuse myocardial disease states, which affect the myocardial extracellular space. The ability to display ECV maps in quantitative units that may be interpreted on an absolute scale offers the potential for simplified detection and measurement of the extent of abnormalities affecting the myocardial ECV. There is a continuous spectrum of spatial heterogeneity between diffuse and focal fibrosis. The use of pixelwise mapping offers a new tool to better assess the heterogeneity of the myocardial tissue and to measure ECV of the diseased regions.

T2 MAPPING

The transverse relaxation time (T2) of myocardial tissue may be altered by disease. Edematous tissue with increased water content has elevated T2[18,19] and may be a by-product of an acute disease process caused by inflammation. Presence or absence of edema is used to differentiate acute and chronic MI,[65] to identify the area at risk,[4] and in assessment of nonischemic disease such as myocarditis.[66] Increased iron concentration leads to a reduction in both T2 and T2* as seen in iron overload (e.g., due to thalassemia).[17] Although T2-weighted imaging may be used to detect focal abnormalities, it is more challenging to detect global changes in T2 caused by diffuse disease where there generally is not a remote healthy point of reference. T2 mapping provides a means of automatic, quantitative measurement of T2 on a pixelwise basis that may be used in diagnosis of disease across a spectrum of heterogeneity from diffuse to focal.

Methods

T2 mapping is performed by acquiring multiple images ($N \geq 2$) with different T2 weightings and estimating the T2 at each pixel by performing a two-parameter curve fit to the measured signal for each pixel $S_n(x, y)$. A mono-exponential model $S_n = PD \exp(-TE_n/T2)$ is used, where T2 is the unknown to be estimated, PD is the unknown proton density, and TE_n (known) is the effective echo time of the individual T2-weighted image for the nth acquisition ($n = 1, 2, ..., N$). T2-weighted images may be acquired by a number of methods. Methods for cardiac MRI T2 mapping include (1) T2-prepared SSFP (T2p-SSFP),[67] (2) multiecho spin echo (MESE),[68] and (3) a hybrid of MESE and either turbo spin echo (TSE)[69,70] or gradient spin echo (GraSE).[71,72]

The most widely used method at this time is the T2p-SSFP. An example of pixelwise T2 mapping for a subject with acute MI is shown in Fig. 2.10 for T2p-SSFP. In this example, three T2-weighted images are acquired with echo times of TE = 0, 25, and 55 ms, where the TE = 0 is acquired without any T2 preparation. The anterior MI is edematous, with elevated T2 approximately 72 ms, and the normal myocardium remote from the MI has a T2 of approximately 48 ms.

The single-shot T2-prepared readout approach acquires each T2-weighted image in a single beat, which has the benefit of being robust to cardiac and respiratory motion. ECG gating is used with acquisition in mid-diastole to minimize cardiac motion; respiratory motion may be mitigated by breath-holding or navigated acquisition. Residual in-plane respiratory motion is typically corrected using nonrigid image registration. Either SSFP or FLASH readout may be used.[67] SSFP readout is most commonly used to maximize SNR, particularly at 1.5 T. Single-shot SSFP readout uses a linear phase-encode order to minimize artifacts caused by eddy currents. It is possible to use

TABLE 2.3	**Summary of Pros and Cons of Various Reported T1-Mapping Protocols**						
	MOLLI 3(3)3(3)5	**MOLLI 5s(3s)3s**	**MOLLI 4s(1s)3s(1s)2s**	**ShMOLLI**	**SASHA 2p-fit**	**SASHA 3p-fit**	**SASHA VFA 2p-fit**
Short breath-hold	−	+	+	+	+	+	+
HR insensitivity	−	+	+	+	++	++	++
Absolute accuracy	−	−	−	−	+	++	+
Precision	++	++	++	+	+	−	+
Few image artifacts	+	+	+	+	−	−	+
Reproducibility	−	+	+	+	−	−	++

HR, Heart rate; *MOLLI,* Modified Look-Locker inversion; *SASHA,* saturation recovery single-shot acquisition; *ShMOLLI,* shortened breath-hold modified Look-Locker inversion; *VFA,* variable flip angle.

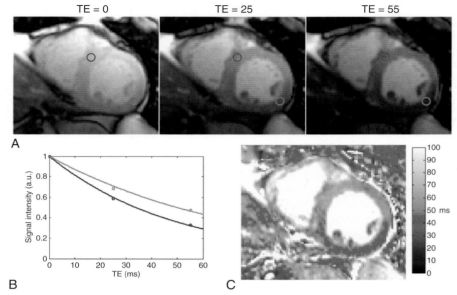

FIG. 2.10 Illustration of T2 mapping approach. T2 mapping approach using T2p-steady-state free precession: (A) acquiring images at three echo times, (B) performing a monoexponential curve fit to signal intensities at each pixel to estimate T2 to (C) produce a pixelwise T2 map.

centric phase encode ordering with a single-shot FLASH readout. By using centric ordering, the center of k-space, which determines the principal contrast, is acquired immediately following the T2 preparation. However, by using linear ordering, there is some delay following the T2 preparation and the center of k-space during which there is T1 regrowth of the magnetization that leads to a T1-dependent bias = PD(1−exp[−TS/T1]), where TS is the time from end of the preparation to the center of k-space.

With the T2p-SSFP approach, it is necessary to have several heartbeats (typically 3 or 4 seconds) between image acquisitions to allow for full magnetization recovery (dependent on T1). If there is insufficient signal recovery, the images will be affected by the preceding image, thus altering the estimated value of T2 and introducing a dependence on T1. Alternatively, it has been proposed to use a saturation preparation to reset the initial condition for each heartbeat to a fixed value.[73] In this way, the number of images acquired may be increased because no recovery beats are required, but there is a significant SNR loss because of the incomplete SR.

The T2 preparation is implemented by tipping the magnetization vector down on the transverse plane for a prescribed duration (TE), followed by tipping the vector back, and crushing any residual transverse magnetization. Refocusing pulses are used between the tip-down and tip-up pulses to avoid dephasing caused by myocardial motion or blood flow, which can result in artifacts. T2 preparations have been designed that are robust to variations in both B_0 (off-resonance) and B_1 (effective transmitted FA). These are based on either composite pulses[20,74] or adiabatic RF designs.[75,76] The minimum TE for the T2 preparation is dependent on the duration and number of refocusing pulses. For designs that use several refocusing pulses, a short TE is not feasible[20] and in this case a readout without any T2 preparation is used for an effective TE = 0. A significant error in FA because of in homogeneity in transmitted B_1+ or calibration error resulting in a reduced signal for the prepared measurements and not the TE = 0 measurement may lead to an underestimate in T2. This may be mitigated using T2 preparation for all measurements and shortening the overall refocusing duration.

The MESE approach acquires the data in a segmented fashion with multiple echoes, with different TEs acquired at each beat for a given phase encode using a spin echo train. This requires a lengthy breath-hold or navigated scan and is included here for completeness of discussion. The MESE is acquired in conjunction with a dark blood preparation to avoid blood flow artifacts, typically double inversion recovery (DIR) applied immediately following the R-wave ECG trigger.

The acquisition of MESE may be accelerated by acquiring multiple phase encodes at each echo time using a hybrid approach such as GraSE,[77,78] which employs a short echo train gradient recalled echo planar imaging (EPI) readout between 180-degree refocusing pulses. In this way, 3 to 7 echoes may be acquired per heartbeat, accelerating the image acquisition for T2 mapping.[71,72] This scheme is also used in conjunction with a DIR dark blood preparation and may be either breath-held or navigated. EPI readout is prone to artifacts caused by off-resonance or fat chemical shift and is often used in conjunction with chemical shift fat saturation. To mitigate ghosting artifacts, a linear interleaved phase-encode order is typically used with echo time shifting to ensure a smooth phase transition across k-space for different EPI echoes.

Spin echo methods are highly motion sensitive. DIR dark blood preparations rely on imaging at the same cardiac phase as the DIR preparation, which is difficult to achieve at higher heart rates or in patients with motion during the imaging interval in diastole. Furthermore, the spin echo readout itself is sensitive to motion. It is common for myocardial wall motion to cause signal loss or complete signal drop out.

Reproducibility: Accuracy, Precision, and Confounding Factors

Similar to the discussion of T1 and ECV mapping, many of the same factors and considerations affect reproducibility. These include blood pool contamination caused by partial volume effects, dependence on off-resonance and transmitted FA, confounding influence of T1, and SNR.

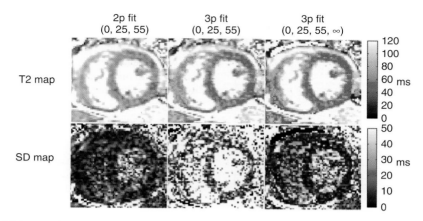

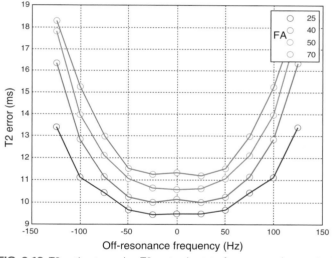

FIG. 2.11 T2 (top row) and corresponding standard deviation *(SD)* maps (bottom row) using T2p- steady-state free precession method with two-parameter fitting (left column), three-parameter fitting including a constant bias term to account for T1-dependent magnetization regrowth (center column), and three-parameter fit with bias term and additional measurement without T2 preparation (TE = ∞) (right column). The two-parameter fit overestimates the T2 because of the bias term. The bias is mitigated using three-parameter fitting but greatly increases the SD unless an additional measurement at TE = ∞ is included.

With the T2p-SSFP approach, there is a T1 bias due to the magnetization regrowth following the T2 preparation and the acquisition of the center of *k*-space. This signal bias can lead to an overestimation of T2 by 5 to 10 ms. Although in theory a three-parameter fit ($S = PD \exp[-TE/T2] + b$) may be used to eliminate this confounding bias variable, b, three-parameter fit with only a few relatively short TE measurements is very noisy. It has been proposed to directly measure the bias term[79] by acquisition of an image using an SR preparation without any T2 preparation, which corresponds to the TE = ∞ image. In this way, a three-parameter fit may be used without incurring a large SNR penalty, thus effectively eliminating this T1-confounder. This is illustrated in Fig. 2.11, which shows the reduced benefit of a three-parameter fit in reducing the T2 bias, and the improvement in SD of the three-parameter fit using the additional TE = ∞ measurement. The SSFP readout itself has image contrast dependent on T1 and T2. To a large extent the image contrast is shared for all of the T2-weighted images and does not affect the fit. However, single-shot imaging is acquired on the approach to steady state, and the contrast depends on the initial conditions, which in turn depends on the TE of the T2 preparation. Thus there is some residual T1 contrast dependent on the readout that may alter the T2 estimate.

The T2-SSFP measurement is sensitive to off-resonance. The SSFP readout has an off-resonance response that is different for the different T2 preparation echo times (TEs). This leads to an overall dependence of T2 measurement on the off-resonance frequency. The T2 error has been characterized experimentally[80] for a specific imaging protocol and found to vary significantly for off-resonance > ±150 Hz, and errors of approximately 5% at ±100 Hz. The frequency dependence of the T2 preparation also contributes to the response. The off-resonance sensitivity is reduced by using a lower excitation FA. The T2 error is shown in Fig. 2.12, which illustrates off-resonance sensitivity and the FA dependence, as well as on-resonance bias described above. The composite hard pulse design is wideband, but the adiabatic designs used for greater independence of FA generally have a narrower bandwidth. Thus care must be taken to ensure the volume is properly shimmed. The T2p-SSFP approach will not work well in the presence of device implants.

Using the GraSE approach, there is also a significant bias.[71] Using a TSE approach, it is difficult to completely eliminate stimulated echo

FIG. 2.12 T2 estimates using T2p–steady-state free precession method are sensitive to off-resonance and flip angle *(FA)*, with increasing errors at higher FA. Significant errors are observed for off-resonance > ± 50 Hz.

pathways, which may also lead to a T1 dependence in the contrast. This bias is not well characterized, and there are no methods for eliminating it.

The precision of the T2 measurement is determined by the SNR, number of measurements, the actual value of T2, and specific echo times used. The SD of the T2 estimate attributed to random noise (Fig. 2.13) was calculated analytically for a myocardial T2 of 45 ms at various SNR for three echo time measurements (solid lines) and four echo time measurements (dotted lines). Measurements were equally spaced at 0, $TE_{max}/2$, TE_{max} for three TEs and 0, $TE_{max}/3$, $2TE_{max}/3$, and TE_{max} for four TEs. These agree well with numerical simulation performed for a specific T2-SSFP protocol[80] with three measurements constrained to be 0, TE, and 2TE, where the best TE was found for normal myocardium at T2 = 45 ms to be in the range of 30 to 40 ms: that is, echo times (0,

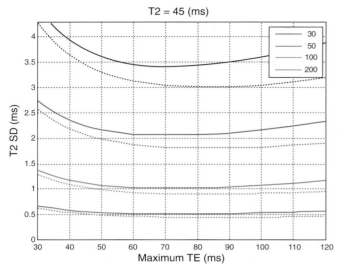

T2 = 45 (ms)

FIG. 2.13 Variation of standard deviation *(SD)* for T2 estimates at SNRs = 30, 50, 100, and 200. Equally spaced echo times are between 0 and the maximum echo time (TE$_{max}$) using three measurements *(solid lines)* and four measurements *(dotted lines)*. Baseline normal myocardium T2 = 45 ms is used in this calculation, and SD is fairly insensitive to TE$_{max}$ over a wide range (50–100 ms).

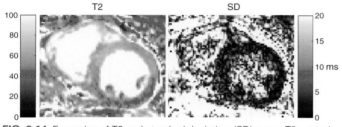

FIG. 2.14 Examples of T2 and standard deviation *(SD)* maps. T2p-steady-state free precession is used for a subject with acute myocardial infarction. SD is increased in the edematous region because of elevated T2.

30, 60 ms) to (0, 40, 80 ms). The SD may be calculated on a pixelwise fashion in a similar manner as for T1[57] or T2*.[81] Examples of T2 and SD maps for the case shown in Fig. 2.10 are shown in Fig. 2.14. The pixelwise noise SD for this case is approximately 2.1 ms in a remote region, with T2 = 44 ms and an SD approximately 3.7 ms in the edematous region with elevated T2 = 68 ms.

Limitations and Potential Pitfalls

The dark blood preparation used in spin echo-based techniques such as GraSE helps to eliminate contamination of myocardial signal caused by partial volume effects. However, spin echo readouts and DIR dark blood preparations are highly motion sensitive and prone to signal loss, particularly at higher heart rates. Off-resonance leads to bias errors in SSFP methods and to artifacts in EPI methods; therefore it is essential to ensure the volume is adequately shimmed.

T1-weighted contrast may confound the T2 measurement caused by magnetization regrowth in the case of T2p-SSFP and stimulated echoes in SE methods. Methods have been proposed to mitigate bias in T2p-SSFP[79] but may not be widely available. This may be avoided by using T2p single-shot FLASH with centric readout, particularly

at 3 T where the SNR of FLASH may be adequate. It is also important to avoid T2 mapping after administering Gd contrast to avoid short T1.

Current imaging protocols have been designed for myocardial T2 measurement and are not suitable for accurate measurement of blood T2. The echo times are much shorter than the T2 of the blood, leading to poorly conditioned fitting and sensitivity to blood signal loss due to dephasing at longer echo times.

Summary

T2 mapping in the heart using 2D imaging is feasible in a clinical environment and has sufficient accuracy and precision to be of value to answer a number of clinical questions. Absolute baseline values will depend on the field strength, and to some extent on the method. T2p-SSFP is the most widely used method and is fairly robust in terms of image quality.

CONCLUSION

Future developments to address the current limitations in quantitative measurement are focused on reduction in partial volume effects, differentiation between edema and fibrosis, establishment of baseline normal values, standardization, and quality control. Quantitative methods of T1, T2, and ECV mapping have been successful in population-based studies. Addressing the remaining issues is key to the reliable application of quantitative methods to the diagnosis of disease in individual patients.

A better understanding of confounding factors such as the effect of T2 on T1 measurement is important for interpretation of measurements. Understanding how scanner adjustments such as off-resonance or FA may affect quantitative measurements is important for the reliable detection of subtle disease. Multiparametric measurements may help differentiate between edema and fibrosis and may also play a role in disentangling the coupling in measurements of T1 and T2.

Partial volume contamination by adjacent blood pool or by intramyocardial fat is an important issue in current protocols. Use of higher spatial resolution or 3D imaging helps mitigate partial volume to some extent. Suppression of blood or fat may be required to further reduce this contamination; however, these methods may introduce other side effects.

Standardization encompasses methods for acquiring quantitative maps, displays, ROI measurements, and reporting. Visualization of parametric maps is most commonly done by color display. However, there is no current consensus on the scale or colormap. The visual display has a significant effect on classification of normal versus abnormal tissue or on the assessment on quality of the map. Use of quality control phantoms may also play a role in standardization.[82]

Quantitative mapping has the potential for increasing the objectiveness of CMR and improving the sensitivity for detecting subtle changes in the global state due to disease processes. Mapping has come a long way in the past decade, and technical developments continue to improve methods and find new and interesting clinical and research applications.

ACKNOWLEDGMENTS

Portions of text and figures have been excerpted and modified from the *Journal of Cardiovascular Magnetic Resonance* Open Access publication.[39,45]

REFERENCES

A full reference list is available online at ExpertConsult.com

3

Cardiovascular Magnetic Resonance Contrast Agents

Eric M. Gale and Peter Caravan

Although currently not approved by the US Food and Drug Administration (FDA) for cardiac imaging, the vast majority of cardiovascular magnetic resonance (CMR) studies use a gadolinium-based contrast agent.[1] The CMR contrast agent typically makes diseased tissue appear brighter (or in some cases darker) than the surrounding tissue. Cardiovascular applications, such as magnetic resonance angiography (MRA), functional imaging of myocardial perfusion, and viability with late gadolinium enhancement (LGE) imaging of fibrosis represent the bulk of CMR scans that use a contrast agent. The first magnetic resonance (MR) approved contrast agent, gadopentetate (Gd-DTPA), appeared in 1988, and several other compounds followed. These first contrast agents were extracellular fluid (ECF) agents. Although frequently used in CMR and an essential component of CMR perfusion and LGE assessment of fibrosis, none of these agents is currently approved by the FDA for cardiac applications. Thus, the use of these agents in CMR is considered "off-label." There are now also an approved hepatobiliary contrast agent and an intravascular agent designed specifically to enhance contrast-enhanced (CE) MRA. At the preclinical stage, there are exciting advancements in molecular imaging agents, including compounds that detect pH changes, enzymatic activity, specific biomolecules such as fibrin or collagen, and magnetically labeled cells.

This chapter focuses first on the general underlying chemistry and biophysics of contrast agents in clinical CMR. The mechanism of action of different classes of contrast agents is described, with examples drawn from CMR applications. Finally, there is a brief survey of novel contrast agents potentially useful for cardiovascular indications that are currently in clinical or preclinical development.

The vast majority of CMR agents in clinical use are small molecules based on chelated gadolinium (Gd). The bulk of this chapter focuses on gadolinium complexes, including their chemistry, biophysics, and applications. Other exogenous compounds have been used to change signal properties in MRI (e.g., iron particles, hyperpolarized nuclei), and these will be discussed as appropriate to CMR. This chapter assumes that the reader has a basic understanding of CMR vocabulary, and the reader is referred to Chapter 1 for further clarification.

INTRODUCTION TO THE BIOPHYSICS OF MAGNETIC RESONANCE IMAGING

All contrast agents shorten both T1 and T2 relaxation times. However, it is useful to classify CMR contrast agents into two broad groups based on whether the substance increases the transverse relaxation rate (1/T2) by roughly the same amount that it increases the longitudinal relaxation rate (1/T1) or whether 1/T2 is altered to a much greater extent. The first category is referred to as "T1 agents" because, on a percentage basis, these agents alter 1/T1 of tissue more than 1/T2 as a result of endogenous transverse relaxation in tissue. With most pulse sequences, this dominant T1-lowering effect gives rise to *increases* in signal intensity, and thus these agents are referred to as "positive" contrast agents. The T2 agents largely increase the 1/T2 of tissue selectively and cause a *reduction* in signal intensity, and thus they are known as "negative" contrast agents. Paramagnetic gadolinium-based contrast agents are examples of T1 agents, whereas ferromagnetic large iron oxide particles are examples of T2 agents.

There are many mechanisms by which contrast agents shorten T1 and T2. Considerable chemistry and biophysics can be applied to understand or predict these mechanisms. However, in many cases, the effect of these mechanisms can be reduced to a single constant, called "relaxivity." Fig. 3.1 shows the effect and definition of relaxivity.

Fig. 3.1A shows the effect of a typical contrast agent on the relaxation time of two hypothetical tissues, one with T1 = 1200 ms (similar to heart muscle at 1.5 T) and one with T1 = 400 ms. At low concentration (left side of the graph), it appears that the contrast agent has a larger effect (change in T1) on the tissue with the longer T1. At higher contrast agent concentrations (right side of Fig. 3.1A), both tissues approach approximately the same T1. A simple way to quantify this effect is to consider the rate of relaxation, 1/T1 (sometimes denoted "R1"). In most cases in medical imaging, the contrast agent increases the relaxation rate proportional to the amount of contrast agent:

$$\frac{1}{T1} = \frac{1}{T1_0} + r_1 [CA] \qquad \text{Eq. 3.1}$$

where T1 is the observed T1 with contrast agent in the tissue, $T1_0$ is the T1 before addition of the contrast agent, [CA] is the concentration of contrast agent, and r_1 is the longitudinal relaxivity, often just "relaxivity." The conventional units for r_1 are $mM^{-1}s^{-1}$ (per millimolar per second, sometimes $L \cdot mol^{-1}s^{-1}$). Thus, the slope of 1/T1 as a function of contrast agent concentration (Fig. 3.1B) shows the relaxivity, in this case, 4 $mM^{-1}s^{-1}$. Fig. 3.1B shows that the effect of the contrast agent on the relaxation rate is independent of the initial T1 of the tissue: that is, in terms of relaxation rate, the contrast agent has the same effect, regardless of initial T1. Transverse, or T2, relaxivity is defined in an analogous way:

$$\frac{1}{T1} = \frac{1}{T2_0} + r_2 [CA] \qquad \text{Eq. 3.2}$$

For all contrast agents, r_2 is larger than r_1. Relaxivity is dependent on magnetic field strength, on temperature, and in some instances can depend on protein binding, pH, or even the presence of enzymes.

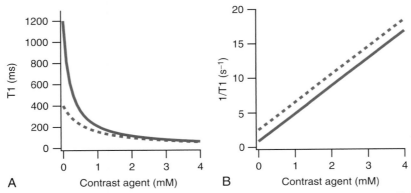

FIG. 3.1 Change in (A) longitudinal relaxation time (T1) and (B) longitudinal relaxation rate (1/T1) for typical myocardial tissue (*solid line*, T1 = 1200 ms at 1.5 T) and short T1 tissue (*dashed line*, T1 = 400 ms).

Contrast agent behavior in vivo is seldom as simple as the pure linear effect relaxation rate shown in Fig. 3.1. Even in the simple case of pure linear relaxation, the effect of the contrast agent on the CMR image is generally nonlinear. In traditional spin echo sequences, non-linearity can be a result of T1 saturation or T2 signal loss. Once the contrast agent reduces T1 < repetition time (TR)/2, increasing contrast agent concentration will have little effect on increasing the available longitudinal magnetization because the tissue will have nearly fully recovered the magnetization before the next radiofrequency (RF) pulse. Furthermore, because contrast agents affect both T1 and T2 relaxation, at high enough concentration, the contrast agent will reduce T2 to the order of the echo time (TE), and will then decrease MR image intensity. These effects are seen in Fig. 3.2, where signal intensity is plotted versus contrast agent concentration for T1- and T2-weighted spin echo sequences. Fig. 3.2 was generated assuming a contrast agent relaxivity of 4 mM^{-1}s^{-1}, typical of most commercial ECF gadolinium agents, and tissue relaxation times typical of myocardium at 1.5 T (T1 = 1200 ms, T2 = 50 ms). For the T1-weighted sequence (TE/TR = 15/600), Fig. 3.2A, signal intensity begins to level out at a contrast agent concentration between 0.5 and 1.0 mM. From Fig. 3.1A, this is the range at which the T1 of the myocardium decreased to approximately 300 ms, or TR/2. At concentrations >1 mM, the T1 effect is saturated, and the only *imaging* effect of the contrast agent is to make T2 shorter and cause signal loss, even on this T1-weighted sequence. Signal is lost because even a T1-weighted sequence has a finite TE, and T2 effects can enter when T2 is short enough.

The signal intensity plateau on the T2-weighted scan (TE/TR = 80/3000), Fig. 3.2B, occurs at much lower contrast agent concentration. Because TR is so long, the only real effect of the contrast agent is to reduce (rather than increase) signal intensity on this T2-weighted scan. However, this negative contrast can also be medically useful, and certain contrast agents (notably, the iron oxide particles) create negative contrast exactly by providing enhanced T2 relaxation, and thus darker images on T2-weighted scans.

Increasing the relaxivity (r_1 or r_2) will have the effect of pushing the simulated curves in Fig. 3.2A to the left, which means that peak signal and subsequent signal loss will occur at *lower* contrast agent concentrations. A more linear response of signal to contrast agent can be achieved with a fast three-dimensional (3D) spoiled gradient recalled echo (GRE) sequence. This is seen in Fig. 3.2C, where signal intensity is plotted versus contrast agent concentration using the same tissue relaxation times and relaxivities as in Fig. 3.2A and B for a typical fast 3D spoiled GRE sequence, TE/TR/flip = 2.2/9.0/40 degrees. The short TR and very short TE ensure that signal intensity increases across the entire concentration range. At high concentration, the effect of the contrast agent is becoming nonlinear, but the signal is still increasing with increasing contrast agent concentration.

Commercial Contrast Agents and Those in Clinical Development

The addition of paramagnetic materials to reduce relaxation times goes back to the earliest days of MR. In the 1940s, Bloch and colleagues used ferric nitrate to enhance the relaxation rate of water.[2] Exogenous contrast was applied to MRI in 1978 when Lauterbur and associates reported using manganese dichloride to differentiate normal from infarcted myocardium in dogs.[3] Carr and colleagues reported the first use of a gadolinium complex, gadopentetate dimeglumine (Gd-DTPA; Magnevist, Bayer, Berlin, Germany), in patients with brain tumors in 1984.[4] By 1988, Gd-DTPA was FDA approved for clinical use.

Extracellular Agents

The most common contrast agents used clinically are ECF agents. Although several are approved for clinical use, as mentioned previously, none is specifically FDA approved for *cardiac* applications. These all behave in a very similar manner, and are typically referred to as "gadolinium" or "gado" agents. Fig. 3.3 shows the chemical structures of several approved ECF agents. Chemically, these compounds exhibit three similar features: they all contain Gd, they all contain an 8-coordinate ligand binding to Gd, and they all contain a single water molecule coordination site to Gd. Nomenclature for contrast agents can be confusing: there is a generic name (e.g., gadopentetate dimeglumine), a trade name (e.g., Magnevist), and usually a chemical code name or abbreviation (e.g., Gd-diethylenetriaminepentaacetic acid or Gd-DTPA). Any of these three names may be used in the scientific literature.

The multidentate ligand is required for safety.[5] The ligand encapsulates the Gd, resulting in a high thermodynamic stability and kinetic inertness with respect to metal loss. This enables the contrast agent to be excreted intact, an important property because these contrast agents tend to be much less toxic than their substituents. For example, the DTPA ligand and gadolinium chloride both have an LD$_{50}$ of 0.5 mmol/kg in rats (LD$_{50}$ = dose that causes death in 50% of the animals), whereas the Gd-DTPA complex has a safety margin that is higher by nearly a factor of 20, with an LD$_{50}$ of 8 mmol/kg for the Gd-DTPA complex.[6]

The Gd ion and coordinated water molecule are essential to providing contrast. The Gd (III) ion has a high magnetic moment and a relatively slow electronic relaxation rate, properties that make it an excellent relaxer of water protons. The proximity of the coordinated water molecule leads to efficient relaxation. The coordinated water molecule is in rapid chemical exchange (10^6 exchanges/s) with solvating water molecules.[7]

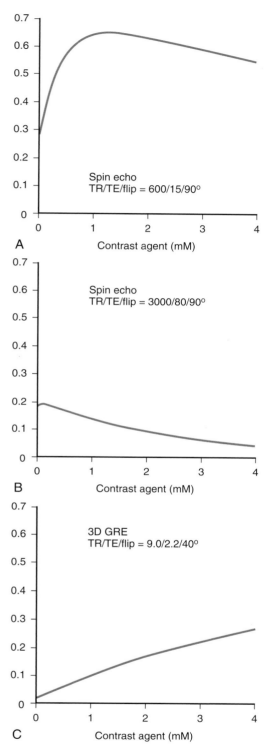

FIG. 3.2 Effect of contrast agent on myocardial image intensity on T1-weighted and T2-weighted spin echo scans. (A) T1-weighted spin echo (repetition time *[TR]* = 600 ms) assumes a patient with 100 beats per minute heart rate and shows a linear increase of signal only for contrast agent concentration <0.5 mM. (B) T2-weighted spin echo images (TR = 3000 ms) show only T2 signal loss effects as a result of contrast agent with no T1 enhancement because of the long TR. (C) Typical short-TR fast spoiled gradient recalled echo *(GRE)* sequence. The very short echo time *(TE)* and short TR give monotonically increased image intensity across the entire range of contrast agent concentrations typically found in clinical scans.

This rapid exchange leads to a catalytic effect whereby the Gd complex effectively shortens the relaxation times of the bulk solution.

The ECF agents have very similar properties, and these are summarized in Table 3.1. They are all very hydrophilic complexes with similar relaxivities and excellent safety profiles. In addition, they can be formulated at high concentrations. On injection, these ECF agents quickly and freely distribute to the extracellular space. Administration of any of these agents (with rare exceptions)[8] yields similar diagnostic information.

There are some differences among the physical properties. The diamide complexes gadodiamide and gadoversetamide have considerably lower thermodynamic stability (log $K \sim 17$ vs. log $K > 21$ for other Gd complexes).[9,10] The nonionic (neutral) compounds gadodiamide, gadoteridol, gadoversetamide, and gadobutrol were designed to minimize the osmolality of the formulation. This was prompted by the distinct reduction in toxicity and side effects brought on by the development of nonionic x-ray contrast media. However, for CMR, the injection volumes are much *smaller* than the volumes used for x-ray angiography or computed tomography (CT) angiography. Thus the overall increase in osmolality after injection of a CMR contrast agent is minimal. Unlike with x-ray contrast, there is no documented safety benefit in using nonionic CMR contrast agents. One benefit of the nonionic compounds is the ability to formulate them at high concentration (1 M)[11] without drastically increasing osmolality or viscosity (see Table 3.1). These high-concentration formulations may be useful in fast dynamic studies, such as dynamic MRA or myocardial perfusion. These ECF agents, as with iodinated preparations used for x-ray and CT, are excreted by the kidneys. As a result, clearance is impaired in patients with impaired/reduced renal function (discussed later).

Blood Pool Agents

Because CMR contrast agents are administered intravenously, they are all potentially capable of imaging the blood lumen. The ECF agents described earlier are used routinely for CE-MRA (see Chapters 25, 26, 44, 45, and 46). One potential drawback of using ECF agents for MRA is their pharmacokinetics. ECF agents rapidly leak out of the vascular space into all the interstitial spaces of the body. Angiography with ECF agents is thus typically limited to dynamic/first-pass arterial studies. There has been considerable effort made toward designing specific blood pool agents that would be tailored for vascular imaging. The ideal blood pool agent should remain in the vascular compartment and not leak out into the extracellular space. It should be capable of being given as a bolus such that a dynamic arterial image can be obtained. At the same time, it should have sufficient relaxivity and blood half-life to allow high-resolution steady-state images to be obtained. MS-325 (gadofosveset, initially marketed as Vasovist; and more recently as Ablavar; in the United States by Lantheus Medical Imaging, Billerica, MA; Fig. 3.4) is approved, and there are several other blood pool agents that have reached various stages of clinical development. However, as this chapter was being written, Lantheus announced that it would no longer produce gadofosveset. Three approaches have been taken to design blood pool agents: protein binding, increased size, and ultrasmall iron oxide particles. These are discussed later.

MS-325 (gadofosveset)[12,13] is a Gd-based compound that binds reversibly to serum albumin. Albumin is the most abundant protein in plasma, and its concentration is high enough (600–700 μM) to reversibly bind most of the MS-325 after injection. Reversible albumin binding serves four purposes: (1) the albumin slows the leakage of the contrast agent out of the intravascular space; (2) the reversible binding still allows a path for excretion—the unbound fraction can be filtered through the kidneys or taken up by hepatocytes; (3) the bound fraction is "hidden" from the liver and kidneys, leading to an extended plasma half-life; and

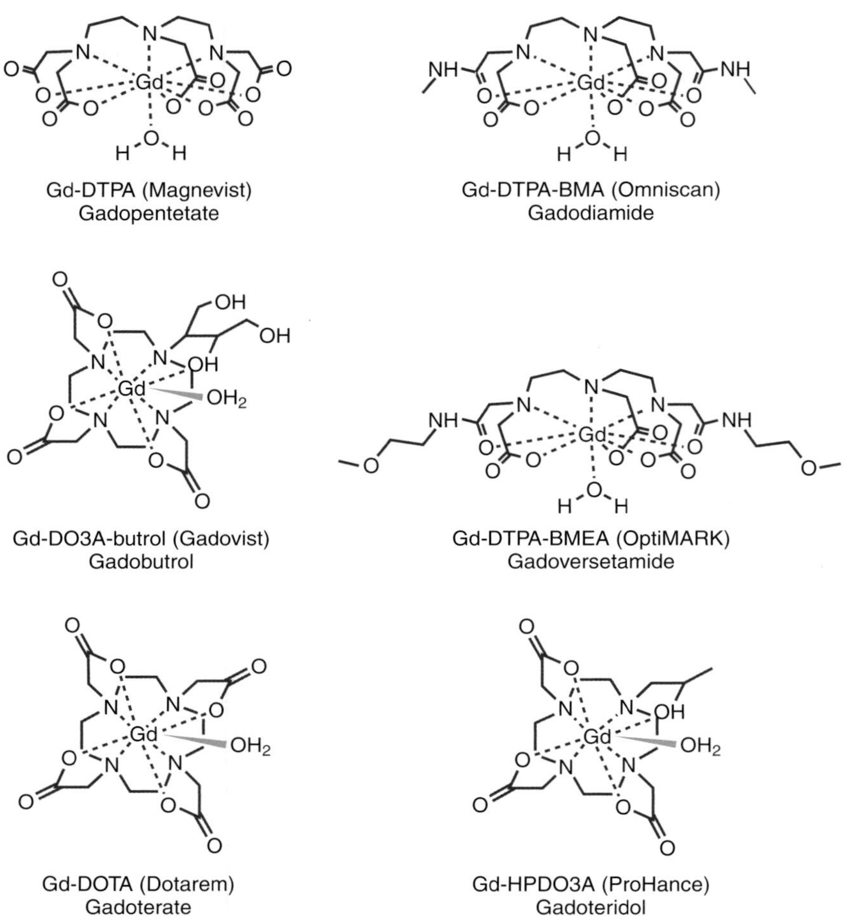

FIG. 3.3 Chemical structures of commercial (United States or Europe) extracellular fluid contrast agents.

TABLE 3.1 Approved (December 2016) Magnetic Resonance Imaging Contrast Agents: Relaxivity,[150] Osmolality, and Viscosity

Generic Name	Product Name	Chemical Abbreviation	r_1, 0.47 T 40°C	r_2, 0.47 T 40°C	Osmolality[a] (Osmol/kg)	Viscosity[a] (cP)
Gadopentetate	Magnevist (Bayer HealthCare Pharmaceuticals)	Gd-DTPA	3.4	4.0	1.96[151]	2.9[151]
Gadoterate	Dotarem (Guerbet Group)	Gd-DOTA	3.4	4.1	1.35[152] (4.02)[152]	2.0[152]
Gadodiamide	Omniscan (GE Healthcare)	Gd-DTPA-BMA	3.5	3.8	0.79[151] (1.90)[152]	3.9[152]
Gadoteridol	ProHance (Bracco Diagnostics, Inc.)	Gd-HPDO3A	3.1	3.7	0.63[152] 1.91[152]	1.3[152] (3.9)[152]
Gadobutrol	Gadovist (Bayer HealthCare, Inc.)	Gd-DO3A-butrol	3.7	5.1	0.57[153] (1.39)[151]	1.4[153] (3.7)[151]
Gadoversetamide	OptiMARK (Mallinckrodt, Inc.)	GD-DTPA-BMEA	4.2	5.2	1.11[154]	2.0[154]
Gadobenate	Multihance (Bracco Diagnostics, Inc.)	Gd-BOPTA	4.2	4.8	1.10[155]	5.3mPas[155]
Gadofosveset	Ablavar (Lantheus Medical, Inc.)	MS-325	5.8	6.7	0.83[156]	3.0[156]
Gadoxetic acid	Eovist (Bayer HealthCare Pharmaceuticals)	Gd-EOB-DTPA	5.3	6.2	0.69[157]	1.2[157]

[a]All concentrations 0.5 M except those in parentheses, which are 1 M.

(4) the relaxivity of the contrast agent is increased 4-fold to 10-fold on binding to albumin (discussed later). Gd-BOPTA (gadobenate; see Fig. 3.4) has weak affinity[14,15] for albumin (~10% bound), which leads to a modest increase in relaxivity relative to the other ECF agents.

The binding and relaxivity features of Gd-based blood pool agents are listed in Table 3.2. Because binding affinity is moderate to weak for these compounds, the fraction bound to albumin will depend on the concentrations of albumin and the contrast agent.[13,16] Immediately after injection, when the concentration of the contrast agent is high relative to albumin, there will be a greater free fraction. As the concentration of the contrast agent begins to stabilize (at ~0.5 mM) the fraction bound will become constant. The observed relaxivity will depend on the fraction bound; unlike ECF agents, the plasma T1 change is not linearly related to contrast agent concentration.[16,17]

Early work on blood pool compounds involved Gd covalently linked to macromolecules, such as polylysine, dextran, or modified bovine serum albumin.[5] The large size of these compounds restricted diffusion out of the vascular space and led to very good vascular imaging properties. However, these compounds cleared very slowly in preclinical studies and there were concerns about a potential immunologic response. An alternative approach is to use a coated iron oxide nanoparticle. So-called ultrasmall superparamagnetic particles of iron oxide (USPIO) are very large (10–30 nm) but still small enough to evade substantial capture by the reticuloendothelial system.[18] Such particles also have strong r_1 relaxivity, especially at lower field strengths. Unlike the Gd-based compounds, which will extravasate to some extent, these iron oxide particles are true intravascular blood pool agents. Currently there are no USPIO commercially available that are approved for MRI, but ferumoxytol (Feraheme) is a carboxymethyldextran-coated USPIO that is approved as an intravenous iron replacement therapy.[19] Ferumoxytol has been used off-label as a blood pool agent and has seen some use in pediatric CMR owing to the long circulating blood half-life which facilitates high-resolution imaging and obviates the need for timing of boluses.[20,21] Ferumoxytol can also be used to image monocytes and macrophages on delayed phase imaging (next day) as accumulation in the reticuloendothelial system is the ultimate fate of these particles.[22,23] The iron oxide particles are not excreted; the iron is eventually resorbed into the body.

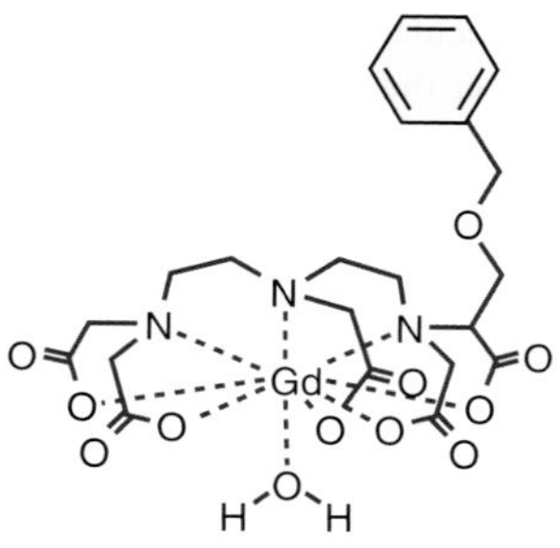

The Guerbet company is developing a new extracellular fluid agent with high relaxivity. The compound P03277 is reported to have relaxivities of 12.8 mM^{-1}s^{-1} at 1.5 T and 11.6 mM^{-1}s^{-1} at 3 T.[24] This Gd chelate contains two water molecules bound to the metal ion, which leads to the high observed relaxivity. P03277 is a low molecular weight (970 Da) contrast agent that distributes in the extracellular space similarly to other ECF agents and has blood elimination kinetics comparable to gadobutrol in animal models. At the time of writing (2017), P03277 is currently undergoing Phase 2 clinical trials.

Gd-BOPTA (MultiHance)
Gadobenate

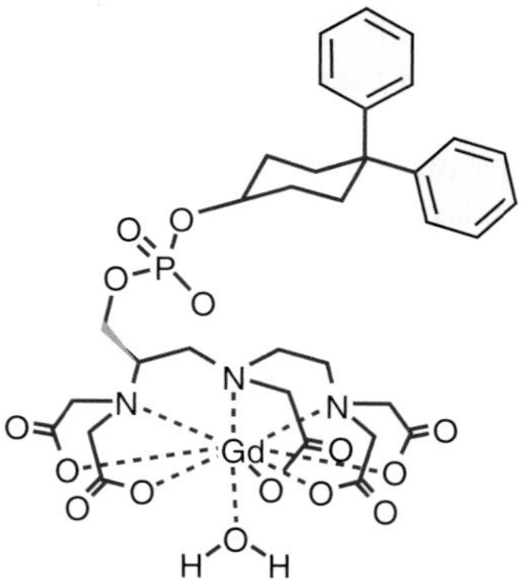

MS-325 (Vasovist; Ablavar)
Gadofosveset

FIG. 3.4 Chemical structures of other commercial contrast agents with weak (Gd-BOPTA) or strong (MS-325) serum albumin binding.

RELAXIVITY

Because their effect is indirect, CMR contrast agents differ from other diagnostic imaging agents. Water and fat are imaged, and it is the action of the contrast agent on the relaxation properties of the water hydrogen nuclei that generates contrast; in x-ray contrast media and nuclear imaging agents, the effect observed is more direct. Because water is present at a very high concentration (55,000 mM) and the contrast agent is typically at a much lower concentration (0.1–1 mM), the contrast agent must act catalytically to relax the water protons for there to be a measurable effect. Relaxivity, r_1 and r_2, thus describes this catalytic efficiency. Some compounds are better magnetic catalysts than others (have higher relaxivity). Moreover, relaxivity is dependent on the external magnetic field, B_0. This section explains these differences and the molecular basis for them. For discrete ions, such as Gd(III) and manganese (Mn[II]), the factors influencing relaxivity are the same; for iron oxide particles, the relaxation mechanism is different and will be treated separately.

TABLE 3.2 Albumin Binding and Observed Relaxivities (20 MHz) of MS-325, B22956, Gd-BOPTA, Gadomer-17, at 37°C		
	MS-325 Gadofosveset	**Gd-BOPTA Gadobenate**	**Gadomer-17[a]**
Agent type	Strong protein binding	Weak protein binding	Increased size
r_1 buffer (mM^{-1}s^{-1})	6.6[12]	4.4[158]	16.5[150]
r_1 plasma (mM^{-1}s^{-1})	50[12]	9.7[159]	19.0[150]
% bound plasma	91[12]		

[a]Relaxivity per gadolinium.

A Gd-based contrast agent specific to type I collagen was described,[72] and this probe was used to show in vivo molecular imaging of fibrosis in a mouse model of healed postinfarction myocardial scarring.[73] Because the extracellular matrix of the heart is very rich in collagen, this compound was used to assess myocardial perfusion in a pig model of coronary artery stenosis. Collagen binding served to retain the probe in the myocardial extracellular matrix for extended periods such that a delayed, high-resolution steady-state image of heart could be obtained that reflected the initial perfusion of the contrast agent.[74] This probe has been also used to stage liver fibrosis in rodents and could be useful in tracking the progress of cardiovascular pathologies with elevated collagen levels.[75–77]

An agent that targets elastin has also been developed. Elastin levels are largely increased following injury to load-bearing tissues. Elastin content in injury or healing cardiovascular tissue is a sufficiently abundant biomarker for monitoring tissue remodeling. The elastin specific magnetic resonance contrast agent Gd-ESMA targets elastin with high affinity and specificity. Fig. 3.8 shows increased Gd-ESMA retention and contrast enhancement in the vessel wall of an aneurysm-bearing artery versus a normal artery. In this study, Gd-ESMA was used to visualize rupture of aortic elastic lamina and monitor the compensatory increase in elastin content of the dilated vessel over the course of weeks in a mouse model of aortic abdominal aneurysm.[78] Gd-ESMA has also been used to visualize the vascular remodeling process at the site of disrupted plaques in rabbit model of atherosclerosis.[79] Changing elastin content postmyocardial infarction in both the infarcted and remote myocardium has serially monitored Gd-ESMA out to 3 weeks in a mouse model.[80] In another study, Gd-ESMA was used to quantify

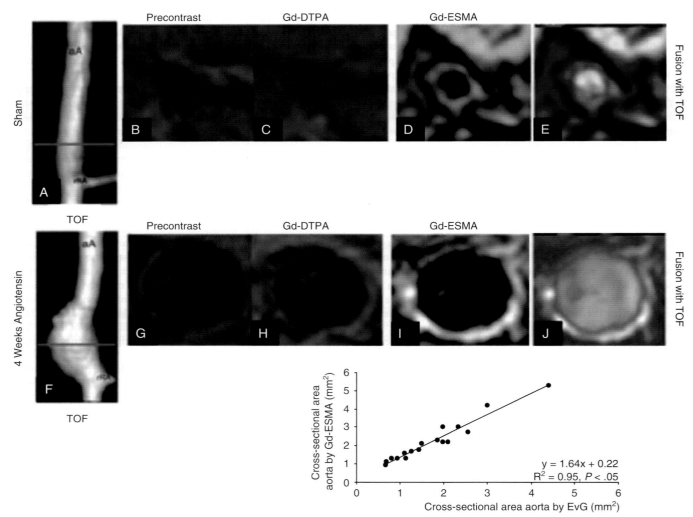

FIG. 3.8 Magnetic resonance images (MRI) of the suprarenal abdominal aorta in sham-treated mice (A–E) and mice bearing a pharmacologically induced abdominal aortic aneurysm (F–J). Time-of-flight *(TOF)* angiograms are shown in (A) and (F), the red lines mark the axial cross sections of the vessels depicted in images (B–E) and (G–J). Images (B–D) and (G–I) were acquired using the same T1-weighted protocol. (B) and (G) were acquired without contrast enhancement, (C) and (H) were contrast-enhanced using Gd-DTPA, (D) and (I) were contrast-enhanced using the elastin-seeking MRI probe Gd-ESMA. The TOF and Gd-ESMA enhanced imaging data are fused in (E) and (J). The aneurysm-bearing vessel is strongly enhanced compared with the vessel in the negative control animal. An increase in elastin content accompanies the compensatory remodeling of vessel wall at the site of the dilation. (K) The cross-sectional area of the aneurysm-bearing arterial wall measured using Gd-ESMA-enhanced MRI correlates closely with cross-sectional area determined by ex vivo histology (Elastica van Gieson staining). (Courtesy Dr. R. Botnar, King's College, London, UK.)

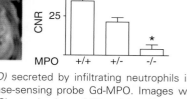

FIG. 3.9 Magnetic resonance image of myeloperoxidase *(MPO)* secreted by infiltrating neutrophils in a mouse model of myocardial infarction using the myeloperoxidase-sensing probe Gd-MPO. Images were acquired 2 hours after intravenous injection of Gd-MPO. (A–C) Short-axis view of T1-weighted images of wild-type (+/+), heterozygous (+/-), and homozygous (-/-) MPO knockout mice, respectively. The infarct in the left ventricle wall is denoted with yellow arrows. (D) Infarct zone versus remote myocardium contrast-to-noise ratio *(CNR)* correlates with MPO activity. (Courtesy Dr. D. Sosnovik, Massachusetts General Hospital/ Harvard Medical School, Boston, USA.)

intrascar elastin out to 3 weeks following myocardial infarction in a mouse model.[81]

The Massachusetts General Hospital group developed a gadolinium-based agent (MPO-Gd) sensitive to myeloperoxidase (MPO) activity. Ischemic injury of the myocardium causes timed recruitment of neutrophils and monocytes/macrophages, which produce substantial amounts of local MPO. MPO forms reactive chlorinating species capable of inflicting oxidative stress and altering protein function by covalent modification. MPO-Gd is first radicalized by MPO and then either spontaneously oligomerizes or binds to matrix proteins, all leading to enhanced spin-lattice relaxivity and delayed washout kinetics. MPO-Gd was used to noninvasively measure inflammatory responses after myocardial ischemia or stroke in murine models,[82,83] and vascular inflammation in a murine modes of Kawasaki disease and a rabbit model of aneurysm.[82–85] Fig. 3.9 shows differing degrees of contrast enhancement at the site of myocardial infarction in wild-type, heterozygous, and homozygous MPO knockout mice. There is a clear correlation between infarct enhancement and local MPO activity.[82]

The Massachusetts General Hospital group also developed a Gd-based contrast agent (Gd-TO) to detect extracellular DNA, which is a useful biomarker of acute necrosis.[86] Gd-TO binds DNA with high specificity and affinity. Gd-TO was used to monitor the clearance of intracellular debris from acutely necrotic cardiac tissue in a mouse model of myocardial infarction.[86]

Manganese (Mn)-based complexes have also been explored as contrast agents. The Massachusetts General Hospital group is developing an Mn-based complex agent as a Gd-free alternative.[87] A lead candidate agent (Mn-PyC3A) provides contrast equivalent to the commercial Gd-based agents. Preliminary biodistribution and clearance studies performed in a mouse model indicate >99% clearance of Mn-PyC3A within 24 hours by mixed renal and hepatobiliary paths.

There is a rich literature describing the use of iron oxide particles as targeted contrast agents. Commercial USPIOs passively accumulate in macrophages. This property has been exploited to provide negative contrast in macrophage-rich atherosclerotic plaques. There appears to be a positive correlation between macrophage uptake and plasma half-life.[88,89]

Iron oxides have also been used to label cells, and then the cells are tracked in vivo using CMR.[90,91] Visualization of mesenchymal stem cells engrafted into the myocardium of a pig has been demonstrated at 1.5 T.[92,93] Injection sites containing >10^5 cells could be detected in vivo.[92] In a mouse model of myocardial infarction, a therapeutic intervention of mouse embryonic stem cells could be followed by visualizing the stem cells and following their effect on left ventricular (LV) function over a period of 4 weeks.[94] Care must be taken in interpreting MRI data to track USPIO-labeled stem cells because the local presence of

USPIO will void the MRI signal, regardless of cell viability. A recent study using MRI and histology to track the fate of USPIO-labeled mesenchymal stem cells implanted into infarcted myocardium provides a cautionary example. Four weeks after implantation of the labeled cells, the injection site remained hypointense but histologic analysis revealed very few viable stem cells. The USPIOs had accumulated in macrophages that infiltrated the injection site.[95]

The Massachusetts General Hospital group has also shown that the iron oxide coating material can be chemically modified to introduce new targeting vectors.[96–98] They termed this contrast agent platform "cross-linked iron oxide (CLIO)." For example, annexin V can be grafted onto a cross-linked iron oxide[99] to detect apoptotic cardiomyocytes in a mouse model of transient left anterior descending artery occlusion.[100] Another CLIO-based probe is targeted to vascular cell adhesion molecule-1 using a peptide specific to this molecule.[101] This probe was used to identify inflammatory activation of cells in a mouse model of atherosclerosis.

The fluorine ^{19}F signal of perfluorocarbon nanoemulsions has been used to image macrophage infiltration during inflammation. ^{19}F resonances are absent from tissues and thus fluorinated molecular imaging probes can report with a high degree of specificity. Intravenously injected perfluorocarbon nanoemulsions can be taken up by circulating monocytes, and monocyte accumulation at the site of inflammation results in a strong, localized ^{19}F signal. These ^{19}F probes have been used to visualize monocyte infiltration into the site of myocardial infarction in explanted porcine hearts 4 days following the ischemic injury, and in vivo in a mouse model of myocarditis.[102,103] Combined ^{19}F MR spectroscopy, T2-weighted MRI, T1-weighted LGE imaging, and cine imaging were applied to monitor changes in monocyte flux, edema, infarct size, and cardiac function over a period of 4 weeks in a mouse model of myocardial infarction.[104] Perfluorocarbon nanoemulsions that seek molecular targets have also been developed. For example, nanoemulsions decorated with polyethylene glycol to avoid macrophage uptake and with α_2-antiplasmin peptide fragments have been shown to selectively accumulate at sites of active thrombosis.[105]

The lack of sensitivity in CMR stems from the very small degree of polarization among the nuclear spins. In a magnetic field there is a net magnetization, but this is small, and approximately 0.0006% of the spins are polarized. A technique called "spin exchange" uses a high-powered laser (also called "optical pumping") to increase the polarization by four to five orders of magnitude (hyperpolarization).[106] Isotopes with long T1 values can be hyperpolarized and used as contrast agents. The long T1 is necessary to maintain the contrast medium in the hyperpolarized state long enough to obtain an image before the spins relax back to the equilibrium value.

Gases often have long T1 values, and isotopes of the noble gases helium (He-3) and xenon (Xe-129) have been used for imaging. Contrast agents with hyperpolarized carbon C-13 have been reported using a C-13-enriched water-soluble compound[107] with long relaxation times (in vitro, T1 = approx. 82 s, T2 = approx. 18 s; in vivo, T1 = approx. 38 s, T2 = approx. 1.3 s). This could be formulated at a C-13 concentration of 200 mM and hyperpolarized to 15%. The authors used this material for CE-MRA in rats and swine.[108]

Hyperpolarized C-13 also offers the potential for investigating metabolic pathways. For instance, Merritt and colleagues studied the metabolism of [1-^{13}C]-pyruvate in a perfused rat heart.[109] [1-^{13}C]-pyruvate metabolism has also been used to serially monitor the metabolic changes that accompany cardiac dysfunction in a rat model of myocardial infarction.[110] Another study using rats temporally tracked [1-^{13}C]-pyruvate metabolism across the entire myocardium throughout and following the course of ischemia/reperfusion.[111] Imaging frameworks have also been optimized for in vivo cardiac imaging of hyperpolarized ^{13}C-labeled metabolites such as acetate and acetylcarnitine.[112]

A major benefit of hyperpolarized contrast media is the excellent sensitivity with no background (high SNR). Challenges include the distribution and availability of the hyperpolarization equipment and imaging hardware compatibility for imaging nonhydrogen nuclei (not available on all clinical scanners). However, there is now a commercial polarizer available.

SAFETY

The safety of CMR contrast agents, which themselves offer no direct therapeutic benefit, is always a question of appropriate medical concern. The Gd-based chelates had initially been considered among the safest injectable compounds in medical use, with a specific reputation for superior safety in patients with renal dysfunction (compared with iodinated preparations used in fluoroscopy and CT). This view has changed with the apparent link between Gd contrast and nephrogenic systemic fibrosis (NSF).

A very rare, but potentially devastating condition affecting patients with acute or chronic kidney disease, NSF has an estimated prevalence of >10% among patients receiving Gd who are on hemodialysis.[113] Although presenting primarily with skin thickening, tethering, hyperpigmentation, and disabling joint flexion contractures, patients with NSF can also have multiorgan/systemic fibrosis, leading to organ dysfunction and even death.[114,115] The universal feature of NSF is Gd administration and acute or chronic kidney disease, most commonly with an estimated glomerular filtration rate of <30 mL/min/1.73 m^2.[115–118] However, NSF-like symptoms have also been reported in patients with apparently normal renal function.[119,120] Gd has been shown to be present in skin biopsy specimens of patients with NSF,[121–126] and also in internal organs.[127] The prevailing hypothesis is that acute or chronic kidney disease results in prolonged exposure to the contrast agent, providing opportunity for the Gd to dissociate from its chelator, and this dissociated Gd is believed to be responsible for the toxic response.[128] The least stable contrast agent, Gd-DTPA-BMA (gadodiamide), is the agent that has been most frequently associated with NSF,[129–131] but it is now established that other Gd compounds also pose a risk.[115,132]

Although ECF agents are similar in terms of their imaging efficacy, they differ in terms of how well they bind Gd. This may prove to be an important risk factor for NSF because both the metal (Gd) and the chelate have potential toxic effects[6] and have shown acute toxicity in animal studies at high enough doses. These various animal studies have been reviewed,[133] and a high-dose study in rats showed NSF-like lesions.[131] Metal complexes such as Gd contrast agents are characterized in terms of their thermodynamic stability and kinetic inertness. Stability is a measure of the affinity of the chelator for the metal ion and is expressed as an equilibrium constant for the association of the

chelator (ligand) with the metal. Stability constants for approved agents have the order Gd-DOTA (gadoterate) > Gd-HPDO3A (gadoteridol) ~ Gd-DO3A-butrol (gadobutrol) ~ MS-325 (gadofosveset) ~ Gd-BOPTA (gadobenate) ~ Gd-DTPA (gadopentetate) > Gd-DTPA-BMA (gadodiamide) ~ Gd-DTPA-BMEA (gadoversatamide).[5] The compounds with lowest thermodynamic stability are the neutral complexes with acyclic chelators: Gd-DTPA-BMA (gadodiamide) and Gd-DTPA-BMEA (gadoversetamide).

Stability constants describe equilibrium values, but do not indicate how quickly equilibrium is reached. In the biologic milieu, protons and other metal ions compete to bind the chelator ligand, whereas there are ions such as phosphate and carbonate that have a high affinity for Gd. Under conditions that favor dissociation of the Gd (e.g., low pH), two complexes with comparable stability may have very different rates of dissociation. For example, the macrocyclic complex Gd-HPDO3A (gadoteridol) is an example of a compound more kinetically inert to Gd loss than Gd-DTPA (gadopentetate), which has a similar stability constant. The rate of acid-assisted Gd dissociation is 20 times faster for Gd-DTPA (gadopentetate) than for Gd-HPDO3A (gadoteridol).[134] Laurent and colleagues measured the rate of Gd loss in the presence of zinc and phosphate under a standard set of conditions for various approved agents.[135,136] The macrocyclic complexes Gd-DOTA (gadoterate), Gd-HPDO3A (gadoteridol), and Gd-DO3A-butrol (gadobutrol) were the most inert with respect to Gd loss. The compound that released Gd the most rapidly was Gd-DTPA-BMA (gadodiamide). These differences in kinetics and thermodynamic stabilities may well translate into safety with regard to patients with chronic kidney disease. For instance, there is a much lower incidence of NSF among patients who received Gd-HPDO3A (gadoteridol),[137] and this may be a result of its combination of stability and inertness.

A series of studies published since 2013 have raised concerns over long-term Gd retention in the brain, bone, and skin of patients receiving multiple contrast-agent-enhanced examinations, including patients with normal renal function. The observation that the dentate nucleus and globus pallidus appear hyperintense in contrast-free T1-weighted scans of patients having received multiple prior contrast-enhanced scans suggested residual gadolinium accumulation in those regions of the brain.[138–139b] Elemental analysis of autopsy specimens collected from patients receiving numerous injections of Gd-based contrast agents confirmed that there was measurable gadolinium in the brain, albeit at low levels.[140] The amount of central nervous system (CNS) Gd deposition may depend on the type of contrast agent received. CNS tissue enhancement by residual Gd appears to be greater after receiving multiple injections of Gd contrast with acyclic chelators.[141] This is evidenced by consistently hyperintense dentate nuclei in patients receiving multiple doses of the Gd complexes with acyclic chelators, whereas the effect is not observed in patients exclusively receiving Gd complexes with macrocyclic chelators. Nonetheless, postmortem elemental analysis detects non-negligible Gd levels in CNS tissue of patients receiving only macrocyclic agents, including healthy patients receiving a single dose in their lifetime,[142] and imaging studies demonstrate retained Gd after high doses of macrocytic agents.[139b] The same study found highly elevated Gd levels in the bone of all patients receiving both acyclic and macrocyclic agents; Gd retention in the skin was also observed.

The speciation of Gd retained in the skin, bone, and CNS remains largely underexplored (chelated vs. unchelated), as do the mechanisms by which Gd is accumulated and the corresponding health risks. A recent study used chromatography coupled with elemental spectroscopy to evaluate Gd speciation in the skin of a patient with healthy kidney function who received 61 contrast-enhanced examination over the course of 11 years.[143] The patient received multiple Gd-based agents including

Gd-DTPA, Gd-BOPTA, Gd-DTPA-BMA, and Gd-HPDO3A. Speciation analysis revealed skin accumulation of intact Gd-DTPA and Gd-BOPTA as well as still uncharacterized Gd-containing species that likely exist in particulate form or are protein bound. In 2015 the FDA announced a formal investigation into the safety risks of Gd retained in the CNS[144] and subsequently recommended against the use of linear agents and have issued a new class warning.[144a]

Regarding other side effects, Kirchin and Runge[145] reviewed the safety record of clinically approved contrast agents as of 2003. The seven approved Gd agents (Gd-DTPA [gadopentetate], Gd-DOTA [gadoterate], Gd-BOPTA [gadobenate], Gd-DTPA-BMA [gadodiamide], Gd-DTPA-BMEA [gadoversatamide], Gd-DO3A-butrol [gadobutrol], and Gd-BOPTA [gadobenate]) appeared indistinguishable with respect to their safety profile. The most common adverse events were headache, nausea, taste perversion, and urticaria (hives). Nearly all adverse events with these agents were transient, mild, and self-limiting. Nevertheless, there are reports of serious adverse reactions, including life-threatening anaphylactoid reactions and death. The best estimate puts the rate of these events at between 1 in 200,000 and 1 in 400,000 patient administrations.[146] The Gd-based ECF contrast agents have been studied, and most are approved for pediatric use in patients older than 2 years, although there are differences in their approval wording. Gd-DO3A-butrol (gadobutrol) is the only Gd-based contrast agent approved for use in patients younger than 2 years of age in the United States.[147] One distinguishing clinical indicator among the Gd-based agents is that patients receiving Gd-DTPA-BMA (gadodiamide) or Gd-DTPA-BMEA (gadoversatamide) often show spuriously low serum calcium levels.[148] These two contrast agents (but not the other Gd-based agents) appear to interfere with the reagent used in the clinical chemistry test for calcium.[149]

The safety profile for current CMR contrast agents of course will not necessarily be the same for future compounds. For all contrast agents, the package insert should always be consulted for the latest safety information.

CONCLUSION

A large number of contrast agents have been approved for MRI in the last 26 years. A significant number of new agents, including tissue-specific agents that are potentially relevant for CMR, are currently in development. The behavior of these agents, which often is summarized by a single effectiveness parameter, r_1, is actually quite complex, in terms of both the underlying chemistry and the biophysics in vivo. Although many elements of that complexity remain active areas of research, both for understanding existing agents as well as for creating new agents and new uses for those agents, the relative safety and ease of use of these agents has brought them into routine use in many medical applications. As clinical CMR expands, no doubt the use of these contrast agents will expand as well, but CMR practitioners need to be cognizant of potential moderate-term complications including NSF in patients with renal dysfunction. The long-term impact of Gd retention in the CNS and elsewhere remains uncertain.

REFERENCES

A full reference list is available online at ExpertConsult.com

4

Myocardial Perfusion Imaging Theory

Michael Jerosch-Herold and Norbert Wilke

INTRODUCTION

The concept of injecting a tracer into the blood stream and detecting its transit and distribution in the heart muscle for the assessment of myocardial perfusion is well established in nuclear cardiology and cardiovascular magnetic resonance (CMR). Both exogenous, injected contrast agents and endogenous contrast mechanisms have been used to assess myocardial perfusion with CMR. The use of a gadolinium (Gd)-based contrast agents for the assessment of myocardial perfusion with CMR has been extensively validated and successfully applied in patient studies (see Chapter 18). Recent developments, in particular the introduction of parallel imaging, and sparse sampling methods (see Chapter 5), have made it possible to combine the requirements for spatial and temporal resolution for myocardial perfusion imaging during the first pass, with multi-slice coverage of the heart. The need for a quantitative, largely observer-independent analysis of perfusion studies has also received increasing support.[1] Several approaches have been developed that allow quantification of myocardial blood flow (MBF) with CMR. Advances in rapid imaging techniques for CMR perfusion imaging (covered in detail in Chapter 5) and the development of methods to obtain reproducible, quantitative measures of myocardial perfusion have established CMR perfusion imaging as an attractive alternative to nuclear perfusion imaging.[2]

THE PHYSIOLOGIC BASIS FOR MEASURING MYOCARDIAL PERFUSION

Coronary circulation blood flow resistance is under normal conditions determined primarily by the myocardial microcirculation, vessels with a diameter less than 300 μm. The adequate supply of oxygen and metabolites to the myocytes is tightly coupled to MBF. The assessment of microcirculatory function has therefore been used as a surrogate marker for the detection of myocardial ischemia, although ischemic conditions are also critically dependent on the workload and metabolic function. For example, under conditions of myocardial hibernation, the degree of ischemia is reduced by a corresponding reduction of the cardiac workload. Adequate and near-constant blood flow is maintained through autoregulation of coronary tone. Compensatory vasodilation can maintain adequate myocardial blood under resting conditions for up to 80% diameter epicardial coronary artery narrowing.[3,4] With more severe narrowing in an epicardial vessel, and in the absence of significant collateral flow, the distal perfusion bed is fully vasodilated even under resting conditions, and no augmentation of blood flow is feasible during periods of increased demand (e.g., if the patient exercises or undergoes pharmacologically induced stress). In healthy subjects, MBF can increase 3- to 4-fold with maximal vasodilation.[5] This means that differences in MBF between a region subtended by a stenosed coronary artery and the territory of a normal coronary artery are significantly amplified with maximal vasodilation.

Myocardial perfusion imaging during pharmacologic vasodilation (e.g., with adenosine, dipyridamole, or regadenoson) rests on the physiologic observation that the hemodynamic significance of an epicardial lesion is most apparent during maximal vasodilation.[3,4] A related measure can be obtained in the catheterization laboratory with an intravascular Doppler flow probe by measuring the coronary flow reserve, to assess lesion severity,[6] or by measuring the fractional flow reserve,[7] defined as mean distal coronary artery pressure divided by the aortic pressure during maximal vasodilatation. These functional tests of coronary resistance and MBF overcome the known limitations of vessel lumen diameter measurements by x-ray angiography for determining the hemodynamic significance of epicardial lesions.

Myocardial perfusion imaging can also be used to assess functional impairments in the coronary microcirculation, when there are no epicardial lesions. Both myocardial perfusion reserve, and coronary flow reserve were found to be abnormally low in women with microvascular dysfunction, and without significant epicardial stenoses.[8,9] There is also evidence from epidemiologic studies that it is feasible with CMR perfusion imaging to detect subclinical disease and silent ischemia in persons without a history or symptoms of atherosclerotic disease. The myocardial perfusion reserve in response to adenosine was found to be associated with coronary artery disease risk factors in patients with a low likelihood of significant epicardial disease.[10] In asymptomatic patients a lower myocardial perfusion reserve is associated with decreased regional left ventricular (LV) function[11] and also with lower regional myocardial strain.[12]

With the development of CMR perfusion imaging, it has become possible to probe with sufficient spatial resolution for more subtle indicators of myocardial ischemia. Blood flow across the myocardial wall is not uniform but instead favors the subendocardium to accommodate the higher workload and higher rate of oxygen consumption in the subendocardial layer.[13,14] Under normal resting conditions the ratio of endocardial to epicardial blood flow is on the order of 1.15:1.[15] With a coronary artery stenosis, blood flow is first diverted away from the subendocardial layer and the endocardial-to-epicardial blood flow ratio is often <1:1, in particular when under stress.[15,16] With myocardial ischemia, the subendocardial layer is accordingly most susceptible to necrosis. The transmural gradient of MBF can only be sufficiently appreciated if the imaging modality provides spatial resolution on the order of ≤2 mm. With CMR it has become feasible to detect flow impairments limited or most accentuated in the subendocardial layer.[17,18] The spatial resolution of conventional imaging modalities such as positron emission tomography (PET) and single photon emission computed tomography (SPECT) was insufficient to detect MBF deficits limited to the subendocardial layer. More specifically, the sensitivity of a myocardial perfusion imaging technique is directly related to its spatial resolution, and the ability to discern transmural variations of flow.[17,19]

CMR offers the unique possibility of quantitatively assessing both perfusion, viability, and function with high accuracy, to distinguish, stunned, hibernating, and infarcted myocardium. Bolli et al. showed that even small differences in blood flow during ischemia result in large differences in postischemic function, suggesting that the ability to quantify flow in the low-flow range is of importance to predict the probability of postischemic recovery.[20] The extent and incidence of microvascular obstruction observed with CMR were associated with the duration of ischemia before coronary intervention.[21]

FIRST-PASS IMAGING WITH EXOGENOUS TRACERS

The success of applying CMR to detect the first pass of an injected contrast agent and detect perfusion abnormalities starts with an understanding of the contrast mechanisms that allow contrast agent detection. The first-pass transit of a contrast agent through the vasculature and tissue leads to changes in the T1 and T2* relaxation time constants for the detected ^{1}H signal: the contrast reagent is not detected directly, but rather through its effects on the signal from ^{1}H nuclei in tissue. The chelates of paramagnetic Gd ions used as contrast reagents have a relatively high magnetic susceptibility, which causes on a microscopic scale magnetic field inhomogeneities and shortens the transverse (T2*) relaxation rate of water (see Chapter 3). The contrast reagent also shortens the longitudinal (T1) magnetization recovery after a radiofrequency pulse has disturbed the equilibrium state.

CMR methods for perfusion imaging can be subdivided into T1- and T2*-weighted techniques: T1-weighted techniques produce signal enhancement during the transit of the contrast agent, whereas T2* techniques cause signal loss. For contrast agents confined to the vascular bed, and in the absence of significant organ motion, T2*-weighted perfusion imaging gives rise to relatively larger signal changes than T1-weighted techniques, because the magnetic susceptibility effects of the contrast agents extend beyond the capillaries. But T2*-weighted imaging techniques have an inherent sensitivity to motion, leading to signal loss in the presence of motion. For myocardial perfusion imaging, T1-weighted techniques such as gradient echo imaging with short echo times, and a magnetization preparation for optimal T1 weighting have therefore steadily gained preference in CMR. We provide here a brief overview of three major sequence techniques for T1-weighted perfusion imaging of the heart. In historical order, they are spoiled gradient echo imaging (e.g., "TurboFLASH" or "turbo field echo" [TFE]); gradient echo imaging with balanced steady-state free precession (bSSFP); and multi-shot T1-weighted echo planar imaging.

Single-shot gradient echo imaging with a magnetization preparation (e.g., TurboFLASH or TFE) is well suited for T1-weighted, quantitative myocardial perfusion imaging. A magnetization preparation for T1 weighting can take the form of an inversion pulse or a saturation pulse; either of them is generally applied in a non-slice-selective mode so that blood flowing into the image plane during the subsequent image acquisition has been subjected to the same T1 preparation as myocardium. In a sequential multi-slice imaging sequence, a saturation preparation can be repeated for each slice, and this will result in the same degree of T1 weighting for each slice. After the magnetization preparation, images for one or more slices are rapidly read out within approximately <200 ms per image, or even less depending on the imaging acceleration technique that is being used. Typical sequence parameters for such rapid readouts are a repetition time per phase-encoding step (TR) of ≤2.5 ms, an echo time (TE) of ≤1 ms, a receiver bandwidth on the order of 400 to 700 Hz/pixel, and an in-plane spatial resolution of 2 to 3 mm. Because of the short TE, the signal is relatively insensitive to flow and magnetic susceptibility variations (e.g., between tissue and blood pool during the first pass). With a linear ordering for the phase-encoding steps, the image acquisition only needs to be delayed by 10 to 20 ms after a saturation recovery preparation. Depending on the effective time after saturation (TS) or time after inversion (TI, if an inversion pulse is used), the signal increases approximately linearly with contrast agent concentration, or as a function of the relaxation rate constant. (Note that the relaxivity of the contrast reagent is not appreciably different between blood and tissue.) Eventually the signal ceases to increase because of the opposite effect of T2* on the signal at higher contrast concentrations, and even in the case of negligible TEs (e.g., with image readouts with ultra-short TE) the signal intensity from a proton density–weighted image represents an effective upper limit for the signal intensity dynamic range. Fig. 4.1 shows an example of a CMR perfusion study with a spoiled gradient echo technique.

The signal-to-noise (SNR) and the contrast-to-noise ratio (CNR) with gradient echo perfusion imaging are relatively low, when short TRs, and wide receiver bandwidths are used. The maximum signal intensity is reached with relatively low flip angles. (The flip angle corresponding to maximum signal intensity is referred to as "Ernst angle.") To overcome this limitation, one can use a bSSFP image readout, which maximizes the preservation of phase coherence of the transverse magnetization between repetition periods (TRs) in the pulse sequence, and efficiently converts magnetization between transverse and longitudinal orientations. With bSSFP, the Ernst angle can approach 90 degrees—that is, one can reach the maximum theoretical signal amplitude after each radiofrequency (RF) excitation, while still repeating the excitations with very short TRs. In fact, the TR should be as short as feasible, because any off-resonance phase shifts increase signal loss, and phase shifts increase with TR, and also with flow.[22] Off-resonance frequency shifts result in dark bands at locations where the frequency shift (in radians/s) times TR (in seconds) equals an odd multiple of $\pi/2$.

The passage of a contrast bolus in the LV cavity can produce a frequency shift as large as approximately 100 Hz at 1.5 T and larger at higher field strengths. As the off-resonance shift varies with changing contrast loading of the blood pool during the first pass, it can induce signal variations over the myocardium, which can mimic perfusion defects (not to be mistaken with dark-rim artifacts, which are discussed later and which have a different appearance). At field strengths of ≥3 T, bSSFP image readouts during first-pass imaging can give rise to quite severe image artifacts, with dark bands appearing over the myocardium. The use of bSSFP readouts has therefore been mostly limited for cardiac perfusion imaging to field strengths of ≤1.5 T. Although the bSSFP readouts can produce appealing image quality,[23] its use has to be approached with caution as the artifacts on bSSFP images can be deceptive.

Echo planer imaging (EPI) eliminates the need for RF excitation before each phase-encoding step, and, as a result, it is one of the fastest imaging methods for freezing heart motion (50–100 ms for single-shot acquisitions). In an EPI pulse sequence, an initial RF excitation creates a coherent precession of transverse magnetization, and a train of gradient echoes is then generated by applying a rapidly oscillating magnetic field gradient along the readout direction. Each of these gradient echoes is preceded by a short, blipped gradient pulse, applied along a direction perpendicular to the oscillating magnetic field gradient. The blipped phase-encoding gradients between echoes advance the trajectory in the frequency acquisition space (k-space) perpendicular to the readout direction. Instead of just a single line, one acquires after each RF excitation a set of parallel lines in frequency space ("k-space"). The T2*-related decay of the gradient echo amplitudes in the echo train

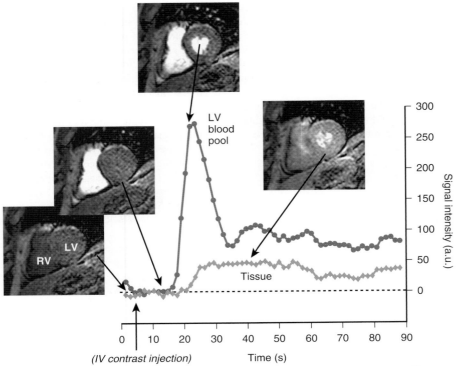

FIG. 4.1 The gradient echo cardiovascular magnetic resonance (CMR) images depict the first pass of an extracellular contrast agent (0.03 mmol/kg of gadodiamide/Omniscan, GE Healthcare) in a healthy subject, with appearance of the contrast first in the right ventricle *(RV)*, followed by the left ventricle *(LV)*, and finally leading to myocardial contrast enhancement. The contrast agent was injected after acquisition of approximately four precontrast images. Images were acquired in the short-axis view at the level of the papillary muscle. The arrows show the correspondence between images and the time course of changes in signal intensity for a region of interest in the LV *(circles)* and a myocardial segment in the inferolateral wall *(diamonds)*. Characteristics of the signal curve for a tissue region such as its increased dispersion, lower amplitude and reduced rate of signal enhancement compared with the ventricle result from transit through the coronary microcirculation, where the volume of distribution is limited to either the extracellular or the intravascular space.

results in an increasing sensitivity of later echoes to T2* and motion and causes blurring. The effective TE can be an order of magnitude longer for EPI sequences compared with fast gradient echo sequences (e.g., 30–40 ms vs. 1.2–2.0 ms for fast gradient echo imaging). Unfortunately, a longer effective TE gives rise to magnetic susceptibility and flow artifacts in the LV cavity. Furthermore, flow- and susceptibility-related artifacts in the LV make it difficult to measure the arterial transit of the contrast agent. To partially capture the speed advantage of EPI, and to minimize T2*- and flow-related artifacts, one reduces the length of the echo trains, and the images are read out with several RF excitations/echo trains.[24] This results in a 30% to 40% speed advantage compared with conventional gradient echo sequences, and is particularly useful at field strengths of ≤1.5 T. (At ≥3 T, any increase of echo time beyond the minimum allowed by the gradient system nearly inevitably gives rise to susceptibility artifacts, in particular during passage of a contrast bolus.)

Ultra-fast T1 measurements (Fig. 4.2) would provide the most accurate estimates of contrast agent concentration, and, with the advent of parallel imaging, this approach may become practical. Chen et al. developed such a T1 Fast Acquisition Relaxation Mapping (T1-FARM) method to obtain single-slice T1 maps of the heart with 1 s resolution.[25,26] With a direct T1 measurement, the problems associated with the saturation of the signal with increasing contrast agent dosage can be avoided. This should allow for a more accurate quantification of blood flow using

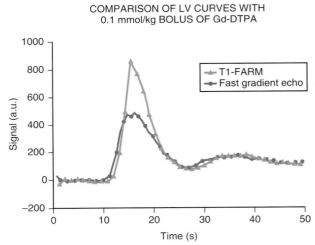

FIG. 4.2 Comparison of signal time curves for left ventricular regions of interest obtained in a canine with quantitative T1 imaging (T1-FARM) and T1-weighted, saturation recovery prepared TurboFLASH (TR/TE = 2.4/1.2 ms; flip angle = 18 degrees) and a Gd-DTPA dosage of 0.075 mmol/kg at 1.5 T. The curves were normalized so the Turbo-FLASH and T1-FARM recirculation peaks were equal. (From Z. Chen, C.A. McKenzie, and F.S. Prato, St. Joseph's Hospital, London, Ontario.)

higher contrast agent dosages. A T1-based estimation of the contrast concentration is particularly advantageous for the blood pool, as saturation of the contrast enhancement is of foremost concern for the arterial input. If instead one measures T1 in the blood pool during the first pass of the contrast agent, the arterial input can be reconstructed from these T1 data rather than the signal intensity because the latter suffers from saturation effects. Chen et al. developed a slice-interleaved radial imaging technique,[27] that runs continuously and can be used for reconstruction of cardiac phase-resolved images, and beat-by-beat estimation of T1 for arterial input sampling.

In its current state, all CMR techniques offer higher spatial resolution than is feasible with nuclear imaging techniques. An illustration of this is shown in Fig. 4.3 from studies in an experimental animal model.

ADVANCED TECHNIQUES FOR PERFUSION IMAGING ACCELERATION

Myocardial perfusion CMR has been at the forefront of developments in image acceleration techniques aimed at increasing coverage of the LV. Increased coverage can translate into a larger number of image slices, or, by switching to three-dimensional image acquisitions, increase spatial coverage of the myocardium. The increased LV coverage should not come at the cost of lower temporal resolution—for example, by increasing the repetition time for each slice location from one to two heart beats—because a lower temporal resolution will affect the accuracy for distinguishing gradual changes in MBF, in particular during stress conditions. Chapter 5 of this book is dedicated to advanced techniques for CMR perfusion imaging that provide increased coverage of the LV, possibly higher in-plane spatial resolution, and suffer from fewer image artifacts (e.g., "dark-rim" artifact). This chapter will instead focus on the underlying theory and principles of CMR myocardial perfusion imaging.

ENDOGENOUS CONTRAST FOR THE ASSESSMENT OF MYOCARDIAL PERFUSION

Approaches have been developed for an assessment of myocardial perfusion that are not based on the use of an exogenous MR contrast agent but instead exploit endogenous contrast mechanisms related to blood flow and blood oxygenation. These approaches fall under the categories of spin labeling,[28] blood-oxygen-level-dependent (BOLD) contrast,[29,30] and magnetization transfer (MT) contrast.[31,32] These techniques have to be considered technically more challenging than measurements with exogenous contrast agents, or offer only an indirect measure of blood flow.

With spin labeling, the spins are either inverted or saturated in a slab that is generally located upstream from the imaged slice.[33–35] The flow-dependent change of signal intensity because of the inflow of saturated or inverted spins into the image slice provides a measure of tissue perfusion. The spin-labeling method generally relies on the assumption that the net arterial blood flow in the myocardium follows the direction from base to apex. Cardiac motion complicates the interpretation of signal changes in a spin-labeling experiment because the labeled spins can be transported into the imaged slice either through blood flow or by through-plane motion of the heart.

BOLD offers a measure of hemoglobin saturation reflecting regional oxygen supply and demand. Deoxyhemoglobin is paramagnetic, whereas oxyhemoglobin is only diamagnetic, which means that deoxyhemoglobin causes a considerably larger reduction of T2* than oxyhemoglobin and therefore a larger signal intensity attenuation in gradient echo images. Deoxyhemoglobin can be used as an endogenous intravascular tracer because of the tight coupling between oxygen demand and blood flow. BOLD contrast changes have been observed in the heart after administration of dipyridamole and dobutamine.[29,30] The link between BOLD contrast and blood flow depends on the balance between blood flow and oxygen metabolism—that is, between oxygen supply and demand.[36]

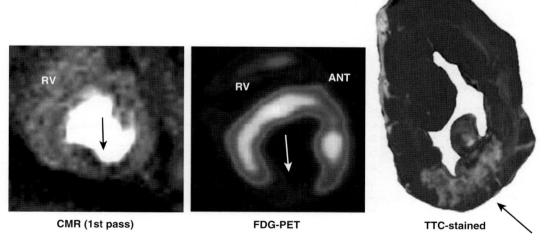

CMR (1st pass)   **FDG-PET**   **TTC-stained**

FIG. 4.3 Images from cardiovascular magnetic resonance *(CMR)*, positron emission tomography *(PET)*, and triphenyltetrazolium chloride *(TTC)* staining in a porcine model in which obtuse branches of the left circumflex coronary artery had been ligated 4 weeks before combined CMR and PET studies. From CMR images acquired during the first pass of an intravascular iron oxide contrast agent (NC100150 Injection, Nycomed), the one shown at left corresponds to the highest peak signal enhancement in tissue and indicates a subendocardial perfusion defect in the posterior segment, in agreement with TTC staining shown at right [13]NH$_2$ PET *(middle image)* was carried out 3 hours before the CMR study and shows a fixed defect in the inferolateral segment, suggesting a transmural infarct. FDG-PET images (not shown) also indicated irreversible damage in the posterior segment, in disagreement with the findings from CMR and TTC staining. *ANT,* Anterior wall; *RV,* right ventricle.

Spin labeling, BOLD, and MT contrast CMR have an advantage in that they can be carried out in the steady state, meaning there is no need to capture with ultra-fast imaging the transient signal changes observable in the myocardium after injection of an exogenous tracer. Ultimately these techniques may allow an assessment of myocardial perfusion with very high spatial resolution (~1 mm or less).

QUANTITATIVE EVALUATION OF MYOCARDIAL PERFUSION

The images acquired in a "first-pass" study of myocardial perfusion—meaning rapid dynamic imaging during the first pass of an injected contrast bolus—can be qualitatively evaluated for differential signal enhancement in the myocardium. With a T1-weighted imaging technique, myocardial segments showing reduced signal intensity enhancement during the first pass, relative to other myocardial segments, are interpreted as hypoperfused. This type of qualitative judgment of signal enhancement differences can suffer from substantial observer bias and small reductions in perfusion may be missed. Although higher dosages of contrast agent would increase the dynamic contrast enhancement, and thereby render myocardial regions with reduced contrast enhancement more apparent, the images are also more likely to be contaminated by artifacts near the endocardial border. Furthermore, global reductions of blood flow because of diffuse microvascular ischemia will be missed by this approach. It then becomes advantageous to evaluate the contrast state during stress or vasodilation, relative to a baseline or resting state to uncover global impairments of perfusion.

With a fast T1-weighted gradient echo sequence and low contrast agent dosages (e.g., 0.03 mmol/kg of Gd-DTPA for an intravenous bolus injection into an antecubital vein) the myocardial contrast enhancement is approximately proportional to the local contrast agent concentration. Under these conditions the signal curves can be interpreted as, or transformed into, contrast agent residue curves. Absolute units do not matter here as much as a faithful reproduction of the relation in contrast concentrations between tissue and blood pool—enhancement in the tissue is interpreted relative to the enhancement in the blood pool. In fact, the tissue is often, for the purpose of quantifying perfusion, viewed as a linear, stationary system, where the enhancement in the tissue can be modeled as a linear response to arterial input of contrast.

Investigators using PET have over the years presented compelling arguments for a quantitative approach to myocardial perfusion imaging, including absolute quantification of MBF.[37] With CMR, a quantitative analysis of contrast enhancement is based on signal intensity curves, which can be generated for user-defined regions of interest (ROI), or at the pixel level. CMR perfusion studies require a careful approach for image segmentation and registration. CMR perfusion studies are not motion-averaged, the endocardial borders are relatively well defined during transit of contrast through the ventricular cavity, and the large signal enhancement in the ventricular cavity requires accurate image segmentation to avoid spill-over effects. Fig. 4.4 shows an example of a CMR perfusion study in a patient for absolute quantification based on model-independent analysis of signal intensity curves.[38]

In the vein of Zierler's[39–41] original work on the central volume principle, we consider here a tissue ROI with a single arterial input and

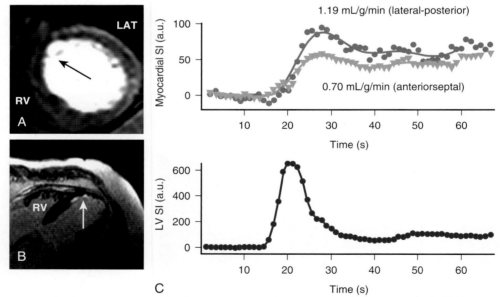

FIG. 4.4 A 71-year-old male patient had presented with a silent non-Q-wave anterior myocardial infarction. (A) Image from a series of 60 dynamic images taken at rest shows the initial contrast enhancement in the myocardium, with reduced contrast uptake in the anterior and anterior-septal segments because of an eccentric 90% stenosis with a lesion length of 10 mm in the proximal left anterior descending (LAD) coronary artery. (B) Late gadolinium enhancement was observed in anterior and anterior-septal segments (highlighted by *white arrow*) from mid level to apex, but not at a more basal level including the level of the slice in shown in A. (C) Myocardial blood flow was quantified by model-independent deconvolution of the myocardial signal intensity *(SI)* curves, using an arterial input measured in the left ventricular *(LV)* blood pool. Blood flow at rest in an anterior-septal segment (highlighted with *arrow* in A) was 0.7 mL/g/min, compared with 1.2 mL/g/min in the inferolateral wall. The anterior and anterior-septal segments appeared hypokinetic on cine cardiovascular magnetic resonance (CMR). After CMR study, the patient was referred for coronary angiography. During percutaneous coronary intervention, a drug-eluting stent was deployed in the proximal LAD. *LAT,* Lateral; *RV,* right ventricle.

a single venous output. The injection of a tracer is described by the variation of tracer concentration at the (arterial) input $c_{in}(t)$. The amount of tracer that remains in the tissue region at any time t, $q(t)$, represents the difference between the amount supplied to the tissue region up to time t, and the total amount of tracer that has exited the region of interest up to the time t:

$$q(t) = F \int_0^t [c_{in}(s) - c_{out}(s)] \cdot dt \qquad \textbf{Eq. 4.1}$$

where F represents the flow blood, for example, in units of mL/min/g of tissue, and c_{out} is the concentration at the output of the region of interest. (We consider here a single arterial input and venous output to the ROI, but this overly restrictive model is assumed here only for the sake of simplifying the presentation. It can be shown that one can generalize the theory to allow for multiple inputs and outputs.[42])

Zierler showed that if the transport within a tissue ROI is assumed to be linear and stationary, then the response to an arbitrary arterial input is given by the convolution of this input with the tissue impulse response[41]:

$$q(t) = \int_0^t c_{in}(t - \tau) \cdot R(\tau) d\tau \qquad \textbf{Eq. 4.2}$$

We denote the impulse response by $R(t)$. The response in a tissue region to an impulse input, the tissue impulse response, has the useful property that its initial amplitude equals the MBF through that region. This can be seen from Eq. 4.1 by considering the special case when the input is a Dirac delta impulse, $c_{in}(t) = \delta(t)$, and requiring that $c_{out}(t = 0) = 0$, that is, the tracer cannot instantaneously reach the output after injection. This property of the impulse response is independent of the vascular and compartmental structure inside the tissue ROI, or the properties of barriers such as their permeability. For example, leakage of a contrast agent from the capillaries into the interstitial space produces a redistribution of the contrast agent within the ROI, but does not contribute to flow in and out of the ROI, as long as transport by diffusion and convection is much slower than by blood flow. For a CMR contrast agent such as Gd-DTPA these assumptions hold up well, but for freely diffusible tracers they may not always apply.

The central volume principle indicates that the blood flow can be determined from the impulse response amplitude. To obtain the impulse response one has to perform a deconvolution of the measured tissue residue curve with the arterial input curve—that is, perform the inverse of the convolution operation shown in Eq. 4.2. The deconvolution analysis is quite sensitive to noise in the data, and one therefore needs to constrain the deconvolution operation. A Fermi function has been used as an empirical model for the impulse response to fit the first-pass portion of the signal curves.[43,44] The Fermi model of the impulse response has the following functional form:

$$R(t) = \frac{A}{1 + \exp[-(t - w)/\tau]} \qquad \textbf{Eq. 4.3}$$

where A, w, and t are model parameters, with no direct physiologic meaning. From an empirical standpoint, the shape of the Fermi function provides a reasonable approximation to the shape of the impulse response of an intravascular tracer. The portion of the signal intensity curves up to the peak has higher sensitivity to flow changes than later phases of the contrast enhancement, and the early enhancement is relatively insensitive to capillary leakage of contrast agent. This part of the signal intensity curve can be approximated well by the Fermi function model to assess blood flow, even when an extravascular,

extracellular Gd-based contrast agent is used. The Fermi model for the quantification of myocardial perfusion and the perfusion reserve was validated by comparison to blood flow measurements with labeled microspheres[45,46] and also by comparison to invasive coronary flow reserve measurements.[44]

The Fermi model, although used in numerous studies, has some well-known limitations. It was initially proposed by Axel[43] for deconvolution analysis of tissue contrast enhancement from an intravascular contrast agent. The shape of the Fermi function cannot reproduce the delayed wash-out of contrast observed with an extracellular contrast agent, which results from leakage of contrast across the capillary barrier into the interstitial space, and the subsequent relatively slow clearance of contrast from the interstitial space—the interstitial space volume in myocardial tissue is two to three times larger than the vascular space volume. In a CMR first-pass perfusion study this slow clearance of contrast from myocardial tissue manifests itself by the fact that after the first pass of the contrast in the arterial input, the signal intensity in the myocardium shows little or a relatively small decline over the approximately 1- to 2-minute time frame that images are typically collected in a cardiac perfusion study. To overcome this shortcoming of the Fermi function model for analyzing perfusion studies where extracellular contrast agents are used, one can add a constant offset term to the Fermi function that accounts for the persistent contrast enhancement. This amounts to assuming that the contrast leaks into the interstitial space, but wash out is negligible.

A more general approach has been developed that is limited to imposing conditions on the impulse response that are consistent with the physiologic basis of the contrast enhancement:

1 The impulse response has to be a monotonically decaying function of time because, by definition of the impulse response, no additional tracer enters the tissue region after the initial contrast input impulse—after this initial impulse input of contrast, the concentration can only remain the same or decline. This constraint by itself can still lead to impulse responses that show sudden step-size changes, which is inconsistent in that the transport of contrast within the region of interest proceeds at steady and finite rates.

2 As a second condition, one can require that the impulse response shape changes smoothly—that is, the aforementioned sudden changes in shape are not consistent with the underlying steady-state transport processes in tissue. Smoothness of the impulse response follows to the degree that the magnitudes of flow, diffusion, and permeation in the heart impose constraints that exclude abrupt signal intensity changes in myocardial tissue after contrast agent injection. To impose such smoothness constraints, one can represent the impulse response as a sum of smooth cubic spline basis functions. The degree of smoothness is then determined by the number of spline components. The number of spline basis functions needs to be empirically determined. For this purpose, it is useful to use simulated data (using the types of models discussed in the next section).[38] One can then verify whether with a certain number of spline basis function components one can estimate without a significant bias the myocardial blood flow over a value range that covers the physiologic range of blood flow in the myocardium. In this context it is particularly the maximum flow that is important because it is associated with the most rapid changes of contrast enhancement.

The deconvolution algorithms that use these physiologic constraints without assuming a specific shape of the impulse response have been termed "model-independent" deconvolution[38] to distinguish them from the approach where a parameterized representation of the impulse response (e.g., Fermi model) is used. The advantage of this more general approach is that it is far less sensitive to the choice of data window that is chosen for deconvolution analysis.

signal covariance from training data. One method of improving this is to incorporate sensitivity encoding information into the reconstruction—this is the k-t SENSE method.[18] A further solution, which allows the use of higher acceleration factors, is to constrain the reconstruction using a standard data compression technique, called principal component analysis (PCA)—this is a commonly used mathematical algorithm that

reduces highly dimensional datasets to lower dimensionality by extracting and exploiting relevant correlations within the data. The extension of k-t BLAST or k-t SENSE methods using PCA in the reconstruction is referred to as k-t PCA.[19]

In the k-t PCA method, the adaptive filter used to remove aliasing is improved by applying PCA to the training data from which the filter is derived. Effectively, PCA is used to transform the images into a new mathematical domain of temporal "basis function" more suitable for reconstruction. The advantage of this new mathematical domain is that it is sparser, even in cases of nonperiodic motion such as respiration or misgating, and therefore the core perfusion data is contained within a few principal components and the rest can be discarded. This mathematical transformation process facilitates the easier separation of overlapping signals before they are converted back into images and accounts for the greater temporal fidelity and relative robustness of k-t PCA to motion.

Non-Cartesian Techniques

Alternative approaches to acceleration involve data acquisition along non-Cartesian patterns such as radial trajectories through the center of k-space (Fig. 5.5). Spatial and temporal redundancy are exploited serially and the altered geometry of k-space coverage facilitates greater efficiency compared with conventional Cartesian techniques by collecting more data with each RF excitation.[2,18,20] Non-Cartesian techniques can also be combined with parallel imaging techniques and hold potential for large gains in spatial–temporal resolution.

In the highly constrained back-projection reconstruction (HYPR) method and other radial acquisition variants, k-space data is acquired with undersampled radial projections and overall rotation of the undersampling pattern at different time points.[20–22] In image reconstruction, a fully sampled composite image is formed by populating missing data from neighboring time frames. This very low temporal resolution

TABLE 5.1	Basic Perfusion CMR Technique
Pulse sequence	Saturation recovery imaging with readout: • Spoiled GRE • GRE-echo planar hybrid • Steady-state free precession
Acceleration method	Parallel imaging, if available
Temporal resolution	Every heartbeat (for ischemia detection)
Readout temporal resolution (= acquisition shot duration)	~100–125 ms or shorter as available
No. of dynamics	Image for 40–50 heartbeats, by which time contrast has passed through the LV myocardium
No. of slices	At least 3 short-axis slices
In-plane spatial resolution	<3 mm
Slice thickness	8 mm
Contrast agent dose and administration regime	0.05–0.1 mmol/kg (3–7 mL/s) followed by at least 30 mL saline flush (3–7 mL/s)
Breath-holding	Breath-hold starts during early phases of contrast infusion before contrast reaches the LV cavity

CMR, Cardiovascular magnetic resonance; *GRE,* gradient echo; *LV,* left ventricular.

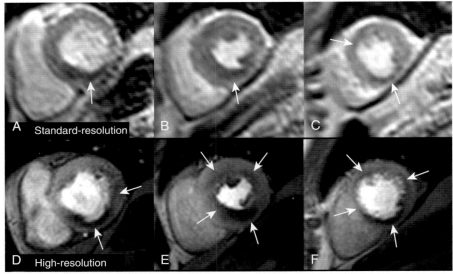

FIG. 5.1 High-resolution perfusion cardiovascular magnetic resonance (CMR). Standard (A–C) and high-resolution (D–F) stress perfusion CMR in a patient with three-vessel coronary artery disease. Standard resolution shows perfusion defects *(arrows)* in the basal-inferior (A), mid-inferior, mid-inferoseptal (B), apical-anterior and apical-inferior segments (C). High resolution shows a similar distribution of perfusion defects but demonstrates additional ischemia in the basal-lateral (D), mid-anterior and mid-anterolateral segments (E) with a circumferential defect in the apical slice (F). Perfusion defects are also better delineated at high resolution and the transmural extent of ischemia more clearly seen. (From Motwani M, Maredia N, Fairbairn TA, et al. Assessment of ischaemic burden in angiographic three-vessel coronary artery disease with high-resolution myocardial perfusion cardiovascular magnetic resonance imaging. *Eur Heart J Cardiovasc Imaging.* 2014;15:701–708.)

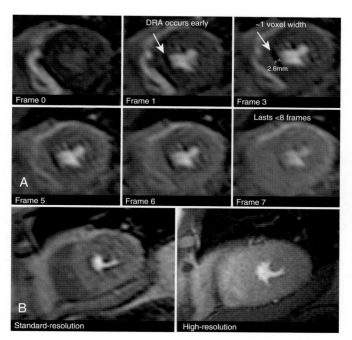

FIG. 5.2 Dark rim artifact. (A) Dark rim artifact *(DRA) (arrows)* is a frequent finding in standard-resolution perfusion cardiovascular magnetic resonance (CMR) and relates to several factors, including cardiac motion, Gibb's ringing, susceptibility and partial volume cancellation between the myocardium and blood pool. Although DRAs may mimic perfusion defects, they can be distinguished by characteristic features: they occur at the arrival of contrast in the left ventricular cavity and before its arrival in the myocardium (Frame 1); they tend to disappear within 8 to 10 frames (Frame 7); their location is usually typical for a particular pulse sequence; and their width roughly equates to the in-plane spatial resolution, which was 2.5 mm in this example (Frame 3). (B) A 60-year-old man with suspected angina underwent stress perfusion CMR at 1.5 T with both standard-resolution (2.5 mm in-plane) and high-resolution (1.5 mm in-plane) acquisition (8 × *k-t* BLAST). There was no perfusion defect seen with either acquisition but there was significant DRA on the standard-resolution images *(arrows)*. X-ray angiography confirmed normal coronary arteries.

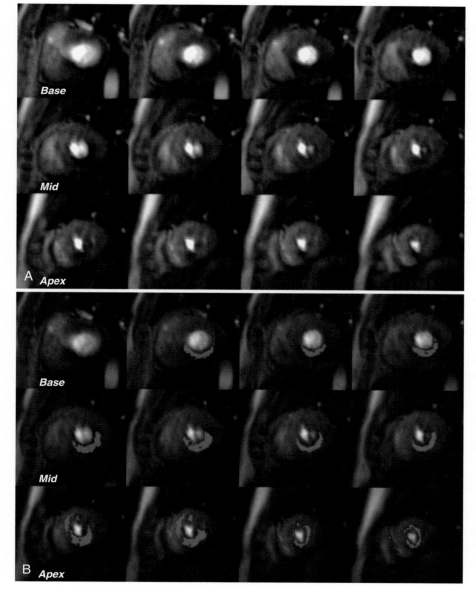

FIG. 5.3 Three-dimensional (3D) perfusion cardiovascular magnetic resonance (CMR). (A) Consecutive slices of a 3D perfusion CMR scan facilitated by *k-t* principal component analysis during adenosine stress in a patient with significant stenoses in the proximal right coronary artery and distal left anterior descending coronary artery. (B) Identical images illustrating volumetry of myocardial hypoenhancement using a signal intensity threshold of 2 standard deviations below remote myocardium *(red areas)*. The volume of myocardial hypoenhancement was 30.4% of total myocardium. (From Motwani M, Jogiya R, Kozerke S, et al. Advanced cardiovascular magnetic resonance myocardial perfusion imaging: high-spatial resolution versus 3-dimensional whole-heart coverage. *Clin Cardiovasc Imaging.* 2013;6:339–348.)

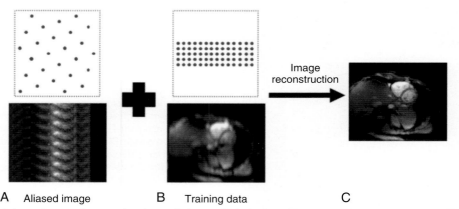

FIG. 5.4 *k-t* undersampling acceleration techniques. (A) In *k-t* broad linear speed-up technique (BLAST) and *k-t* sensitivity encoding (SENSE), data acquisition is accelerated by undersampling along the spatial encoding *(k)* and time *(t)* axes, which leads to an aliased image. (B) Low-resolution "training data" is also obtained to determine data correlations: that is, "prior-knowledge." (C) Finally, a nonaliased full image series is reconstructed using a statistical model derived from the training data. (From Motwani M, Jogiya R, Kozerke S, et al. Advanced cardiovascular magnetic resonance myocardial perfusion imaging: high-spatial resolution versus 3-dimensional whole-heart coverage. *Clin Cardiovasc Imaging.* 2013;6:339–348.)

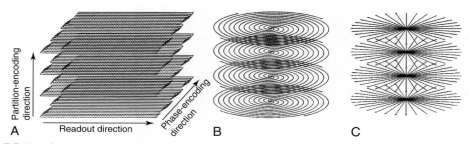

FIG. 5.5 Non-Cartesian trajectories. Examples of three potential alternate trajectories discussed in the text: (A) echo planar imaging demonstrated with an echo train length of 4; (B) a spiral trajectory with 4 interleaves; and (C) a radial projection design. Partition encoding direction in (B) and (C) is the same as for (A). (From Fair MJ, Gatehouse PD, DiBella EV, et al. A review of 3D first-pass, whole-heart, myocardial perfusion cardiovascular magnetic resonance. *J Cardiovasc Magn Reson.* 2015;17:68.)

composite is then used to constrain back projection of the undersampled data acquired for each individual time frame.[20,22]

To date, perhaps because other approaches are already well established, radial imaging has not been widely applied to two-dimensional (2D) perfusion CMR, other than for specific research purposes such as multiple samples through the center of *k*-space to calculate the arterial input function (AIF) or to capitalize on its inherent motion robustness for developing free-breathing techniques.[23,24] Radial sampling does, however, lend itself to combination with compressed sensing methods (see later) and may therefore see greater future application in 3D perfusion CMR techniques requiring particularly high acceleration factors.[5]

Spiral imaging is another non-Cartesian technique in which data is acquired spiraling outward from the central raw data through *k*-space.[25–28] Spiral pulse sequences have some inherent efficiency and SNR advantages over the radial technique, but are also more sensitive to off-resonance effects. However, careful selection of readout duration, flip angle strategy, and other sequence characteristics have been shown to compensate for spiral-related artifacts to produce high-quality high-resolution perfusion images.[25] Most commonly, for 3D data acquisition, a stack of spiral planes with Fourier encoding in the third direction is used to achieve whole-heart coverage in a cylindrical distribution (Fig. 5.6).[5,26]

Compressed Sensing

Non-Cartesian trajectories have reduced cardiac motion-induced dark rim artifact compared with conventional Cartesian acquisition strategies.[5,28] In addition, the acquisition efficiency and benign aliasing artifacts enable acquisition of higher-resolution images for a given acquisition time. However, both radial and spiral techniques require accurate scanner calibration and special image reconstruction techniques. An alternative method for reconstruction of undersampled data is compressed sensing (CS), which is based upon the principle that an image with a sparse representation in a known transform domain can be recovered from randomly undersampled *k*-space data using a nonlinear reconstruction (Fig. 5.7).[29,30] Sparsity in this context describes a matrix of pixels with predominantly zero values in a single image or series of images. CS is therefore readily applicable to perfusion CMR because the signal is sparse in the combined temporal and spatial domain with only portions of the field of view requiring full temporal bandwidth and the other regions having only static information or at low temporal frequencies. The additional CS requirement of incoherence (i.e., that undersampling artifacts look like additive noise) can be achieved in perfusion CMR by randomly omitting phase-encoding lines *(k_y)* with a different pattern for each time point *(t)*, generating a random undersampling pattern in *k_y-t* space. Compared with *k_y*-only random

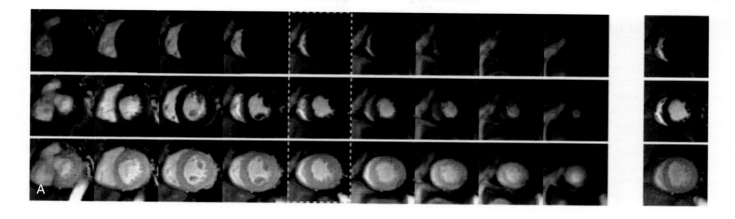

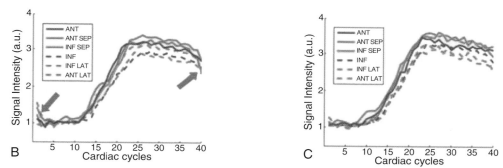

FIG. 5.6 (A) Stack-of-spirals three-dimensional perfusion cardiovascular magnetic resonance. Illustrative images acquired through stack of spirals during right ventricle blood pool *(top)*, LV blood pool *(middle)*, and LV myocardial *(bottom)* enhancement. Dotted lines indicate the middle slice, which was used for comparison with the corresponding single-slice two-dimensional (2D) Cartesian acquisition (not shown). (B–C) The corresponding myocardial signal–time curves for this and its corresponding 2D slice are shown, demonstrating good agreement, except for *k-t* parallel imaging artifacts in the early and late frames. (From Shin T, Nayak KS, Santos JM, et al. Three-dimensional first-pass myocardial perfusion MRI using a stack-of-spirals acquisition. *Magn Reson Med*. 2013;69:839–844.)

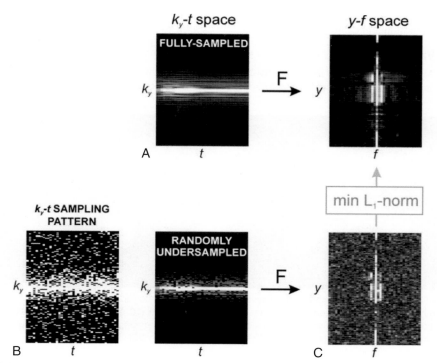

FIG. 5.7 Compressed sensing. Conceptual illustration of the compressed sensing technique for cardiac perfusion magnetic resonance imaging. (A) Sparsity: the fully sampled k_y-t data is sparse in y-f space. (B) Incoherence: k_y-t pseudo-random undersampling preserves the original sparse representation in y-f space and presents artifacts that look like additive noise (pseudo-noise). (C) Nonlinear reconstruction: the sparse coefficients in y-f space can be recovered with a nonlinear reconstruction that minimizes the number of nonzero coefficients (minimum L_1-norm). *F*, Fourier transform. (From Otazo R, Kim D, Axel L, et al. Combination of compressed sensing and parallel imaging for highly accelerated first-pass cardiac perfusion MRI. *Magn Reson Med*. 2010;64:767–776.)

undersampling, k_y-t random undersampling increases the incoherence, because the undersampling artifacts are incoherently distributed along two dimensions rather than one.

Unlike k-t BLAST and k-t SENSE, CS does not require training data, and, as a result, it may be less sensitive to inconsistencies between training and imaging data. Application of CS to dynamic CMR has been presented in methods such as k-t SPARSE and k-t FOCUSS, using the temporal fast Fourier transform (FFT) as the sparsifying transform, and k_y-t random undersampling.[29,31–33] Maximum acceleration rate in CS is determined by image sparsity, and in practice, the number of required samples is approximately three to five times the number of nonzero coefficients in the image.[29,32] Similar to the other advanced acceleration methods discussed, CS can be combined with parallel imaging techniques when multiple receiver coils are employed to obtain higher accelerations (Fig. 5.8).

HIGH-RESOLUTION PERFUSION CARDIOVASCULAR MAGNETIC RESONANCE

There is no clear definition of "high-resolution perfusion CMR," but an in-plane spatial resolution better than 2 mm, which is comparable with that of other common CMR methods such as late gadolinium enhancement (LGE) or cine imaging, is generally considered high. The rationale for pursuing high-resolution CMR is to facilitate comparison with cine and LGE images, to improve the detection of subendocardial ischemia and transmural ischemic gradients, and to reduce dark rim artifacts. These artifacts are a common finding in conventional perfusion CMR and are thought to be caused by magnetic susceptibility effects, Gibbs ringing, and cardiac motion during acquisition.[34] Because these artifacts are directly proportional to voxel size, high-resolution perfusion CMR leads to a reduction of dark rim artifact (see Fig. 5.2).[6,10,11] As discussed, non-Cartesian sampling techniques such as radial or spiral imaging have shown particular benefits in minimizing dark rim artifact reduction because of their robustness to motion and Gibbs ringing effects.[34,35]

Methods and Clinical Validation

High-resolution perfusion CMR was first described in a feasibility study using 5-fold k-t SENSE to achieve an in-plane spatial resolution of 1.5 mm.[17] The study reported similar overall image quality as standard-resolution (in-plane spatial resolution: 2.6 mm) SENSE-accelerated acquisition, but there was a significant reduction in the extent of dark rim artifact (mean thickness: 1.7 vs. 2.4 mm; $P < .01$) and SNR corrected for pixel size was higher for the k-t method. In a subsequent small study by Maredia et al.,[11] different tradeoffs between spatial resolution and shot duration were explored and a reduction in dark rim artifact with the highest in-plane spatial resolution was confirmed.

Following the first feasibility studies in volunteers, high-resolution perfusion CMR has been validated in several small patient studies (Table 5.2).[6–8,11] Plein et al. used an identical sequence to their previous volunteer study (1.5 T, 5-fold k-t SENSE, in-plane resolution 1.4 mm) in 51 patients with known or suspected coronary artery disease (CAD).[6] High-resolution acquisition was found to have high image quality and a high diagnostic accuracy (area under the curve, AUC: 0.85) compared with quantitative coronary angiography (QCA) with similar performance in single-vessel and multivessel disease (AUC: 0.87 vs. 0.82). Manka et al.[8] used k-t SENSE with 8-fold acceleration at 3 T to achieve an in-plane spatial resolution of 1.1 mm, reporting an AUC of 0.94 in 20 patients with suspected CAD against QCA. Lockie et al.[9] validated high-resolution perfusion CMR (5-fold k-t BLAST, in-plane resolution 1.2 mm) against invasive fractional flow reserve (FFR) and in 42 patients reported a high diagnostic accuracy (AUC: 0.92) for the detection of hemodynamically significant lesions (FFR < 0.75). In a study by Salerno et al.,[28] a saturation recovery interleaved variable-density spiral pulse sequence achieving 2 × 2 mm in-plane spatial resolution for three short-axis slices was used in 41 patients listed for QCA. The sensitivity, specificity, and accuracy were 89%, 85%, and 88%, respectively, to detect coronary stenosis >50%. Finally, a variant of the HYPR method known as sliding-window conjugate gradient HYPR (6 contiguous slices, 1.6 mm in-plane spatial resolution), has been shown to be clinically feasible in a single-center study ($n = 50$) and demonstrated high diagnostic accuracy (sensitivity 96%, specificity 82%).[22] Radial perfusion CMR has also been shown to be effective in eliminating the need for ECG gating and has the potential to achieve high diagnostic accuracy in arrhythmic patients (Fig. 5.9).[36]

Although these clinical validation studies show good diagnostic performance of high-resolution perfusion CMR against anatomical

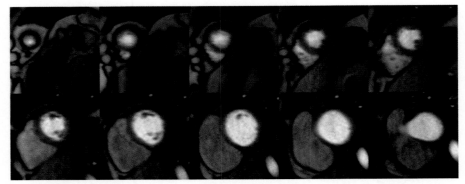

FIG. 5.8 Compressed sensing three-dimensional perfusion cardiovascular magnetic resonance. An example of breath-held, 8-fold accelerated whole-heart perfusion acquisition (10 short-axis slices) is achieved by a combination of compressed sensing and parallel imaging. In this example, compressed sensing and parallel imaging are combined by merging the k-t SPARSE technique with SENSE reconstruction to substantially increase the acceleration rate for perfusion imaging. These k-t SPARSE-SENSE reconstructed images exhibited good image quality. Image acquisition matrix = 128 × 128, spatial resolution = 3.2 × 3.2 mm², and temporal resolution = 38.4 ms. The reconstruction time per slice was approximately 15 minutes, which represented a total reconstruction time of approximately 2.5 hours for the 10 slices using Matlab (The MathWorks, Natick, MA) on a 64-bit quad core workstation. (From Otazo R, Kim D, Axel L, et al. Combination of compressed sensing and parallel imaging for highly accelerated first-pass cardiac perfusion MRI. *Magn Reson Med.* 2010;64:767–776.)

TABLE 5.2 Clinical Validation of Advanced Accelerated Perfusion Cardiovascular Magnetic Resonance

	No.		Advanced Acceleration Method	In-Plane Resolution	Spatial Coverage	Reference Standard	Diagnostic Accuracy
High Resolution							
Plein et al. 2008[6]	51	1.5 T	5 × k-t-SENSE	1.4 mm	4 slices (NC)[b]	QCA > 50%	0.85[c]
Plein et al. 2008[7]	33	1.5 T	5 × k-t SENSE	1.5 mm	4 slices (NC)[b]	QCA > 50%	0.80[c]
Plein et al. 2008[7]	33	3.0 T	5 × k-t SENSE	1.3 mm	4 slices (NC)[b]	QCA > 50%	0.89[c]
Manka et al. 2010[8]	20	3.0 T	8 × k-t SENSE	1.1 mm	3 slices (NC)	QCA > 50%	0.94[c]
Lockie et al. 2011[9]	42	3.0 T	5 × k-t BLAST	1.2 mm	3 slices (NC)	FFR < 0.75	0.92[c]
Lockie et al. 2011[9]	42	3.0 T	5 × k-t BLAST	1.2 mm	3 slices (NC)	FFR < 0.75	0.89[c] [MPR][a]
Motwani et al. 2012[10]	100	1.5 T	8 × k-t BLAST	1.6 mm	3 slices (NC)	QCA ≥ 50%	0.93[c]
Ma et al. 2012[22]	50	3.0 T	SW-CG-HYPR	1.6 mm	6 slices (WH)	QCA ≥ 50%	0.90[d]
Chirbiri et al. 2013[40]	67	3.0 T	5 × k-t SENSE	1.2 mm	3 slices (NC)	FFR < 0.80	0.86[c] [TPG][a]
Salerno et al. 2014[28]	41	1.5 T	8 × VD Spiral	2.0 mm	3 slices (NC)	QCA > 50%	0.88[d]
3D							
Manka et al. 2011[13]	146	3.0 T	6 × k-t SENSE	2.3 mm	16 slices (WH)	QCA ≥50%	0.83[d]
Manka et al. 2012[14]	120	1.5 T	10 × k-t PCA	2.0 mm	16 slices (WH)	FFR < 0.75	0.87[d]
Jogiya et al. 2012[15]	53	3.0 T	10 × k-t PCA	2.3 mm	12 slices (WH)	FFR < 0.75	0.91[d]
Jogiya et al. 2014[43]	33	3.0 T	10 × k-t PCA	2.3 mm	12 slices (WH)	QCA ≥ 70%	0.88[d]
Manka et al. 2015[49]	150	3.0 T	10 × k-t PCA	2.3 mm	16 slices (WH)	FFR < 0.80	0.87[c]
Motwani et al. 2014[46]	20	3.0 T	10 × k-t PCA	2.3 mm	12 slices (WH)	QCA ≥ 70%	0.95[b] [sMBF][a]

[a]These data refer to quantitative analysis rather than visual analysis.
[b]In these studies, temporal resolution was 2 R-R intervals.
[c]In these studies, diagnostic accuracy was calculated by receiver-operating characteristic analysis.
[d]In these studies, diagnostic accuracy was expressed as the proportion of correctly classified subjects.
3D, Three-dimensional; *BLAST*, broad linear speed-up technique; *FFR*, fractional flow reserve; *HYPR*, highly constrained back-projection reconstruction; *MPR*, myocardial perfusion reserve; *NC*, noncontiguous; *PCA*, principal component analysis; *QCA*, quantitative coronary angiography; *SENSE*, sensitivity encoding; *sMBF*, stress myocardial blood flow; *SW-CG-HYPR*, sliding-window conjugate-gradient HYPR; *TPG*, transmural perfusion gradient; *VD*, variable density; *WH*, whole-heart.

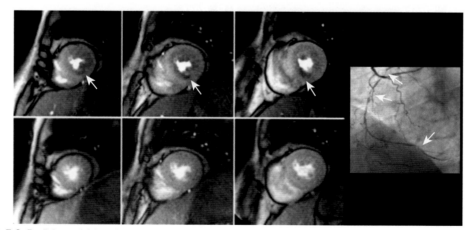

FIG. 5.9 Radial acquisition all-systolic nongated high-resolution perfusion cardiovascular magnetic resonance (CMR). Non-Cartesian perfusion CMR performed using a non–electrocardiogram (ECG) gated continuous radial sampling enables systolic imaging of all slices at 3 T at stress *(top)* and rest *(bottom)* at high-resolution (1.4 × 1.4 mm²) in a patient with a history of coronary artery disease and prior revascularization. A transmural perfusion gradient with hypoperfused subendocardium in the inferior wall is consistent with the severe disease throughout the right coronary artery by angiography *(arrows, right panel)*. Continuous radial acquisition can achieve high-resolution systolic imaging without ECG gating, which is free of dark rim artifact. (From Sharif B, Arsanjani R, Dharmakumar R, et al. All-systolic non-ECG-gated myocardial perfusion MRI: feasibility of multi-slice continuous first-pass imaging. *Magn Reson Med.* 2015;74:1661–1674.)

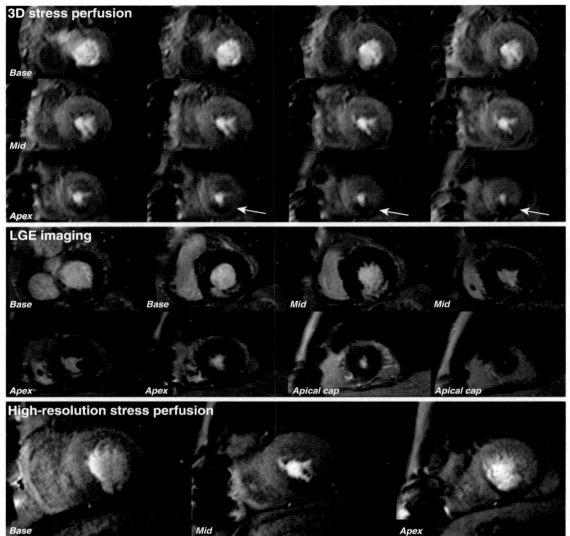

FIG. 5.12 Case example 1. A 62-year-old man with a history of prior bypass surgery presented with angina recurrence. The top panel dimensional shows three-dimensional (3D) perfusion cardiovascular magnetic resonance (CMR) at stress (2.5 mm in-plane resolution, 12 slices); the middle panel shows late-gadolinium enhancement *(LGE)* imaging (1.5 mm in-plane resolution), and the bottom panel shows high-resolution stress perfusion CMR (1.1 mm in-plane resolution, 3 slices), all performed on the same patient at 3.0 T. Both 3D perfusion and high-resolution techniques show inferior perfusion defects from base to apex. The benefit of whole-heart coverage with the 3D technique is demonstrated in this case because hypoperfusion is seen to extend beyond the scar into the apical cap *(top panel, arrows)* which is not covered by the 3-slice high-resolution technique. On the other hand, the perfusion defects and their transmural extent are better delineated with the high-resolution technique, particularly at the mid-ventricular level. By virtue of their similar in-plane spatial resolution, it is easier to correlate LGE images with high-resolution perfusion CMR on a per slice basis, compared with the 3D technique. (From Motwani M, Jogiya R, Kozerke S, et al. Advanced cardiovascular magnetic resonance myocardial perfusion imaging: high-spatial resolution versus 3-dimensional whole-heart coverage. *Clin Cardiovasc Imaging.* 2013;6:339–348.)

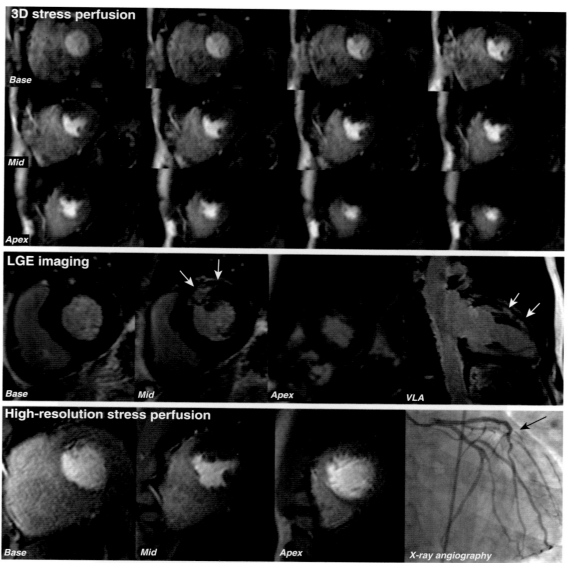

FIG. 5.13 Case example 2. A 45-year-old man with prior percutaneous coronary intervention (PCI) to the left anterior descending (LAD) presented with significant angina. The top panel shows 3D perfusion cardiovascular magnetic resonance (CMR) (12 slices) at stress; the middle panel shows late-gadolinium enhancement *(LGE)* imaging, and the bottom panel shows high-resolution (1.1 mm in-plane) stress perfusion CMR, all performed at 3.0 T. Three-dimensional (3D) perfusion CMR shows stress-induced hypoperfusion throughout the anterior wall from base to apex—that is, well beyond the area of scar seen in the mid-anterior wall on LGE imaging *(arrows)*. This example shows the benefit of whole-heart coverage with the 3D acquisition, as the 3-slice high-resolution techniques did not demonstrate any significant ischemia beyond the established scar in the mid-ventricle. Invasive coronary angiography confirmed a subtotal occlusion of a large diagonal branch, accounting for the anterior ischemia *(black arrow)*. *VLA,* Vertical long axis. (From Motwani M, Jogiya R, Kozerke S, et al. Advanced cardiovascular magnetic resonance myocardial perfusion imaging: high-spatial resolution versus 3-dimensional whole-heart coverage. *Clin Cardiovasc Imaging.* 2013;6:339–348.)

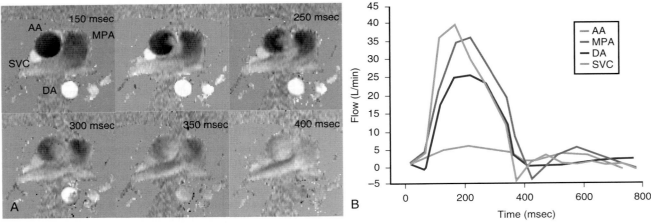

FIG. 6.3 (A) Flow velocity images of a transverse slice at the level of the right pulmonary artery showing head/foot flow velocities at six times in the cardiac cycle. (B) Plot of measured volume flow versus time for the ascending aorta *(AA)*, descending aorta *(DA)*, main pulmonary artery *(MPA)*, and superior vena cava *(SVC)*.

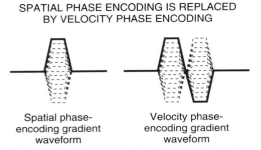

FIG. 6.4 Gradient waveforms required for spatial and velocity phase encoding.

colleagues[26] described a development of this method in which the signal from stationary tissue was saturated and the sequence was repeated much more rapidly. The issue of time precluding the use of spatial phase encoding remains a problem, although 2D RF pulses have been used successfully to locate signals within a column.[27,28] More recently, Luk Pat and associates[29] showed a method of real-time Fourier velocity imaging that used an excited column to localize the signals. In vivo aortic flow waveforms were presented with a temporal resolution of only 33 ms.

IMPROVING THE ACCURACY OF PHASE CONTRAST VELOCITY MEASUREMENTS

The vast majority of MR flow imaging applications have used the method of phase contrast velocity mapping. The accuracy of this method is highly dependent on such factors as flow pulsatility, velocity, and size and tortuosity of the vessel. One simple approach to improving the overall accuracy of the method is to adjust the velocity sensitivity of the sequence so that the velocity-related phase shift is close to 2π for the maximum expected velocity. Buonocore[30] extended this approach by varying the velocity sensitivity during the cardiac cycle, based on the knowledge that the arterial flow velocity is high in systole but low in diastole. The accuracy can be improved further by allowing a velocity-related phase

shift greater than 2π that will result in aliasing that can be corrected by use of a phase unwrapping algorithm (Fig. 6.5).[31]

Another approach to improving accuracy has been suggested by Bittoun and associates.[32] The method is a combination of phase contrast velocity mapping and Fourier velocity imaging with a small number of velocity phase-encoding steps. The final phase contrast velocity map is calculated from the best fit through the Fourier velocity encoded result. One potential problem with this method that can also affect conventional phase contrast velocity imaging occurs if there is any beat-to-beat variation in flow velocity. As a result of the high-velocity phase sensitivity used with this method, significant phase variations can occur, with resulting ghosting artifacts and loss of flow information.

Another method that was originally described to give a measure of velocity and flow quantification was phase contrast angiography. This technique again involves acquiring two image datasets with sequences having opposite phase velocity sensitivities, although in this case, the raw data are subtracted before reconstruction. This technique has the advantage of subtracting out signal from stationary tissue, which removes errors caused by partial volumes where voxels contained a mixture of flowing and stationary tissue. The method is, however, generally less accurate because the signal and hence the velocity measurement can be affected by factors such as in-flow enhancement and intravoxel dephasing (signal loss). In the mid-1990s, Polzin and colleagues[33] suggested combining this method with phase contrast velocity mapping, which they showed to be more accurate in a number of phantom studies. The methods are yet to be fully validated in vivo, however, and are likely to be affected by problems of signal loss and motion, particularly when imaging is performed on small mobile vessels, such as the coronary arteries.[34]

One of the most significant factors affecting the accuracy of the flow measurement methods is flow-related signal loss. This is normally the result of loss of phase coherence within a voxel, and eventually it results in an inability to detect the encoded phase of the flow signal above the random phase of the background noise. Even if a velocity-compensated imaging sequence is used, the acceleration and even the higher orders of motion present in complex flows can result in loss of phase coherence. Fig. 6.6 shows an example of a long-axis image of a patient with a mitral valve stenosis in which the valve is also regurgitant. In this case, a region of blood signal is lost from the ventricle during

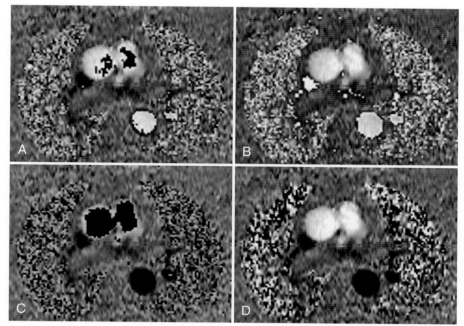

FIG. 6.5 Method of phase unwrapping. (A) Systolic image in which high velocities result in aliasing in both the positive and negative directions. (B and C) Adjustment of the velocity window to remove aliasing in the positive and negative directions, respectively. (D) The same image data after processing by the antialiasing algorithm.

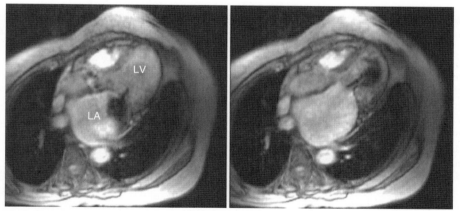

FIG. 6.6 Systolic and diastolic long-axis frames from cine datasets acquired in a patient with a stenotic and regurgitant mitral valve. Signal loss can be seen in the left atrium *(LA)* during systole and the left ventricle *(LV)* during diastole.

diastole as a result of the stenosis generating complex flows and from the atrium during systole because of a regurgitant jet of flow through the valve. Partial signal loss, however, does not greatly affect the accuracy of the phase contrast velocity mapping measurement unless it is accompanied by partial volume errors. When signal loss is the result of a spread of phase within a voxel, the mean phase will be detected, although this will be affected by differential saturation effects.[35] The phase contrast velocity mapping techniques are most susceptible to signal loss of one form or another, although this can normally be minimized by

appropriate gradient profile design. A good way to reduce signal loss is to use a symmetrical gradient waveform that nullifies phase shifts caused by all of the odd-order derivatives of position and then to shorten the sequence as much as possible to reduce the effects of the even-order derivatives.[36] Signal loss of the type described is much less of a problem with the Fourier flow imaging method. In this case, the Fourier transform is used to separate out constituent velocities.

Errors can be caused by phase differences for reasons other than the velocity encoding pulses, resulting in the phase map velocity values being offset from zero, even for stationary tissues.[37] This background phase offset generally varies gradually with position across the image, and it also varies with image plane orientation and other sequence parameters that affect the gradient waveforms, such as V_{enc}. Distortion of the requested magnetic field gradients is unavoidable because of the fundamental laws of electromagnetism, and these are known in MR imaging as *Maxwell*, or *concomitant*, gradients. These background phase shifts become more significant when high-amplitude gradients are used and also when imaging is performed at lower main magnetic field strengths. However, with the latest gradient systems, Maxwell gradient effects are certainly a factor for phase velocity mapping at 1.5 T. However, these velocity map offsets can be corrected precisely and automatically in software, with no user intervention required.[38] A second common reason for background phase shifts is the presence of small uncorrected side effects of the gradient pulses in the magnet, known as *eddy currents*. These phase shifts became more of a problem with the advent of higher-performance gradients, although more recently the problem appears to have been reduced. Software is sometimes provided that allows the user to place markers identifying stationary tissues so that this background phase error can be calculated and removed from the entire image. Sometimes, however, if the phase shifts are nonlinear or if there is little signal from stationary tissue, then the only way to correct for them is to acquire an additional set of images of a large static phantom using the same sequence parameters as those used in vivo, and then to subtract out the phase errors on a pixel-by-pixel basis.[39]

Pixels without any signal in velocity maps have a random phase or show the phase of a weak ghost that may not be visible on the magnitude image with normal brightness settings. Particularly for poststenotic jet images, it is important to check that the magnitude image pixels of the jet are not affected by signal loss. Avoiding the inclusion of noise pixels can be problematic in regions of interest around the great vessels, and ideally, the image analysis software enables the user to set the velocity to zero for pixels whose magnitude is below a user-defined threshold.

Provided that the sequence parameters are carefully chosen such that the potential errors and artifacts discussed earlier can be minimized or avoided, phase velocity mapping has been shown to be accurate and reproducible. Validation has been reported in phantoms by comparison with true measured flow and with Doppler[36,40,41] in animal models by comparison with in vivo flow meter measurements.[42] Validation has also been reported in humans by comparison with methods such as Doppler ultrasound or catheterization.[43–45] Perhaps the most convincing forms of validation were those performed initially by comparing the aortic flow with the left ventricular stroke volume and later flow in both the aorta and pulmonary artery with left and right ventricular stroke volumes in normal subjects.[22,46,47] For the latter, the four measurements should be the same except for small differences caused by coronary and bronchial flow, and it can be calculated that flow measurements in large vessels are accurate to within 6%.

The effect of breath-holding on flow measurement is another factor that could affect more recent studies. Sakuma and associates showed a significant change in both pulmonary and aortic cardiac output during a large lung volume breath-hold.[48] Conversely, flows measured during a small volume breath-hold were found to be similar to those measured during normal breathing.

There are other potential sources of error that have been reported. These include misalignment of the vessel with the direction of velocity encoding and misregistration of flow signal caused by flow between excitation and readout. Because of these and the other sources of errors discussed earlier, care is required when setting up the scan parameters, to minimize their effect.

Rapid Phase Flow Imaging Methods

With the very rapid scanning hardware available today, it is possible to repeat a phase contrast velocity sequence so fast that low-resolution images can be acquired in 100 ms or high-resolution images can be acquired in a breath-hold. The major problem is for pulsatile flow where the accuracy of the measurements and the temporal resolution can be limited if the acquisition period per cardiac cycle is too long. Also, if high spatial resolution is required, the cardiac motion of structures, such as coronary arteries, can cause blurring, with subsequent errors in flow measurement.[49] For this reason, it is likely that more efficient *k*-space coverage methods, such as interleaved spirals, will be important.

Ultra-fast flow imaging techniques have also been developed, either by combining a phase-mapping type approach with imaging methods, such as single-shot echo planar and spiral imaging,[50,51] or by imaging only one spatial dimension.[52] A compromise generally has to be made in temporal or spatial resolution and probably also in the signal-to-noise ratio. However, taking into account these constraints, the methods have generally been shown to be accurate. One complication with the echo planar sequence is flow signal loss because of its inherent phase sensitivity, even when additional flow compensation is applied. However, this has been used to advantage for more qualitative flow imaging showing flow disturbances, for example.[53]

The one-dimensional rapid acquisition mode, real-time acquisition and velocity evaluation (RACE),[52] can be used to measure flow perpendicular to the slice. The technique can be repeated rapidly throughout the cardiac cycle to give near-real-time flow information. One problem with this type of approach is that data are acquired from a projection through the patient; this means that any signal overlapping with the flow signal will combine and introduce errors to flow measurement. Several strategies have been suggested for localizing the signal to avoid this: they include spatial presaturation, projection dephasing (applying a gradient to suppress stationary tissue), and collecting a cylinder of data and multiple oblique measurements.

Yang and colleagues used a 2D RF excitation scheme to excite a narrow rectangular X-section column and used only 16 echoes to spatially resolve the other dimension in high resolution.[54] This approach allowed real-time flow measurements to be acquired. The authors used the method to show the effect of controlled breathing on flow in the ascending aorta and superior vena cava (Fig. 6.7).

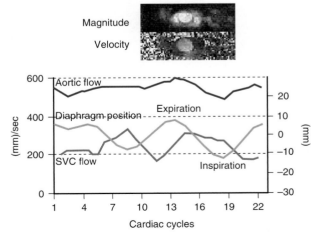

FIG. 6.7 Real-time magnitude and flow images from the excited region containing the aorta and the superior vena cava *(SVC)*. The plot shows the variation in flow during a period of respiratory maneuver.

Visualizing Flow and Flow Parameters

The method used to visualize MR flow data has depended on the method used for acquisition. For Fourier velocity measurement, each voxel may contain a range of measured velocities, and the Fourier velocity image normally takes the form of a plot of velocity versus time or velocity versus position in one direction. Fig. 6.8 shows an example in which velocity images were acquired from a column of excited tissue, including the descending aorta.[55] The front edge of the aortic pulse wave can be seen on successive frames as it travels down the vessel.

Phase contrast velocity images contain only one velocity measure per image voxel. Historically, these have been shown with a gray scale such that flow in one direction tends toward white, flow in the other direction tends toward black, and stationary material is mid-gray, as shown previously in Fig. 6.3A. When flow is measured in more than one direction, more sophisticated methods of display can be used. Fig. 6.9 shows a vector map of flow in the root of the aorta of a patient with an atherosclerotic aneurysm. This systolic image, shown alongside a pressure map (described later), shows high-velocity flow impinging on the wall of the aneurysm. An alternative type of representation would be to use the cine velocity images to calculate the path of a seed over time.[56]

The ability to study flow in such detail and at any site in the body is unique to MR imaging. For this reason, a large amount of interest is being generated from those who wish to understand the physiology of blood flow and its interaction with blood vessels and the cardiac chambers. Despite the relatively poor spatial resolution, a number of groups have studied methods of extracting a measure of the wall shear stress from the MR images. Both Oshinski and colleagues and Oyre and associates developed fitting methods to derive the velocity profile at subpixel distances from the vessel wall.[57,58] Both groups presented expected values of stress, although it is difficult to suggest a method of validating the accuracy of these measurements. Frayne and Rutt suggested an alternative approach that potentially gave more information about the flow within a voxel that straddled the vessel wall.[59] Their method used Fourier velocity encoding to distinguish the distribution of flow velocities, so that only the spatial location had to be considered.

There has also been considerable interest in the possibility of deriving pressure measurements from MR images. Urchuk and coworkers considered vessel compliance and the flow pulse wave to calculate the pressure waveform and showed a good correlation with catheter pressure measurements made in a pig model.[60] In contrast, Yang and colleagues derived flow pressure maps from the cine phase contrast velocity maps using the Navier-Stokes equations.[61] Fig. 6.10 shows an example of the changing flow pressure around the aortic arch during the first half of the cardiac cycle. Fig. 6.11 shows an interesting example of a flow pressure map, showing the descending aorta in a patient who underwent polyester fiber (Dacron, Dupont, Wilmington, DE) graft repair of aortic coarctation. In contrast to the rest of the aorta, no pressure gradient can be seen in the repaired region, possibly because of the reduced compliance.

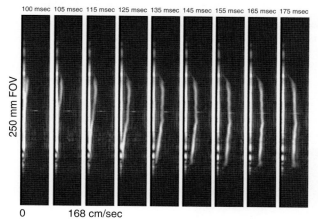

ECG Gate Delay

100 msec 105 msec 115 msec 125 msec 135 msec 145 msec 155 msec 165 msec 175 msec

250 mm FOV

0   168 cm/sec

FIG. 6.8 Series of nine Fourier velocity images at 10-ms intervals showing the velocity pulse wave propagating down the descending aorta. *ECG,* Electrocardiogram; *FOV,* field of view.

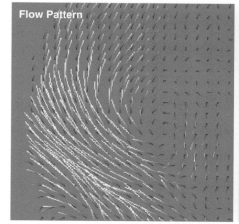
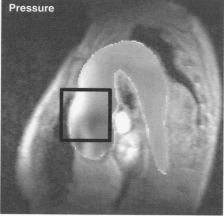

Flow Pattern

Pressure

FIG. 6.9 Flow vector map showing the systolic flow pattern in the aortic root of a patient with an atherosclerotic aneurysm. The associated image shows the corresponding pressure distribution.

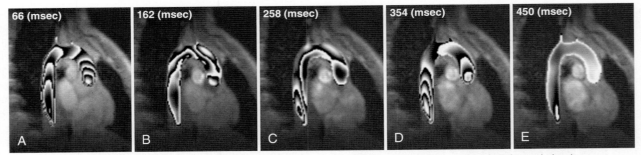

FIG. 6.10 Selected frames from a cine series of calculated flow pressure maps showing the variation in pressure at different times in the cardiac cycle (A to E). Each gray-scale band from white to black represents a pressure gradient of 1 mm Hg. A positive pressure gradient during systole (A) reverses during the deceleration phase of diastole (D).

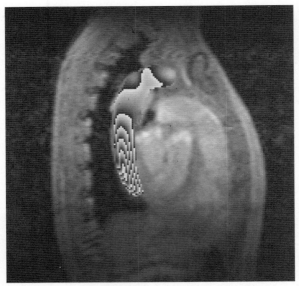

FIG. 6.11 Systolic pressure map of the aortic arch in patient with a polyester fiber (Dacron, Dupont, Wilmington, DE) repair. No pressure gradient is seen in the region of the repair.

Pathlines emitted from the mitral valve at approx. time of peak A-wave (left panel) and traced to early systole (right panel)

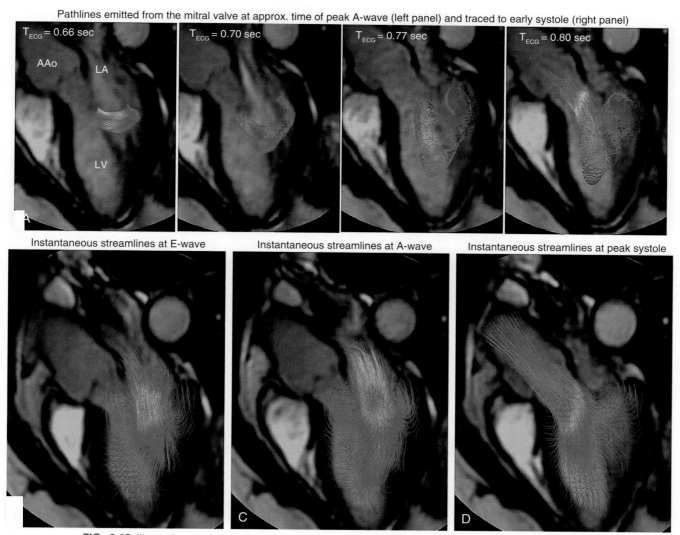

FIG. 6.12 Illustrative examples of four-dimensional flow cardiovascular magnetic resonance visualization techniques in the normal heart. In these examples, flow visualization is overlaid onto a two-dimensional bSSFP acquisition in a three-chamber view. Pathlines, the trajectories that massless fluid particles would follow, allow the study of the path of pulsatile blood flow over time. (A) The transit of blood through the left ventricle *(LV)* is shown by pathlines emitted from the mitral valve at the timepoint of the peak of the A-wave and traced to the time point of early systole. *AAo,* Ascending aorta; *LA,* left atrium. (B–D) Streamlines generated in a long-axis plane show parts of the intracardiac velocity field at the timepoints of peak early filling *(E-wave)*, peak late filling *(A-wave)*, and peak systole.[86] (From Dyverfeldt P, Bissell M, Barker AJ, et al. 4D flow cardiovascular magnetic resonance consensus statement. *J Cardiovasc Magn Reson.* 2015;17:72.)

Four-Dimensional Phase Contrast Flow Velocity Mapping

To fully understand, visualize, and measure flow parameters in blood vessels, a method of acquisition is required that measures velocity in three dimensions and three directions over time, with high spatial and temporal resolution. This has presented a significant problem in terms of acquisition and data handling, but methods have been developed and are now used routinely in clinical research applications. Following early implementation by Firmin et al.[62] in 1993 and then improvements by Wigstrom et al. in 1996,[63] particularly more recently, there has been considerable work to speed up the acquisition by a variety of acceleration techniques.[64,65]

Although the clinical importance of the four-dimensional (4D) approach is still not entirely clear, a number of studies have shown that similar quantitative measures of volume flow are made when compared with 2D.[66–74] 4D flow measurements share the same problems as 2D with regard to background phase errors;[75,76] however, there are a number of advantages with regard to volume flow measurement. One important advantage is that several volume flow measures from the same or different vessels can be made from the same acquisition dataset, and this enables the employment of the principle of conservation of mass to check the internal consistency of the data.[67,73,77–85] Another advantage is that analysis planes can be retrospectively placed and located at will during the time of analyzing the flow data and this can be particularly

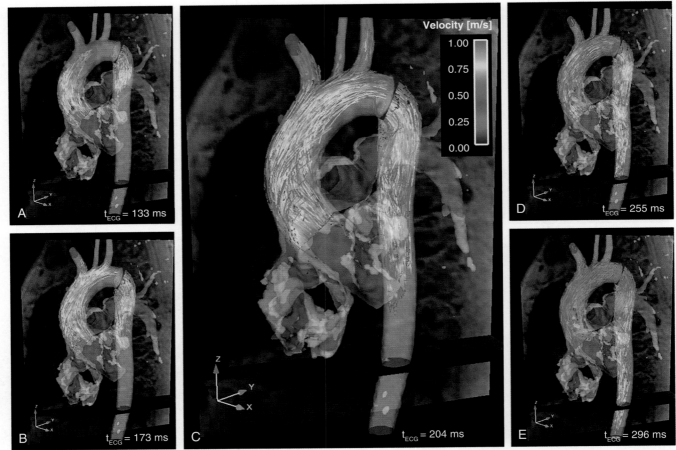

FIG. 6.13 (A–E) Visualization of multidirectional flow structures in a normal thoracic aorta illustrating the temporal evolution of blood flow at five different time points in systole. Pathlines were repetitively emitted at successive instants and originate from two emitter planes, one in the ascending aorta and one in the proximal descending aorta. Color coding reflects the local absolute velocity.[90] (From Markl M, Kilner PJ, Ebbers T. Comprehensive 4D velocity mapping of the heart and great vessels by cardiovascular magnetic resonance. *J Cardiovasc Magn Reson.* 2011;13:7.)

advantageous when a large number of flow planes are required.[71] Unlike with 2D flow measurement, where great care and expertise can be required during the scan for the placement of the flow imaging planes, the three-dimensional volume of the 4D dataset can be more simply positioned. An additional potential advantage is that with the improved coverage available through the third spatial dimension, the chances of capturing the peak velocity through a valve jet should be increased.[72] However, contradictory studies have shown lower velocities measured by the 4D approach,[70] a finding that might be explained by the relatively low temporal resolution (50–55 ms).[86]

The most striking feature of 4D flow imaging is in its use to intuitively visualize multidirectional flow structures and how these are affected by different cardiovascular diseases.[56,87–90] Studies have reported applications in the heart chambers and connecting valves[3,79,91–106] (Fig. 6.12), the great vessels[77,106–124] (Fig. 6.13), carotid and intracranial arteries and veins,[125–136] hepatic arterial and portal venous systems of the liver,[82,122,137–139] renal arteries,[140,141] and peripheral arteries.[142] Additionally, in complex congenital heart disease there are also promising applications.[74,122,143,144]

REFERENCES

A full reference list is available online at ExpertConsult.com

7

Use of Navigator Echoes in Cardiovascular Magnetic Resonance and Factors Affecting Their Implementation

David Firmin and Jennifer Keegan

Respiration has been shown to be an important factor influencing the quality of cardiovascular magnetic resonance (CMR) images. In addition to cardiac motion, which can be addressed reasonably well by electrocardiographic (ECG) triggering, respiratory motion moves the position and distorts the shape of the heart by several millimeters between inspiration and expiration. In 1991, Atkinson and Edelman[1] showed the detrimental effects of breathing on the quality of cardiac studies by showing improved detail (fast low angle shot) in breath-hold segmented fast gradient echo images compared with conventional non–breath-hold images. Although breath-holding produces images that are free of respiratory motion artifact, it is not without problems. The breath-hold position may vary from one breath-hold scan to the next, giving rise to misregistration effects, and it may also vary during the breath-hold period itself,[2] resulting in image blurring and artifacts. In addition, the scan parameters are limited by the need to perform imaging within the duration of a comfortable breath-hold period, and for a number of patients, this period may be very short.

An alternative to breath-holding is to monitor respiratory motion throughout the data acquisition period and to correct the data for that motion, either in real time or through postprocessing, with the efficacy of both techniques being strongly dependent on the accuracy of the method of motion assessment. During normal tidal respiration, the superior-inferior (SI) motion of the diaphragm is approximately four to five times the anterior-posterior motion of the chest wall,[3] and consequently, diaphragm motion is the most sensitive measure of respiratory motion. In 1989, Ehman and Felmlee[4] were the first to introduce navigator echoes for measuring the displacement of a moving structure and to demonstrate their use in determining diaphragm motion during respiration. The navigator echo is the signal from a column of material oriented perpendicular to the direction of the motion to be monitored. On Fourier transformation, this signal results in a well-defined edge of the moving structure. The navigator echoes may be interleaved with the imaging sequence and, consequently, enable the motion to be determined throughout the data acquisition period.

In CMR, there have been a number of developments in the use of navigator measurement to reduce the problems of respiratory motion. This chapter discusses these developments, considers the various choices that have been studied in the implementation of navigators, and discusses their importance. There are many variables in the application and use of navigator echoes, and although there have been some attempts to study these, it is unlikely that we are close to optimizing their application.

USE OF NAVIGATOR INFORMATION

There are two distinct ways of using navigator echoes to reduce the problems of respiratory motion in CMR, which are multiple breath-holding with feedback and free-breathing methods. The first of these uses the navigator information to provide visual feedback on the diaphragm position to subjects to allow them to hold their breath at the same point repeatedly.[5] The second uses the navigator echo measurement as an input to some form of respiratory gating algorithm while the patient breathes normally. Fig. 7.1 shows actual respiratory trace data in a subject when performing multiple breath-holds and when free breathing. In both cases, a navigator acceptance window, typically 5-mm wide, is defined, and all data acquired when the navigator is outside of this window are ignored. The resulting image therefore consists of data acquired over a narrow range of respiratory positions. The respiratory or scan efficiency is defined as the percentage of ECG triggers that fall within the navigator acceptance window and is a measure of the data rejection rate, which in turn determines the overall scan duration. As the navigator acceptance window is reduced, the rejection rate increases and the scan efficiency decreases. Fig. 7.2 shows the residual diaphragm displacements that occurred during data acquisitions performed during conventional breath-holding, breath-holding with navigator feedback, and navigator free-breathing in normal subjects.[6] Both navigator techniques result in images acquired over a reduced range of diaphragm displacement compared with those acquired using repeated conventional breath-holding. In addition, they allow a longer overall scan time. This allows for averaging of data to improve the signal-to-noise ratio, increasing the k-space coverage for improved spatial resolution, and increasing the temporal resolution by reducing the number of individual image views acquired per cardiac cycle.

Multiple Breath-Hold Methods

Wang and colleagues[7] were the first to show the use of a respiratory feedback monitor to reduce misregistration artifacts in consecutive breath-hold segmented fast gradient echo coronary artery images and to show improved image quality from averaging scans acquired over multiple breath-holds. When used in informed healthy volunteers, this technique has been shown to produce good results with reasonable scan efficiency.[8] However, a period of training is required, and the process can be problematic, particularly with patients who have difficulty holding their breath because of a combination of illness and anxiety.[6] Although it might be expected that breath-holding with respiratory feedback would enable the completion of a cardiac study much more quickly

selection that enables the highly efficient acquisition of high-quality coronary artery images without the need for a predefined acceptance window.[18] 3D motion-adapted gating[19] is a similar technique that yields images comparable with standard prospective navigator gating, with significantly improved scan efficiency.[20] A further development of these ideas, termed continuously adaptive windowing strategy (CLAWS), was described by Jhooti et al. in 2010.[21] This novel and dynamic acquisition strategy ensured all potential navigator acceptance windows are possible and acquires an image with the highest possible efficiency regardless of variations in the respiratory pattern. Unnecessary prolongation of scan durations due to respiratory drift or navigator acceptance window adjustments are avoided. Because CLAWS requires no setting of the acceptance window, nor monitoring of the navigator traces during the scan, operator dependence is minimized and ease of use improved. This method has been applied by Keegan et al.[22] to improve the respiratory efficiency of 3D late gadolinium enhancement imaging and by Jhooti et al.,[23] who combined it with biofeedback to increase the navigator efficiency for imaging the thoracic aorta.

NAVIGATOR ECHO IMPLEMENTATION

Method of Column Selection

Two methods have been used for the generation of a navigator echo.

With the spin echo technique, a spin echo signal is generated from the column of material formed by the intersection of two planes, one excited by a 90-degree radiofrequency (RF) pulse and the other by a 180-degree RF pulse. The column cross section may be either rectangular or rhombic, depending on the orientation of the two planes. This approach is very robust and produces an extremely well-defined column. However, it cannot be repeated rapidly, and care must be taken to ensure that the column selection planes do not impinge on the region of interest.

The alternative approach is to use a selective two-dimensional (2D) RF pulse to excite a column of approximately circular cross section.[24] Although this technique is much more sensitive to factors such as shimming errors, which can potentially cause blurring and distortion of the column, with a reduced flip angle, it can be repeated more rapidly and the navigator artifact is less extensive.

Both methods are used routinely for research studies on coronary imaging, without any reported problems.

Correction Factors

In CMR, navigator echoes are most frequently used to measure the position of the diaphragm. However, the motion of the heart is not straightforward, and only the inferior border that sits on the diaphragm will move to the same extent, whereas superiorly, the relative motion will be reduced. This was first studied by Wang and associates,[3] who measured the displacement of the right coronary artery root, the origin of the left anterior descending artery, and the superior and inferior margins of the heart relative to the diaphragm in 10 healthy subjects. For the right coronary artery origin, the mean (± standard deviation) relative displacement (or correction factor [CF]) was 0.57 (± 0.26). McConnell and coworkers[25] first used this CF to track the position of the imaging slice during breath-holding and showed improved image registration relative to untracked acquisitions. In free-breathing studies, the CF was first applied by Danias and colleagues,[26] who showed that tracked image quality was maintained as the navigator acceptance window increased from 3 mm to 7 mm, whereas in untracked images, it decreased significantly. This technique, called *real-time prospective slice following,* or *slice tracking,* is now used routinely for both 2D and 3D methods of acquisition. Of note, however, is the relatively high standard deviation of the CF discussed earlier, which reflects considerable intersubject

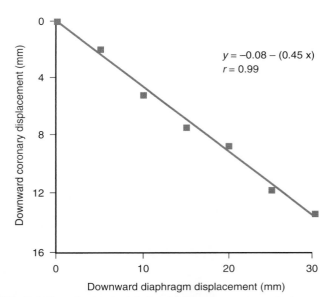

FIG. 7.4 Plot of superior-inferior right coronary artery displacement against superior-inferior diaphragm displacement for a single subject. The gradient of the linear regression line is the subject-specific correction factor. (From Taylor AM, Keegan J, Jhooti P, Firmin DN, Pennell DJ. Calculation of a subject-specific adaptive motion-correction factor for improved real-time navigator echo-gated magnetic resonance coronary angiography. *J Cardiovasc Magn Reson.* 1999;1:131–138.)

variation in the degree of cardiac motion with respiration. This was also observed by Danias and coworkers, who used real-time 2D echo planar imaging to study the SI motion of the heart as a function of navigator position.[27] The accuracy of slice-following techniques will obviously depend on the accuracy of the CF implemented. In 1997, Taylor and colleagues[28] showed how a subject-specific factor could be measured rapidly with end-inspiratory and end-expiratory breath-hold scans before the coronary imaging protocol. Fig. 7.4 shows the relationship between the motion of the right hemidiaphragm and the coronary ostia measured in one subject, with the slope of the graph giving the CF. Fig. 7.5 shows two examples of subjects with very different CFs, showing how a wider acceptance window can be used, thus improving scan efficiency. The need for a subject-specific CF has further been confirmed in 3D coronary angiography, where its use was found to yield optimal image quality.[29] In 2002, Keegan and associates further developed this area of work by studying the variability of CFs in the SI, anterior-posterior, and right-left directions for both breath-holding and free-breathing.[30] The study concluded that subject variability in CFs, together with within-subject differences between breath-holding and free-breathing, is such that slice following should be performed with subject-specific factors determined from free-breathing acquisitions.

An additional or alternative approach to the real-time slice following described earlier is to use a postprocessing adaptive motion correction technique[4] to correct an image retrospectively for movement occurring during data acquisition. This technique, which can be used to correct a 2D acquisition for in-plane displacement or a 3D acquisition for in-plane and through-plane displacement, may not appear to be an attractive option initially, but it has the advantages of allowing the CF to be optimized for each individual patient and provides an alternative approach to those centers with scanners that do not have a real-time decision-making capability. This approach has been implemented with

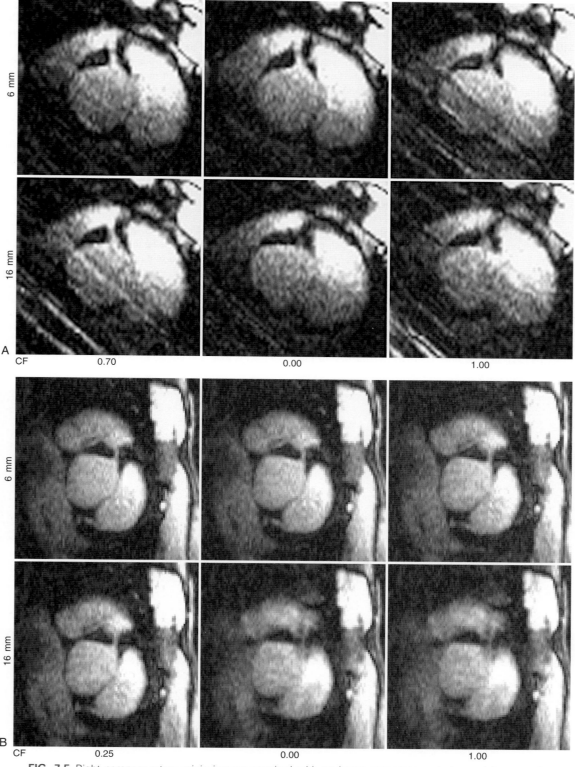

FIG. 7.5 Right coronary artery origin images acquired with navigator acceptance windows of 6 mm and 16 mm in subjects with subject-specific correction factors *(CF)* of 0.7 (A) and 0.25 (B). For both subjects, images were also acquired with CFs of 0 and 1. In the absence of slice following (CF = 0), image quality is reduced as the navigator acceptance window increases from 6 mm to 16 mm. When slice following with a subject-specific CF is used, however, image quality is maintained. (From Taylor AM, Keegan J, Jhooti P, Firmin DN, Pennell DJ. Calculation of a subject-specific adaptive motion-correction factor for improved real-time navigator echo-gated magnetic resonance coronary angiography. *J Cardiovasc Magn Reson*. 1999;1:131–138.)

both segmented gradient echo[31] and interleaved spiral[32] coronary artery acquisitions, with promising results.

Column Positioning

The degree of diaphragm motion detected by the navigator echo is dependent on the positioning of the navigator column. The dome of the right hemidiaphragm is higher than that of the left, and the two move coherently with respiration, but to differing degrees.[33] Motion of the diaphragm is also greater posteriorly than anteriorly (anterior and dome excursions are 56% and 79%, respectively, of posterior excursions), and at the level of the dome, it is greater laterally than medially.[34] The CF implemented in real-time slice following or postprocessing adaptive motion correction, as described earlier, is strongly dependent on the positioning of the navigator column and further supports the use of a subject-specific factor, as described in the previous section.

McConnell and colleagues[35] studied the effects of varying the navigator location on the image quality of coronary artery studies. Navigators were positioned through the dome of the right hemidiaphragm, through the posterior portion of the left hemidiaphragm, through the anterior and posterior left ventricular walls, and through the anterior left ventricular wall, as shown in Fig. 7.6. The advantage of the latter navigator position is that it would eliminate the need for a CF, as described in the previous section, relating the navigator-echo-measured displacement to the coronary artery motion. The results are summarized in Table 7.2 and show no significant differences in the image quality scores obtained with varying navigator location. There was a tendency for the anterior left ventricular wall navigator scans to be longer in duration, but the difference did not reach statistical significance. One of the problems with monitoring the heart itself is the complex anatomy, making it more difficult to find a suitable position for the navigator column. More sophisticated methods of positioning the column may further improve this method of monitoring cardiac motion.

MULTIPLE COLUMN ORIENTATIONS

There is a linear relationship between the SI and anterior-posterior motions of the heart, with the SI motion being approximately five times that of the anterior-posterior motion.[3] For this reason, the real-time slice-following methods first used by McConnell and colleagues[25] and by Danias and associates[26] included a correction for anterior-posterior motion of the heart, assuming it to be equal to 20% of the SI motion. Unfortunately, there is not always such a strong relationship between the directions of motion of the heart with respiration. Sachs and colleagues showed this by using three navigators to measure the SI, anterior-posterior, and right-left motions of the heart.[36] Fig. 7.7 shows an example from this study illustrating the scatter of SI, right-left, and anterior-posterior measurements, made over a period of approximately 10 minutes. The group went on to compare the use of one, two, and three navigators for imaging the right coronary artery and showed an improvement when multiple directions of motion were considered. This improvement in image quality, however, must be offset against the main disadvantage, which is that scan efficiency is reduced, potentially introducing more

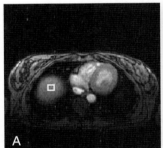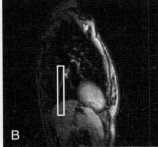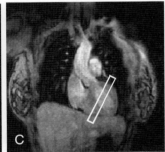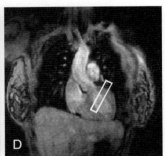

FIG. 7.6 Navigator column locations positioned on transverse, coronal, and sagittal pilot images: (A) through the dome of the right hemidiaphragm, (B) through the posterior left hemidiaphragm, (C) through both anterior and posterior left ventricular walls, and (D) through the anterior left ventricular wall.

TABLE 7.2   Image Quality Scores, Registration Errors, and Total Scan Times[a]

Parameter	Right Diaphragm Navigator	Left Diaphragm Navigator	LV Navigator	Anterior LV Wall Navigator
Image quality score (0–4)	2.3 ± 0.1	2.3 ± 0.1	2.4 ± 0.1	2.2 ± 0.2
Registration error (mm):				
Craniocaudal	0.5 ± 0.1	0.4 ± 0.1	0.6 ± 0.1	0.4 ± 0.1
Anteroposterior	0.3 ± 0.1	0.3 ± 0.1	0.3 ± 0.1	0.4 ± 0.1
Total scan time[b] (s)	294 ± 28	314 ± 30	342 ± 62	427 ± 111

[a]Image quality scores (0 = very poor, 4 = excellent), registration errors, and total scan times for different navigator column positions during free-breathing magnetic resonance coronary angiography. There were no significant differences between the navigator column locations. Data are presented as mean ± standard error of the mean.
[b]Total scan time is the time from start to finish for six scans.
LV, Left ventricle.
Modified from McConnell MV, Khasgiwala VC, Savord BJ, et al. Comparison of respiratory suppression methods and navigator locations for MR coronary angiography. *Am J Roentgenol.* 1997;168:1369.

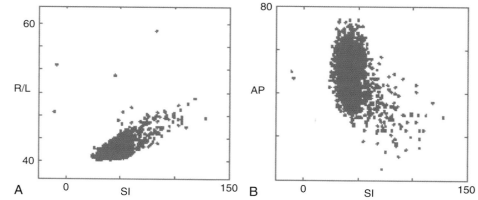

FIG. 7.7 Anteroposterior *(AP)* (A) and right-left *(R/L)* (B) navigator echo measurements as a function of superior-inferior *(SI)* navigator echo measurements in a healthy subject. (Data from Todd Sachs, Stanford University.)

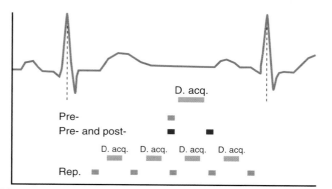

FIG. 7.8 Timing of the navigators for pre-, pre- and post-, and repeated *(Rep.)* navigator echo-controlled data acquisition *(D. acq.)*.

problems associated with long-term drift in the breathing pattern. A more recent study by Jahnke and coworkers used a new cross-correlation-based approach and showed the potential advantage of combining three orthogonal navigators.[37]

Navigator Timing

Navigator timing is one of the more important parameters; however, flexibility to alter this is often limited by the computing architecture of the scanner being used (discussed later). Fig. 7.8 shows the three main alternatives: (1) prenavigators, (2) prenavigators and postnavigators, and (3) navigators repeated regularly throughout the cardiac cycle. A simple prenavigator provides the highest scan efficiency when a navigator acceptance window is used, but may not be reliable if there is a sudden change in breathing between the navigator measurement and image data acquisition. Prenavigators and postnavigators overcome this problem, but of course, they also reduce scan efficiency. In our experience, the use of prenavigators only produces acceptable results for free-breathing studies, whereas multiple breath-hold acquisitions certainly require both prenavigators and postnavigators. An important factor that depends on the computer hardware and architecture is the time required after the navigator acquisition before the start of the imaging sequence. Particularly, if prenavigators only are being used, the longer this interval, the greater the potential for errors caused by respiratory motion. Also, for ECG R-wave-triggered scans, this may also have implications for the minimum gating delay that can be obtained and for

short gating delay or cine scans, post-only navigators can be used as an alternative. This approach was recently implemented in left ventricular function studies, where it was found that image quality in a group of patients with heart failure was significantly improved over conventional breath-hold scans.[38]

Repeated navigators allow for improved cine or multislice imaging and also provide some potential for estimating internavigator respiratory motion. The potential problem with this is that the navigator signal-to-noise ratio could be reduced and this may affect the accuracy of navigator edge detection. In addition, as the time for navigator output increases, the time for imaging decreases and the number of phases or slices that can be acquired is reduced.

Precision of Navigator Measurement

Commonly, a spatial resolution of 1 mm is used along the navigator echo column, for example, having a field of view of 512 mm and sampling 512 points on the navigator readout. However, the precision of the measurement is dependent to a large extent on the signal-to-noise ratio of the navigator measurement. The most important factor affecting the signal-to-noise ratio is the coil arrangement. If, for example, a single coil is used for imaging and navigator detection, it must be large enough to cover both the imaging area of interest and the region of navigator detection. On the other hand, if phased array coils are used, it is possible to position one coil specifically for navigator detection, possibly over the region of the right diaphragm. Another important factor in the precision of the measurement is the quality of the edge on the navigator trace. To obtain a well-defined edge of the diaphragm, for example, have a reasonably small column cross section and position it through the dome of the diaphragm, so that the column is perpendicular to the diaphragm edge, rather than more posteriorly, where motion is greatest. Finally, the diaphragm edge may be detected by edge detection, correlation, or least-squares fit algorithms. For rapid tracking (repetition time <100 ms) or narrower columns, the signal-to-noise ratio in the diaphragm trace could be too poor for simple edge detection methods to succeed. Of the remaining two techniques, the least-squares fit method has been shown to be more resistant to the effects of noise and to the diaphragm profile deformation that occurs during respiration than the correlation method and therefore would be the technique of choice.[39] However, most navigator techniques acquire only one or two navigators per cardiac cycle, and in such cases, the signal-to-noise ratios are usually relatively high and edge detection algorithms are generally adequate.

8

Cardiovascular Magnetic Resonance Assessment of Myocardial Oxygenation

Rohan Dharmakumar, Sotirios A. Tsaftaris, Hsin-Jung Yang, and Debiao Li

MYOCARDIAL OXYGENATION: SUPPLY VERSUS DEMAND

Under physiologic conditions, myocardial blood flow (MBF), myocardial oxygen consumption (MVO_2), and myocardial mechanics are intimately related. Therefore it is not surprising that the key disease processes involving the heart manifest from imbalances between myocardial oxygen supply and demand. Consequently, the noninvasive assessment of imbalances in myocardial oxygen supply and demand, particularly on a regional basis, is of critical importance in both clinical cardiology and for cardiovascular research. The noninvasive quantification of MVO_2 was not possible until it was shown that positron emission tomography (PET), using ^{11}C-acetate, permits accurate quantification of MVO_2.[1-4] Using this approach, numerous studies have demonstrated the salutary effects of restoring nutritive perfusion on MVO_2 and cardiac function and the importance of preserving MVO_2 as a descriptor and probable determinant of myocardial viability in both acute and chronic ischemic disease.[5-8] However, PET studies are limited by relatively poor spatial resolution, limited availability mainly due to short-life radiotracers, and potentially harmful ionizing radiation, especially when repeated examinations are needed.

Magnetic resonance imaging (MRI) has become an important clinical imaging modality because it is noninvasive, does not require iodinated contrast media or ionizing radiation, and is widely available. MRI can also provide structural and functional information as well as report on several important biomarkers in the same setting. To date, multiple cardiovascular magnetic resonance (CMR) applications have been developed, including anatomic imaging of the heart and great vessels, coronary artery imaging, methods to characterize myocardial infarction with or without gadolinium (Gd) contrast media, methods for characterizing extracellular space, methods for evaluating myocardial wall motion, and first-pass perfusion (FPP) for the identification of perfusion defects in the myocardium. Over the past two decades, efforts have also been made to use CMR to determine regional myocardial blood oxygenation levels.[9-30] The blood oxygenation state of the myocardium reflects the combined effects of MBF and oxygen extraction (which together reflect MVO_2). Thus a change in myocardial blood oxygenation secondary to imbalances in oxygen supply and demand would be useful in evaluating disease processes such as coronary artery disease (CAD) or microvascular disease (MVD), which can lead to impaired myocardial perfusion reserve. Noninvasive assessment of myocardial venous blood oxygenation may permit the measurement of oxygen extraction. When coupled with flow, these data would allow for measurement of MVO_2. Anatomic, functional, and metabolic information can then be obtained in a single CMR study, thereby providing a comprehensive examination for the diagnosis of ischemic heart disease and the evaluation of therapies for improving the balance between MBF and oxygen demand.

If we assume that the blood oxygen saturation of hemoglobin in the arterial blood is 100% and is Y in the venous pool, then the MVO_2 can be estimated to first order by Fick's law as

$$MVO_2 = F \times Hct \times (1-Y)$$

where F (in mL/g/min) is the blood flow to the myocardium and Hct (in percent) is the hematocrit of the blood.[31] Hence if F, Y, and Hct are known, it is possible to estimate MVO_2.

Furthermore knowledge of myocardial venous blood oxygenation can permit noninvasive evaluation of myocardial perfusion reserve, defined as the ratio between the peak myocardial perfusion rate at maximum vasodilation and rest.[32] Under pharmacologic vasodilation, such as that in response to dipyridamole or adenosine, normal coronary blood flow increases several fold, whereas the oxygen consumption remains relatively unaltered, leading to an increase in myocardial venous blood oxygen saturation. However, with progressive coronary lumen narrowing or with microvascular dysfunction, the maximal increase in MBF under vasodilatory stress is blunted proportionately relative to the healthy myocardium. This is illustrated in the case of CAD in Fig. 8.1. Such perfusion abnormalities lead to regional differences in myocardial venous blood oxygenation, allowing for the assessment of the functional significance of CAD. Extensive clinical support now exists for imaging myocardial perfusion research with CMR using Gd-based contrast agents (GBCAs).[33-36] However, it is contraindicated in severe chronic kidney disease (CKD, stage 4 or 5). According to the National Institutes of Health (NIH) and the United States Renal Data System (USRDS), the prevalence and the cost of treating new cases of CKD has more than doubled in the past 10 years and this trend is predicted to grow given the increasing prevalence of diabetes and its contribution to the development of CKD.[37] Moreover, recent imaging/autopsy studies from Italy,[38] the United States,[39] and Japan[40] have shown that even in patients with normal kidney function, there are retained Gd deposits in the brain—a finding that is contrary to the widely held belief that Gd is fully cleared from the body within hours of infusion.[41] These observations are central to the growing interest and emphasis on non–Gd-based approaches for studying myocardial perfusion, particularly based on changes in blood oxygenation, in all subjects suspected of having ischemic heart disease.

In this chapter, we provide an overview of the basic biophysical concepts that allow for the assessment of myocardial changes in blood oxygenation. We then summarize the preclinical and clinical literature to date in the assessment of myocardial oxygenation. This is followed by growing literature on image-processing methods that have the capacity

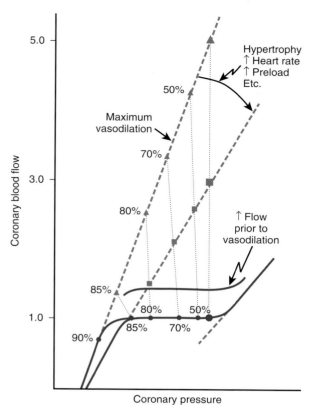

FIG. 8.1 A schematic showing the relationship between the coronary flow and coronary arterial pressure. The solid curve represents the normal relationship. At a constant level of myocardial metabolic demand, coronary artery flow is maintained constant over a wide range of coronary artery pressures, between the bounds of maximum coronary vasodilation and constriction (dashed curves). The solid circle represents the normal operating point under basal conditions; the solid triangle is the flow observed at the same pressure during maximum vasodilation. Myocardial flow reserve is the ratio of flow during vasodilation to that measured before vasodilation. Note that the flow reserve decreases in a nonlinear manner with reduction of coronary pressure (or coronary artery stenosis). Also note that hypertrophy, increased heart rate, and increased preload all decrease the coronary flow reserve. (Modified from Klocke FJ. Measurements of coronary flow reserve: defining pathophysiology versus making decisions about patient care. *Circulation*. 1987;76:1183–1189.)

to enable accurate visualization and quantification of blood-oxygen-level-dependent (BOLD) signal changes in the myocardium. Finally, we review the emerging methods that show promising evidence into how BOLD CMR can become a reliable tool for examining ischemic heart disease in the clinical arena and conclude with a brief outlook on the future of myocardial BOLD CMR.

BIOPHYSICS OF MYOCARDIAL BOLD CONTRAST

Blood is a magnetically inhomogeneous medium in which the magnetic susceptibility of red blood cells is strongly dependent on the blood oxygen saturation ($\%O_2$), defined as the percentage of hemoglobin that is oxygenated.[42,43] Because the susceptibility of blood plasma is generally invariant, the cooperative binding of oxygen to the heme molecules within the red blood cells results in a detectable susceptibility difference between plasma and the red blood cells. This susceptibility variation gives rise to local magnetic field inhomogeneities, resulting in local frequency variations that lead changes in T2* and apparent T2 of whole

blood.[44,45] This observation has allowed for the acquisition of oxygen-sensitive images permitting the discrimination between arteries and veins.[46] Its utility for detecting chronic mesenteric ischemia[47] and the identification and quantification of cardiac shunts associated with congenital abnormalities have also been demonstrated.[48]

An extension of this phenomenon into the microcirculation opened the door for assessing myocardial oxygenation changes. In the myocardium, nearly 90% of the blood volume is within the capillaries[49]; accordingly, our discussions will be limited to capillary beds. A change in blood oxygenation in the capillary bed leads to changes in magnetic field variations between the red blood cells and plasma and between the intravascular and extravascular spaces. Following the excitation of the magnetization onto the transverse plane, these field variations cause the spins to lose coherence, leading to a decay of the magnetic resonance (MR) signal.[50–55] In particular, the severity of the field variation due to changes in blood oxygen saturation directly determines the rate of loss of the spin coherence (MR signal). This phenomenon, referred to as the BOLD effect, implies that when the capillaries contain deoxygenated blood, with all else remaining the same, the MR signal associated with the deoxygenated state (rest) will be lower than that of the hyperemic state (vasodilation) when the capillary oxygenation is substantially higher (~30% [resting] vs. ~80% [hyperemic]). This allows for detecting regional myocardial oxygen differences as regions of signal loss with imaging sequences sensitive to local field inhomogeneities.[9] In addition, the sensitivity of the MR signal to the BOLD effect is dependent on the blood volume, hematocrit, and choice of pulse sequences used.[50–55] Both gradient and spin echo sequences as well as balanced steady-state free precession (bSSFP) methods have been used to probe these effects.[50,55]

BOLD effect was first demonstrated in the brain,[56–59] before being adopted for cardiac applications.[9–15] However, there are important biophysical differences between BOLD CMR of the heart and brain. Specifically, the heart has a larger blood volume fraction than the brain (~10% vs. ~4%) and the venous blood oxygen saturation in the heart is approximately 30%, compared with approximately 60% in the brain.[9] This allows for a wider range of signal change with vasodilator-induced flow in the myocardium compared with the brain, which provides greater BOLD sensitivity in the heart. However, in contrast to brain imaging, the challenge for myocardial BOLD CMR has been imaging artifacts from motion (cardiac, respiratory, and pulsatile blood flow), as well as bulk susceptibility shifts between heart and lung interface.

VASODILATORS IN THE ASSESSMENT OF MYOCARDIAL OXYGENATION

Common Pharmacologic Vasodilators

Presently, vasodilators appear to be essential for assessing myocardial blood oxygenation, especially in the context of ischemic heart disease. Their importance was first demonstrated in human subjects with multigradient echo methods using two different pharmacologic stress agents: dipyridamole and dobutamine.[14,16] Both agents induce hyperemia, but with different effects on myocardial venous blood oxygenation. Dipyridamole is a potent coronary vasodilator that typically induces a 3- to 4-fold increase in MBF with minimal effect on MVO_2.[60] Consequently, myocardial venous blood oxygen saturation *increases* as oxygen supply (blood flow) exceeds demand (oxygen consumption). In contrast, dobutamine is a potent beta-agonist with a primary pharmacologic effect to increase cardiac work.[60] This results in a concomitant *increase* in MVO_2, which triggers an increase in MBF. Thus oxygen supply and demand remain largely balanced, and there is little to no change in myocardial venous blood oxygen saturation.[61]

Vasodilators have also facilitated direct demonstration of the in vivo correlation between BOLD CMR response (via changes in R2* [or 1/T2*]) and venous blood oxygen saturation. In a well-controlled canine model, a wide range of global myocardial venous blood oxygen saturation levels were created. Hyperemic conditions were induced by the intravenous administration of dipyridamole and dobutamine. To induce hypoxemia, the oxygen content of the inspired gas was reduced by ventilating dogs with a mixture of 10% oxygen and 90% nitrogen, which reduced the oxygen saturation in both arteries and veins. To correlate myocardial R2* with global venous blood oxygenation, venous blood oxygen saturation levels were measured directly by coronary sinus sampling. MBF was quantified invasively by the administration of radio-labeled microspheres. Measurements of myocardial R2* were obtained at baseline, during and after infusion of dipyridamole and dobutamine, and when the dogs were ventilated with hypoxic air. Paired arterial and coronary sinus blood samples were withdrawn at the six different stages of the study. Blood oxygen saturation levels were measured by using a blood gas analyzer interfaced with an oximeter. Coronary sinus blood oxygen saturation levels ranged from 9% to 80% with experimental interventions with dipyridamole, dobutamine, or hypoxic air. Administration of dipyridamole and dobutamine and ventilation of hypoxic air all increased MBF significantly, but significant decrease in myocardial R2* was observed only with dipyridamole infusion, which indicates that myocardial R2* is a reflection of MBF only when myocardial oxygenation demand is not significantly altered between rest and hyperemia. The relationship between the changes of myocardial R2* from baseline and the %O$_2$ in the coronary sinus showed a linear regression ($r = 0.84$), indicating a strong correlation between myocardial R2* and %O$_2$ in the coronary sinus.

These studies also showed that both dipyridamole and hypoxic air increased myocardial blood volume (MBV) fraction in excess of 50%. However, their effects on R2* are manifested differently. With administration of dipyridamole, %O$_2$ in coronary sinus increases, which leads to a decrease in R2*. However, the blood volume fraction in the myocardium also increases, which increases the hematocrit content of a voxel, which tends to increase myocardial R2*; this is the opposite of the effect of increased oxygen saturation. Because a decrease in myocardial R2* was observed in these studies, increased oxygen saturation clearly has the dominant effect over increased blood volume, but the apparent R2* change as a function of %O$_2$ is reduced because of the accompanied blood volume effect. In contrast, during hypoxia, both %O$_2$ in coronary sinus and the blood volume fraction increase, and their effects enhance each other. As a result, the apparent change in R2* as a function of %O$_2$ is greater than that if blood volume fraction remained the same. These studies showed that by measuring MBV fraction changes using technetium-99m-labeled (^{99m}Tc-labeled) red blood cells at each of the interventions and correcting their effects on myocardial R2*, a more linear relationship was found between R2* and the blood oxygen saturation. Thus an accurate assessment of myocardial oxygen saturation using CMR will probably require a correction for blood volume.

Hypercapnia as a New Potent Coronary Vasodilator

It has long been known that carbon dioxide (CO_2) may act as a vasodilator in the heart, but its sensitivity to impart sufficient coronary vasodilation to assess regional changes in MBF has not been clear. Recent studies, enabled by prospective gas control allowing for rapid and independent control of arterial CO_2 and O_2, have made it possible to directly relate the influence of arterial CO_2 on coronary vasodilation. The use of targeted increases in arterial CO_2 to vasodilate the coronary arteries and invoke changes in myocardial oxygenation and its relation to adenosine in the preclinical models and healthy human subjects has been demonstrated (Fig. 8.2).[62] However, its utility to assess changes in myocardial oxygenation in patients with ischemic/nonischemic heart disease has not been demonstrated.

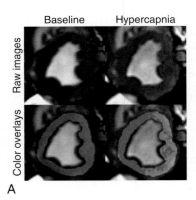
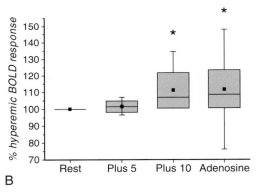

FIG. 8.2 Effect of changing arterial carbon dioxide (CO_2) on blood-oxygen-level-dependent *(BOLD)* cardiovascular magnetic resonance signal intensities in healthy humans. (A) Representative short-axis BOLD cardiovascular magnetic resonance images collected from a healthy human at baseline (end-tidal CO_2 [PETCO$_2$] = 37 mm Hg) and hypercapnia (PETCO$_2$ = 47 mm Hg). BOLD signal intensity increased during hypercapnia. For ease of visualization, color overlays of the left ventricle (with color bar showing BOLD signal intensity in arbitrary units [a.u.]) corresponding to the gray-scale images are shown directly below. (B) Box plot showing the dependence of % hyperemic BOLD response on PETCO$_2$ and standard dose of adenosine: % hyperemic response increased at higher PETCO$_2$ values; response at Plus 10 did not differ from that because of standard adenosine infusion. % hyperemic BOLD response for adenosine is from reported values in the literature.[80] Asterisk denotes statistically significant difference relative to rest ($P < .05$). Top and bottom of boxes indicate upper limit +1 standard deviation (SD) and lower limit −1 SD, respectively; error bars *(whiskers)* are maximum and minimum of data. The mean and median are represented as a point and a band within the box, respectively. For adenosine, the whiskers represent the boundaries of 1st and 99th percentile of the data. (Modified from Yang HJ, Yumul R, Tang R, et al. Assessment of myocardial reactivity to controlled hypercapnia with free-breathing T2-prepared cardiac blood-oxygen-level-dependent MR. *Radiology.* 2014;272:397–406.)

An alternate approach for modulating $PaCO_2$ is through breathing maneuvers, where a subject is asked to hyperventilate, typically for 30 seconds, and then suspend breathing during imaging to invoke a hyperemic response. The combined hyperventilation/suspension of breathing is expected to provide a significant change in $PaCO_2$ to invoke a hyperemic blood flow response in the heart. To date, the value of this approach in modulating the BOLD CMR response has been demonstrated in healthy human subjects.[63] Comparative studies between this approach and prospective gas control methods to probe myocardial oxygenation changes in response to hypercapnia are yet to be conducted.

MYOCARDIAL BOLD CMR: PRECLINICAL STUDIES

T2*- and T2-Prepared Methods

To date, a number of isolated heart and animal studies have demonstrated that vasodilator interventions that alter the blood oxygenation levels result in BOLD signal changes.[9–13,21,22,24–30] One of the first studies to demonstrate the feasibility of assessing myocardial oxygenation on the basis of the BOLD effect was performed in a rat model. This study showed significant signal loss in both the left ventricular chamber and the myocardium during apnea.[9] A subsequent study in an isolated rabbit heart model confirmed a substantial correlation between the gradient echo image intensity of the myocardium and deoxyhemoglobin concentration levels.[13] In large animal models, gradient echo myocardial signal enhanced significantly after the infusion of dipyridamole,[11] presumably because of an increase in MBF in the absence of a corresponding increase in oxygen demand, resulting in a *decrease* in myocardial venous blood oxygen saturation. Several studies have now independently validated these studies in large animal models with T2-prepared methods.[22,27,28] Canine studies also suggest that it is possible to derive myocardial oxygen extraction fraction and quantitative perfusion reserve values with BOLD CMR.[24–26]

Perhaps the greatest expectation of BOLD CMR imaging is in detecting regional differences in myocardial oxygenation caused by focal CAD. Fig. 8.3[18] shows a schematic of the coronary vessels that supply the different myocardial territories of the mid left ventricle in humans.[18] Luminal narrowing of the coronary vessels can lead to regional perfusion deficits in the associated myocardial territories during pharmacologic stress. Whereas vasodilators are effective at increasing blood flow to the myocardium perfused by healthy coronary vessels, MBF to territories distal to the coronary artery stenosis is limited. The reduction in blood flow to the affected region decreases the oxygen saturation of hemoglobin and aids in delineating regional perfusion differences. Over the past two decades, both clinical and preclinical animal studies have demonstrated BOLD CMR may be an alternative to FPP methods. Some of the earliest studies of the utility of BOLD CMR to understand the perfusion deficits associated with coronary occlusion were performed with gradient echo sequences. These studies showed that the occlusion of the left anterior descending artery (LAD) resulted in signal reduction in corresponding regions of the myocardium perfused by the LAD.[11,12] These initial studies were followed by T2* mapping of the myocardium, which demonstrated that the myocardial regions with perfusion deficits also show preferential reduction in T2* under vasodilation. T2-prepared gradient echo methods in canine models demonstrated that it may be possible to extend the myocardial BOLD technique to three-dimensional (3D) imaging and acquire multiple slices with BOLD contrast.[21] However, poor image quality and signal-to-noise ratio (SNR), long scan times, and inadequate sensitivity are notable limitations of the gradient echo technique at 1.5 T.

T2-prepared methods have been proposed as an alternative to T2*-based methods. Whereas T2-prepared methods employing spiral readouts showed the capability to capture the BOLD contrast, off-resonance-based blurring was a key limitation.[22,23] A subsequent T2-preparation method with a bSSFP readout showed significant improvements in SNR, image quality, and scan times over the gradient echo techniques[29,30] and good sensitivity for evaluating myocardial BOLD signal changes. This technique has been employed in canine models with varying degrees of stenosis of the left circumflex coronary arteries (LCXs) in the presence of systemic adenosine infusion to demonstrate the effect of perfusion abnormalities with BOLD effect.[30] Results showed a visually discernible BOLD signal drop in the inferior and inferolateral walls supplied by the LCXs as well as a close correspondence between flow reductions in the same region as identified by the FPP images and microsphere flow maps (Fig. 8.4).

Prospective, targeted control of arterial partial pressure of CO_2 ($PaCO_2$), as discussed earlier, has been shown to be valuable in modulating coronary blood flow. Recent studies using T2-prepared bSSFP-based BOLD CMR demonstrated the capability of physiologically tolerable hypercapnia to induce myocardial hyperemia, and compared this response with intravenous adenosine. These studies showed that repeat targeting of a desirable hypercapnic stimulus punctuated by return of arterial CO_2 levels to baseline leads to a reproducible BOLD response. These findings provide early evidence into novel means of examining myocardial oxygenation through a benign/repeatable coronary vasodilator.

Most studies to date have employed 2D methods, with the majority of them using T2*- or T2-based (weighted or mapping) methods. These approaches often require suspension of breathing and cannot provide full ventricular coverage over the time period over which adenosine is typically delivered. To overcome these limitations, a fast, free-breathing 3D T2-mapping technique that uses near-perfect imaging efficiency, with insensitivity to heart-rate changes which take place in the presence of vasodilator stress, allowing for full coverage of the whole left ventricle within 5 minutes, has been developed. This approach demonstrated in preclinical studies promises to offer a more refined BOLD CMR method with the 3D free-breathing T2-mapping technique and has the capability to map the hyperemic BOLD response throughout the left ventricle during adenosine administration.

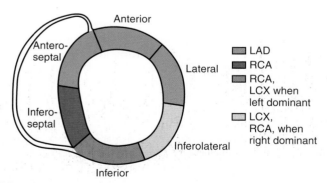

FIG. 8.3 A schematic representation of the myocardial segments of the mid ventricular section with the assigned coronary territories. *LAD*, Left anterior descending coronary artery; *LCX*, left circumflex coronary artery; *RCA*, right coronary artery. (Modified from Friedrich MG, Niendorf T, Schulz-Menger J, Gross CM, Dietz R. Blood oxygen level-dependent magnetic resonance imaging in patients with stress-induced angina. *Circulation.* 2003;108:2219–2213.)

Steady-State BOLD CMR: Cardiac Phase–Resolved Imaging of Myocardial Oxygenation

To date, systematic studies have demonstrated that bSSFP imaging can be used in the assessment of oxygen-sensitive imaging. Controlled in vitro

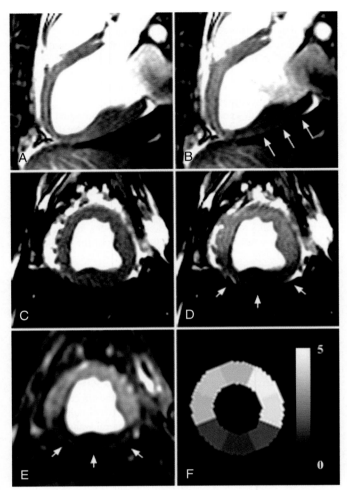

FIG. 8.4 Preclinical studies for detecting perfusion defects using T2-prepared balanced steady-state free precession cardiovascular magnetic resonance. Comparison of blood-oxygen-level-dependent (BOLD) magnetic resonance images acquired with T2-prepared steady-state free precession (T_R/T_E = 3.0/1.3 ms, 40-ms T2 preparation) at rest (A and C) and during stress stenosis (B and D), with corresponding first-pass image (E) (saturation recovery steady-state free precession, T_R/T_E = 3.0/1.5 ms) and microsphere flow image (F). Arrows indicate the region of reduced perfusion due to stenosis in the BOLD stress stenosis and first-pass images. Note the clear delineation of the myocardial region fed by the stenosed artery in the BOLD images, as well as the excellent matchup of the stress stenosis BOLD image with the first-pass image and microsphere flow map. (The microsphere flow map was generated by calculating flow ratios in each segment in relation to one reference segment. The scale indicates black for 0 flow ratio and white for a 5-fold flow ratio.) (Modified from Shea SM, Fieno DS, Schirf BE, et al. T₂-prepared steady-state free precession blood oxygen level-dependent MR imaging of myocardial perfusion in a dog stenosis model. *Radiology.* 2005;236:503–509.)

studies with blood samples oxygenated to various levels revealed that when the off-resonance effects are minimized through the appropriate choice of flip angle and phase-cycling scheme, oxygen-sensitive contrast can be realized in whole blood in a repetition time (TR)-dependent manner.[64] The results showed that relatively long TRs (compared with those that are used in conventional bSSFP imaging) are necessary to establish oxygen-sensitive contrast in bSSFP images in blood. This was subsequently used to demonstrate that arteries and veins can be

separated, based on %O₂ differences.[65] The advantages of the bSSFP method over other BOLD CMR methods is increased in SNR. In the heart, however, there are other advantages, including cardiac phase–resolved (CP) imaging allowing one to capture potential BOLD effects as well as function in one acquisition. This was first demonstrated in canines with and without coronary stenosis. Two-dimensional (2D) cardiac phase–resolved BOLD (CP-BOLD) bSSFP with a relatively long TR (6.3 ms) was used to demonstrate that occlusion of the LCX leads to regional myocardial oxygen deficit in the coronary territory supplied by LCX. The results were compared with the FPP technique and validated with microsphere-based perfusion analysis. 2D CP-BOLD CMR accurately predicted the regional MBF deficit region identified by the first-pass technique employing an exogenous contrast media. The benefits of CP-BOLD CMR with this approach permits increased confidence for evaluating myocardial BOLD signal changes in the presence of a coronary artery stenosis. Canine studies by Vöhringer et al.[66] have demonstrated that CP-BOLD CMR can identify changes in myocardial oxygenation and flow in the presence of intracoronary infusion of acetylcholine, an endothelium-dependent vasodilator, and adenosine, an endothelium-independent vasodilator. These studies showed that CP-BOLD CMR has the capability to report on oxygenation changes in the setting of CAD or MVD.

Several noncardiac studies have shown that BOLD contrast is directly tied to field strength, and this was demonstrated in the heart as well as through theoretical simulations, and animal studies have also established this in the heart.[67] These studies showed that at 3 T, a 3-fold increase in oxygen sensitivity could be expected in comparison to 1.5 T in theory. Experimental canine studies showed that a 2.5-fold ± 0.2-fold increase in BOLD sensitivity is possible at 3 T relative to 1.5 T (Fig. 8.5).[67] On the basis of the relationship between BOLD signal changes and microsphere perfusion, it was found that the minimum regional perfusion differences that can be detected with CP-BOLD CMR at 1.5 T and 3.0 T were 2.9 and 1.6, respectively. These findings suggest that CP-BOLD CMR at 3 T may have the necessary sensitivity to detect the clinically required minimum flow difference of 2.0 that is achievable with FPP methods.

Vasodilatory stress is the standard paradigm for probing myocardial oxygenation (O₂) changes due to coronary artery stenosis on the basis of BOLD MRI. However, because vasodilation is typically achieved with provocative stress, approaches that can identify the presence of stenosis on the basis of microvascular alterations at rest are highly desirable. It is known that MBV varies throughout the cardiac cycle; MBV *increases* during diastole and *decreases* during systole.[68,69] It has also been shown that changes in MBV lead to increased O₂ extraction by cardiomyocytes.[70] Thus MBV and O₂ are expected to vary at different parts of the cardiac cycle. In particular, in diastole, it is expected that MBV and O₂ extraction are maximal, whereas in systole, MBV and O₂ extraction are minimal. In addition, as MBV increases, even at a stable level of O₂, the number of deoxygenated hemoglobin molecules within a voxel increases, causing a proportionate elevation in the local magnetic field inhomogeneities.[71] Moreover, with increasing grade of stenosis, the MBV in the myocardial territory supplied by a stenotic artery increases in systole.[19,72–74] Thus the relative MBV and O₂ changes between systole and diastole are expected to be different between myocardial territories supplied by healthy and stenotic coronary arteries. Moreover, it is also known that T1 of myocardium is dependent on MBV and that the apparent T2 is dependent on blood O₂. Because bSSFP signals are approximately T2/T1 weighted, it was expected that CP-BOLD signal intensities at systole and diastole may reflect changes in MBV and blood O₂. In addition, because stenosis leads to an increase in systolic MBV and is accompanied by a reduction in blood O₂, it was hypothesized that systolic and diastolic CP-BOLD signal intensities may be used to

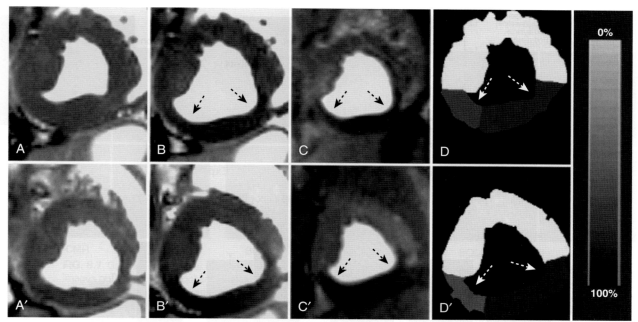

FIG. 8.5 Demonstration of increased myocardial blood-oxygen-level-dependent sensitivity at 3 T. Short-axis two-dimensional balanced steady-state free precession (bSSFP) cardiovascular magnetic resonance images obtained at 1.5 T (*top row*, A–C) and at 3 T (*bottom row*, A'–C') in canines. Images A and A' are bSSFP images obtained without stenosis, images B and B' are bSSFP images at systole under severe stenosis of the left circumflex coronary artery (LCX), and images C and C' are the corresponding first-pass perfusion (FPP) images acquired under stenosis of similar extent as in B and B'. Images D and D' represent the spatial map (scale provided by the gray-scale bar) of percent difference in microsphere-based regional flow between prestenosis and severe stenosis in the presence of adenosine infusion at 1.5 T and 3 T, respectively. The arrows subtend the suspected regions (LCX territory), where the perfusion deficits are expected to develop as a result of LCX stenosis in dogs. Note the discriminating signal loss in these regions in images B and B' and the close correspondence between the FPP (C and C') and microsphere-based flow difference maps (D and D'). (Modified from Dharmakumar R, Mangalathu Arumana J, Tang R, et al. Assessment of regional myocardial oxygenation changes in the presence of coronary artery stenosis with balanced SSFP imaging at 3.0 T: theory and experimental evaluation in canines. *J Magn Reson Imaging.* 2008;27:1037–1045.)

detect the ischemic territories at resting states. These hypotheses were shown to be accurate with simulations and canine experiments with maximal coronary stenosis using a 2D CP-BOLD sequence (Fig. 8.6) designed to mitigate against flow-mediated phase changes, which otherwise would appear as "ghost" artifacts.[75] Although these results are encouraging, further validation of the proposed method is required. Moreover, technical advances in sequence development for 3D CP-BOLD (for minimizing potential signal variations due to through-plane motion), methods to overcome image artifacts in bSSFP images at 3 T, improvements in image processing, along with additional preclinical studies at more modest coronary stenosis may be necessary before clinical translation.

CLINICAL EXPERIENCE WITH BOLD CMR

Successful demonstrations of the BOLD effect in animal models have provided the impetus for myocardial BOLD CMR in patients with CAD. In the past decade, there has been an extensive number of studies in ischemic and nonischemic patients.

T2*-Based BOLD CMR in Patients

In one of the first and pioneering studies, T2*-weighted BOLD CMR method was compared against single-photon emission computed tomography (SPECT) with the aim of visualizing regional oxygen deficits under pharmacologic stress. This study was performed in 25 patients (23 patients with >50% stenosis, 10 of whom had severe stenosis, i.e., >75%). Results demonstrated that significant changes in suspected regions of the myocardium were apparent in patients with severe stenosis. Receiver operating characteristic (ROC) analysis of both BOLD CMR and thallium SPECT methods showed that the area under the ROC curve is 0.66 and 0.73, respectively. These results indicated that both methods have limitations in identifying regional perfusion deficits and that the limitations are attributable to suboptimal resolution of SPECT images and the well-known image artifacts associated with gradient-recalled T2*-weighted methods in the heart, as discussed earlier. In addition to demonstrating the feasibility of the BOLD method for studying CAD in patients (Fig. 8.7),[18] these studies demonstrated that improved CMR methods are needed.

Another clinical study by Wacker and colleagues[19] examined the possibility of evaluating oxygen-sensitive changes in patients with CAD without pharmacologic stress. Their study included a control group of 16 healthy subjects (age 31 ± 10 years old) with no history of cardiovascular disease and 16 patients (63 ± 9 years old) with single-vessel CAD (degree of stenosis >70%) identified by x-ray coronary angiogram. Within the control group, T2* mapping of the mid left ventricular myocardium was homogeneous (35 ± 3 ms) and increased

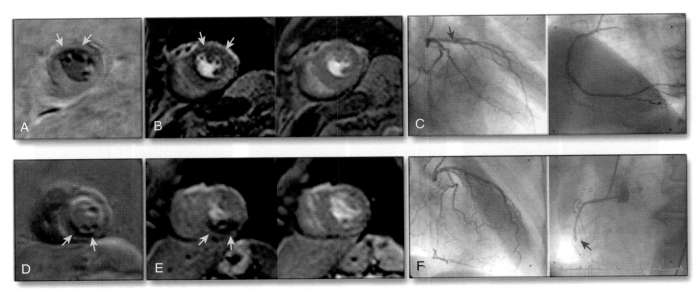

FIG. 8.8 Representative cardiovascular magnetic resonance examples of blood-oxygen-level-dependent (BOLD) and first-pass perfusion (FPP). *Upper row,* Subtracted BOLD image (A), stress and rest FPP (B), and corresponding invasive angiogram of the left and right coronary artery (RCA) (C) in a patient with known coronary artery disease and prior stenting of the RCA. Subtracted BOLD and FPP imaging show a stress-induced deficit in the anterior/anterolateral myocardial segments *(yellow arrows).* Invasive coronary angiography confirmed severe stenosis of the left anterior descending (LAD) coronary artery *(blue arrow)* (quantitative coronary angiography 63%). *Bottom row,* Subtracted BOLD image (D), stress and rest FPP (E), and corresponding invasive angiogram of the left and right coronary artery (F) in a patient with suspected coronary artery disease. Subtracted BOLD and FPP imaging detected a stress-induced deficit in the inferoseptal/inferior wall *(yellow arrows).* Invasive coronary angiography revealed a complete occlusion of the RCA *(blue arrow)* (100%) with retrograde filling of the distal RCA via extensive collaterals. (Modified from Jahnke C, Gebker R, Manka R, et al. Navigator-gated 3D blood oxygen level-dependent CMR at 3.0-T for detection of stress-induced myocardial ischemic reactions. *JACC Cardiovasc Imaging.* 2010;3:375–384.)

or severely affected. Segmental bSSFP signal intensities at rest and stress were measured, and the signal intensity ratio (stress/rest) was calculated. Statistical results showed that there are significant differences in stress/rest values computed from healthy, mildly affected, and severely affected segments ($P < .05$). More recently this approach has been studied in 37 CAD patients with FFR measurements as the ground truth, which showed that in subjects with FFR <0.8, the sensitivity and specificity for detecting the presence of diminished vasodilator response in affected segments was 86% and 92%, respectively.[89] However, because of poor image quality, a large minority (~40%) of segments had to be excluded. Improved CP-BOLD CMR strategies such as those that can overcome flow/motion artifacts may help to overcome this limitation but remain to be studied in the clinical setting.[90]

VISUALIZATION AND QUANTIFICATION OF BOLD EFFECTS VIA IMAGE PROCESSING

Maximal BOLD CMR response from healthy myocardial segments is typically on the order of 15% to 20% and segments with disease are significantly lower. Without proper windowing, visualizing these BOLD signal changes is difficult. Manual windowing requires significant time (several minutes), is subjective, and can introduce large intraobserver and interobserver variability. Until recently, the evaluation of myocardial BOLD CMR relied on measuring the relative mean signal intensity changes in segments of interest under rest and pharmacologically induced vasodilation. This paradigm assumes that all pixels within the entire

segment are equally affected, which need not be the case because the epicardial coronary artery supplying a given segment is not well defined and can vary among individuals and within a segment.[18] Because it overemphasizes the magnitude of intensity changes over the regional extent of the BOLD effect at rest and vasodilation, it may contribute to the reduced sensitivity and specificity reported by a number of studies.[18,22,30,67] To date, several attempts have been made to identify new ways to visualize and evaluate the BOLD effect, including the simultaneous acquisition of BOLD and cine wall motion assessment.[90a]

Detecting and Quantifying Pixel-Level BOLD Changes Under Vasodilator Stress With ARREAS

One of the early efforts to improve the visualization and quantification of myocardial BOLD, area-based biomarker for characterizing coronary stenosis (ARREAS) aimed to provide pixel-level assessment of ischemia on the basis of a statistical model of myocardial intensity distribution.[91] ARREAS relies on the combination of a statistically derived threshold and connectivity analysis to identify the territories affected by the stenosis. It assumes that the myocardial intensity distribution under rest conditions can be represented as a unimodal scaled distribution (e.g., Student's *t*). On the other hand, under stress conditions, the distribution is the same but because of the increase in BOLD contrast (attributed to vasodilation), a different mean is used. In the case of disease, the distribution becomes bimodal (one representing healthy myocardium, and the other, affected myocardium) but because the contrast change is within the deviation, these underlying distributions are not separable. Thus the ARREAS approach, with the aid of a Student's

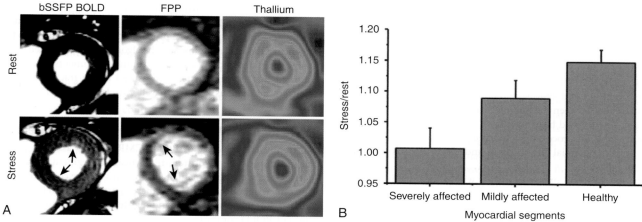

FIG. 8.9 Patient studies with two-dimensional balanced steady-state free precession *(bSSFP)* blood-oxygen-level-dependent *(BOLD)* cardiovascular magnetic resonance at 1.5 T. Midventricular short-axis steady-state free precession BOLD, first-pass perfusion *(FPP)*, and thallium single-photon emission computed tomography (SPECT) images obtained from a patient with 70% stenosis of the left anterior descending (LAD) coronary artery at rest and stress (A). The windowing and leveling of images obtained at rest and stress are the same. Myocardial signal in the rest BOLD, FPP, and SPECT images are relatively homogeneous. However, under stress, the territory supplied by the LAD (larger arc subtended by *arrows*) does not increase in the BOLD images as expected. This pattern of regional signal differences is also evident in the FPP and SPECT images. Statistical results from the myocardial BOLD signal analysis showed that significant differences in stress/rest values exist between healthy and affected regions (B). In comparison to healthy segments, the stress/rest values of affected regions are lower, consistent with previous findings in animals that bSSFP signals obtained under pharmacologic stress are significantly reduced in myocardial territories supplied by stenotic arteries. (Modified from Dharmakumar R, Green JD, Flewitt J, et al. Blood oxygen-sensitive SSFP imaging for probing the myocardial perfusion reserves of patients with coronary artery disease: a feasibility study. *J Cardiovasc Magn Reson.* 2008;10[suppl 1]:A101.)

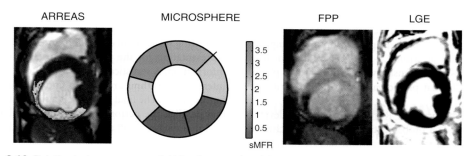

FIG. 8.10 Relation between myocardial blood-oxygen-level-dependent (BOLD) image processed using area-based biomarker for characterizing coronary stenosis *(ARREAS)*, segmental myocardial flow ratio *(sMFR)* bull's eye plot, first-pass perfusion *(FPP)*, and late gadolinium enhancement *(LGE)* images. FPP image obtained under adenosine stress with critical (70%) left circumflex coronary artery stenosis and the corresponding BOLD image (processed with the ARREAS) are shown for comparison. LGE image confirms the absence of any infarction. (Modified from Tsaftaris SA, Tang R, Zhou X, et al. Detecting clinically significant coronary stenosis by inducing changes in microcirculatory oxygenation: an experimental study in canines using oxygen-sensitive magnetic resonance imaging. *J Magn Reson Imaging.* 2012;35:1338–1348.)

t distribution, fitted on myocardial intensities at rest, establishes an intensity threshold. This threshold is used to find, in rest and stress images, pixels that have intensity higher than the threshold (termed, for simplicity, "affected" pixels). The ratio of affected pixels over the area of the myocardium is termed as *affected fraction*, the ratio of which defines a biomarker called *ischemic extent* that aims to characterize how many more pixels can be identified as hypoperfused following vasodilatory stress.

This was demonstrated in canines using microsphere as gold standard—an example of visualization with ARREAS and comparison to microsphere analysis and FPP is shown in Fig. 8.10. This study showed that ischemic extent is exponentially related to microsphere flow and increases with the severity of surgically implemented coronary stenosis. This indicated that the extent of epicardial narrowing likely affects the supplied territories in a graded fashion; that is, with a greater narrowing of a given epicardial coronary artery, a greater fraction of

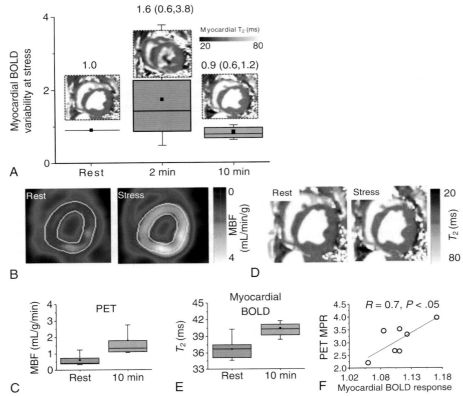

FIG. 8.11 Myocardial blood-oxygen-level-dependent *(BOLD)* variability at stress relative to rest. Box plot of myocardial BOLD variability and representative images at rest and from 2 and 10 minutes post regadenoson are shown. Large myocardial BOLD variability is observed at 2 minutes post regadenoson compared with rest and is markedly reduced at 10 minutes post regadenoson administration. ^{13}N-ammonia positron emission tomography *(PET)* myocardial blood flow *(MBF)* and BOLD. Both PET and BOLD images showed significant increase in *MBF* and BOLD response, at 10 minutes postregadenoson administration compared with rest (A–E). Results from regression analysis showed good correlation between PET myocardial perfusion reserve *(MPR)* (MBF[stress]/MBF[rest]) and myocardial BOLD response ($R = 0.7$, $P < .05$; panel [F]). *MPR,* Myocardial perfusion reserve. (Modified from Yang HJ, Dey D, Sykes J, et al. Towards reliable myocardial blood-oxygen-level-dependent (BOLD) CMR using late effects of regadenoson with simultaneous ^{13}N-ammonia PET validation in a whole-body hybrid PET/MR system. *J Cardiovasc Magn Reson.* 2016;18[suppl 1]:O19.)

or oxygenation is expected to be of paramount importance, because it can enable the detection of myocardial oxygenation changes in patients with all forms of CAD, especially those with balanced ischemia secondary to multivessel CAD. Successful adoption of recent advances through clinical studies and additional technical improvements can propel myocardial BOLD CMR toward becoming a powerful noninvasive diagnostic method in the early detection and posttreatment monitoring of ischemic heart disease.

ACKNOWLEDGMENT

This work was supported in part by National Institutes of Health R01 HL91989.

REFERENCES

A full reference list is available online at ExpertConsult.com

9

Cardiac Magnetic Resonance Spectroscopy

Stefan Neubauer and Christopher T. Rodgers

INTRODUCTION

Cardiovascular magnetic resonance (CMR) imaging uses the ^{1}H nucleus in water (H_2O) and fat (CH_2 and CH_3 groups) molecules as its only signal source, and therefore offers little insight into the biochemical state of cardiac tissue. In contrast, MR spectroscopy (MRS) of the heart allows the study of many other nuclei. It is the only available method for the noninvasive assessment of cardiac metabolism without needing the application of external radioactive tracers. Information on the major nuclei of interest for the metabolic study of cardiac tissue by MRS is given in Table 9.1, including ^{1}H, ^{13}C, ^{23}Na, and ^{31}P. Although, theoretically, many clinical questions can be answered with cardiac MRS, the main reason why MRS has not yet fulfilled its potential in clinical cardiology is related to the fundamental physical limitations of the method. MRS is often used to study nuclei other than ^{1}H, which have a much lower intrinsic MR sensitivity than ^{1}H. Furthermore, metabolite concentrations in vivo are typically in the mM (millimolar) range, which is several orders of magnitude lower than for water (approximately 80 M) or fat (often >1 M). Therefore the temporal and spatial resolution of MRS has so far remained far behind that of CMR imaging. Successful applications of MRS are those in which the unique metabolic insights of MRS are more important than obtaining high spatial or temporal resolution.

Although this chapter focuses on clinical cardiac MRS, some explanation of the experimental principles of MRS is important even for the clinical reader: MRS has been a widespread method in experimental cardiology, ever since the first ^{31}P-MR spectrum from an isolated heart was obtained by Radda's group in the 1970s,[1] and since then experimental MRS studies have offered numerous fundamental insights into cardiac metabolism. Furthermore, only with an understanding of the major implications of experimental MRS studies are we able to fully appreciate the potential of the method and extrapolate to clinical cardiac MRS applications that should become feasible in the future, once the technical challenges presently limiting the clinical utility of MRS have been overcome. For those interested in greater detail on experimental MRS and methodological background, comprehensive reviews of the subject are available elsewhere.[2–4] Complementary clinical reviews are also available.[5,6]

PHYSICAL PRINCIPLES

The basic principles of MRS (see the reference list for textbooks on the general physical principles of CMR and MRS[7–9]) are best explained from the most extensively studied nucleus, ^{31}P, and from the most widely used animal model, the isolated buffer-perfused rodent heart. These principles apply to MRS of all nuclei. An MR spectrometer consists of a high-field superconducting magnet (currently up to 23.5 T, where tesla [T] is the unit of magnetic field strength) with a bore size ranging between ~5 cm and ~1 m. The nucleus-specific probe head with the radiofrequency (RF) coils, which are used for MR excitation and signal reception, is seated within the magnet bore. The magnet is interfaced with a computer, a pulsed magnetic field gradient system, an RF transmitter, and RF receivers. MRS requires a much higher magnetic field homogeneity than CMR; therefore, before any MRS experiment, the magnetic field must first be homogenized with shim gradients. Spin excitation is achieved by transmitting a radiofrequency pulse through the RF coils into the subject. The resulting MR signal, known as the free induction decay (FID), is then received from the subject by RF coils and recorded by the scanner. The signal (or FID) oscillates with time but within an overall exponentially decaying "envelope." It typically reaches negligible levels after tens of milliseconds. An MR spectrum is then computed from the FID (by applying the discrete Fourier transform formula[10]). The MR spectrum describes the signal intensity as a function of resonance frequency. Because of the low sensitivity of MRS, in practice, many FIDs are averaged to obtain MR spectra with an adequate "signal-to-noise ratio" (SNR; i.e., the height of a peak in the spectrum after "matched filtering" divided by the standard deviation of baseline noise[11]). The required number of averages depends on the concentration of the metabolite under investigation, its MR relaxation times (T1, T2, T2*), the "filling factor" (the mass of the heart relative to the coil size), the natural abundance of the nuclear isotope studied, its relative MR sensitivity (see Table 9.1), the pulse angle, and the pulse repetition time (TR). For a perfused rat heart experiment at ≥7 T, 100 to 200 FIDs are typically acquired. To quantify metabolite concentrations from MR spectra, it is vital to correct for partial saturation, which depends on the selected pulse angles and TR. This is because the maximum MR signal is only obtained when nuclei are excited from a fully relaxed spin state, that is, when a time of at least 5 × T1 has passed since a previous excitation (e.g., T1 of phosphocreatine [PCr] at 7 T is ~3 s requiring TR of ≥15 s, at 1.5 T the PCr T1 ~4.4 s requiring TR of ≥22 s); acquisition of fully relaxed MR spectra therefore requires long TRs, leading to prohibitively long acquisition times. In practice, we take advantage of the fact that the initial part of the FID contains most of the signal. Use of shorter TRs therefore yields spectra with higher SNR for a given acquisition time, but some of the signal is lost because of saturation. Such spectra are termed "partially saturated." The extent of saturation also varies for different ^{31}P-resonances, because the T1s of ^{31}P-metabolites such as PCr and adenosine triphosphate (ATP) are significantly different (T1 of PCr is 2–3 × longer than T1 of ATP). Therefore for metabolite quantification from partially saturated spectra, the spectral peak areas are determined (e.g., fitted using the Advanced Method for Accurate, Robust, and Efficient Spectral Fitting [AMARES][12] or LCModel[13]), and then correction factors are applied to obtain the metabolite concentration. By comparing fully relaxed and saturated spectra, these factors can be determined for each metabolite. In practice, TRs and pulse flip angles for MRS are chosen to yield acceptable measurement times at

deoxygenation can be measured.[55] Technical challenges for ^{1}H-MRS include the need for suppression of the strong ^{1}H signal from water and the complexity of ^{1}H spectra with overlapping resonances, many of which remain to be characterized, and which means that excellent shimming and motion compensation are needed.[56,57]

^{13}C-MRS

The ^{13}C nucleus has a low natural abundance (~1%), and for a classical ^{13}C-MRS experiment, the heart has to be supplied with ^{13}C-labeled compounds such as, for example, 1-^{13}C-glucose. Cardiac substrate utilization,[58] citric acid cycle flux, pyruvate dehydrogenase flux or beta-oxidation of fatty acids can then be quantified.[59,60] Clinical cardiac studies have yet to be reported because of the low sensitivity of ^{13}C-MRS and the requirement for high concentrations of exogenous ^{13}C-labeled precursors.

However, the technique of hyperpolarization can increase the SNR of ^{13}C experiments by a factor of up to 10,000× for a few minutes, until the magnetization decays by T1 relaxation back to thermal equilibrium.[32,33] This is a very active area of research as new pulse sequences, analysis methods, and injectable hyperpolarized agents are developed to capitalize on this extraordinary but brief burst of enhanced signal-to-noise. Pyruvate[61,62] is a particularly attractive molecule to hyperpolarize because it plays a pivotal role in substrate uptake before oxidative phosphorylation, enabling fluxes into acetyl acetate, lactate, and bicarbonate to be quantified. These enable experimental assessment of the balance between fats, carbohydrates, and ketone bodies being metabolized by the heart, a balance which may well be disturbed in disease. Hyperpolarization studies in animal models are revisiting many of the systems previously characterized by ^{31}P-MRS to obtain further insight, for example, ischemia-reperfusion models.[63]

[23]Na-CMR

[23]Na-CMR can evaluate changes in total and intracellular and extracellular Na$^+$ during cardiac injury.[64] A cardiac [23]Na spectrum shows a single peak representing the total Na$^+$ signal. To split the intracellular and extracellular Na$^+$ pools into two resonances, paramagnetic shift reagents, such as [TmDOTP]$^{5-}$, are added to the perfusate. This method has been used experimentally to examine the mechanisms of intracellular Na$^+$ accumulation in ischemia-reperfusion injury,[65] but [23]Na-MR shift reagents are not yet available for clinical use. Experimental CMR of total [23]Na shows that in acute ischemia, the total myocardial [23]Na CMR signal increases because of the breakdown of ion homeostasis

and the formation of both intracellular and extracellular edema (see Kim et al.[66] and Horn et al.[67]). Furthermore, [23]Na remains significantly elevated during chronic scar formation post coronary ligation[67] because of the expansion of the extracellular space in scar, and the area of elevated [23]Na signal correlates closely with histologically determined infarct size. Importantly, [23]Na content is not elevated in stunned or hibernating myocardium.[67] Thus [23]Na CMR may allow detection of myocardial viability without the use of external contrast agents. Significant improvements in image quality were made at 3 T,[68–70] and, recently, high-quality human [23]Na images and retrogated cine movies have been acquired at 7 T in the human heart.[71,72] An example of the high spatial and temporal resolution from 7 T is shown in Fig. 9.4. Furthermore, Umathum et al. have recently presented the first results from a whole-body [23]Na birdcage coil at 7 T, which can image from the pelvis to the heart in one scan.[73] The outlook for cardiac sodium CMR has recently been reviewed by Bottomley.[74]

Other Nuclei

The availability of ultra-high field (7 T) CMR scanners is making it possible to perform human in vivo spectroscopy and imaging also of fluorine (^{19}F), which is not present naturally in the body in mobile form and therefore makes an attractive CMR tracer to study, for example, in drug uptake. Imaging of chlorine ([35]Cl) and potassium ([39]K) has also been demonstrated at 7 T,[75–78] which makes it possible to map cell membrane potential in vivo.[78]

CLINICAL MAGNETIC RESONANCE SPECTROSCOPIC STUDIES

Methodologic Considerations

Historically, almost all human cardiac MR spectroscopy studies have interrogated the ^{31}P nucleus. The main reason for the slow progress with clinical cardiac MRS is that the method poses major technical challenges. In practice, total examination time should not be more than 60 minutes, and time for signal acquisition is therefore limited. The heart is a rapidly moving organ, currently requiring gating to the electrocardiogram (ECG), and, when resolution is further improved, ultimately to respiration as well.[79] Most clinical MRS studies were performed at 1.5 T until the early 2000s, and since then mostly at 3 T; the first 7 T studies are now being published.[80,81] Although the field strength of animal scanners continues to increase, the latest 7 T human systems

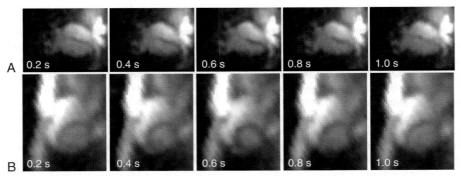

FIG. 9.4 [23]Na-cardiovascular magnetic resonance of the human heart. (A) A four-chamber view with field of view (FOV) zoomed to (210 × 273) mm^2 and (B) a short-axis view (FOV = [180 × 150] mm^2). The ventricles and the septum are clearly visible in A and B. The left and right atriums are delineated from the ventricles in the four-chamber views. The rib cartilage shows the highest signal intensity because of the high sodium concentration. The temporal resolution is 200 ms, nominal spatial resolution (6 mm)^3. The images were acquired with the ST acquisition scheme (10,000 projections) and reconstructed with a Hanning filter. (From Resetar A, Hoffmann SH, Graessl A, et al. Retrospectively-gated CINE (23)Na imaging of the heart at 7.0 tesla using density-adapted 3D projection reconstruction. *Magn Reson Imaging.* 2015;33:1091–1097.)

have comparable field strength with that used historically for many important animal studies. The cardiac muscle lies behind the chest wall skeletal muscle, which creates a strong ^{31}P signal that must be suppressed by spectral localization techniques, outer volume suppression,[82] or surface spoiling gradient coils.[83] Such localization methods include depth-resolved surface coil spectroscopy (DRESS), rotating frame one-dimensional chemical shift imaging (1D-CSI), image-selected in vivo spectroscopy (ISIS), and three-dimensional (3D)-CSI (Fig. 9.5). These methods are reviewed in detail elsewhere.[84] Bottomley et al.[85–87] have pioneered most of the early methodological development of human cardiac MRS. Most MRS studies have been performed in prone position rather than supine because this reduces motion artifacts and may slightly reduce the distance of the heart from the surface coil, thereby improving sensitivity. Most spectroscopic techniques require a stack of ^{1}H scout images to be obtained first, which are used to select the spectroscopic volume(s). The low sensitivity of ^{31}P-MRS requires relatively large voxel sizes, typically about 20 to 70 mL (and often rather larger if one considers the "true" integrated point-spread-function volume).[80] A set of ^{31}P-MR spectra acquired from a healthy volunteer with 3D-CSI at 1.5 T, 3 T, and 7 T is shown in Fig. 9.6. Compared with the rat heart spectrum in Fig. 9.1, the signal-to-noise is lower at 1.5 and 3 T, and two additional resonances are detected: 2,3-diphosphoglycerate (2,3-DPG), because of the presence of erythrocytes in the interrogated voxel, and phosphodiesters (PDE), a signal caused by membrane as well as serum phospholipids. The 2,3-DPG peaks overlap with the Pi resonance, which is therefore challenging to discriminate in blood-contaminated human ^{31}P-MR spectra. Thus intracellular pH is hard to determine; early results[87a] suggest that Pi and pH become detectable in human myocardium when spatial resolution and signal-to-noise are increased by scanning at 7 T. By calculating the PCr/ATP and PDE/ATP peak area ratios, relative quantification of human ^{31}P spectra is simple. PCr/ATP is a powerful index of the energetic state of the heart (see Experimental Foundations section), whereas the meaning of the PDE/ATP ratio is poorly understood, and this ratio probably does not change with cardiac disease. ^{31}P resonances must be corrected for partial saturation, as described for experimental MRS. Appropriate T1 values have been summarized.[2,80] Intrinsic ^{31}P-T1 values are believed to remain constant in the presence of cardiac disease,[88] although observed T1 values can change because of the effects of chemical exchange in the CK system.[89] Furthermore, ^{31}P spectra require correction for blood contamination: blood contributes signal to the ATP, 2,3-DPG and PDE resonances. Because human blood spectra have an ATP/2,3-DPG area ratio of ~0.11 and a PDE/2,3-DPG area ratio of ~0.19, for blood correction, the ATP resonance area of cardiac spectra is reduced by 11% of the 2,3-DPG resonance area, and the PDE resonance area is reduced by 19% of the 2,3-DPG resonance area.[90] ^{31}P-metabolite ratios in blood also change in the presence of disease,[91] which should be taken into account.

Absolute quantification of PCr and ATP is technically challenging, but is desirable because the PCr/ATP ratio does not detect simultaneous decreases of both PCr and ATP, which occur in the failing heart[92] or in infarcted nonviable myocardium.[93] Absolute ^{31}P-metabolite levels can be obtained by acquiring signal from a ^{31}P standard as well as estimates of myocardial mass from CMR.[86,94] A different approach calibrates the ^{31}P signal to the tissue water proton content, measured by ^{1}H-MRS.[87] Signals can be calibrated to an electronically synthesized reference signal using the "electronic reference to access in vivo concentrations" (ERETIC) method.[95] Modern "non-Fourier" methods solve for the metabolite concentrations using the powerful "inverse problem" mathematical formulation. For example, spectral localization with optimum pointspread (SLOOP)[96] postprocessing can deliver concentrations in noncuboidal compartments (e.g., myocardium). Spectroscopy with linear algebraic modeling (SLAM)[97,98] accelerates the acquisition steps to focus the scan

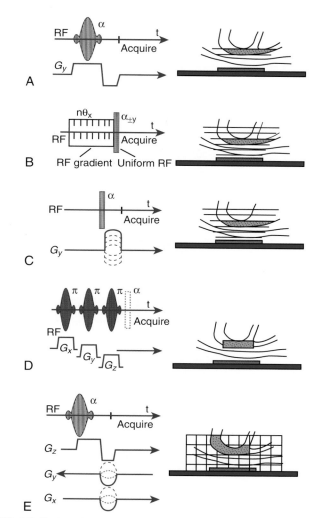

FIG. 9.5 Basic pulse sequences for localized cardiac spectroscopy with surface coils. (A) "Depth-resolved surface coil spectroscopy." A single section parallel to the plane of the surface coil is selected by applying a magnetic resonance (MR) imaging gradient G in the presence of a modulated radiofrequency *(RF)* excitation pulse of flip angle α. (B) The "rotating frame" MR method uses the gradient inherent in a surface coil to simultaneously spatially encode spectra from multiple sections parallel to the surface coil by means of application of a θ flip angle pulse, which is stepped in subsequent applications of the sequence. (C) The "one-dimensional chemical shift imaging" method similarly encodes multiple sections but uses an MR imaging gradient whose amplitude is stepped. (D) The "image-selected in vivo spectroscopy" method localizes to a single volume with selective inversion pulses applied with G_x, G_y and G_z MR imaging gradients. All eight combinations of the three pulses must be applied and the resultant signals added and subtracted. (E) A section-selective "three-dimensional chemical shift imaging" sequence employs MR imaging section selection in one dimension and phase encoding in two dimensions. (From Bottomley P. MR spectroscopy of the human heart: the status and the challenges. *Radiology.* 1994;191;593–612.)

time most effectively to find concentrations in a predetermined compartment, for example, myocardium segmented from a ^{1}H image. A variety of non-Cartesian acquisition methods, such as compressed sensing (CS) spectroscopy[99] or spiral ^{31}P-MRS,[100] also enable a smooth tradeoff between acquisition time, spatial resolution, and spectral resolution.

A long-term goal for human cardiac MRS is to combine ^{31}P- and ^{1}H-spectroscopy to measure free ADP and ΔG of ATP hydrolysis, as

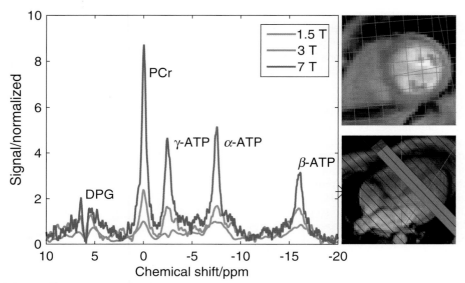

FIG. 9.6 *Left,* ^{31}P-magnetic resonance spectra from the interventricular septum of the same volunteer recorded at 1.5 T, 3 T, and 7 T using a three-dimensional chemical shift imaging (3D-CSI) sequence. Field-of-view 240 × 240 × 200 mm³ with a 12 × 8 × 8 matrix with 32 averages in 22 minutes at 1.5 T; a 16 × 16 × 8 matrix with 10 averages in 28 minutes at 3 T and 7 T. *DPG,* 2,3-Diphosphoglycerate (from blood); *PCr,* phosphocreatine; *γ-, α-, β-ATP,* the three phosphorus atoms of adenosine triphosphate. To facilitate comparison the spectra are normalized to the baseline noise level, apodized, and the 1.5 T spectrum is scaled to account for its larger voxel size and shorter acquisition. *Right,* Corresponding short-axis and four-chamber localizer images recorded by [1]H-cardiovascular magnetic resonance at 3 T. The 3D-CSI voxel grid is overlaid. The voxel corresponding to the ^{31}P spectra is highlighted.

described in canine myocardium by Bottomley et al.[48] Another highly relevant energetic parameter is the rate and extent of ATP transfer ("CK rate k_f" and "CK-flux"; see Experimental Foundations section). Bottomley et al.[101] developed the four-angle saturation transfer (FAST) method, which allows measurement of creatine kinase rates in ~30 minutes at 1.5 T. More recently, Bottomley et al. have introduced the triple repetition time saturation transfer (TRiST)[35] and two repetition time saturation transfer (TwiST)[88] methods to measure CK flux at 3 T based on dual-TR T1 measurements[102] during saturation (illustrated in Fig. 9.7), and we have introduced Bloch-Siegert four angle saturation transfer (BOAST) to measure 3D-resolved CK rates at 7 T.[36]

The methods of ^{31}P-MRS are still being improved significantly. Nevertheless, a major effort to standardize protocols and to make routinely available advanced RF coils and pulse sequences at ultra-high field strengths will be required to bring cardiac MRS into clinical practice.

Healthy Volunteers

Because of differences in the MRS methods used, the range of "normal" human heart PCr/ATP ratios reported in the literature is considerable, from about 1.1 to 2.4, with an overall average of about 1.8.[2] This attests to the need for development of methodologic standards for MRS. SLOOP values for absolute PCr levels in normal human myocardium are 9.0 ± 1.2 mmol/kg wet weight, and ATP levels are 5.3 ± 1.2 mmol/kg wet weight.[103] There is an accumulation of evidence that high-energy phosphate levels decrease slightly with advanced age,[104–107] perhaps because of increasing mitochondrial dysfunction.[27,108] During stress, PCr/ATP ratios stay normal for all but extreme levels of inotropic stimulation, when there is a small decrease.[109] Using FAST (see earlier), high-energy phosphate turnover rates (CK reaction rates) were found to be 0.29 ± 0.06 s⁻¹ in healthy volunteers at rest and did not change during doubling of the cardiac rate–pressure product.[53]

Athlete's Heart and Hypertension

In patients with hypertension, Lamb et al.[110] demonstrated reduced PCr/ATP ratios both at rest and during dobutamine stress, and PCr/ATP ratios also correlated inversely with indices of diastolic function (E deceleration peak). In contrast, two other studies showed no significant changes of cardiac energetics in patients with hypertension.[92,104] Differences in patient characteristics—for example, severity and duration of hypertension—may be responsible for this discrepancy. Experimental data clearly suggest that cardiac energetics are impaired in long-standing hypertension.[111] In contrast, physiologic hypertrophy in the athlete's heart does not lead to a decrease of the myocardial PCr/ATP ratio, either at rest or during stress[112]; experimental studies in exercise-trained rats had predicted this finding.[113] In the future, it will be important to unravel the molecular mechanisms responsible for these differences in energy metabolism between physiologic and pathologic hypertrophy.

Diabetes and Obesity

Other than via the well-recognized secondary mechanisms (e.g., accelerated coronary disease), diabetes has numerous deleterious effects on cardiac metabolism that may lead to cardiomyopathy. For example, the diabetic heart is insulin resistant and glucose utilization is impaired. Plasma free fatty acid levels are elevated, leading to increased expression of mitochondrial uncoupling proteins and reduced expression of glucose transporters (GLUT4). Several studies have examined cardiac energy metabolism in patients with maintained left ventricular (LV) ejection fraction and type 2[114–116] or type 1[117,118] diabetes mellitus and have uniformly shown reduced PCr/ATP ratios. Van der Meer et al.[119] observed no change in PCr/ATP in 78 type 2 diabetes mellitus men given either pioglitazone or metformin for 24 weeks, despite improvements in LV function. PCr/ATP ratios were found to correlate inversely with plasma free fatty acid levels[114] and with indices of diastolic function.[115,117] Shivu

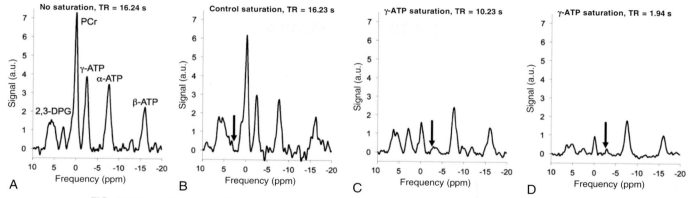

FIG. 9.7 Illustration of raw data used to measure the creatine kinase rate constant k_f at 3 T with the two repetition time saturation transfer (TwiST) protocol. (A) A 9-minute acquisition without any saturation used to determine M_0 from the peak height of the phosphocreatine (PCr) peak. This spectrum is also used to determine the saturation frequency of the γ-adenosine triphosphate (ATP) peak in the heart. (B) A 9-minute acquisition with control saturation at the frequency indicated by the arrow used to determine $M_0^{control}$. (C) A 22-minute acquisition with γ-ATP saturation *(arrow)* and long TR used to determine M_0' in the TwiST experiment, and $M'(TR_{long})$ in the triple repetition time saturation transfer (TRiST) experiment. (D) This 9-minute acquisition is only used in TRiST but not in TwiST. It is acquired with γ-ATP saturation *(arrow)* and short repetition time and used to determine $M'(TR_{short})$. TwiST uses acquisitions shown in B and C; TRiST uses acquisitions shown in B, C, and D; Q-corrected TwiST uses acquisitions shown in A, B, and C; and Q-corrected TRiST uses acquisitions shown in A, B, C, and D. (From Schar M, Gabr RE, El-Sharkawy AM, Steinberg A, Bottomley PA, Weiss RG. Two repetition time saturation transfer (TwiST) with spill-over correction to measure creatine kinase reaction rates in human hearts. *J Cardiov Magn Reson.* 2015;17:70.)

et al.[118] showed that in 25 asymptomatic type 1 diabetic patients, PCr/ATP was reduced (1.6 ± 0.2 vs. 2.1 ± 0.5 in controls) within 5 years of diagnosis and that this changed little more than 10 years after diagnosis (to 1.5 ± 0.4), whereas microvascular dysfunction worsened in diabetics over time (myocardial perfusion reserve index 1.7 ± 0.6 vs. 2.3 ± 0.4, $P = .005$). We recently showed in a study of 31 type 2 diabetic patients that exercise further reduced the PCr/ATP ratio (resting PCr/ATP was 1.74 ± 0.26 in patients vs. 2.07 ± 0.35 in controls, and dropped to 1.54 ± 0.26; $P = .005$), and that this correlated with myocardial perfusion reserve index from adenosine stress CMR imaging.[116]

Initial evidence also suggests reduced PCr/ATP ratios in patients with uncomplicated obesity and elevated free fatty acid levels.[120] For example, Rider et al.[121] demonstrated cardiac energetic differences between obese and normal-weight subjects by ^{31}P-MRS at rest: the obese group had a 15% lower PCr/ATP ratio (1.73 ± 0.40 vs. 2.03 ± 0.28; $P = .048$). During dobutamine stress, a further reduction in PCr/ATP occurred in the obese group (from 1.73 ± 0.40 to 1.53 ± 0.50; $P = .03$) but not in normal-weight subjects (from 1.98 ± 0.24 to 2.04 ± 0.34; $P = .50$). Together, these results suggest that early cardiac metabolic derangement as observed in diabetes and obesity may contribute to the later development of heart failure, suggesting a possible explanation for the increased incidence of heart failure in diabetes and obesity. However, intriguingly, it is also observed that obese patients with heart failure survive longer than normal-weight patients with heart failure, a phenomenon termed the "obesity paradox."[122,123]

Proton spectroscopy (^{1}H-MRS) is an established method to monitor triglyceride (TG) concentration ("fat fraction") in the liver[124–127] and heart.[128] Van der Meer et al.[129] investigated the effect of drinking 800 mL cream for 3 days on healthy young men, observing a more than doubling of hepatic TG concentration, but no significant effects on cardiac TG, function, or energetics. Holloway et al.[130] compared the effect of a 5-day high-fat or normal-fat diet in healthy males, observing a 9% ($P < .01$) reduction on cardiac PCr/ATP in the high-fat group. Recently, Levelt et al.[131] demonstrated that myocardial triglyceride content is an independent predictor of LV concentric remodeling and cardiac systolic strain in a study of 46 patients with type 2 diabetes.

Heart Failure

Experimental studies have firmly established altered energy metabolism as a hallmark of the chronically failing myocardium (see above). Initial clinical ^{31}P-MRS studies, however, which included mild stages of heart failure, did not find significant reductions of PCr/ATP ratios.[132–134] Hardy et al.[135] first reported that the myocardial PCr/ATP ratio is significantly reduced (from 1.80 ± 0.06 to 1.46 ± 0.07) in patients with symptomatic heart failure of ischemic or nonischemic etiology. Subsequently, we found that the decrease of PCr/ATP ratios in dilated cardiomyopathy (DCM) correlated with the New York Heart Association (NYHA) class[90] and with LV ejection fraction.[136] Thus PCr/ATP ratios decrease in advanced stages of heart failure (Fig. 9.8) but initially remain normal. This pattern was observed also by Leme et al. in a study of 39 patients with Chagas disease, whose PCr/ATP ratios at rest correlated with NYHA class[137] and where PCr/ATP dropped further during isometric handgrip exercise, consistent with the involvement of ischemia in Chagas disease.[138] PCr/ATP ratios also hold prognostic information on survival of patients with heart failure. We showed that in DCM, the myocardial PCr/ATP ratio was a better predictor of long-term survival than LV ejection fraction or NYHA class[139] (Fig. 9.9). It is known from experimental work that in heart failure, both PCr and ATP levels decrease in parallel,[140] and this cannot be detected by measurement of PCr/ATP ratios. Accordingly, using SLOOP (see above) in patients with heart failure because of DCM (ejection fraction 18%), Beer et al.[141] reported that absolute PCr levels were reduced by 51%, ATP levels by 35%, whereas the PCr/ATP ratio decreased by 25% only. Furthermore, significant correlations between LV volumes/ejection fraction and energetics were found, with the strongest correlations observed for PCr and the weakest for the PCr/ATP ratio. Thus ATP levels are reduced in human heart failure, and the true extent of changes in energy metabolism in heart failure is underestimated when PCr/ATP ratios rather than absolute

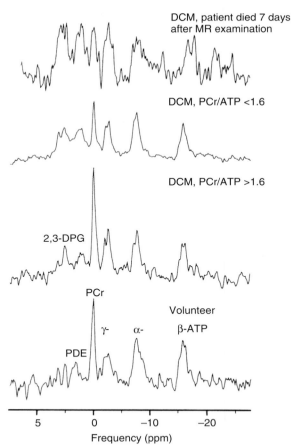

FIG. 9.8 Cardiac ^{31}P-magnetic resonance (MR) spectra. From bottom to top: volunteer; dilated cardiomyopathy with normal phosphocreatine/adenosine triphosphate (ATP) ratio; dilated cardiomyopathy with reduced phosphocreatine/ATP ratio; dilated cardiomyopathy with severely reduced phosphocreatine/ATP ratio; this patient died 7 days after the MR examination. *2,3-DPG*, 2,3-Diphosphoglycerate; *PDE*, phosphodiesters; *PCr*, phosphocreatine; γ-, α-, and β- are P atoms of adenosine triphosphate *(ATP)*. (From Neubauer S, Horn M, Cramer M, et al. Myocardial phosphocreatine-to-ATP ratio is a predictor of mortality in patients with dilated cardiomyopathy. *Circulation.* 1997;96:2190–2196.)

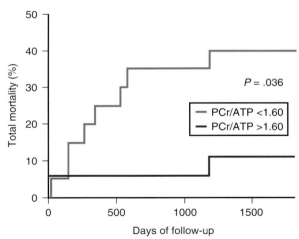

FIG. 9.9 Kaplan-Meier life table analysis for total mortality of dilated cardiomyopathy patients. Patients were divided into two groups, split by the myocardial phosphocreatine/adenosine triphosphate *(PCr/ATP)* ratio (<1.60 vs. >1.60). Patients with an initially low PCr/ATP ratio showed increased mortality over the study period of, on average, 2.5 years. (From Neubauer S, Horn M, Cramer M, et al. Myocardial phosphocreatine-to-ATP ratio is a predictor of mortality in patients with dilated cardiomyopathy. *Circulation.* 1997;96:2190–2196.)

years, and showing that CK flux was a significant predictor of heart failure outcomes even after correction for NYHA class, LV ejection fraction, and race. For each increase in CK flux of 1 μmol/g/s, risk of heart failure–related composite outcomes decreased by 32% to 39%.[44] Overall, therefore, ^{31}P-MRS may be valuable for prognosis evaluation in heart failure.

Heart failure trials from the past two decades show that energy-costly treatment, such as beta-receptor mimetics or phosphodiesterase inhibitors, increases mortality, whereas energy-sparing treatment, such as beta-blockers, angiotensin-converting enzyme (ACE) inhibitors, or angiotensin II receptor blockers, improves survival.[123] Thus one of the most promising future applications of clinical ^{31}P-MRS is monitoring of the cardiac energetic response to new forms of heart failure treatment, and it is likely that the PCr/ATP ratio or absolute concentrations of PCr and ATP are powerful surrogate parameters for mortality in this situation. For example, in 6 patients with DCM treated with ACE inhibitors, digitalis, diuretics and beta-blockers for 3 months, PCr/ATP ratios improved significantly during clinical recompensation, from 1.51 ± 0.32 to 2.15 ± 0.27.[90] However, no systematic controlled study has so far used ^{31}P-MRS to monitor cardiac energetics during heart failure treatment. A treatment trial using ^{31}P-MRS to monitor cardiac energetics has been reported for Friedreich ataxia. This primarily neurological disease is often associated with cardiomyopathy, as lack of the mitochondrial protein frataxin leads to deficient mitochondrial respiration and increased free radical damage. In patients with Friedreich ataxia treated with antioxidants (coenzyme Q and vitamin E) for 6 months, Lodi et al.[146] reported that the myocardial PCr/ATP ratio increased from 1.34 ± 0.59 to 2.02 ± 0.43, demonstrating that cardiac energy metabolism was markedly improved by antioxidative treatment. Hirsch et al. demonstrated that 600 mg allopurinol (a xanthine oxidase inhibitor) improved cardiac energetics in patients with heart failure (i.e., PCr/ATP increased by 11%, P < .02), and CK flux increased by 39% (from 2.07 ± 1.27 μmol/g/s to 2.87 ± 1.82 μmol/g/s, P < .007).[54] However, the 253 patient multicenter randomized controlled Xanthine Oxidase Inhibition for Hyperuricemic Heart Failure Patients (EXACT-HF) trial failed to observe any improvement in outcomes after 24-week administration

concentrations are measured. In a later study, Beer et al.[142] applied SLOOP ^{31}P-MRS before and after exercise training in a study involving 24 DCM patients. They demonstrated that exercise training improves LV function without causing deterioration in cardiac energetics. Similar results were obtained by Holloway et al.[143] in a study of 15 DCM patients using 3 T ^{31}P-MRS at rest and during exercise, where LV function improved but no significant changes in PCr/ATP were observed. Nakae et al.[144] used ^{1}H-MRS to demonstrate significant reductions of total creatine levels and a correlation of creatine and LV ejection fraction in patients with DCM.

Weiss et al.[53] showed a 50% reduction of CK reaction rates in mild-to-moderate heart failure, indicating that energy turnover rates are depressed to a greater extent than steady-state levels of PCr and ATP. Weiss et al.[145] subsequently measured the CK flux (i.e., ATP synthesis rate) in failing hypertrophied myocardium, suggesting that the kinetics of ATP turnover through CK distinguish failing from non-failing hypertrophic hearts more clearly than the relative or absolute CK metabolite pool sizes. Weiss et al. subsequently performed a prospective study following 58 heart failure patients for a median of 4.7

of allopurinol,[147] suggesting that effective treatment requires modification of more than this one aspect of the cardiac nitroso-redox balance.[148,149]

Frenneaux et al.[123] investigated the application of the antianginal drug perhexiline to treat heart failure in a series of studies. Perhexiline is believed to inhibit the metabolism of free fatty acids. In heart failure patients, perhexiline increased the rate of PCr recovery in skeletal muscle after exercise, indicating improved mitochondrial capacity.[150] Recently, Frenneaux et al.[151] published the results of a clinical trial in 50 patients with nonischemic heart failure, observing that treatment with perhexiline 200 mg once daily for 1 month was associated with a 30% increase in PCr/ATP (from 1.16 ± 0.39 to 1.51 ± 0.51; $P < .001$).[152]

Specific Gene Defects With Cardiac Pathology

Clinical cardiac ^{31}P-MRS has major potential for the noninvasive phenotyping of cardiomyopathies because of specific gene defects, which may eventually be identifiable by a specific metabolic profile. Most of the work in this area has been on hypertrophic cardiomyopathy (HCM), which is, in most cases, because of specific gene mutations associated with structural disarray of myofibrils and often with substantial increases of left ventricular wall thickness. Energetic derangement has been suggested as the common pathophysiologic mechanism underlying all forms of HCM,[153] and experimental studies of transgenic models of HCM confirm this.[154] Human studies in HCM[134,155–157] have uniformly shown reduced PCr/ATP ratios. For example, Jung et al.[158] demonstrated that in young, asymptomatic patients with HCM, PCr/ATP ratios were reduced, indicating that energetic imbalance occurs early in the disease process. They also reported that HCM patients with a familial history of the disease showed a more pronounced derangement of energetics than those patients without a family history.[159] Abraham et al.[160] observed a 24% reduction in myocardial PCr, 26% reduction in CK k_f, and 44% reduction in forward CK flux in patients with HCM caused by a point mutation of Arg403Gln compared with volunteers. They argue that the energetic deficit, even in patients without changes in cardiac function, means that the energetic deficit results from the mutation and is not simply a consequence of mechanical dysfunction.[160] Larger studies at 3 T have confirmed the derangement of energetics in HCM.[161,162] Dass et al.[163] demonstrated that in 35 patients with HCM, leg exercise further reduced PCr/ATP (1.56 ± 0.29 vs. 1.71 ± 0.35 at rest; $P = .02$), whereas there was no change on exercise in normal (2.16 ± 0.26 vs. 2.14 ± 0.35 at rest; $P = .98$). Frenneaux et al.[164] showed that treatment of HCM patients with perhexiline for 4.6 ± 1.8 months improved PCr/ATP (from 1.27 ± 0.02 to 1.73 ± 0.02, $P = .003$). Using ^{1}H-MRS, Nakae et al.[144] reported reduced total creatine content in patients with HCM. In the future, large patient groups with HCM and known specific gene defects will have to be studied to establish whether metabolic phenotyping by ^{31}P- and ^{1}H-MRS can identify the underlying genetic mutation.

Becker muscular dystrophy, an X-chromosome linked disease associated with the absence or altered expression of dystrophin in cardiac and skeletal muscle, may lead to the development of cardiomyopathy and heart failure. Clarke et al.[165] showed that both patients (PCr/ATP ratio 1.55 ± 0.33) and female gene carriers (1.37 ± 0.25) had significantly lower PCr/ATP ratios than control subjects (2.44 ± 0.33), although all of the carriers and most of the patients showed preserved left ventricular function. Thus energetic imbalance occurs early in the disease process and may contribute to the development of contractile dysfunction in Becker disease. Altered cardiac energetics have also been demonstrated in hereditary hemochromatosis,[166] in familial hypercholesterolemia,[167] where PCr/ATP ratios returned to normal after treatment with statins, and in Fabry disease where PCr/ATP in 23 patients was 1.68 ± 0.43 compared with 1.92 ± 0.50 in volunteers.[168]

Valvular Heart Disease

Experimental studies have shown impaired cardiac energy metabolism in advanced left ventricular hypertrophy.[169] Similarly, in patients with left ventricular hypertrophy resulting from aortic stenosis or incompetence, Conway et al.[170] detected reduced PCr/ATP ratios (1.1 ± 0.32 vs. 1.5 ± 0.2 in volunteers; mean $\pm$ standard deviation) when patients were in clinical heart failure, but PCr/ATP ratios were normal (1.56 ± 0.15) for clinically asymptomatic stages. Likewise, in patients with aortic valve disease, we showed reduced PCr/ATP ratios only for NYHA classes III and IV but not for classes I and II.[171] When matched for the degree of heart failure, energy metabolism was more affected in aortic stenosis (pressure overload) than in aortic incompetence. We also showed that in aortic stenosis, altered energetics correlated with left ventricular end-diastolic pressures and with end-diastolic wall stress.[171] We reported unchanged absolute ATP concentrations and a 28% decrease of PCr concentrations in aortic stenosis using SLOOP.[141] The time course of recovery of cardiac energetics during regression of hypertrophy after surgical valve replacement can also be monitored by ^{31}P-MRS.[172] When patients with aortic valve stenosis were studied before and 40 weeks after surgery, the PCr/ATP ratio increased from 1.28 ± 0.17 to 1.47 ± 0.14 (control subjects 1.43 ± 0.14); that is, energetic impairment was completely reversed 9 months after valve replacement. Energetics in aortic stenosis patients (1.45 ± 0.21 vs. 2.00 ± 0.25 in controls, $P < .001$) have been shown to correlate with perfusion, oxygenation, and LV functional defects, and to improve markedly 8 months after aortic valve replacement energetics (PCr/ATP 1.86 ± 0.48).[173] A recent multicenter randomized control trial of perhexiline to augment myocardial protection in patients with left ventricular hypertrophy undergoing cardiac surgery was halted early when it became clear that perhexiline did not provide an additional benefit in hemodynamic performance or attenuate myocardial injury in the hypertrophied heart secondary to aortic stenosis (AS).[174] Nevertheless, long-term prospective clinical studies of the role of energetics in valvular disease remain the best strategy to determine whether ^{31}P-MRS provides clinical information on the optimum timing of valve replacement.

Ischemic Heart Disease
Magnetic Resonance Spectroscopy Stress Testing to Detect Ischemia

Within seconds after reduction of oxygen supply, PCr levels decrease and inorganic phosphate increases; that is, these changes are extremely rapid indicators of myocardial ischemia (see above). If it were feasible to detect these metabolites in human myocardium with high temporal and spatial resolution, a ^{31}P-MRS-based "biochemical stress test" would be a powerful diagnostic tool for detecting exercise-induced regional ischemia, only requiring low levels of stress and without the need for intravenous agents or radiation. In selected patients with large anterior wall territories, which become ischemic on exercise, the feasibility of this principle has been demonstrated: Weiss et al. (Fig. 9.10) showed that in patients with high-grade stenosis of the left anterior descending or left main coronary arteries, PCr/ATP ratios were normal at rest, decreased during handgrip exercise (leading to a 30%–35% increase of cardiac work) from 1.5 ± 0.3 to 0.9 ± 0.2, and returned toward normal during recovery.[175] After revascularization, PCr/ATP ratios remained constant during exercise. These findings were reproduced by Yabe et al.,[176] who also demonstrated that a decrease of PCr/ATP ratios was only detected in patients with reversible defects on thallium scintigraphy (viable myocardium) but not in those with fixed thallium defects (scar), where PCr/ATP was already reduced at rest.[93] Najjar et al.[177] applied ^{31}P-MRS stress testing to investigate potential cardioprotective effects of RSR13 (an allosteric modifier of hemoglobin's affinity for oxygen)

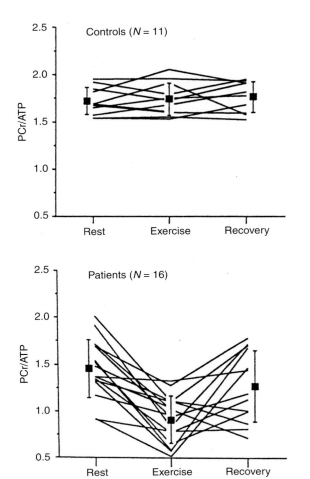

FIG. 9.10 Phosphocreatine/adenosine triphosphate *(PCr/ATP)* ratios. At rest, during handgrip exercise, and during recovery in controls and in patients with stenosis of the left anterior descending coronary artery. PCr/ATP decreased in patients but not in healthy volunteers. *ATP,* Adenosine triphosphate; *PCr,* phosphocreatine. (From Weiss RG, Bottomley PA, Hardy CJ, Gerstenblith G. Regional myocardial metabolism of high-energy phosphates during isometric-exercise in patients with coronary-artery disease. *N Engl J Med.* 1990;323:1593–1600.)

in seven subjects with coronary artery disease but did not observe significant changes in energetics,[177] in contrast to successful results in canine models.[178] Exercise testing has also been performed at 3 T.[116,179] With a ^{31}P-MRS stress test, we would also be able to test the efficacy of revascularization procedures or of established or new antianginal medication. It is conceivable that a "PCr threshold" may become a clinically relevant parameter as the level of exercise achievable without a decrease of myocardial PCr concentrations. This may in the future allow objective fine-tuning of antianginal therapy.

The pathophysiologic mechanisms of exercise-induced chest pain in women with a normal coronary angiogram remain unclear, but microvascular dysfunction and subsequent tissue ischemia in the absence of epicardial coronary stenoses has been postulated. Pohost's group[180] showed that in 7 out of 35 women with chest pain and normal coronary arteries, the PCr/ATP ratio decreased by $29 \pm 5\%$ during handgrip exercise, providing direct evidence of exercise-induced myocardial ischemia. In a subsequent study, they showed that, at 3-year follow-up, an initially abnormal ^{31}P-MRS stress test was a strong predictor of future cardiovascular events.[181] ^{31}P-MRS stress testing may facilitate the development and monitoring of treatment for this ubiquitous condition.

Myocardial Viability Assessment

Akinetic myocardium, supplied by a stenotic coronary artery, may be nonviable (scarred), or it may be viable, that is, stunned or hibernating. By readjusting the balance between oxygen supply and demand, hibernating myocardium has downregulated its contractility to reduce energy needs. Stunned myocardium shows transient contractile dysfunction following reperfusion after reversible ischemia. ^{31}P-MRS studies of animal ischemia-reperfusion models[182–186] have shown that in stunned and hibernating[187] myocardium, ATP levels remain close to normal, whereas myocardial scar tissue contains negligible amounts of ATP (<1% of normal levels). Thus a noninvasive diagnostic test that allows measurement of myocardial ATP levels with high spatial (1–5 mL) and acceptable temporal resolution (<30 minutes) should be attractive for viability assessment. For example, Kalil-Filho et al.[188] studied 29 patients with anterior myocardial infarction (MI) 4 days and 39 days after MI. All patients showed akinetic anterior myocardium, which had recovered function at the time of the second examination. PCr/ATP ratios were normal in stunned myocardium (1.51 ± 0.17 vs. 1.61 ± 0.18 in volunteers) and did not change during the recovery of contractile function (1.51 ± 0.17 vs. 1.53 ± 0.17). These observations were confirmed by Beer et al.,[189] who also showed that in patients with nonviable infarcts, failing to recover regional contractile function after 6 months, ^{31}P-spectra showed complete absence of PCr. The same group later reported the detection of inferior infarcts by "acquisition-weighted" ^{31}P-MRS.[190] However, loss of myocardial tissue because of necrosis and scar formation primarily leads to a reduction of both PCr and ATP, and the extent of viable tissue loss can therefore not be detected using the PCr/ATP ratio. Instead, measurement of absolute concentrations of high-energy phosphates is necessary. Yabe et al.[93] showed that absolute myocardial ATP content was significantly reduced in patients with fixed thallium defects (nonviable), but was unchanged in patients with reversible defects (viable myocardium). Bottomley et al.[191] also reported that the CK flux drops in infarcted tissue. Although these initial results are promising, substantial improvement in spatial resolution is necessary if ^{31}P-MRS evaluation of viability is to become competitive with current imaging methods of assessment.[192]

Viability detection may also be feasible by measuring total creatine content by localized ^{1}H-MRS[48–51] or potentially by CrCEST imaging,[52] because creatine concentrations in scar tissue are negligible. Due to the higher MR sensitivity of ^{1}H and because the concentration of CH_3-creatine protons is ~10-fold higher than ^{31}P-concentrations of ATP, the resolution of ^{1}H-MRS is superior to ^{31}P-MRS, currently at ~1 mL vs. ~70 mL. However, several methodologic hurdles (see earlier) remain to be overcome before clinical ^{1}H-MRS can be more widely applied.

Because the myocardial [23]Na signal is elevated in both acute necrosis and in chronic scar (see above), [23]Na-CMR may allow detection of myocardial viability without the use of external contrast agents. Due to 100% natural abundance, relatively high MR sensitivity (9.3% of ^{1}H) and tissue concentration (~140 mM extracellular, ~10 mM intracellular) of [23]Na, and due to its short T1 (~30 ms at 1.5 T), allowing for short TR, [23]Na yields the second-highest CMR resolution of all MR-detectable nuclei. [23]Na-CMR has been demonstrated with a resolution of up to 216 µL with 100 ms cine temporal resolution during a 19-minute scan in volunteers at 7 T,[72] which is a dramatic improvement compared with 392 µL resolution (in patients[193]) using an ECG-triggered 3D spoiled gradient echo sequence, in ~1 hour, at 1.5 T. In patients studied days and again more than 6 months after acute MI, Sandstede et al.[194] obtained the first in vivo [23]Na-MR images of infarcted human myocardium. All patients after subacute infarction and 12 out of 15 patients with chronic infarction showed an area of elevated [23]Na signal intensity that significantly correlated with wall motion abnormalities. In a follow-up study, we demonstrated that the total Na[+] signal remained significantly elevated in scar over a time period of at least 1 year.[195] Bottomley recently summarized the status of [23]Na-CMR as a potential clinical imaging modality.[74] He identified the primary challenge for [23]Na-CMR as being a need to demonstrate unique insight beyond that available, for example, by [1]H-CMR extracellular volume mapping.[196]

Thus ^{31}P-MRS, ^{1}H-MRS, and ^{23}Na-CMR/MRS provide an array of methods that might in the future become the preferred approach for viability assessment, if substantially higher spatial resolution can be achieved. Unlike currently used techniques, such as dobutamine stress echocardiography, nuclear imaging, or delayed enhancement CMR, the MRS approach provides intrinsic contrast for distinction between viable and nonviable myocardium, is radiation-free, does not require intravenous agents, and can avoid stress testing.

Hypoxia/Altitude

Volunteers exposed to normobaric hypoxia (80% O_2 saturation) for 20 hours showed PCr/ATP of 1.7 versus 2.0 before exposure (a 15% reduction).[197] A group of 14 healthy volunteers scanned 4 days after a 17-day trek to Mount Everest Base Camp (5300 m) showed an 18% ($P < .01$) reduction in cardiac PCr/ATP, which suggests that reduced cardiac PCr/ATP ratios may be a general response to hypoxia, whether that be because of the environment or disease.[198] However, a similar study in skeletal muscle observed no significant change in exercising energetics in subjects who had climbed Mount Everest.[199]

MAGNETIC RESONANCE SPECTROSCOPY AT 3 T AND 7 T

The most promising route for the improvement of spatial and temporal resolution of MRS is the use of higher magnetic field strengths, because MRS methods are fundamentally still signal-to-noise limited.

Early attempts to increase the field strength[200,201] were limited by the technical prototype nature of the magnets available at that time. From 2009, significant (~2×) gains were demonstrated for ^{31}P-MRS at 3 T compared with 1.5 T in volunteers[82,202,203] and in HCM patients.[161] Proton ^{1}H-MRS also improves significantly at 3 T.[128,204] In the last decade, methods for absolute quantitation[102] for measuring the creatine kinase forward rate constant k_f and ATP flux[35,88] have also been developed. 3 T ^{31}P-MRS has been used in tens of patient studies in Oxford and elsewhere to date.

Since 2011, we have pioneered the use of ultra-high field 7 T scanners for cardiac ^{31}P-MRS. We have observed further 2.8× gains in SNR (compared with 3 T) in volunteers,[80] and a similar 2.6× gain in DCM patients.[81] We have already demonstrated adiabatic excitation[205] and made the first 3D-resolved cardiac creatine kinase k_f measurements[36] using the 7 T system. Realizing the potential of 7 T scanners will require significant continuing methodologic development[83,205a] to use the increased SNR, while avoiding excessive RF heating, line broadening, or spatial inhomogeneity. Nevertheless, non-^{1}H MR spectroscopy and imaging is expected to be one of the principal beneficiaries of ultra-high field MR systems, as exemplified in Figs. 9.4 and 9.6.[206,207]

MODELING STUDIES

The changes seen in ^{31}P spectra reflect the latter part of the cardiac energy supply through the creatine kinase shuttle. Human hyperpolarized [13]C

studies should be able to probe some of the earlier substrate utilization steps. Technologies for genetic manipulation of animal models, for optical and electron microscopy, and computer modeling of biologic systems have all advanced considerably since Bessman and Geiger proposed the compartmentalized creatine kinase shuttle[18] (reviewed in references[208–211]).

Several recent experiments are challenging our understanding of the role of the CK shuttle in the heart. For example, genetically manipulated mouse models with selective knockout[212–215] or overexpression[216] of the various components of energy metabolism have demonstrated the crucial role of cardiac energetics in normal and failing heart.

Bottomley et al.[217] performed diffusion-weighted ^{31}P spectroscopy confirming a b-value for PCr consistent with the CK shuttle hypothesis in skeletal muscle.

However, studies using a combination of high-resolution 3D electron microscopy, optical fluorescence microscopy, and focused ultraviolet UV laser destruction of mitochondria are lending fresh impetus to the notion of a mitochondrial reticulum[218–221] capable of delivering energy to myofibrils in the form of a mitochondrial electrochemical gradient $\Delta\Psi$.

It will be exciting in the years ahead to see how the results from these many methods can be synthesized into an improved understanding of cardiac energetics, and particularly the roles of creatine kinase,[20,222] as a temporal and spatial energy buffer.[26–28,223–225]

PERSPECTIVE AND GENERAL CONCLUSIONS

MR spectroscopy allows for the noninvasive assessment of many aspects of cardiac metabolism in the normal and diseased heart, providing a wealth of information that should, in theory, be clinically relevant for patient management. The main obstacle for the widespread implementation of cardiac MRS is its technical complexity and limited resolution, and a major technological effort is required to substantially improve spatial and temporal resolution. Also, to reduce measurement variability to less than 5%, high signal/noise spectra need to be acquired. Finally, standardized acquisition and quantification protocols will have to be developed and agreed upon to provide clinicians with reliable measurements, which are also comparable among different centers. These goals should be achievable in the coming years by a major dedicated technical development effort on coil design, sequence design, and in particular on high-field magnets and hyperpolarization methods. High-resolution metabolic imaging would then finally become a reality in patients with ischemic heart disease, heart failure, valve disease, and genetic cardiomyopathy.

ACKNOWLEDGMENTS

S.N. acknowledges support from the Oxford NIHR Biomedical Research Centre and from the Oxford British Heart Foundation Centre of Research Excellence. C.T.R. is funded by a Sir Henry Dale Fellowship from the Wellcome Trust and the Royal Society (098436/Z/12/Z).

REFERENCES

A full reference list is available online at ExpertConsult.com

10

Special Considerations for Cardiovascular Magnetic Resonance: Safety, Electrocardiographic Setup, Monitoring, and Contraindications

Pieter van der Bijl, Victoria Delgado, and Jeroen J. Bax

During the last three decades, cardiovascular magnetic resonance (CMR) has developed into an important diagnostic clinical tool in cardiology. Not only the anatomy of the heart but also its function, metabolism, and perfusion, as well as the coronary arteries, can be evaluated with CMR. There are advantages of CMR over other diagnostic imaging methods: first, CMR does not use ionizing radiation; second, the radiofrequency (RF) radiation penetrates bony and air-filled structures without attenuation; third, CMR gives additional diagnostic information about tissue characteristics; and, finally, CMR provides three-dimensional (3D) images or images of arbitrarily oriented slices.

However, when performing CMR, particular precautions must be taken. Because CMR operates with high static and gradient magnetic fields, special safety regulations must be taken into account and certain contraindications must be considered. This chapter reviews the safety, electrocardiographic (ECG) setup, patient monitoring, and contraindications to CMR; in particular, the issue of devices (pacemakers, implantable cardioverter defibrillators [ICDs]) as well as coronary stents and prosthetic heart valves, is addressed.

SAFETY OF CARDIOVASCULAR MAGNETIC RESONANCE

General Issues

CMR generally takes longer than other diagnostic modalities (although the time is significantly shortened with real-time imaging[1]), and the confined space in which the patient is placed is rather narrow, which some patients find uncomfortable. During CMR, communication with the patient may be difficult because of interfering noise from the gradient coils. On the other hand, CMR is entirely noninvasive. Overall, the safety issues during CMR that may pose potential safety concerns can be summarized as follows[2]:

1. Biologic effects of the static magnetic field
2. Ferromagnetic attractive effects of the static magnetic field on certain devices
3. Potential effects on the relatively slow time-varying magnetic field gradients
4. Effects of the rapidly varying RF magnetic fields, including RF power deposition concerns
5. Auditory considerations of noise from the gradients
6. Safety considerations concerning superconducting magnet systems
7. Psychological effects

8. Possible effects of the intravenous use of magnetic resonance (MR) contrast agents
9. Patient safety during stress conditions

The safety concerns inherent to these issues are discussed.

Biologic Effects

Concerning the biologic effects of a static magnetic field, many structures in animals and humans are affected by magnetic fields. Many potential biologic effects and different magnitudes of magnetic fields have been examined, including the effect of the field on cardiac contractility and function. Gulch and colleagues concluded that static magnetic fields used in CMR do not constitute any hazard in terms of cardiac contractility.[3] These magnetic fields do not increase ventricular vulnerability, as assessed by the repetitive response threshold and the ventricular fibrillation threshold.[4] In one of the investigations, however, cardiac cycle length was shown to be altered.[5] Two studies reported that lymphocytes from blood samples obtained in humans exposed to a 1.5 tesla (T) field demonstrated DNA double-strand breaks and changes consistent with mild inflammation.[6,7] However, these studies have significant limitations and four recent reports have found no such DNA damage.[8–11] Another area of concern is CMR during pregnancy, for example, teratogenicity (cellular effects, for example on differentiation, have been demonstrated in animals), damage to the fetal inner ear due to noise exposure and tissue heating effects, although none have been documented to cause harm.[12] A recent study of CMR in pregnancy (including first trimester) found CMR to be safe.[13] Furthermore, 7 T scanners are becoming more common (although currently very rarely used for CMR), and have been associated with transient dizziness upon movement of the subject into the scanner (postulated to be due to induced currents affecting vestibular hair cells in the inner ear), as well as a metallic taste in the mouth in up to 11% of patients.[14] Numerous biologic effects on other systems have been investigated extensively, and it may be concluded that no deleterious biologic effects from static magnetic fields used in CMR have yet been established.

Ferromagnetism

The physical effect of the static magnetic field consists of a potential health hazard from the attractive effect on ferromagnetic objects. Ferromagnetic objects can be defined as those in which a strong intrinsic magnetic field can be induced when they are exposed to an external magnetic field. The existence of different kinds of scanners with different

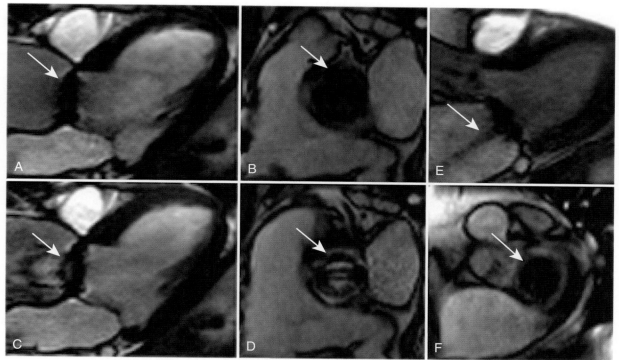

FIG. 10.1 Bileaflet, tilting disc, mechanical aortic valve prosthesis *(arrow)* during diastole on steady-state free precession (SSFP) imaging (A). Short-axis view of the same prosthesis *(arrow)* as in A during diastole, clearly demonstrating an artifact (B). Systolic image of the prosthesis *(arrow)* in A (C). Systolic, short-axis view of the same prosthesis *(arrow)* as in B, with both leaflets visible in the open position (D). Bileaflet, tilting disc, mechanical mitral valve prosthesis during systole on an SSFP image, demonstrating a regurgitant jet *(arrow)* (E). Short-axis view of the same prosthesis *(arrow)* as in E (F). (From Von Knobelsdorff-Brenkenhoff F, Trauzeddel RF, Schulz-Menger J. Cardiovascular magnetic resonance in adults with previous cardiovascular surgery. *Eur Heart J Cardiovasc Imaging.* 2014;15(3):235–248.)

shielding makes the discussion about this topic even more crucial. When dealing with a static magnetic field, two types of physical concerns exist.

First, there are concerns about forces exerted on ferromagnetic objects within, on, or distant from the patient. These forces result in rotational (torque) or translational (attractive) motion of the object. Within the human body, a ferromagnetic metallic structure may be sufficiently attracted, or have a sufficient amount of torque exerted, to create a hazardous situation. These factors should be carefully considered before subjecting a patient with a ferromagnetic implant or material to CMR, particularly if the device is located in a potentially dangerous area of the body, where movement or dislodgment of the device could injure the patient. Another potentially injurious effect is known as the *projectile,* or *missile,* effect. This refers to the fact that ferromagnetic objects have the potential to gain sufficient speed during attraction to the magnet that the accumulated kinetic energy could be injurious or even lethal if the object were to strike a patient. Numerous studies have been performed to assess the ferromagnetic qualities of various metallic implants and materials.[15–19] The results indicate that patients with certain metallic implants or prostheses that are nonferromagnetic or are minimally deflected by static magnetic fields can safely undergo CMR. The literature on this topic has been extensively reviewed and compiled.[17] However, there are common misconceptions about what types of objects are ferromagnetic. The most important misconception is that stainless steel is ferromagnetic, when it is not. Patients with stainless steel implants can therefore be imaged safely, except for a small number of well-described exceptions, as discussed later. The implant will interfere locally with the images; for example, signal loss occurs around metallic prosthetic valves (Fig. 10.1) and sternal wires (Fig. 10.2) after bypass surgery, but this does not make the imaging hazardous.[20] Nonstainless steel, which may be ferromagnetic, is not used for human implants, but is commonly used for oxygen cylinders, for example. Finally, batteries are typically attracted to the magnet, and this is one of the problems of imaging pacemakers.

The second type of physical concern deals with magnetically sensitive equipment, the functioning of which may be adversely affected by the magnetic field. The most common of these is the cardiac pacemaker. Most pacemakers include a reed relay switch whereby the sensing mechanism can be bypassed and pacing in the asynchronous mode can occur. This switch is activated when a magnet of sufficient strength is held over the pacemaker.[21] In addition, the function of cardiac pacemakers may be influenced by field strengths as low as 17 gauss.[21] In practice, reed switch closure can be expected in all pacemakers placed in the bore of the scanner. Pacemaker and ICD function is considered again later in this chapter.

Effect of Rapidly Switched Magnetic Fields

CMR exposes the patient to rapid variations of magnetic fields by the transient application of magnetic gradients during imaging. The effect of rapidly switched magnetic fields may be the induction of currents within the body or any other electrical conductor, according to Faraday's law. The current is dependent on the time rate of change of the magnetic field (dB/dt), the cross-sectional area of the conducting tissue loop, and the conductivity of the tissue. Biologic effects of induced currents can be caused either by power deposition by the induced currents (thermal

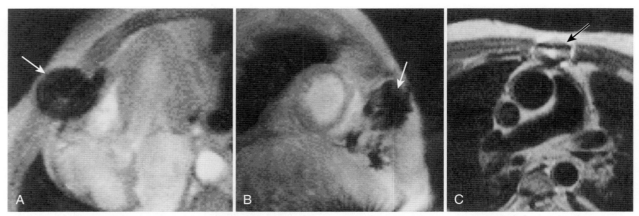

FIG. 10.2 Cardiovascular magnetic resonance image of a patient with sternal wires after bypass grafting. The artifact is clearly seen *(arrows)* on the horizontal long-axis (A) and short-axis (B) gradient echo cine images, and to a much lesser extent, on the transaxial spin echo image (C). (Courtesy Dr. Dudley Pennell, Royal Brompton Hospital, London.)

effects) or by direct effects of the current (nonthermal effects). Thermal effects as a result of switching gradients are not believed to be clinically significant.[22–24] Possible nonthermal effects include stimulation of nerve or muscle cells. The threshold currents for nerve stimulation and ventricular fibrillation are known to be much higher than the estimated current densities induced under clinical CMR conditions. The echo planar imaging method, however, involves more rapidly changing magnetic field gradients, and peripheral muscle stimulation in humans has been reported.[25] Such considerations have become more important as new technology has allowed the introduction of commercially available ultrafast gradient switching systems, and guidelines for maximum magnetic field variation are under development.

Radiofrequency Time-Varying Field

The transmitted RF time-varying field induces electrical currents within the tissue of the patient. The majority of this power is transformed into heat within the patient's tissue as a result of ohmic heating. The time-varying magnetic gradients have the potential to cause either thermal or nonthermal biologic effects. The distinction between these two is a matter of frequency, waveform shape, and magnitude. The discussion about nonthermal effects from RF magnetic fields is controversial because of questions about the relationship between chronic exposure to electromagnetic fields over many years and the causation of cancer or developmental abnormalities. The most recent evidence suggests that proximity to power lines is not injurious.[26] Clearly, acute exposure of a patient to short-term RF fields for a diagnostic CMR examination is different from chronic exposure. The induced currents from RF magnetic fields are unable to cause nerve excitations. One of the difficulties faced by medicine is proving that a procedure is not injurious because of anecdotal case reports of adverse events and publication bias toward nonneutral reports.[27] This issue is also faced by such a well-established technology as ultrasound, where safety concerns have been raised over acoustic exposure.[28]

In contrast to the insignificant thermal effects caused by switched gradients, however, thermal effects as a result of RF pulses are of significant concern. The main biologic effects induced by RF fields are therefore related to the thermogenic qualities of the RF field. A general point of discussion is the appropriate safety regulations for levels of magnetic field strength in CMR imaging. Application of the fundamental law of electrostimulation is well established, both on theoretical and experimental grounds. Application of this law, in combination with Maxwell's law, yields an equation called the *fundamental law of*

magnetostimulation, which has the hyperbolic form of a strength-duration curve and allows an estimation of the lowest possible value of the magnetic flux density capable of stimulating nerves and muscles. Calculations have shown that the threshold for heart excitation is more than 200 times higher than for nerve and muscle stimulation, depending on pulse duration.[29] However, in clinical practice, some precautions are necessary. First and most importantly, the specific absorption rate of the imaging sequence being operated is monitored by the scanner software and must be kept below limits set by such bodies as the US Food and Drug Administration (FDA). Second, circumstances that could enhance the possibility of heating injury should be avoided. This includes ensuring the prevention of loops that could act as aerials within the scanner and enhance the heating effect locally. Therefore, patients should not be allowed to cross their legs (loop via the pelvis) or clasp their hands (loop via the shoulder and upper chest). The simple use of pillows prevents such problems. Other possible loops include the ECG leads, which should always be run out of the scanner parallel to the main field, and not looped across the chest. Finally, pacemaker and ICD leads make excellent aerials. The pacemaker lead can heat significantly during CMR and become a potential hazard (discussed later). Another consideration in patients after cardiac surgery is the effect of retained epicardial pacemaker leads. These leads can be left in place after surgery, and they may therefore act as an antenna during CMR. Studies have suggested that such short retained epicardial wires do not pose a significant problem.[30,31]

Finally, the use of ECG electrodes, which are essential for cardiac gating, must be considered. Metallic ECG electrodes may cause burns during CMR, but this risk can be reduced with the use of carbon fiber electrodes, and these have now become standard.[32,33]

Auditory Considerations

During CMR, the gradient coils and adjacent conductors produce a repetitive sound because they act essentially as loudspeakers, with current being driven through them while they are in a magnetic field. Auditory considerations should therefore be taken into account when imaging a patient. The amplitude of this noise depends on factors such as the physical configuration of the magnet, the pulse sequence type, timing specifications of the pulse sequence, and the amount of current passing through these coils.[34] In general, the amplitude of the generated noise from the clinical CMR scanners remains between 65 and 95 dB. However, there have been reported instances of temporary hearing impairment as a result of CMR. Magnet-safe headphones or wax earplugs are readily available and have been shown to prevent hearing loss, and these are in common use.[35] Systems combining sound attenuation with the facility to play music of the patient's choice are also available. Research on the reduction of noise in MR scanners is ongoing, and the use of antinoise is one area of interest.[36]

Superconducting System Issues

Most superconducting CMR scanner systems use liquid helium. The helium maintains the magnet coils in their superconducting state. Helium achieves the gaseous state at approximately −269°C (4 K). If for any reason the temperature within the cryostat rises, or in a system quench, the helium will enter the gaseous state. This means a marked increase in volume and thereby pressure within the cryostat. A pressure-sensitive valve is designed to give way to the gaseous helium, which is always vented outside the CMR scanner room. However, it is possible that some helium gas is released into the imaging room should the system not work perfectly. Asphyxia and frostbite are potential hazards if a patient is exposed to helium vapor for a prolonged time, although there are no reports of such an occurrence in the medical community. For older scanners that still use a buffer of liquid nitrogen within the system (boils at 77 K), an oxygen monitor is recommended in the scanner room. Cryogenic dewars should be stored away from the scanner and in well-ventilated areas.

Psychological Effects

Claustrophobia or other psychological problems may be encountered in up to 10% of patients undergoing CMR, although on average, the incidence is closer to 2% to 4%, and this can be reduced further to a small number of intractably anxious patients by the use of explanation, reassurance, and where necessary, light sedation with, for example, 2 to 5 mg intravenous (IV) diazepam.[37,38] The development of shorter magnets and open designs are promising, although 39% of patients experienced some level of claustrophobia in a short-bore scanner and 26% in an open-bore scanner in a direct comparison.[39]

Such problems are related to a variety of factors, including the restrictive dimensions of the scanner, the duration of the examination, the noise, and the ambient conditions within the magnet bore.[40] Fortunately, adverse psychological effects with CMR are usually transient. In a study reported by Weinreb and colleagues, based on the experience of 450 patients undergoing CMR and computed tomography (CT) examinations, it was clearly shown that patients often prefer the CMR study, although CMR took longer.[41] Furthermore, the patient is placed into a confined space and there are difficulties in communicating with the patient during CMR scanning because of the noise from the gradient coils and the necessity of eliminating all extraneous RF sources from the examination room. To a certain extent, this can be avoided when the patient assumes a prone position in the scanner, facilitating communication with the outside surroundings.[42] Simple maneuvers, such as using mirrors, also help in allowing the patient a clear view of the scanning room. Allowing the anxious patient to visit the scanner before the appointment gives the patient an opportunity to become familiar with the facility and staff.

Safety Considerations Associated With CMR Contrast Agents

The safety profile of the contrast agents containing gadolinium currently on the market is extremely good. Their safety profile is well documented.[43,44] The median lethal dose of gadopentetate dimeglumine (Gd-DTPA) is roughly 10 mmol/kg, which is 100 times the diagnostic dose and exemplifies the wide safety margin that these contrast agents enjoy. Patient tolerance is also high, and the prevalence of adverse reactions is approximately 2%. Among the reactions related to the IV

administration of gadolinium contrast agents are headache, nausea, vomiting, local burning or cool sensation, and hives. There have been reported incidents of anaphylactoid reactions associated with IV injection, although the frequency of this appears to be approximately 1 per 100,000 doses.[45] The safety margins with these agents appear to be considerably better than with x-ray contrast agents, although issues of nephrogenic systemic fibrosis are a concern in patients with severely impaired renal function, and there are differences in safety between the commercially available gadolinium contrast agents favoring the tighter-bound chelates (see Chapter 3). Evidence of cerebral deposition (especially globus pallidus and dentate nucleus) of gadolinium-based contrast agents has emerged from animal and human studies, although the mechanism(s) and clinical implications are currently unknown.[46,47] The risk of cerebral deposition appears related to the number of administrations of gadolinium-based contrast.[48] The use of gadolinium in pregnancy depends on the risk-benefit ratio, as in general contrast agents are best avoided. Gadolinium can be used and safety appears good, but with a possible small increase in adverse outcomes, the interpretation of which is limited by small numbers.[13] For CMR, these agents are used to increase contrast between blood and soft tissue for cine imaging for functional studies or angiography, to enhance cardiac tumors and cysts, to assess myocardial perfusion, and to examine for myocardial infiltration. In summary, FDA-approved gadolinium complexes can be safely used in patients with cardiac disorders.

Multiple new CMR contrast agents are being developed and investigated. These are mainly gadolinium complexes, sometimes with novel binding molecules for special actions, but in addition, iron-based compounds are being developed. Some of these agents (e.g., gadofosveset) bind to albumin and are retained in the vascular system and do not leak into the extravascular space. The adverse-effect profile of gadofosveset appears similar to other gadolinium-based agents, although a prolongation of the corrected QT interval (without any dysrhythmias) has been reported. These agents may have clinical utility for angiography, possibly in the coronaries, and for functional imaging. Hyperpolarized CMR—executed with tracers such as 1-^{13}C pyruvate—has only recently been introduced to humans and safety data are limited.[49] Molecular imaging employs "probes," which bind to molecular targets either actively or passively by accumulation, and trace various anatomical and functional processes, such as thrombus formation, angiogenesis, atherosclerotic plaque, and fibrosis development.[50,51] Most of these techniques have only been tested in animals, and safety data in humans are scarce.

Patient Safety During Stress Conditions

A concern with stress CMR scans has been the ability to handle emergency situations. Patient monitoring during stress conditions is a critical issue because myocardial ischemia can be provoked in patients with coronary artery disease. Commercial equipment is available for noninvasive monitoring of blood pressure, heart rate, oxygen saturation, and other vital parameters in CMR scanners. The most crucial difference compared with conventional exercise testing outside a magnetic field is the lack of a diagnostic ECG, in particular, at high levels of stress, precluding the proper assessment of stress-induced ST-segment changes. This holds for both conventional exercise using a specially adapted bicycle ergometer and pharmacologically induced stress. Under these circumstances, only heart rate can be monitored reliably. When performing pharmacologic stress CMR (e.g., with dipyridamole, adenosine, regadenoson, or dobutamine), an experienced physician should be present during the examination, and appropriate treatments for complications should be in direct proximity. Dipyridamole (half-life 30 minutes), adenosine (half-life 10 seconds) and regadenoson (half-life 3 minutes) are vasodilators. These agents have similar side effects, such as hypotension, arrhythmias, and bradycardia. During adenosine infusion, atrioventricular (AV) heart block may develop in a small percentage of patients (0.7%–2.8%), although this is usually asymptomatic and self-limited. When patients are symptomatic, the short physical half-life of adenosine means that heart rhythm and symptoms can be restored very quickly by halting the infusion. As a suitable antagonist to dipyridamole, adenosine, and regadenoson, aminophylline may be given slowly at an initial dose of 50 mg IV up to a maximum dose of 250 mg if necessary. In the case of persisting advanced heart block, 0.5 mg atropine IV should be administered up to a total dose of 3 mg. Dipyridamole and adenosine should not be administered to patients with asthma, whereas regadenoson is safe in patients with asthma and chronic obstructive pulmonary disease, because of its more selective action on A_{2A} receptors. Adenosine, and dipyridamole indirectly (by inhibiting the degradation of adenosine), acts on A_1, A_{2A}, A_{2B}, and A_3 receptors. A_{2A} receptors mediate coronary and peripheral vasodilation, whereas A_1, A_{2A}, A_{2B}, and A_3 receptors cause bronchoconstriction and AV block.[52] A further advantage of regadenoson is the fact that it can be administered as a bolus, therefore not requiring a CMR-compatible infusion pump.[52] Dobutamine (half-life 2 minutes) is a beta-agonist leading to an increase in cardiac inotropy (contractility) and chronotropy (heart rate). Common side effects are palpitations, and less commonly, arrhythmias, such as supraventricular tachycardia and (nonsustained) ventricular tachycardia. Dobutamine can be safely administered to patients with asthma.[53] The actions of dobutamine can be counteracted by IV administration of a short-acting beta-blocking agent, such as esmolol. In the case of cardiac arrest or ventricular fibrillation, the recommendations should be followed according to published guidelines, such as those proposed by the European Resuscitation Council.[54] In every CMR facility, an alarm system and a written flow chart should be visually available, with the necessary instructions in case of emergency. It is necessary to be able to remove the patient from the examination room quickly (preferably within 20 seconds) to an area where emergency treatment can be performed safely, away from the hazards of the magnetic field. A nonferromagnetic stretcher stored in the scanner room or a detachable scanner table is ideal. A cardiac arrest trolley must be maintained in close proximity to the scanner room, and all staff should undergo regular training in cardiopulmonary resuscitation techniques. Regular checks should be made of both the resuscitation equipment and the alarm system.

PATIENT MONITORING AND ELECTROCARDIOGRAPHIC SETUP

Patient monitoring during CMR poses problems that will not be familiar to users of other technologies, such as echocardiography. Ferrous metal, which is present in most monitoring equipment, can distort the magnetic field, and such an item has the potential to become a projectile. In addition, monitoring wires that are attached to the patient, leaving the scanner, and passing to another room may act as an antenna for stray RF signals. Electrical equipment in the scanner room also can act as a source of RF noise. All of these disturbances may result in image degradation. Therefore, specific solutions to these problems have been designed.

Commercially available CMR-compatible monitoring equipment, including that used to measure ECG, blood pressure, and chest wall movements, as well as for general anesthesia, has been tested in several studies.[55,56] Satisfactory monitoring can be obtained and images obtained during its use can be evaluated adequately.[57] For some monitoring, simple solutions work, such as that reported by Roth and associates, who measured arterial blood pressure outside

the CMR scanner by lengthening the rubber tubing connected to a blood pressure cuff.[57] The newest monitoring equipment eliminates the need for wires and tubes to leave the scanning room by using a microwave transmitter communicating with a slave display unit in the operating room.

The CMR procedure depends on a high-quality ECG signal for routine imaging, and each manufacturer has developed its own solution to the problems posed. Fiberoptic transmission of ECG signals for gating is now common, and this significantly reduces RF pulse artifacts in the ECG. Felblinger and coworkers showed that this type of system could yield signals almost free from interference, during both conventional and high gradient activity sequences, such as during echo planar imaging.[58–60] From this signal, the authors also developed a method for respiration monitoring during MR sequences. Third-party ECG solutions are also now being incorporated into the latest generation of scanners, and these come with specific ECG recommendations for lead placement. Carbon fiber electrodes are required to eliminate the risk of burning that has been reported with standard metallic ECG electrodes.[32] Typical lead placement is the result of compromise. A better signal results from widely spaced electrodes, but this results in more artifact from the gradients. In general, therefore, the leads are kept relatively close together, and on the left side, which reduces the magnetohydrodynamic effect (the effect of systolic aortic flow causing surface potentials on the ECG that distort the ST segment; Fig. 10.3). A typical lead placement that is commonly adopted is shown in Fig. 10.4. Some centers have found ECG gating using electrodes on the back to be successful, but this is not widely used. The ECG leads should not be allowed to form loops, which could present a burning hazard, and they should be braided together and brought out of the magnet while aligned parallel to the bore to reduce electrical interference. Keeping the electrical cables short is helpful, and fiberoptic conversion modules are therefore often very close to the patient's chest. Switching between the ECG traces sometimes allows flexibility to reduce gating errors from tall T-waves or electrical interference. One thing is certain, however, and that is that time spent ensuring that the ECG is stable and working correctly at the start of the scan is time very well spent.

An alternative technique to routine surface ECG recording has been described by Fischer and colleagues using vectorcardiography, and has been widely implemented.[61] The system examines the 3D orientation of the ECG signal and uses the calculated vector of the QRS complex as a filter mechanism to ignore electrical signals, which are of similar

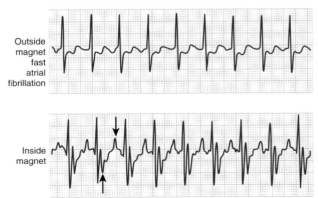

FIG. 10.3 The magnetohydrodynamic effect. The top trace was recorded in a patient with atrial fibrillation outside of the magnet, and the bottom trace, inside. Note the distortion of the ST segment *(arrows)* caused by added potentials arising from systolic flow in the aorta. (Courtesy Dr. Dudley Pennell, Royal Brompton Hospital, London.)

Outside magnet fast atrial fibrillation

Inside magnet

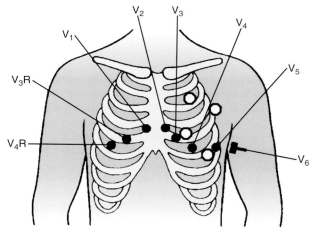

FIG. 10.4 Typical electrode placement for cardiovascular magnetic resonance. The conventional chest leads *(black circles)* are shown for comparison, and the positions of the four carbon electrocardiographic electrodes over the left chest are indicated *(white circles)*. (Courtesy Dr. Dudley Pennell, Royal Brompton Hospital, London.)

timing and similar magnitude in the cardiac cycle, but a different vector. The system as reported identified the QRS complex correctly in 100% of cases, with 0.2% false-positive findings. In a subsequent study in normal individuals and patients with supraventricular extrasystoles, the same authors showed that vector cardiography-based triggering provided nearly 100% triggering performance during CMR examinations.[62] This system represents a significant improvement for CMR in stabilizing this important gating signal.

Should interpretation prove impossible for technical reasons, a standard vascular Doppler can be used to monitor heart rate during CMR. The Doppler and telemetric ECG do not contain enough ferromagnetic material to cause visible image degradation. Jorgensen and associates evaluated whether patients could be monitored during CMR with 1.5 T machines in a manner that complies with monitoring standards.[63]

The high magnetic field can interfere with normal functioning of equipment, not only monitoring equipment but also smaller items such as infusion pumps used for stress testing. In general, the influence of the CMR scanner on nearby equipment depends on several factors, such as the strength of the CMR magnetic field, the proximity of the equipment to the scanner, the amount of ferromagnetic material in the equipment, and the design of the electrical circuitry.

Finally, simple devices, such as closed-circuit television and a two-way intercommunication system, also aid in monitoring by allowing a constant view of the patient and easy communication if the patient is in discomfort. However, the latter may be impaired during imaging as a result of the noise of the gradients. Because sequences are now commonly being reduced in duration to a breath-hold, however, this limitation is becoming much less important.

CONTRAINDICATIONS TO CARDIOVASCULAR MAGNETIC RESONANCE

In general, there are potential hazards with artifacts of ferromagnetic and nonferromagnetic materials in CMR, for example, neurosurgical clips and ocular implants.[64–66] The (relative) contraindications of these materials for CMR are dependent on factors such as the degree of ferromagnetism, the geometry of the material, the gradient (for force), and the field strength (for torque) of the imaging magnet and many other factors.

General Contraindications to Cardiovascular Magnetic Resonance

There are a number of circumstances in which CMR is better avoided. This is because of reports of death or harm that have occurred. Prominent among these are patients with cerebral aneurysm clips, which have become dislodged by MR, causing fatal cerebral hemorrhage. Modern clips are not ferromagnetic and are safe, but the problem is establishing the type of clip with certainty before performing CMR. In general, therefore, CMR should be avoided in these patients unless written information is available and appropriate advice from a neurosurgical center is obtained. There have been cases of bleeding in the eye in patients with previous injury with metallic shards (usually metal workers), and again a history of this should be sought. A skull x-ray can be helpful in cases of doubt. Electronic implants are the other major problem. These may dysfunction or may be damaged by CMR, which is therefore best avoided. This applies to cochlear implants, neurostimulation systems, non-MR conditional pacemakers/implantable cardioverter-defibrillators (ICDs), and a number of other modern implants. In general, the main rule to observe is to determine the risk-benefit ratio for the proposed procedure. If the information can only be obtained by CMR, and if it is very important, then the risk-benefit ratio may be positive for some patients (as has been shown in some patients with pacemakers). In many clinical circumstances, however, the information required can be obtained by other means. Reference texts on the safety of specific devices are available (e.g., http://www.mrisafety.com/).

For CMR, a number of other specific device issues require mention. Swan-Ganz catheters and temporary pacing wires, in general, preclude CMR, but sternal wires and vascular clips on grafts do not present safety problems, although localized artifacts occur on the images. Three specific areas are discussed in more detail: namely, coronary stents, valvular prostheses and structural heart disease intervention devices, and cardiac implantable electronic devices. Many of them are not considered absolute contraindications for CMR. However, timing and scanning protocol should be adjusted in each clinical scenario.

Coronary Stents

The first intracoronary stents were implanted in human coronary arteries in 1986 by Sigwart and colleagues.[67] The reduced restenosis rate compared with conventional balloon angioplasty has resulted in routine use of stent placement for treatment of coronary stenoses.[68–71]

Most coronary stents are metallic structures that remain in situ for life. As a result, there have been concerns about stent dislodgment during CMR as well as concern about possible heating effects. Several factors determine the risk of placing these materials in a magnetic field. These factors include the ferromagnetism of the material, the strength of the static and gradient magnetic fields, the metal mass, and the geometry of the material.[19,72] It is generally recommended that 6 to 8 weeks elapse before CMR imaging to allow for tissue ingrowth, although this is not based on robust data.[73] The most commonly used stents are made of stainless steel or nitinol, which is not ferromagnetic.[74] Metallic stents have been exposed to field strengths up to 7 T in vitro, without significant heating.[75] Large studies have subsequently confirmed the safety of stent imaging with CMR. Gerber and coworkers evaluated 111 patients with CMR within 8 weeks of stent implantation (median 8 days; range 0 to 54 days); during follow-up, 4 noncardiac deaths occurred as well as 3 revascularization procedures.[76] These events were not related to the CMR procedure. This finding agrees with widespread clinical experience in which stent imaging has been performed on the day after implantation, or soon afterward.[77,78] Moreover, assessing changes in coronary flow reserve after percutaneous intervention with stenting was shown to be feasible.[79]

Another issue regarding CMR procedures in patients with coronary stents is the image distortion caused by the ferromagnetic properties of the stent. Generally, the greater the ferromagnetism of a metallic implant, the greater its magnetic susceptibility artifact. However, studies have shown that CMR angiography could reliably be used for noninvasive imaging and evaluation of blood flow after stent placement.[80,81] Bioabsorbable vascular scaffolds (BVS) are constructed from polymers, which are hydrolyzed and metabolized to CO_2 and H_2O.[82] They have a number of potential advantages compared with metallic stents, such as more physiologic vasomotion postplacement, facilitation of percutaneous or surgical reintervention, and little or no artifact with CMR, allowing imaging of the stent lumen.[82,83] BVS do sometimes contain metallic, radiopaque markers, for example, platinum, with the same potential effects as metallic stents when exposed to a strong magnetic field (i.e., heating and physical motion of the stent).[82] An in vitro study conducted at 3 T led to no heating (1.6°C, equivalent to the maximum background change) and no torque or deflection (0 degrees).[82]

Valvular Prostheses and Structural Heart Disease Intervention Devices

Heart valve prostheses are all safe for CMR.[84] These are the most recent recommendations, and they supersede those that suggested that pre-model 6000 series Starr-Edwards valves might cause problems during MR. This conclusion is backed up by numerous data. Studies up to 3 T static magnetic fields have shown that for a number of prosthetic valves there is no hazardous deflection during exposure of the magnetic field.[85–87] In general, a waiting period of 6 weeks is advocated for valvular prostheses and structural heart disease devices (allowing tissue to heal) before CMR evaluation.[73] Heating of small metallic implants was tested in a study reported by Davis and associates.[64] The authors found no significant increase in temperature in steel and copper clips that were exposed to changing magnetic fields 6.4 times as strong as those expected to be used in the CMR scanner. As a result, there is no contraindication to CMR in patients with the currently used prosthetic valves.[88–90] However, prosthetic material may lead to artifacts on CMR images. To evaluate the influence of prosthetic valves on the interpretation of CMR images and the capability of functional valve analysis, in a group of 89 patients and 100 heart valve prostheses, Bachmann and colleagues showed convincingly that all patients could be imaged with CMR without any risk and that prosthesis-induced artifacts did not interfere with image interpretation.[89] In particular, physiologic valvular regurgitation was easy to differentiate from pathologic or transvalvular regurgitation. Di Cesare and coworkers studied 14 patients who were surgically treated with nine biologic and seven mechanical aortic and mitral valves.[90] Three classes of artifacts were distinguished and graded as minimal, moderate, or significant. The biologic valves produced minimal artifacts and the mechanical valves showed only moderate artifacts. In all 16 prosthetic valves, CMR allowed adequate semiquantitative analysis of flow over the valve.

Transcatheter aortic valve replacement (TAVR) is frequently performed for patients with calcific, aortic stenosis who are considered high risk for conventional, surgical valve replacement. An in vitro study has been conducted on a TAVR device (containing nitinol) at 3 T, which demonstrated no torque, minimal (3 degrees) deflection and a low-grade heating effect (temperature rise of 2.5°C), leading the authors to conclude that scanning the particular device in question at a high field strength is likely to be safe in vivo.[91] A number of studies have evaluated paravalvular leaks post-TAVR with CMR, demonstrating safe scanning at a field strength of 1.5 T in humans.[92–94] Even though an artifact is created, the lumen of the TAVR device can be visualized (Fig. 10.5).[95] Percutaneous closure of the left atrial appendage has become an option

for patients with atrial fibrillation and contraindications or intolerance to oral anticoagulants. Left atrial occluder devices contain metal, such as nitinol mesh, but have been safely scanned at 1.5 T and 3 T.[73,96,97] Artifacts are minimal, even allowing qualitative and quantitative evaluation of residual leaks (see Fig. 10.5).[98]

Severe mitral regurgitation can be successfully treated with percutaneous, mitral valve repair in high-risk patients, and CMR has been safely performed at 1.5 T and 3 T.[99,100] The MitraClip device contains cobalt and chromium, which creates a significant artifact in the mitral valve area, disallowing accurate evaluation of the mitral valve leaflet morphology and residual mitral regurgitation postimplant (see Fig. 10.5).[101]

Use of septal occlusion devices has become widespread, and such devices containing nitinol and cobalt have been tested in vitro at 3 T, showing no torque, maximum deflection of 4 degrees, and a temperature increase of 0.4°C.[100] These devices may therefore be considered safe for CMR, but do cause large artifacts in the region of the interatrial septum.[100]

Cardiac Implantable Electronic Devices

The issues surrounding CMR of pacemakers are complex. In general, three hazardous MR interactions with pacemakers and ICDs should be considered. First, the static magnetic fields exert mechanical forces on the ferromagnetic components of the devices, including the pacemaker and shock leads; the static magnetic fields can also induce asynchronous pacing. Second, a pulsed RF field may result in oversensing or may induce currents in the leads, resulting in thermal damage at the tissue-electrode interface. Third, the gradient magnetic fields may induce voltages on leads, resulting in over- and undersensing. Combined fields may also result in device damage and failure.

Finally, pacemaker leads may serve as an antenna, which could result in pacing the heart during scanning at the frequency of the applied imaging pulses. This could potentially lead to hypotension and dysrhythmias. This effect was shown in experiments and in several patients while positioned in a CMR system, but this effect must be separated from excitation caused by the pulse generator.[102,103] Battery depletion is another concern—primarily occasioned by activation of telemetry circuitry.[104,105]

It is estimated that 50% to 70% of patients with a cardiac implantable electronic device (CIED) will require MR imaging during the lifetime of the device, making a rational and safe approach to this issue imperative.[104,106] Asynchronous mode is recommended in pacemaker-dependent patients, because temporally varying gradient fields may mimic cardiac electricity and lead to inhibition of pacing output.[107] This is not without risk, because competitive intrinsic and pacing rhythms may be dysrhythmogenic.[105] Sense-only mode is preferred in patients with high intrinsic heart rates, precisely to avoid competitive pacing if pacemaker tracking of electromagnetic interference occurs.[105,106] Studies of CIEDs and MR imaging at 1.5 T (only studies with >100 patients included) are summarized in Table 10.1. A limitation shared by many studies is that few CMR scans were performed (in contrast to MR scans of extracardiac anatomy).

In the largest study of CIEDs in MR, 438 scans were performed in 555 patients (54% pacemakers and 46% ICDs) who were subjected to MR scans at 1.5 T.[107] In this study, asynchronous mode was selected in pacemaker-dependent patients, and careful monitoring of vital signs during scanning was performed. Two power-on resets (reversion to a default programming mode—usually an inhibited pacing mode) were documented in pacemakers, and one in an ICD.[107] Two studies of CIEDs at 3 T have been reported (primarily brain imaging), with no serious adverse effects on pacemaker function noted in either (total of 58 patients in both studies).[105,108] A "burning" sensation was noted by one patient

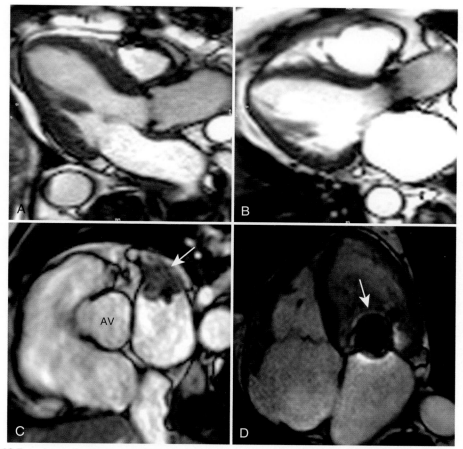

FIG. 10.5 Images of valvular prostheses and structural heart disease intervention devices. An aortic bio-prosthesis is demonstrated in (A), with a transcatheter aortic valve replacement (TAVR) device in (B). A left atrial occlusion device (Watchman) is shown in situ in the left atrial appendage *(arrow)* (C). The arrow in (D) identifies a MitraClip device, causing an artifact in the mitral valve area on a steady-state free precession image in a four-chamber view. *AV,* Atrioventricular. (A and B, From Crouch G, Tully PJ, Bennetts J, et al. Quantitative assessment of paravalvular regurgitation following transcatheter aortic valve replacement. *J Cardiovasc Magn Reson.* 2015;17:32. C, From Hong SN, Rahimi A, Kissinger KV, et al. Cardiac magnetic resonance imaging and the WATCHMAN device. *J Am Coll Cardiol.* 2010;55(24):2785. D, From Lurz P, Serpytis R, Blazek S, et al. Assessment of acute changes in ventricular volumes, function, and strain after interventional edge-to-edge repair of mitral regurgitation using cardiac magnetic resonance imaging. *Eur Heart J Cardiovasc Imaging.* 2015;16(12):1399–1404.)

in the above-mentioned study, but no evidence for pacemaker dysfunction could be uncovered in the subject in question.[108] Sixteen percent of patients experienced a power-on reset in a 3 T study by Naehle et al., but no emergencies arose as a consequence.[105]

Even though concern has been raised about potential coronary sinus (CS) lead dislodgment in cardiac resynchronization therapy (CRT) devices, because of the fact that they do not possess active fixation mechanisms, no such dislodgment was noted in a study of 40 patients with nonconditional CS leads, who were scanned at 1.5 T.[109] In addition, no evidence was found for lead dysfunction or dysrhythmogenesis.[109] Inclusion of patients with CRT devices in other trials also did not signal alerts.[104,107]

The largest trial of CIEDs in MR to date included 201 ICD devices at 1.5 T.[107] One power-on reset occurred in an ICD (with no attempt by the ICD to deliver antitachycardia therapy, which is a potential consequence).[107] It has been suggested that formal defibrillation testing be performed after CMR imaging of an ICD device.[108] In the Evera trial,

150 MR conditional ICDs were evaluated.[110] A fast gradient echo sequence delivered moderate-to-good images of the left ventricle in 74% of cases, and moderate-to-good images of the right ventricle in 84% of cases, which can be explained by the fact that the generator is generally placed closer to the left ventricle, and causes more significant artifacts than the right ventricular lead.[111]

Loop recorders may be safely scanned, although substantial artifacts are generated (more pronounced with gradient echo than spin echo sequences).[112] Rhythm artifacts may be produced, and the theoretical risk of electromagnetic fields impacting stored data requires all data to be downloaded from the loop recorder before MR imaging.[113,114]

MR conditional pacemakers have been developed, with adaptations to hardware (minimization of ferromagnetic components and changes in lead design) and software (substitution of a reed switch with Hall sensor, which will not close or open unexpectedly when exposed to a magnetic field, thereby switching to asynchronous pacing or inhibition). Promising safety profiles of such devices have been demonstrated in

TABLE 10.1   **Summary of Studies of Cardiac Implantable Electronic Devices and Magnetic Resonance Imaging at 1.5 T (Only Studies With >100 Patients Are Included)**

Trial	Year Published	No. of Scans	No. of Patients Scanned	Type of Device(s) and % of Patients or Scans	CMR %	Adverse Effects
Higgins et al.[117]	2015	256	198	PPM (DC) 87.9% of scans ICD 2.3% of scans	Unknown	9 power-on resets
Bailey et al.[118]	2015	229	229	PPM (SC) 10.5% of patients PPM (DC) 89.5% of patients	0%	No significant
Higgins et al.[117]	2015	512	398	Unknown	Unknown	1 significant lead threshold change
Gold et al.[110]	2015	156	156	ICD (SC) 52.6% of patients ICD (DC) 47.4% of patients	Unknown	No significant
Gimbel et al.[116]	2013	150	150	PPM (DC) 100% of patients	Unknown	No significant
Cohen et al.[104]	2012	125	109	PPM (SC) 4% of scans PPM (DC) 63% of scans CRT-P 2% of scans ICD (SC) 3% of scans ICD (DC) 16% of scans CRT-D 13% of scans	4%	Battery voltage decrease in 4% of scans, lead threshold change in 3% of scans, and lead impedance change in 6% of scans
Nazarian et al.[107]	2011	555	438	PPM 54% of patients ICD 46% of patients CRT-D 12% of patients	16%	3 power-on resets
Mollerus et al.[119]	2010	127	103	Unknown	Unknown	1 device reset requiring reprogramming

CMR %, Percentage of cardiac magnetic resonance studies; *CRT-D*, cardiac resynchronization therapy with defibrillator function; *CRT-P*, cardiac resynchronization therapy with pacemaker function; *DC*, dual chamber; *ICD*, implantable cardioverter defibrillator; *PPM*, permanent pacemaker; *SC*, single chamber.

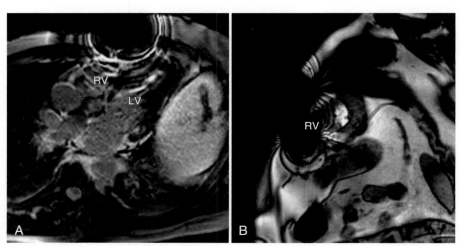

FIG. 10.6 A significant imaging artifact created by a cardiac implantable electronic device in a four-chamber view (A) and a short-axis view (B). *LV*, Left ventricle; *RV*, right ventricle. (From Nordbeck P, Ertl G, Ritter O. Magnetic resonance imaging safety in pacemaker and implantable cardioverter defibrillator patients: how far have we come? *Eur Heart J.* 2015;36(24):1505–1511.)

trials.[110,115,116] With appropriate selection, programming, monitoring and follow-up, CIEDs may therefore be subjected to CMR with an acceptable risk, with the possible exclusion of pacemaker-dependent patients.[109] Pacing dependency may be temporally variable, and it is therefore challenging to define.[108] The European Society of Cardiology guideline on cardiac pacing and cardiac resynchronization therapy provides a class IIb recommendation for nonconditional CIED systems, and a class IIa recommendation for conditional devices.[106] CIEDs can cause significant artifacts, which may hamper image interpretation (Fig. 10.6).[115]

CONCLUSION

In general, CMR is safe and no long-term ill effects have been reported. Very rapidly changing gradients may induce nerve excitations that may result in muscle twitching. However, clinical scanners operate below the threshold for such effects. The threshold of excitation of the myocardium is approximately 200 times higher than that for other muscles, and so the heart will not be stimulated by the rapidly changing gradients. Pharmacologic CMR stress testing can be performed safely with appropriate monitoring. Most metallic implants, such as intracoronary stents, prosthetic valves, structural heart disease intervention devices and sternal sutures, present no hazard because most materials used are nonferromagnetic. MR-conditional pacemakers may be safely scanned, whereas patients with other CIEDs may be considered for CMR if the risk-benefit ratio is in favor of imaging.

REFERENCES

A full reference list is available online at ExpertConsult.com

11

Pacemaker and Implantable Cardioverter-Defibrillator Safety and Safe Scanning

Esra Gucuk Ipek and Saman Nazarian

Magnetic resonance imaging (MRI) has gained popularity over the last decade because of its excellent soft tissue imaging capability and superior spatial resolution as well as lack of ionizing radiation. These properties have led to expanded indications for MRI. At the same time, with the aging of the US population, the need for cardiac implantable electronic devices (CIEDs) is increasing in parallel to that for MRI indication. Despite its advantages, MRI is relatively contraindicated in individuals with CIEDs because of the possibility for heating, induction, and electromagnetic interference. This is a public health issue because it limits diagnostic access to MRI for millions of CIED recipients and ever-increasing trends for device implantation.[1,2] According to a recent 61-country survey, there was a significant rise in the use of implantable cardioverter-defibrillators (ICDs) by the year 2009 compared with 2005, with most implants occurring in the United States (434 new implants per million population).[3] Moreover, the high prevalence of comorbidities in the same population indicates potential benefits from MRI. Within 1-year post implant, 17% of the CIED recipients have an MRI indication, and estimates indicate a lifetime need for MRI in up to 75% of recipients.[4–6]

Owing to an increased awareness of the public health importance of this issue, device manufacturers have focused on the development of MRI conditional CIEDs, device systems that demonstrate no known hazards in a specified MRI environment with specified conditions of use. Most important, to be considered MRI conditional, all implanted CIED components must be tested together for electromagnetic compatibility and approved for such use by the US Food and Drug Administration (FDA). Other CIED systems are considered to be "legacy" systems or "nonconditional" for MRI.

A decade ago, the presence of a CIED was considered an absolute contraindication for MRI. However, this approach was challenged with numerous case series demonstrating no significant safety issues when MRI was performed with specific protocols to minimize electromagnetic interference.[7] Today, we know that MRI examination is feasible and can be performed with minimal risk as long as a well-defined and tested safety protocol is followed. According to current guidelines, MRI examination should be avoided in CIED recipients, but, if necessary, it can be done in experienced centers under specific protocols.

In this chapter, we review the current data on nonconditional and conditional CIEDs and experiences with MRI examination, summarize the Johns Hopkins protocol for MRI safety in the setting of nonconditional CIED systems, and review associated MRI-related artifacts.

CARDIAC IMPLANTED ELECTRONIC DEVICES AND MAGNETIC RESONANCE IMAGING INTERACTIONS

Owing to potential interactions with the electromagnetic environment, CIEDs are classified as MRI unsafe or MRI conditional based upon the intended design and prior experience with the CIED in an MRI environment (Table 11.1). Potential interactions between CIED systems and the MRI environment are summarized in Table 11.2. The static magnetic field, in addition to radiofrequency (RF) energy generated during MRI, may interact with the CIED and lead to adverse effects. The magnetic field strength, RF power, patient position/orientation within the scanner, CIED type, and patient characteristics are all important variables that help quantify the magnitude of interaction.[8]

CLINICAL STUDIES WITH NONMAGNETIC RESONANCE IMAGING CONDITIONAL DEVICES

Up to 1.5 T

Clinical studies of MRI in the setting of nonconditional devices are summarized in Table 11.3. The first study was performed in 1984 by Fetter et al.,[9] who examined the in vivo effects of MRI on CIED function.[9] Although device parameters did not change, an asynchronous pacing mode was activated during MRI scanning in one patient. After this initial experience, in 1996, Gimbel et al.[10] examined five patients with pacemakers undergoing 0.5 T MRI scan and observed a 2-second pause in a pacemaker-dependent patient. In 2000, Sommer et al.[11] evaluated the effects of 0.5 T MRI on pacemaker generators and leads in vitro, then examined 44 non–pacemaker-dependent patients in vivo, and reported no adverse events. The following year, the same group reported a prospective study that investigated safety at 0.5 T in 32 pacemaker patients undergoing MRI.[12] Lead impedance, sensing thresholds did not change after MRI. They showed overall safety; however, battery voltage decreased immediately after MRI, and returned to baseline at the 3-month follow-up.

In the last decade, several studies have examined the interaction of nonconditional CIED systems with MRI. Roguin et al.[13] studied CIED behavior and changes in system parameters in vitro and in vivo in animal models. Older (pre-2000) ICD systems were damaged following MRI, but no significant changes were observed in newer (2000 and later) systems. Pathologic examination showed limited necrosis or fibrosis adjacent to the lead tip that was not different than that observed in animals that were not exposed to MRI. Later, Martin et al. performed 62 MRI examinations in 54 pacemaker patients. There were no adverse events; but changes in pacing threshold were observed in 10 leads, 2 of which required a change in programmed output.[7]

Because of significant adverse events reported with older-generation ICDs, it was first thought that MRI was an absolute contraindication in the setting of ICD systems.[14] Junttila et al.[15] performed three serial cardiac MRI scans in 10 ICD recipients. In that series, patients reported no symptoms during the MRI examination, and none of the examinations required early termination. No adverse event or change in device/

TABLE 11.1 American Society for Testing and Materials Categorization of Medical Devices in a Magnetic Resonance Imaging Environment

Category	Description
MR safe	No known hazards in an MR environment
MR conditional	No known hazards in a specified MR environment with specified conditions
MR unsafe	Known to pose hazards in all MR environments

MR, Magnetic resonance.

TABLE 11.2 Potential Interactions Between a Cardiac Implantable Electronic Device and Electromagnetic Interference

Force and torque	• Magnetic fields can attract ferromagnetic materials within the CIEDs that may lead to generator dislodgment
	• The torque is directly related to ferromagnetic content, distance between ferromagnetic material and magnetic source, and field strength of the magnetic field
	• In vitro studies showed that maximum torque is 0.98 Newton with a 1.5 T scanner[13]
Induced electrical current	• Electrical currents induced by MRI-related electromagnetic components may theoretically initiate ventricular or atrial arrhythmias[61]
Heating and tissue damage	• The pacing leads can act as an antenna under an electromagnetic field, resulting in heating and tissue damage around the tip of the lead. The eventual tissue damage may change pacing, sensing, or capture thresholds[29]
	• Retained/abandoned or epicardial leads may carry a higher risk of local heating
Reed switch activity	• Reed switch activity of CIED may lead to asynchronous pacing[62]
Inappropriate function	• Radiofrequency energy pulses may lead to inappropriate inhibition of demand pacing, tracking, or programming changes
	• Sensing of electromagnetic interference may be interpreted as an arrhythmia and may lead to attempts by the device to deliver antitachycardia therapies

CIED, Cardiac implantable electronic device; *MRI,* magnetic resonance imaging.

lead parameters was observed during short-term and long-term follow-up. Similarly, in another small cohort of 10 ICD recipients, there were no adverse events after 1.5 T MRI.[16] Naehle et al.[17] performed 1.5 T MRI in 18 ICD recipients. Although no significant pacing threshold and lead impedance changes were observed, battery voltage significantly decreased. In a subset of patients, the voltage recovered completely; however, in the remaining patients, decreased battery voltage persisted. Moreover, RF noise was oversensed as ventricular fibrillation (VF), but no therapies were initiated. There was no evidence of overheating or tissue damage as assessed by troponin level.

Sommer et al.[18] performed 115 nonthoracic 1.5 T MRI examinations in 85 patients with CIED. There were no arrhythmias, but pacing capture threshold increased significantly. After four MRI examinations, serum troponin levels increased, which was associated with the increased pacing threshold in one case. Decreased battery voltage was again noted immediately after the MRI; but this drop was transient in most cases and returned to baseline at follow-up. Naehle et al.[19] evaluated the effects of serial MRI in 47 CIED recipients. There was a statistically significant decrease in battery voltage and pacing capture threshold after two or more MRI examinations, but no clinically relevant or cumulative changes that would affect device longevity were noted. In 2011, the same group reported another series pacemaker and ICD patients that underwent safe cardiovascular magnetic resonance (CMR) imaging without any change in pacing capture threshold, lead impedance, or troponin levels.[20]

Cardiac resynchronization therapy and coronary sinus leads also appear to be safe.[21] Little is known about the safety of epicardial leads. In a study by Pulver et al.,[22] 11 patients with pediatric and adult congenital heart disease underwent 1.5 T MRI, including 6 patients with epicardial leads. There were no adverse events such as symptoms that could be related to lead heating. Of note, three patients with epicardial leads underwent CMR without any safety issue.

Cohen et al.[23] performed 125 clinically indicated MRI examinations in 109 patients with CIED, including ICD systems, and compared the outcomes with 50 CIED recipients who did not have an MRI. The authors did not report MRI-related adverse events; however, they did observe small nonsignificant changes in device parameters after MRI that were similar to their control group. Such insignificant changes may be unrelated to MRI itself and reflect random physiologic variations in the interaction CIED tissue interface.

Muehling et al.[24] also examined 356 CIED recipients who underwent 1.5 T cranial MRI. There was no significant change in device parameters, and troponin levels were stable immediately after MRI. Moreover, patients were followed for 1 year and device interrogations were performed at 2 weeks, 2 months, 6 months, and 12 months after the MRI. No significant change was observed in device-related parameters during follow-up.

Finally, the MagnaSafe Registry is a multicenter, prospective cohort study designed to evaluate the safety of non-MRI conditional CIED systems following nonthoracic 1.5 T MRI.[25] The MagnaSafe Registry included 1500 cases in which patients had a nonthoracic MRI with a pacemaker ($n = 1000$) or ICD ($n = 500$) implanted after 2001. Patients with abandoned or inactive lead were excluded. There were no deaths, lead failures, losses of capture, or ventricular arrhythmias during the index MRI. Prespecified changes in lead impedance, pacing threshold, battery voltage, and P-wave and R-wave amplitude were exceeded in a small number of cases. Repeat MRI was not associated with an increase in adverse events.[25]

In addition, another large study from our Johns Hopkins group reported on MRI safety at 1.5 T in 1509 patients who had a pacemaker (58%) or ICD (42%) and underwent 2103 thoracic and nonthoracic MRI. The pacing mode was changed to asynchronous mode for pacing-dependent patients and to demand mode for others. No long-term clinically significant adverse events were reported. In 9 (0.4%) MRI examinations, the device reset to a backup mode, which was transient in all but one device. An acute decrease in P wave amplitude occurred in 1% of studies that increased to 4% of patients on long-term follow-up. The observed changes in lead parameters were not clinically significant and did not require device revision or reprogramming.[25a]

There are limited data on high-risk groups such as pacemaker-dependent patients. Gimbel et al.[26] examined 10 pacemaker-dependent patients who underwent 1.5 T MRI. There were no clinical adverse events; however, minor capture threshold changes were observed in 7 patients. Higgins et al.[27] reviewed 198 CIED recipients who underwent 1.5 T MRI. Power-on reset events occurred in 8 patients, all patients having older-generation devices. Importantly, devices reset to an inhibited pacing mode. Finally, 137 (9%) of the 1509 patients in the previously

TABLE 11.3 Clinical Studies With Nonmagnetic Resonance Imaging Conditional Devices

Study Group	Year	Patient No.	Device	MRI Scanner	Findings
Gimbel et al.[10]	1996	5	Pacemaker	0.5 T	Pause detected in a pacemaker-dependent patient with unipolar lead
Sommer et al.[11]	2000	44	Pacemaker	0.5 T	No adverse events; no change in device and lead parameters
Vahlhaus et al.[12]	2001	32	Pacemaker	0.5 T	Battery voltage decreased after MRI that turned back to baseline in 3 months; reed switch deactivation was observed in 37.5% of the patients
Martin et al.[7]	2004	54	Pacemaker	1.5 T	Pacing threshold was changed in 9.4% of the leads
Del Ojo et al.[33]	2005	13	Pacemaker	2.0 T	No adverse events; no change in device and lead parameters
Gimbel et al.[63]	2005	7	ICD	1.5 T	Power-on reset occurred in 1 patient
Gimbel et al.[26]	2005	10	Pacemaker	1.5 T	Minor changes in capture thresholds
Nazarian et al.[40]	2006	55	Pacemaker and ICD	1.5 T	No adverse events; no change in device and lead parameters
Sommer et al.[18]	2006	82	Pacemaker	1.5 T	Capture threshold was increased; increased troponin levels in 4 cases. One of the capture threshold increases was associated with elevated troponin levels
Gimbel et al.[35]	2008	14	Pacemaker, ICD and loop recorder	3.0 T	No change in device and lead parameters. One patient reported chest pain
Naehle et al.[34]	2008	44	Pacemaker	3.0 T	No adverse events; no change in device and lead parameters
Mollerus et al.[64]	2008	37	Pacemaker and ICD	1.5 T	No adverse events; no change in device and lead parameters
Naehle et al.[17]	2009	18	ICD	1.5 T	A decrease was observed in battery voltage; electromagnetic interference was interpreted as VF in 2 cases
Naehle et al.[19]	2009	47	Pacemaker	1.5 T	Pacing threshold and battery decreased after serial MRI
Pulver et al.[22]	2009	11	Pacemaker	1.5 T	Minimal change in device voltage; lead threshold; lead impedance in 6 patients
Mollerus et al.[65]	2009	52	Pacemaker and ICD	1.5 T	No adverse events; no change in device and lead parameters
Halshtok et al.[66]	2010	18	Pacemaker and ICD	1.5 T	Power-on reset occurred in 2 patients
Strach et al.[32]	2010	114	Pacemaker	0.2 T	No adverse events; no change in device and lead parameters
Burke et al.[16]	2010	38	Pacemaker and ICD	1.5 T	No adverse events; no change in device and lead parameters
Mollerus et al.[67]	2010	103	Pacemaker and ICD	1.5 T	Sensing amplitudes and pacing impedances decreased significantly
Nazarian et al.[6]	2011	438	Pacemaker and ICD	1.5 T	Power-on reset in 1.5% of the patients
Juntilla et al.[15]	2011	10	ICD	1.5 T	No adverse events; no change in device parameters
Naehle et al.[20]	2011	32	Pacemaker and ICD	1.5 T	No adverse events; no change in device and lead parameters
Cohen et al.[23]	2012	109	Pacemaker and ICD	1.5 T	Battery voltage decreased in 4%; pacing threshold increased in 3%; pacing lead impedance changed in 6%
Muehling et al.[24]	2014	356	Pacemaker	1.5 T	No adverse events; no change in device and lead parameters
Higgins et al.[27]	2015	198	Pacemaker and ICD	1.5 T	Power-on reset in 8 patients
Sheldon et al.[21]	2015	42	CRT-D, CRT-P, pacemaker	1.5 T	No adverse events; no change in device and lead parameters
Russo et al.[25]	2017	1500	Pacemaker and ICD	1.5 T	No deaths or lead failures; one ICD generator was replaced because it could not be interrogated after MRI
Nazarian et al.[25a]	2017	1509	Pacemaker and ICD	1.5 T	No deaths or lead failures; one pacemaker needed replacement because it could not be reprogrammed; no clinically significant change in lead parameters

CRT-D, Cardiac resynchronization therapy defibrillator; *CRT-P,* cardiac resynchronization therapy pacemaker; *ICD,* implantable cardioverter defibrillator; *MRI,* magnetic resonance imaging.

mentioned study of Nazarian et al.[25a] were pacer-dependent (including 22 of whom had an ICD with asynchronous programming mode capability). There was similar safety as in the overall study. Thus MRI examination should be carefully considered and closely monitored in pacemaker-dependent patients with older (pre-2000) devices.

Retained/Orphaned Leads

Patients with retained/orphaned leads constitute another high-risk group, because of the possibility of increased heating. An in vitro study compared retained/orphaned leads with pacemaker-attached leads, and showed that heating of the retained lead was significantly higher, and the risk was significantly correlated with lead length.[28,29] In another study by Higgins et al.,[30,31] the safety of retained pacemaker lead was evaluated in 19 patients who underwent nonthoracic 1.5 T MRI. There were no adverse events and in a subset of patients who had their devices reconnected to the retained leads, lead parameters were unchanged. The

same study group evaluated troponin levels in 348 patients, including 22 patients with abandoned leads. There was no change in troponin levels in these patients, which may serve as a surrogate for myocardial thermal damage. Finally, low-field (0.2 T) MRI was performed in 114 CIED patients who required MRI examination for urgent indications, including pacemaker-dependent patients and patients with abandoned leads.[32] No adverse events or changes in device parameters were reported.

High-Field Magnetic Resonance

There are limited studies with high-field MRI. Del Ojo et al.[33] performed 2 T MRI in 13 patients with pacemakers. This is one of the initial studies that showed MRI can be safely performed in CIED recipients, even though the magnetic field is relatively high. 3 T MRIs are most commonly used in neurologic imaging. Because of the increased magnetic field strength, some risks are theoretically higher. However, neurologic imaging with transmit-receive head coils decreases power deposition upon the CIED and mitigates the risk of heating and current generation. In contrast, the CIED will be exposed to more force and torque. Naehle et al.[34] evaluated brain 3 T MRI in CIED recipients. No safety issues, changes in device parameters, or changes in troponin levels occurred in the 44 patients who underwent 55 brain examinations at 3 T. Similarly, Gimbel et al.[35] safely performed 3 T MRI in 14 patients without adverse effects or changes in device parameters. However, in the following year, Gimbel et al.[36,37] reported two cases of pacing inhibition with 3 T MRI.

Recommendations

According to current guidelines, patients with MRI nonconditional devices may undergo 1.5 T MRI if the benefit of the MRI overweighs the risk of the procedure, provided that the CIED is a new-generation device and appropriate supervision is provided.[8,38,39] The following are recommended by the guidelines.[38]

1. MRI can be performed if there is no alternative imaging modality, the CIED is a new-generation system that has been implanted for at least 6 weeks, and there are no abandoned or epicardial leads.
2. The CIED should be interrogated *before* examination, and system parameters should be adjusted according to patient and device characteristics.
3. During the MRI examination, experienced personnel should perform continuous monitoring.
4. Device interrogation should be performed after the scan.

THE JOHNS HOPKINS PROTOCOL

Our institutional safety protocol is based upon our experience with over 2000 MRI examinations since 2003. The protocol has been published previously and is summarized in Fig. 11.1.[40] First, we acquire all the CIED-related information, such as the implantation date, type of the device, number of leads, and presence of abandoned or epicardial leads, and assess pacemaker dependence. We exclude patients with epicardial and/or abandoned leads. In all examinations, an electrophysiologist or an experienced registered nurse prepared to respond to device malfunction needs to be present. The pacemakers are programmed to an inhibited mode (DDI/VVI) or, if the patient is pacemaker dependent, to asynchronous mode (DOO/VOO). Other pacemaker functions such as rate response or tachyarrhythmia therapies are deactivated. The electrocardiogram and pulse oximetry signals are monitored carefully during MRI, and pacemaker interrogation is performed after the examination.

Using this protocol, we initially reported on 55 patients with CIED, all of whom underwent MRI without safety issues.[40] Later, we reported on 555 1.5 T MRI examinations (16% cardiac) in 438 patients (12% pacemaker dependent) with CIED (54% pacemakers, 46% defibrillators) systems. The major adverse event was power-on reset, which occurred in 0.7% of the patients.[6] Minor changes were observed in lead sensing and capture thresholds, but none of these required system revision or reprogramming. Our most recent report included MRI safety at 1.5 T in 1509 patients who had a pacemaker (58%) or ICD (42%) and underwent 2103 thoracic and nonthoracic MRI. No long-term clinically significant adverse events were reported. In 9 (0.4%) MRI examinations, the device reset to a backup mode, which was transient in all but one device. An acute decrease in P wave amplitude occurred in 1% of studies that increased to 4% of patients on long-term follow-up. The observed changes in lead parameters were not clinically significant and did not require device revision or reprogramming.[25a]

MAGNETIC RESONANCE IMAGING CONDITIONAL DEVICES

Given the increased need for MRI examinations in CIED recipients, device companies have introduced MRI conditional systems. The

TABLE 11.4 Magnetic Resonance Imaging Conditional Cardiac Implantable Electronic Devices and Leads

Company	Device	Lead
Medtronic	Revo MRI SureScan	CapSureFix/CapsureSense
	Advisa MRI	Medtronic Sprint Quattro
	Evera MRI SureScan	Secure MRI
St. Jude Medical	Accent MRI	Tendril MRI
Biotronik	ProMRI	Safio S53/Safio S60
	Lumax 740	Setrox
	ProMRI ICD	Linoxsmart
Boston Scientific	Ingenio	Ingevity
	Advantio	
Sorin	Kora 100	Beflex

ICD, Implantable cardioverter defibrillator; *MRI,* magnetic resonance imaging.

currently available MRI conditional systems are summarized in Table 11.4. Those systems pose no known hazards when MRI is performed under specific monitoring conditions. The use of ferromagnetic materials is limited when possible; and lead construction materials and internal circuits are modified. Instead of a reed switch, a Hall sensor is used. Inappropriate sensing is prevented by filters. There is also a specific device module for MRI mode that enables limited interaction with electromagnetic field. With these systems, 1.5 T MRI can safely be performed by following manufacturer specific instructions (class IIa, level of evidence B).[38]

The cumulating experience with conditional MRI devices is summarized in Table 11.5. In the randomized study performed by Wilkoff et al.[41] the safety and efficacy of the EnRhythm MRI SureScan and CapSureFix leads was tested under 1.5 T MRI. A total of 464 patients were randomized to either MRI (n = 258) versus control (n = 206) groups. There were no MRI-related complications, and electrical parameters before and after MRI were similar between the two groups. No MRI-induced power-on reset was observed. Of note, the EnRhythm MRI SureScan and CapSureFix leads were designed for 1.5 T MRI with a maximum specific absorption rate (SAR) value of 2 W/kg. Accordingly, the FDA approved the EnRhythm MRI SureScan Pacing System (Medtronic, Minneapolis, MN) in 2011. The SureScan and CapSureFix leads are not approved at higher field strengths.

Forleo et al.[42] evaluated the safety and feasibility of the EnRhythm MRI SureScan and CapSureFix leads in 50 patients and compared the results with a conventional CIED group. The implantation success rates and complication rates were similar in both groups, and during follow-up there were no significant changes in pacing thresholds. In the MRI conditional group, cephalic veins were less likely to be accessed because of the thickness of conditional leads. Later, the same study group reported their experience with MRI-conditional CIED systems with a larger cohort of patients (n = 250). In this study, MRI conditional CIED systems from three different manufacturers were implanted in 250 patients without a significant difference in complication rates compared with conventional devices.[43]

Rickard et al.[44] compared the procedural and long-term performance of the 5086 MRI conditional leads (n = 466) with conventional leads (n = 316). Acute lead dislodgment was higher with MRI conditional leads (2.6% vs. 0.6%). At 12-month follow-up, ventricular sensing was lower and ventricular capture threshold was higher with MRI conditional leads compared with controls. In a smaller study by Elmouchi et al.,[45] 65 patients implanted with MRI conditional leads were compared with 92 patients with conventional leads. Complication rates were higher in

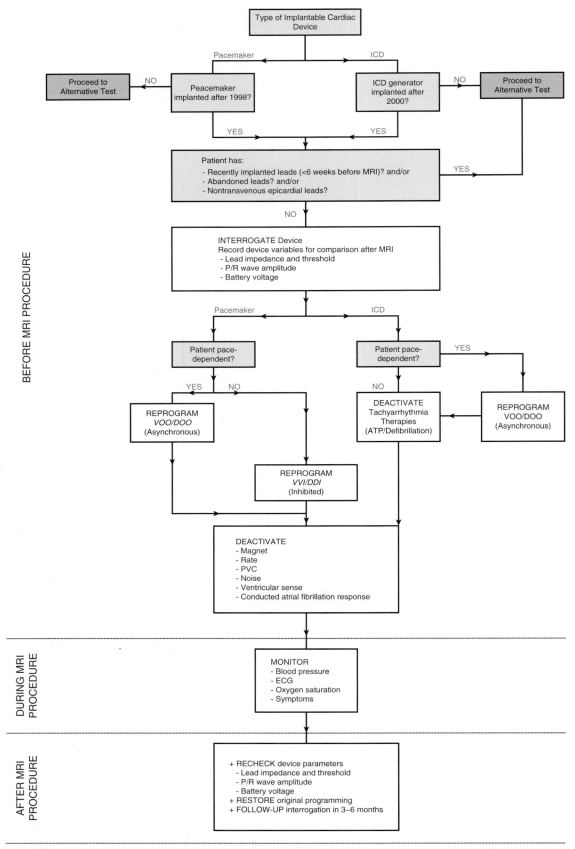

FIG. 11.1 The safety protocol of Johns Hopkins Hospital for magnetic resonance imaging *(MRI)* scanning of the patients with a cardiac implantable electronic device. *ATP,* Antitachycardia pacing; *DDI,* dual-chamber inhibited pacing without atrial tracking; *DOO,* dual-chamber asynchronous pacing; *ECG,* electrocardiogram; *ICD,* implantable cardioverter defibrillator; *PVC,* premature ventricular contraction; *VOO,* ventricular asynchronous pacing; *VVI,* ventricular inhibited pacing.

TABLE 11.5	Previous Studies With Magnetic Resonance Imaging Conditional Devices				
Study Group	**Year**	**Patient No.**	**Device**	**MRI Scanner**	**Findings**
Forleo et al.[42]	2010	107	MRI conditional (EnRhythm) vs. conventional dual chamber pacemaker	None	Successfully implanted without significant procedural complications
Wilkoff et al.[41]	2011	464	MRI conditional (EnRhythm)	1.5 T	There were no scan-related events or safety issues
Forleo et al.[43]	2013	250	MRI conditional pacemaker	None	Successfully implanted without significant procedural complications
Gimbel et al.[47]	2013	263	MRI conditional pacemaker (Advisa MRI)	1.5 T	There were no scan-related events or safety issues
Rickard et al.[44]	2014	466	MRI conditional pacemaker (CapSureFix) vs. conventional leads	None	MRI conditional leads had lower ventricular sensing, higher ventricular capture threshold, and higher acute dislodgment rate
Elmouchi et al.[45]	2014	157	MRI conditional pacemaker (CapSureFix) vs. conventional leads	None	Lead-related complications were higher with CapSureFix leads
Wollman et al.[50]	2014	36	MRI conditional pacemaker (Advisa MRI)	1.5 T	There were no scan-related events or safety issues
Acha et al.[46]	2015	492	MRI conditional pacemaker (CapSureFix) vs. conventional leads	None	Lead-related complication were higher with CapSureFix leads
Klein-Wiele et al.[51]	2015	24	MRI conditional pacemaker	1.5 T	There were no scan-related events or safety issues
Savouré et al.[68]	2015	29	MRI conditional pacemaker (Kora 100)	1.5 T	There were no scan-related events or safety issues
Awad et al.[54]	2015	153	MRI conditional ICD (ProMRI ICD)	1.5 T	There were no scan-related events or safety issues; one patient demonstrated decreased R-wave amplitude in 1 month follow-up
Shenthar et al.[52]	2015	266	MRI conditional pacemaker (Advisa MRI)	1.5 T	There were no scan-related events or safety issues
Gold et al.[53]	2015	275	MRI conditional ICD (Evera MRI)	1.5 T	One patient experienced atrial tachycardia during scanning
Bailey et al.[48]	2015	272	MRI conditional pacemaker (ProMRI)	1.5 T	There were no scan-related events or safety issues
Bailey et al.[49]	2016	245	MRI conditional pacemaker (ProMRI)	1.5 T	Pericardial effusion in one patient that required lead positioning

ICD, Implantable cardioverter defibrillator; *MRI,* magnetic resonance imaging.

the MRI conditional group, including perforation, pericarditis, and lead dislodgment. Acha et al.[46] observed similar results in another study where higher lead perforations (5.5%) with MRI conditional leads (0.5%) were reported. Interestingly, MRI conditional leads tended to cause delayed perforations, occurring over 3 weeks after the implantation. It is likely that the stiffer lead design, shorter length of the lead, and increased diameter were responsible for the observed differences.

Another MRI conditional system was tested under 1.5 T MRI in a prospective randomized multicenter trial.[47] A total of 263 patients were randomized to MRI versus no MRI at 9 to 12 months after implantation. Notably, the MRI sequences included head and thoracic regions. There were no adverse events during MRI, and device interrogation after the MRI showed no significant change in system parameters compared with the control group. Following this trial, the FDA approved the Advisa SureScan MRI (Medtronic, Minneapolis, MN) pacemaker system in 2013.

The ProMRI system (Biotronik, Berlin, Germany), another MRI conditional pacemaker, was tested in two sequential studies. In the first study, 272 patients were enrolled, 226 of whom underwent head and lumbar 1.5 T MRI.[48] There were no adverse events immediately after scan, or during 1-month follow-up; and no significant change was observed in device parameters. Later, ProMRI systems were tested under 1.5 T thoracic spine and CMR.[49] Of 221 patients studied, one patient presented with pericardial effusion, in whom lead positioning was required. In others, no adverse events were reported. Based on these results, ProMRI systems were approved by the FDA in March 2015. Another MRI conditional CIED, the ImageReady MR-Conditional Pacing System (Boston Scientific) has received FDA approval in April 2016 for full-body 1.5 T MRI.

In a small single-center study, Advisa SureScan MRI was tested under 1.5 T CMR.[50] Clinical adverse events were not observed, but there were small changes in system parameters after MRI, which were clinically irrelevant. In a recent study, adenosine stress perfusion CMR was successfully performed in 24 patients with MRI conditional CIED systems.[51] No significant adverse events were observed.

To expand MRI conditional status to previously implanted nonconditional MRI CapSureFix Novus 5076 leads, a randomized trial was designed.[52] In 266 patients, Advisa SureScan MRI devices and CapSureFix Novus 5076 leads were implanted, or previously implanted CapSureFix Novus 5076 leads were connected to newly implanted Advisa SureScan MRI generators. The patients were randomized to MRI versus control groups. There were no MRI-related complications or arrhythmias, and the proportions of the patients with changes in device parameters were similar in the two groups. This study showed that previously implanted conventional CapSureFix Novus 5076 pacemaker leads may safely undergo MRI if connected to the Advisa SureScan MRI conditional generator.

Recently, device manufacturers have also introduced MRI conditional ICD systems. The performance of MRI conditional ICD, Evera MRI SureScan (Medtronic, Minneapolis, MN) was evaluated in a multicenter randomized trial.[53] A total of 263 patients were randomized to full-body MRI versus control groups. In the MRI group, one patient experienced atrial tachycardia during the examination. The scan was stopped and the rhythm was converted noninvasively through the CIED; then the scan was continued without any further safety issues. There were minor changes in system parameters in the MRI group, which did not differ from the control group. Accordingly, FDA approved the Evera MRI SureScan system in September 2015.

Lastly, another MRI conditional ICD, ProMRI ICD system (Biotronik, Berlin, Germany), was granted FDA approval in December 2015 after safety and efficacy was demonstrated under 1.5 T thoracic and CMR in a large prospective study.[54]

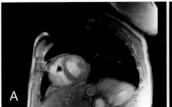
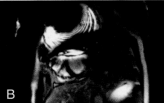

FIG. 11.2 Susceptibility artifact due to a left-sided implantable cardio-verter defibrillator generator in a patient undergoing 1.5 T cardiovascular magnetic resonance. (A) Short-axis cine image: lead artifact can be seen in right ventricle. Generator artifact did not affect the overall diagnostic quality. (B) Short-axis late gadolinium enhancement sequence. Suscep-tibility artifact has severely affected the interpretability of the image of the anterior segment of the left ventricle.

CARDIAC IMPLANTABLE ELECTRONIC DEVICE–RELATED ARTIFACTS

The potential of image artifacts should be considered when deciding to perform an MRI examination in CIED recipients, and the benefit-risk ratio should be determined based on the need of the MRI, the location of the suspected disease, as well as the location of the implanted CIED generator. Susceptibility artifacts are more common with inver-sion recovery and balanced steady-state free precession (bSSFP) sequences. In our experience, selecting imaging planes that are perpendicular to the device generator, shortening echo times, or using spin fast echo sequences may reduce the artifacts. Specialized artifact reduction sequences have also been developed, which can greatly improve the image quality in the setting of CIED systems.[55]

Kaasalainen et al.[56] performed 1.5 T CMR in 16 patients. Overall, CMR was adequate for diagnostic purposes. In all patients with a right-sided generator, there was no compromise in any of the sequences; however, in left-sided generators, the artifacts were visible in several of the sequences, and those were typically observed in apical, anterior, and anteroseptal left ventricular (LV) segments, especially during myo-cardial late gadolinium enhancement (LGE) imaging.

Similarly, we were able to diagnose patients in 100% of the nontho-racic MRIs, and in 93% of the thoracic MRIs.[40] We also showed that the type of CIED (ICDs are more likely to cause artifacts than pacemakers), side of the device generator (left higher than right), indirect param-eters such as body mass index (BMI) and LV end-diastolic volumes that indicate cardiac distance from the device, and the CMR sequence, all affect the presence and amount of the artifact.[57] We observed that artifacts were mainly present in LGE sequence, and in short-axis view, with the anterior and apical LV regions most commonly affected (Fig. 11.2). Lead artifacts did not affect the overall interpretability.

Junttila et al.[15] also reported ICD-related artifacts, especially in the anterior and septal LV segments, and most commonly in the apical region in the LGE sequences that limited the diagnostic capabilities of the CMR. Naehle et al.[20] performed CMR in 32 patients with permanent pacemakers and ICDs. With right-sided implantations, the image quality and diagnostic value were better compared with left-sided CIED (100% vs. 35%). With left-sided devices, the image quality is impaired, specifi-cally in anterior and anterolateral LV segments. In the subanalysis of the Advisa MRI pacemaker trial that was performed with 1.5 T CMR, both right and LV acquisitions had enough diagnostic quality to facilitate quantitative cardiac assessment.[58]

Implantable Long-Term Loop Recorders

Although limited data are available on implantable loop recorders com-pared with pacemakers and ICDs, current data suggest that those patients can safely undergo MRI, albeit with a potential for electromagnetic

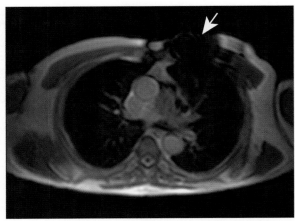

FIG. 11.3 Axial thoracic gradient echo image in a patient with a Medtronic Reveal LINQ long-term monitoring device. Note the anterior image artifact (*arrow*).

noise recordings that may be misinterpreted as an arrhythmia.[35,59] In a case report, two patients with implanted loop recorders were safely examined with MRI.[60] Importantly, several implantable recorders are considered to be MRI conditional by the FDA. Given the small size of these devices, the local artifact is also smaller (Fig. 11.3).

FUTURE DIRECTIONS

MRI conditional CIED systems have been a welcome addition in recent years. However, several questions remain to be answered. Should we implant MRI conditional devices in all patients? If not, how should we select the suitable candidate? Because it is likely that legacy leads will pose minimal hazards, should MRI conditional generators be implanted when a generator replacement is needed? Long-term follow-up, addi-tional analyses of safety, cost-effectiveness, and accumulating experience will answer these questions.

Device-related image artifacts seem to affect the decision to order an MRI in CIED recipients. Based on our current knowledge, type and location of the device, as well as MRI sequence characteristics, may affect the presence and quantity of CIED-related artifacts. Ultimately, newer designs addressing the large local artifact produced by the ICD transformer are necessary to mitigate artifacts.

CONCLUSION

The public health importance of the ability to perform MRI in CIED recipients has led to laudable efforts by device manufacturers to develop MRI conditional systems, and by investigators to develop safety protocols for improved access in patients with legacy systems. Current guidelines suggest that MRI may be performed in legacy CIED recipients using a strict protocol if there is no alternative imaging and the benefits of the MRI outweigh the risk of the examination.

CONFLICT OF INTEREST

Esra Gucuk Ipek has no conflict of interest. Saman Nazarian is a sci-entific advisor to CardioSolv, St. Jude Medical, Spectranetics, and Biosense Webster Inc. and principal investigator for research funding to Johns Hopkins University from Biosense-Webster Inc.

REFERENCES

A full reference list is available online at ExpertConsult.com

12

Special Considerations: Cardiovascular Magnetic Resonance in Infants and Children

Mark A. Fogel

Clinical cardiovascular magnetic resonance (CMR) had been in use for nearly 35 years and has become firmly established in the evaluation of congenital heart disease (CHD) in many ways, including anatomy, physiology, ventricular function, blood flow, and tissue characterization.[1-29] In many instances, it is used as an adjunct to other imaging modalities such as noninvasive echocardiography and invasive angiography; however, in a number of areas such as vascular rings,[25-29] blood flow, as well as ventricular volumes and mass,[30,31] it has become the clinical "gold standard." In addition, CMR offers several advantages over other imaging modalities, including lack of ionizing radiation, which is extremely important for infants and children who are more susceptible to DNA breakage leading to neoplastic disease and have more time to manifest cancer symptomatology than adults. Furthermore, with capabilities such as exquisite soft tissue contrast, a capacity for *true* three-dimensional (3D) imaging in many areas (e.g., anatomy, ventricular function, blood flow), accurate flow quantification, tissue characterization such as myocardial viability, T1 mapping for diffuse fibrosis and perfusion imaging, noninvasive labeling of the myocardium or blood (tagging), coronary imaging and freely selectable imaging planes without limitations to "windows" or overlapping structures make CMR the "one-stop-shop" for noninvasive imaging in children. There are also unique characteristics to CMR, such as building images over many heartbeats so that long-term function and flow are "built into the image" (instead of the imager having to do this mentally by visualizing hundreds of heartbeats), four-dimensional (4D) flow imaging or internal checks to flow (e.g., the flows in the branch pulmonary arteries must sum to the flow measured in the main pulmonary artery) that make hemodynamics especially accurate. These advantages, and continued advances in CMR hardware, software, and imaging techniques, are bringing CMR into even more widespread use in pediatric cardiology. With the advent of relatively new techniques—such as "real-time" cine[32] and flow imaging,[33] dark blood 3D sampling perfection with application-optimized contrasts using different flip angle evolution (SPACE)[34] and fully navigator accepted coronary imaging—CMR is poised to become a first-line imaging modality in many situations in pediatric cardiology and CHD.

Although the application of CMR to CHD uses nearly all of the techniques discussed in the various chapters of this book, it nevertheless stands on its own as a separate discipline in the world of CMR. The multiple reasons for this can be divided into a few broad categories.

1. Technical challenges: imaging infants and children is very demanding because they require both increased spatial resolution as a result of their small size as well as increased temporal resolution because of higher heart rates as compared with adults. CMR in adults makes many tradeoffs to make imaging quicker and simpler without sacrificing diagnostic accuracy, such as obtaining spatial resolution at the cost of temporal resolution and vice versa. Because many pulse sequences are made to image adult patients, the tradeoffs that can be performed in children can only be taken advantage of to a limited degree. In addition, children under 10 years of age usually need some form of sedation, which make sequences designed for breath-holding useless unless the child is paralyzed, intubated, and mechanically ventilated under anesthesia. Because the breath-holding technique is the mainstay of adult CMR, "work-arounds" have been developed to successfully image the pediatric patient. These modifications, or new approaches to CMR, must be understood for children to be imaged successfully.

2. Anatomy of CHD: the anatomy of native CHD is very different from adult cardiology and demands a rigorous and systematic approach to make the correct diagnosis. In addition, because many CHDs rely on surgical as well as an increasing number of catheter-based therapies, the anatomic and physiologic information extracted from the CMR examination needs to keep these approaches in mind. As a corollary, the postoperative/interventional anatomy and hemodynamics in CHD must also be familiar to the physician performing the examination to assess for adequacy of the therapy and follow-up. For example, the connections between the major cardiac segments (atria, ventricles, and great vessels) along with venous anatomy can and are altered in many types of the diseases encountered in CHD (e.g., transposition of the great arteries [TGA]). Communications are present where they should not be (e.g., ventricular septal defects [VSD]), blood vessels from fetal life may still be present (e.g., patent ductus arteriosus), and some cardiac structures might not even be present or present in a markedly hypoplastic form (e.g., hypoplastic left heart syndrome). In the evaluation of CHD after surgery, conduits and baffles constructed to separate the circulations have little parallel in the adult world.[8] As such, anatomy and morphology must be delineated by CMR in ways that are not required in adult heart disease and the physician interpreting the study needs to be schooled in the nuances of both the preoperative and postoperative anatomy of CHD.

3. Physiology: the unique physiology of CHD is most often a result of the altered anatomy. Evaluation of shunts (e.g., VSD) plays a critical role in assessment of any disease entity in pediatrics and yet has a minor role in the adult world. CMR has recently become the only imaging modality to quantify aortic to pulmonary collateral flow development in single ventricles, again, a unique province of CHD.[35-37] Determination of ventricular function in ventricles with strange and unusual shapes (single ventricles, L-looped ventricles) is routine in the practice of CMR in children and demands unique solutions. Assessment of the postoperative/interventional physiology where the surgeon, for example, creates

a systemic to pulmonary artery shunt or creates an anastomosis between the cava and the pulmonary artery must be dealt with. CMR in CHD and in pediatrics must be adapted to fit these needs and the physician interpreting the study needs to understand the complex physiology.

Similar to other imaging modalities, CMR has limitations and challenges in the CHD population. Sedation, and in some instances, general anesthesia for infants and children to hold still for a 45- to 60-minute scan is always a consideration. Even if remaining motionless in the scanner is not an issue, cooperation by the preteen or teen may be problematic (e.g., breath-holding). In addition, intravascular coils, wires, stents, and clips may all cause artifacts if they are near the structure of interest and are found in a number of cases of CHD where catheter and surgical intervention has occurred. The lack of portability of CMR is disadvantageous, especially for the critically ill infant or child who would need to be moved to the CMR suite. And finally, patients with arrhythmias may not allow proper data acquisition; other patients may have bizarre T-waves or bundle branch blocks, which may not allow for proper triggering. This is becoming less of an issue now that "single shot" CMR, "real-time" CMR, and sequences with "arrhythmia rejection" are realities. Pacemakers are still a problem and remain a "relative contraindication"; though safety of MRI in adult patients with non-MRI conditional/legacy pacemakers and implanted cardioverter-defibrillators has been demonstrated,[37a] safety data specific to infants and children are currently lacking. Patients with them usually do not undergo CMR unless it is the only imaging modality that can obtain the data and change management (see Chapter 11).[38]

This chapter discusses the present state-of-the-art of CMR in CHD and some of the newer techniques available. For simplicity, the imaging techniques discussed will be generic; however, some of the "lingo" of CMR will be related to the Siemen's CMR scanners. The reader should understand that other manufacturers, for the most part, have similar sequences but under a different name.

GENERALIZED PROTOCOL OF CMR FOR CONGENITAL HEART DISEASE

CMR for CHD is a technique that constantly requires fine tuning during an examination, in general, because unexpected findings turn up frequently, especially in pediatrics. Nevertheless, certain basic principles exist that can be formulated into a generalized protocol of CMR in CHD (Fig. 12.1). The author does not claim this to be the only way to think about the process, but it is, in the author's opinion, the most efficient and complete. It should be noted that the protocol needs to be individualized to the patient and the disease process.

- Static SSFP-axial
- HASTE
- Cine
- Dark blood
- Gadolinium
- T1 mapping
- Velocity mapping
- Viability
- Coronary imaging } Specialized techniques
- Tagging } Specialized techniques
- Perfusion } Specialized techniques
- 4D flow } Specialized techniques

FIG. 12.1 Generalized protocol for cardiovascular magnetic resonance imaging of congenital heart disease. This is a generalized protocol and should be individualized to the patient and the specific disease. *HASTE,* Half-Fourier acquisition single-shot turbo spin echo; *MPR,* multiplanar reconstruction; *SSFP,* steady-state free precession.

In this section, each step of the protocol will demonstrate a different form of CHD, giving the reader a broad overview of the spectrum of lesions encountered.

Anatomic Imaging (Noncontrast)

After localizers, anatomic data are acquired not only to survey the cardiovascular anatomy and make the "anatomic diagnosis" but also to act as localizers themselves for future physiologic and functional imaging. This is important in that physiologic and functional data must be interpreted in light of the prevailing anatomy. A full contiguous set of axial images from the diaphragm to the thoracic inlet is obtained (typically 40–50 images, Figs. 12.2 and 12.3); the author prefers "static" balanced steady-state free precession (bSSFP) images. This must be extended outside the thorax for special cases such as to the neck if arch anatomy is being evaluated (e.g., innominate artery branches in the neck) or if total anomalous pulmonary venous connections are suspected (e.g., connection below the diaphragm). Imaging that uses bSSFP depends on contrast between blood and the surrounding tissue, which is enhanced by using a high flip angle, and therefore the practice is to allow the scanner to select the highest flip angle possible. These axial images form the basis of examining the anatomy.

One disadvantage to using "static" bSSFP is that turbulence may present on the image as an absence of a structure (signal loss) as in the case of the pulmonary arteries in a single ventricle patient after a Blalock-Taussing shunt; typically, these are very difficult to visualize by this technique because the turbulence creates a major signal loss. This drawback can be compensated for by performing half-Fourier acquisition single-shot turbo spin echo (HASTE) imaging, which yields a set of dark blood images rapidly (or another type of dark blood imaging such as 3D SPACE, although HASTE is the quickest) and is performed while multiplanar reconstruction (MPR) is being done (see later). Alternatively, a set of axial cines can be performed to visualize these structures in the hope that a phase of the cardiac cycle will demonstrate the "missing" structure.

MPR, also called multiplanar reformatting, is a technique where a set of contiguous images (in this case, axial) are stacked atop each other and any plane can be reconstructed. This can be used after the axial stack above is obtained. The exact slice orientation and position can therefore be obtained for any future imaging during the study. In addition, the anatomy can be inspected from multiple views from just the set of axial images as a first pass. It can be used for any type of imaging. Finally, MPR can be used to demonstrate the salient point of the anatomy in instances where the scan needed to be terminated prematurely because of patient instability or technical issues after the stack of contiguous axial images had been obtained. "Curved cuts" can be used to delineate the important parts of the anatomy as well (see Fig. 12.3).

If needed, dark blood imaging can complement the bright blood imaging as in instances of vascular rings to visualize the trachea, coarctation of the aorta (Fig. 12.4) or a systemic to pulmonary artery shunt. This type of imaging is used judiciously because it requires relatively long scanning times. A set of high-resolution double-inversion recovery dark blood images can be obtained or, if available, 3D SPACE, which can obtain a high-resolution slab in 5 minutes or less.

Function/Anatomy: Cine CMR (Fig. 12.5)

Either bSSFP or spoiled gradient recalled echo (GRE) sequences are used and are tailored to the lesion under study. Cine, along with phase

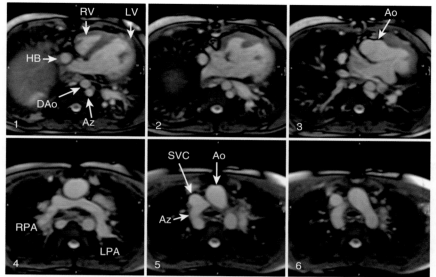

FIG. 12.2 Stack of contiguous static balanced steady-state free precession images. This is a set of selected axial images of a patient with heterotaxy syndrome, tricuspid stenosis with pulmonary atresia (S,D,X) with a hypoplastic right ventricle *(RV)* and interrupted inferior vena cava with azygous continuation to the right superior vena cava *(SVC)* who is imaged after a Kawashima operation (SVC to pulmonary artery connection in the presence of an interrupted inferior vena cava with azygous continuation) and a hepatic baffle to the pulmonary arteries. Images progress from inferior to superior as the panels go from left to right and from top to bottom (numbers 1–6). *Ao,* Aorta; *Az,* azygous vein; *DAo,* descending aorta; *HB,* hepatic baffle; *LPA,* left pulmonary artery; *LV,* left ventricle; *RPA,* right pulmonary artery.

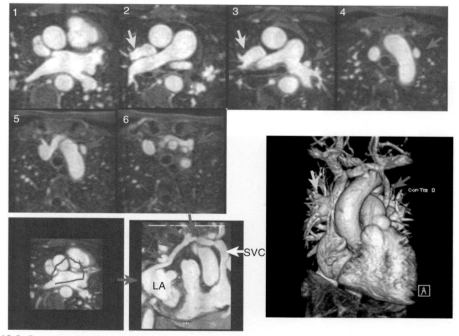

FIG. 12.3 Curved cuts using multiplanar reconstruction. This patient has a partial anomalous right pulmonary venous connection to the superior vena cava *(SVC)* but also a persistent levo-atrio-cardinal vein connecting the left atrium *(LA)* to the innominate vein. The top and middle 6 panels are static bright blood images following the levo-atrio-cardinal vein *(red arrows)* and progress from inferior to superior, going from 1 to 6. The partial anomalous pulmonary venous connection is outlined by the yellow arrows. When the set of static axial bright blood images are stacked one atop the other, a curved plane can be drawn *(lower left panel)* tracing the course of this levo-atrio-cardinal vein in one image *(lower middle panel, red arrows)*. The panel in the lower right demonstrates a three-dimensional reconstruction from the bright blood images showing the levo-atrio-cardinal vein *(red arrows)* and the anomalous pulmonary venous connections *(yellow arrows)*.

it has been demonstrated that surgically placed patches and valves[43] can become bright with this technique.

Perfusion

The same patient population who are candidates for LGE imaging are also candidates for myocardial perfusion imaging (see Fig. 12.14), which, similar to LGE, is not only a consideration for the adult with heart disease.[42] It is a gadolinium-based procedure and is typically imaged with vasodilator (e.g., adenosine ["stress"] at 140 µg/kg/min for 4–6 minutes) followed 20 minutes or so later without adenosine ("rest") and then followed approximately 10 minutes later by LGE imaging similar to adults. This can also be done with dobutamine stress.[45] In CHD, using adenosine stress perfusion is more common.

Myocardial Iron

The T2* technique is used to assess myocardial iron and hematologists use this in conjunction with other parameters such as liver and blood iron to adjust chelation therapy. This applies to children with thalassemia, sickle cell disease, and other hematologic disorders of red blood cell destruction.

Myocarditis

Although there are a paucity of data in the pediatric age group for the CMR assessment of myocarditis, it is not an uncommon diagnosis to entertain in an adolescent with chest pain and elevated troponins. Similar to the adult assessment, the Lake Louise criteria are used, including T2 imaging (edema), T1 imaging before and after gadolinium administration (hyperemia and capillary leak), and LGE (see Chapter 35).

T1 Mapping

The ability to quantify the T1 of the myocardium, both before and after gadolinium contrast administration, has facilitated determination of diffuse fibrosis within the heart with a disproportionate amount of collagen. This may be quantified by native T1 time, partition coefficient, and extracellular volume fraction. There is emerging evidence to suggest that this may be of value clinically in CHD (e.g., in tetralogy of Fallot, the LV and RV T1 mapping values may be different than in normal individuals).[46]

OTHER IMPORTANT TECHNIQUES USED IN CONGENITAL HEART DISEASE

Real-Time Cine Imaging and Phase Contrast CMR

Real-time cine imaging acquires single-shot images at a temporal resolution of ~40 to 50 ms and can be used in exercise CMR (see later), in patients with arrhythmias, or in those who have a problem remaining motionless in the scanner. In addition, real-time cine CMR can be performed interactively using a "real-time window" and three other localizer windows controlled with a cursor and sweeping the ventricle to assess ventricular function or finding small atrial septal defect (ASD) and VSD. In addition, these sweeps can be used to survey the cardiovascular anatomy in conjunction with the static bSSFP imaging.

Real-time PCMR acquires single-shot flow images and can have a similar temporal resolution to real-time cine images. This also may be used for exercise CMR, patients with arrhythmias, or simply to speed up the examination.

Deployment of these two technologies is still limited and analysis tools for real-time PCMR are still in their infancy.

Coronary Artery Imaging[44,47,48]

Using T2-prepared bSSFP imaging combined with the navigator technique[47] or the IR-GRE technique mentioned in the gadolinium section

earlier, coronary imaging (Figs. 12.15–12.17) is indicated in a variety of CHD similar to those who obtain LGE imaging (coronary manipulation such as TGA after arterial switch[44] or with native or acquired coronary disease such as anomalous left coronary artery from the pulmonary artery or in Kawasaki disease to assess for aneurysms). In children with fast heart rates (RR intervals <500 ms), minimizing coronary artery motion by acquiring lines of K-space at the quiescent phase of the cardiac cycle may require obtaining data at end systole rather than mid to late diastole, as in adults.

Exercise Cardiovascular Magnetic Resonance

With the advent of CMR-compatible ergometers, the patient can exercise in the CMR environment with subsequent imaging of function and flow, generally with "real-time" techniques. This is useful in children with chest pain where perfusion at exercise can be assessed, hypertrophic cardiomyopathy (HCM) with poor echocardiographic windows to visualize the LV outflow tract, and adolescents with poor exercise performance to assess ventricular function. For example, it was discovered that poor exercise performance of single-ventricle patients after Fontan was related to increased power loss in the systemic venous pathway in this manner.[49]

Myocardial and Blood Tagging

In limited use now, myocardial tagging such as spatial modulation of magnetization (SPAMM) divides the ventricle noninvasively into "cubes of magnetization" and local deformation of the myocardium can be visualized and strain calculated. In patients where there is a question of regional wall motion abnormalities (e.g., cardiomyopathy such as in Duchenne muscular dystrophy[50] or single ventricle[11,22,23]) or whether or not a focal piece of myocardium is even contracting (e.g., tumor or HCM), myocardial tagging can be used to assess this both qualitatively and quantitatively. With blood tagging, if there are questions about the presence of an ASD or VSD, a saturation band can be laid down on the blood to "tag" it as dark on a gradient echo image[51] and this dark blood can be followed so that shunting can be visualized; this has been largely supplanted by in-plane PCMR.

Tumor/Mass Characterization[52] (see Fig. 12.14)

Although cardiac tumors are relatively rare, they do occur in pediatrics. Many cardiac tumors and masses can be differentiated from each other not only by where they occur in the heart, what symptoms they cause, and at what age they occur but also by their tissue characteristics on CMR. For example, a fibroma will accumulate gadolinium and be signal intense on LGE imaging and T1-weighted images after gadolinium administration, whereas lipomas will be signal intense on T1-weighted images and become signal poor after fat saturation. Tumor characterization procedures by CMR are a protocol in themselves and typically include T1- and T2-weighted images, images with fat saturation, GRE imaging (e.g., for thrombus), perfusion (e.g., for hemangiomas), LGE imaging, T1-weighted images after gadolinium administration, and SPAMM. If time permits, functional imaging can be used to assess for effects of the tumor such as obstruction to flow and decreased cardiac output.

Arrhythmogenic Right Ventricular Cardiomyopathy

Arrhythmogenic right ventricular cardiomyopathy (ARVC) is the replacement of myocardium by fatty or fibrofatty tissue[53] and imaging fulfills only one of the criteria set forth in the revised 2010 Task Force manuscript.[54] CMR has been successfully used in adults for this disease; however, in pediatrics, there is a question as to its usefulness.[55] The findings by CMR in adults with ARVC studies are highly variable[56] but, in general, there is: (1) fatty substitution of the myocardium, which is

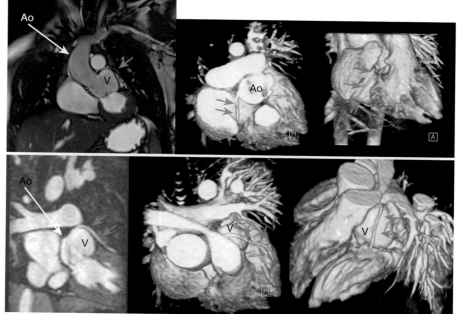

FIG. 12.15 Coronary artery imaging in congenital heart disease. A 2-year-old child with a dilated sinus of Valsalva aneurysm *(V)* with the left main coronary artery originating from it. Top left panel is a cine image showing the dilated sinus. Top middle and right panels are three-dimensional (3D) volume renderings of the right coronary artery origin *(arrows)*. Lower panels are 3D inversion recovery contrast-enhanced gradient recalled echo images of the dilated sinus and the origin of the left coronary artery with the raw data *(lower left)* and 3D volume renderings *(lower middle and right)*. *Ao,* Aorta.

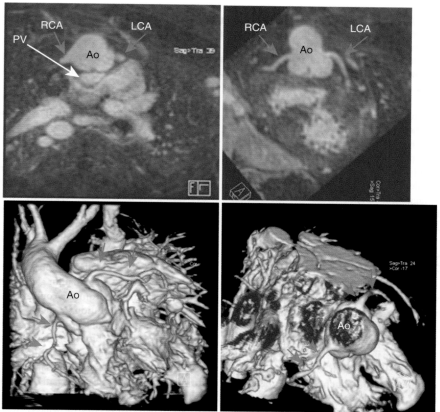

FIG. 12.16 Coronary artery imaging in congenital heart disease. A 4-year-old child with double outlet right ventricle (S,D,D) with left juxtaposition of the atrial appendages after Fontan. The top two panels demonstrate the origins of the coronaries from a three-dimensional (3D) inversion recovery contrast-enhanced gradient echo sequence in the off-axis axial *(left)* and off-axis coronal views *(right)*. The right coronary artery *(RCA)* originates from the right and posterior facing sinus while the left coronary originates from the left posterior facing sinus. The bottom two panels are 3D volume-rendered images of the coronary origins and courses from both anteroposterior *(left)* and off-axis transverse views *(right)*. Arrows in lower panels point to the coronaries. *Ao,* Aorta; *LCA,* left coronary artery; *PV,* pulmonary valve.

13

Human Cardiac Magnetic Resonance at Ultrahigh Fields: Technical Innovations, Early Clinical Applications and Opportunities for Discoveries

Thoralf Niendorf, Till Huelnhagen, Lukas Winter, and Katharina Paul

The development of ultrahigh field magnetic resonance (UHF-MR, B_0 $\geq$ 7 T, $f \geq$ 298 MHz) is moving forward at an amazing speed that is breaking through technical barriers almost as fast as they appear. UHF-MR has become an engine for innovation in experimental and clinical research.[1-11] With nearly 40,000 magnetic resonance (MR) examinations already performed, the reasons for moving UHF-MR into clinical applications are more compelling than ever. The value of high field MR at 3 T has already proven itself many times over at lower field strengths; now 7 T has opened a window on tissues, organs, and (patho)physiologic processes that have been largely inaccessible in the past. The lion's share of UHF-MR examinations today covers neuroscience applications where enabling technology has revealed new aspects of the anatomy, functions, and physiometabolic characteristics of the brain at an unparalleled quality.

The growing number of reports referring to cardiovascular applications is an inherent testament to the advancements of UHF-MR and documents the progress in imaging the heart and large vessels at 7 T.[1-45] These technical and early feasibility studies in healthy subjects and patients respond to unsolved problems and unmet needs of today's clinical cardiovascular magnetic resonance (CMR). These developments are fueled by the signal-to-noise ratio (SNR) advantage and the promise of enhanced relative spatial resolution (voxel per anatomy), and are enabled by novel MR technology. Transferring UHF-CMR into the clinic remains a challenge though.[8] Arguably, the benefits of UHF-MR are sometimes offset by concomitant physics-related phenomena and by practical obstacles. These impediments include magnetic field inhomogeneities, off-resonance artifacts, dielectric effects, radiofrequency (RF) nonuniformities, localized tissue heating, and RF power deposition constraints. It is no surprise that these effects can make it a challenge to even compete with the capabilities of CMR at clinical field strengths of 1.5 T and 3 T.[8] If these impediments can be overcome, the promises of UHF-CMR will open new avenues for MR-based myocardial tissue characterization and imaging of the myocardial macromorphology and micromorphology. The benefits of UHF-MR will catalyze explorations that go beyond conventional ^{1}H MR of the heart. This includes imaging and spectroscopy of [23]Na, ^{19}F, ^{31}P, ^{13}C, and other X nuclei to enable a better insight into inflammatory, metabolic, and (nano)molecular processes of the heart.

Realizing the progress and challenges of UHF-CMR, this chapter provides an overview of the state of the art of cardiac MR at 7 T. It discusses the clinical relevance of what has been already observed and what can be clearly foreseen. The chapter is devoted to surveying technical innovations, practical considerations, safety topics, frontier studies in healthy subjects, early clinical application in small patient cohorts, opportunities for discoveries, and future directions of UHF-CMR. At the moment some of these new concepts and applications are merely of proof-of-principle nature, but they are compelling enough to drive the field forward with the goal to advance the capabilities of cardiac imaging. As they are developed, the boundaries of MR physics, biomedical engineering, and biomedical sciences will be pushed in many ways, with the implications and potential uses feeding into basic cardiology research and clinical sciences.

In the sections that follow, encouraging developments into multiple channel RF concepts are reviewed. Advances in imaging methodology and progress in RF pulse design are discussed. Early applications for imaging of cardiac anatomy, cardiac chamber quantification, myocardial mapping, angiography of the large vessels, and real-time imaging of the heart are surveyed. Clinical opportunities for high spatial resolution MR and parametric tissue characterization (all being facilitated by the traits of UHF-MR) are also discussed. Physiometabolic CMR applications are explored, including sodium MR and phosphorus MR. Practical and safety considerations for cardiac MR in humans at 7 T are outlined. Current trends in CMR are considered, together with their clinical implications. A concluding section ventures a glance beyond the horizon and explores an even further step into the future, with something called extreme field magnetic resonance (EF-MR).

ENABLING TECHNICAL INNOVATIONS FOR UHF-CMR

At ultrahigh fields the crux of the matter is that the RF wavelength in tissue λ becomes sufficiently short ($\lambda_{myocardium} \approx$ 12 cm) versus the size of the upper torso. The heart, being a deep-lying organ surrounded by the lung within the comparatively large volume of the thorax, is a target region that is particularly susceptible to nonuniformities in the RF transmission field (B_1^+). These detrimental transmission field phenomena can cause shading, massive signal drop-off, or even signal void in the images, and hence bear the potential to offset the benefits of UHF-CMR because of nondiagnostic image quality. These constraints are not a surprise as it might appear at the first glance, because transmission field nonuniformities, although somewhat reduced, remain significant in CMR at 3 T.[46] Further to the challenges imposed by B_1^+ nonuniformities, magnetohydrodynamic effects severely disturb the electrocardiogram (ECG) commonly used for cardiac triggering at clinical field strengths. This challenge evoked the need for novel ancillary hardware that supports synchronization of MR data acquisition with cardiac activity.

To address the practical obstacles of UHF-CMR, technical innovations in RF antenna design have evolved in recent years. Novel pulse sequences for transmission field mapping and shaping as well as innovative RF pulse designs along with multichannel RF transmission were reported with the common goal to overcome the detrimental B_1^+ phenomena at 7 T to enable cardiac imaging. Novel triggering techniques that are immune to electromagnetic fields have been established as an alternative to ECG. In this light, this section surveys enabling technical innovations tailored for UHF-CMR.

Enabling Radiofrequency Antenna Technology

A plethora of reports eloquently refer to the development of enabling RF technology tailored for CMR at 7 T. Research directions include local transceiver (TX/RX) arrays and multichannel transmission arrays in conjunction with multichannel local receiver arrays.

Multichannel RF coil designs tailored for UHF-CMR involve rigid, flexible, and modular configurations. The gestation process revealed a trend toward a larger number of transmit and receive elements[5,11,13,14,18,28,41] to improve anatomic coverage and to advance the capabilities for transmission field shaping.[47] Pioneering developments

made good use of building blocks that include stripline elements,[1,2,48–50] electrical dipoles,[22,41,50–54] dielectric resonant antennas,[29] and loop elements,[5,11,13,14,18,28] with up to 32 independent elements.

Loop element-based CMR optimized 7 T transceiver configurations were reported for a 4-channel TX/RX[11] (Fig. 13.1A), an 8-channel TX/RX[18] (Fig. 13.1B), and a two-dimensional (2D) 16-channel TX/RX design (Fig. 13.1C).[13] The 2D approach was extended to a more sophisticated modular 32-channel TX/RX array shown in Fig. 13.1D.[28]

Various stripline element-based 7 T transceiver configurations were proposed for cardiac UHF-MR. In a pioneering 8-element transverse electromagnetic field (TEM) transceiver array design, each element was independently connected to a dedicated RF power amplifier.[1] Other stripline array configurations run flexible designs consisting of a pair of 4 or 8 stripline elements.[2,48] Another practical solution comprising an 8-channel stripline transceive array that uses sophisticated automated tuning with piezoelectric actuators was accomplished.[33]

Electric dipole configurations have been shown to benefit MR of the upper torso and the heart at 7 T.[22,41,51,53,54] Electric dipoles run the trait of a linearly polarized current pattern, where RF energy is directed perpendicular to the dipole along the Poynting vector to the subject, resulting in a symmetrical, rather uniform excitation field with increased depth penetration.[51] Early implementations include straight dipole elements.[51] The need for densely packed multichannel transceiver coil arrays tailored for UHF-CMR has inspired explorations into electric dipole

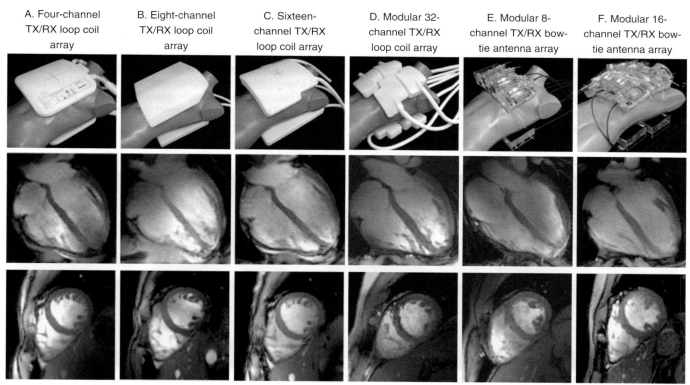

FIG. 13.1 Examples of multichannel transceiver arrays tailored for cardiovascular magnetic resonance at 7 T. *Top row,* Photographs of cardiac optimized 7 T transceiver coil arrays including *(left to right)* a 4-channel, an 8-channel, a 16-channel, and a 32-channel loop array configuration together with an 8-channel and 16-channel bow-tie antenna array. For all configurations, the coil elements are used for transmission and reception. Four-chamber *(middle row)* and short-axis *(bottom row)* views of the heart derived from two-dimensional CINE fast low angle shot acquisitions using the radiofrequency coil arrays shown on top and a spatial resolution of (1.4 × 1.4. × 4) mm³. (From Niendorf T, Paul K, Ozerdem C, et al. W(h)ither human cardiac and body magnetic resonance at ultrahigh fields? Technical advances, practical considerations, applications, and clinical opportunities. *NMR Biomed.* 2016;29(9):1173–1197.)

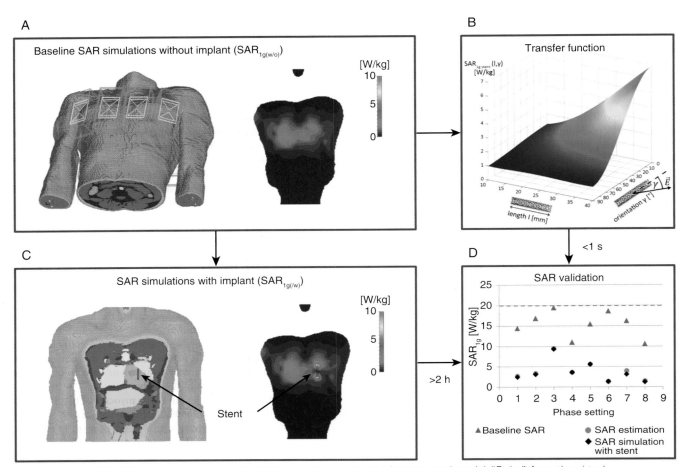

FIG. 13.6 Electromagnetic field (EMF) simulations using the human voxel model "Duke" from the virtual family and an 8-channel transmit/receive bow-tie electric dipole array. (A) Schematic views of the positioning of the anterior bow-tie radiofrequency antennas on the anterior chest of the human voxel model and coronal view of specific absorption rate $(SAR)_{1g\ baseline}$ distribution for a plane through the target position without the stent equivalent being present. (B) Surface plot of SAR_{1g} stent derived from the transfer function for baseline SAR_{1g} for an input power of 1 W/kg. A stent length ranging from 10 to 40 mm and a stent rotation versus the main E-field vector ranging from 0 to 90 degrees was applied. (C) Coronal view of $SAR_{1g\ stent}$ distribution for a plane through the target position with the stent equivalent being present. (D) Simulated maximum baseline $SAR_{1g\ baseline}$ and $SAR_{1g\ stent}$ for the stent equivalent using eight randomly generated phase settings compared with the SAR estimation deduced from the analytical approach (see Eq. 13.3). Although conservatively overestimating SAR, SAR estimation using Eq. 13.3 was able to predict the induced SAR_{1g} levels without the need to perform extra time-consuming EMF simulations with a stent being present in the simulation model. (From Niendorf T, Paul K, Oezerdem C, et al. W(h)ither human cardiac and body magnetic resonance at ultrahigh fields? Technical advances, practical considerations, applications, and clinical opportunities. *NMR Biomed.* 2016;29(9):1173–1197.)

are included. Benchmarking the analytical approach versus EMF simulations showed a good conservative estimation of induced SAR_{1g} peak levels. A practical example is shown in Fig. 13.6 using an 8-channel bow-tie antenna RF coil array optimized for CMR at 7 T (see Fig. 13.1E). EMF simulations including the stent consumed more than 2 hours central processing unit (CPU) and graphics processing unit (GPU) time per phase setting (not including RF shim field combining and SAR calculations) while the analytical approach can be calculated in real time. This example underscores the value of the proposed analytical approach based upon a transfer function for obeying regulatory RF power limits.[99] The approach of using a transfer function is conceptually translatable to other implant configurations, which is in particular suitable for short implants ($\leq\lambda_{tissue}/3$) where the influence of the phase distribution of the RF transmit field is negligible.[115] Furthermore, it

can be conveniently incorporated into state-of-the art SAR prediction concepts[116,117] to provide SAR estimations induced by coronary stents and other conductive implants for arbitrary RF pulses used for transmission field shimming[24,118] or parallel transmission.[89,90] To generalize, this approach provides a novel metric or design criteria for RF coils: for example, to design RF coils (1) with low SAR levels in the vicinity of the stent or (2) with SAR levels during the presence of the stent which do not exceed SAR levels without the presence of the stent.[39] The transfer function approach should not end at SAR estimation, but should move toward temperature or CEM43 estimations. In particular, for short implants like coronary stents, maximum induced SAR levels in the implant are much more restrictive to the allowed input power than maximum temperature or CEM43 values would be. It was shown that even though maximum induced local SAR at the stent tip was by a factor >2 higher than in surface regions, the eventual temperature after 6 minutes of RF heating was by >6°C lower at the stent tip region.[39] This temperature saturation effect at the stent tip originates from a strong temperature gradient toward colder tissue regions at the stent center and is even more pronounced by physiologic parameters such as blood flow in the stented vessel. These findings are heartening; they will accelerate further research on safety assessment of coronary stents and other implants common in clinical practice and will help to relax current UHF-CMR limitations.

EARLY APPLICATIONS AND CLINICAL STUDIES

This section surveys proof-of-principle and feasibility studies of UHF-CMR in healthy human subjects and in small patient cohorts. Early UHF-CMR applications include anatomic imaging using black-blood techniques, cardiac chamber quantification employing 2D CINE techniques, first-pass myocardial perfusion imaging, parametric mapping of the effective transversal relaxation time T2* and the longitudinal relaxation time T1, fat-water imaging, coronary artery angiography, vascular imaging, and real-time imaging of the heart.

Black-Blood Imaging

Transfer of rapid acquisition with relaxation enhancement imaging (RARE) (also known as fast spin-echo [FSE] imaging)-based black-blood imaging to 7 T is of high relevance for advancing the capabilities of UHF-CMR for explorations into cardiac morphology. The feasibility of cardiac RARE imaging at 7 T using an 8-channel transceiver array of bow-tie antennas is demonstrated in Fig. 13.7. A spatial resolution as good as $(0.8 \times 0.8 \times 5)$ mm^3 was applied, which represents an order of magnitude improvement versus standardized protocols of today's clinical CMR practice.[119] The blood suppression inherent to RARE variants works well in most regions of the heart. Only slow-flowing blood in areas close to the endocardium remains visible. The refinement of black-blood preparation modules—including double-inversion recovery preparation—tailored for 7 T is anticipated to further improve the image quality of RARE at 7 T. Also, RARE imaging at 7 T presents an RF power deposition challenge because of the train of high-peak RF power refocusing pulses ($\alpha \leq 180$ degrees). Notwithstanding its utility for improving B_1^+ uniformity in UHF-RARE imaging, recent studies on using adiabatic pulses for UHF-RARE reported long inter-echo times of up to 15 ms[120]; an approach that does not meet the requirements of CMR taking advantage of breath-hold scans to deal with respiratory motion.

Cardiac Chamber Quantification

Early studies demonstrated the feasibility and usefulness of 2D CINE spoiled gradient echo imaging (fast low angle shot [FLASH]) for cardiac chamber quantification of the left ventricle (LV)[6,9,12] and right ventricle (RV)[20] at 7 T. 2D CINE FLASH provides high-quality images with uniform signal intensity distribution and high blood/myocardium contrast over the entire heart, as demonstrated for a 32-channel loop element RF coil array and for a 16-channel bow-tie antenna array in Fig. 13.8. Fig. 13.9 shows long-axis and short-axis views of an exemplary volunteer and underlines the signal uniformity and superb blood-to-myocardium contrast. The latter is competitive with the blood-to-myocardium contrast obtained for 2D CINE steady-state free precession (SSFP) imaging at 1.5 T.[6,9,12] Imaging the right ventricle at 7 T using fast gradient echo (FGRE) provided RV dimensions and function comparable with SSFP imaging at 1.5 T (Fig. 13.10).[20] Cardiac chamber quantification at 7 T agrees closely with LV and RV parameters derived at 1.5 T.[9]

The baseline SNR gain at 7 T can be translated into spatial resolution enhancements versus the kindred counterparts at lower field strengths. Fig. 13.11 surveys four-chamber and short-axis views of the heart obtained with a standardized CMR protocol[119,121] and with an enhanced spatial resolution protocol. This protocol reduced the voxel size from 19.4 mm^3 to 1.6 mm^3, equivalent to a 12-fold improvement in the spatial resolution versus a standardized clinical CMR protocol. This fidelity approaches an effective anatomical spatial resolution—voxel size per anatomy—which resembles that demonstrated for animal models.[122,123] The overall image quality and improvement in spatial resolution enabled the visualization of fine subtle anatomic structures, including the compact layer of the free RV wall and the remaining trabecular layer. Pericardium, mitral and tricuspid valves—and their associated papillary muscles and trabeculae—are identifiable.

To put the spatial resolution enhancements to clinical use, a UHF-CMR study was performed in a small cohort of patients with hypertrophic cardiomyopathy (HCM)[40] (Fig. 13.12). Cardiac chamber quantification of the left ventricle at 7 T was in accordance with the results derived from the 3 T LV assessment of the same HCM patient group as well as from the age and body mass index (BMI)-matched healthy control group. Thanks to the spatial resolution enhancement at 7 T, hyperintense regions were detected in 54% of the HCM patients within late gadolinium enhancement (LGE) positive regions and were identified as myocardial crypts (Fig. 13.13). These crypts were not detectable at 3 T using a clinical 2D CINE SSFP protocol.[40]

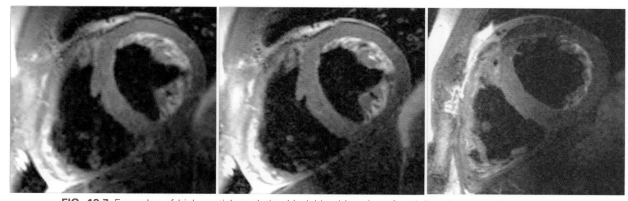

FIG. 13.7 Examples of high spatial resolution black-blood imaging of end-diastolic short-axis views of the heart at 7 T using a rapid acquisition with relaxation enhancment imaging technique. The images exhibit a spatial resolution of *(left)* $(1.2 \times 1.2 \times 5)$ mm^3, *(center)* $(0.9 \times 0.9 \times 4)$ mm^3, and *(right)* $(0.8 \times 0.8 \times 5)$ mm^3, which is by a factor of 2.7 *(left)* or 6 *(center, right)* superior versus the clinical protocols used in today's cardiovascular magnetic resonance practice.

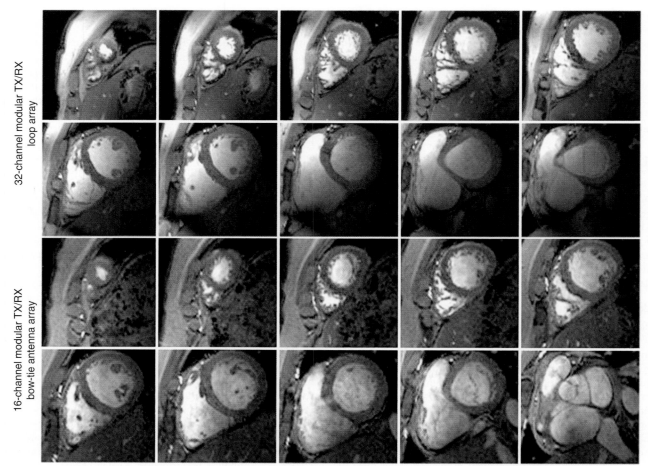

32-channel modular TX/RX loop array

16-channel modular TX/RX bow-tie antenna array

FIG. 13.8 End-diastolic short-axis views covering the heart from the apex to the base derived from two-dimensional CINE fast low angle shot imaging (in-plane resolution 1.1 × 1.1 mm², slice thickness 2.5 mm, generalized autocalibrating partial parallel acquisitions reduction factor 2), using *(top)* a 32-channel modular transceiver (TX/RX) loop array and *(bottom)* a 16-channel modular TX/RX bow-tie antenna array. Both array configurations provided rather uniform signal intensity and no major signal voids for slices covering the heart from the apex to the base. (From Niendorf T, Paul K, Oezerdem C, et al. W(h)ither human cardiac and body magnetic resonance at ultrahigh fields? Technical advances, practical considerations, applications, and clinical opportunities. *NMR Biomed.* 2016;29(9):1173–1197.)

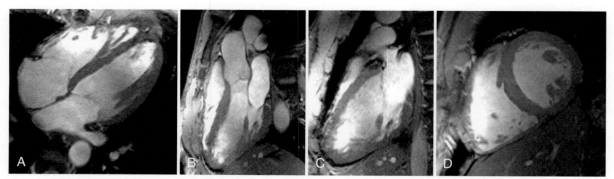

FIG. 13.9 Two-dimensional CINE fast low angle shot images acquired with a 16-channel transceiver (TX/RX) coil array (see Fig. 13.1C) with an in-plane resolution of 1 × 1 mm² (slice thickness 4 mm) using 2-fold acceleration showing a four-chamber view (A), a three-chamber view (B), a two-chamber view (C), and a mid-ventricular short-axis view of the heart (D). (From Thalhammer C, Renz W, Winter L, et al. Two-dimensional sixteen channel transmit/receive coil array for cardiac magnetic resonance imaging at 7 T: design, evaluation, and application. *J Magn Reson Imaging.* 2012;36(4):847–857.)

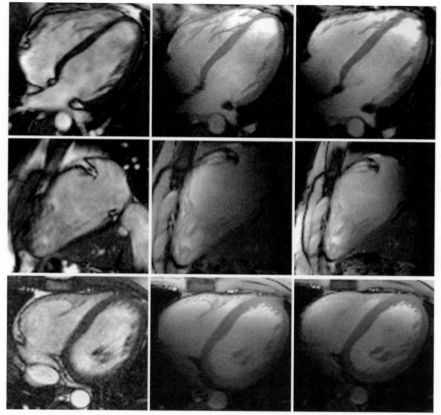

FIG. 13.10 Four-chamber view *(top)*, right ventricle long-axis view *(middle)*, and mid-ventricular transverse view *(bottom)* obtained *(left)* by steady-state free precession at 1.5 T with voxel size 1.2 × 1.2 × 6 mm³ *(left)*, *(center)* by fast gradient echo (FGRE) at 7 T with voxel size 1.2 × 1.2 × 6 mm³ and *(right)* by FGRE at 7 T with voxel size 1.3 × 1.3 × 4 mm³. (From von Knobelsdorff-Brenkenhoff F, Tkachenko V, Winter L, et al. Assessment of the right ventricle with cardiovascular magnetic resonance at 7 tesla. *J Cardiovasc Magn Reson.* 2013;15:23.)

First-Pass Myocardial Perfusion Imaging

Clinical CMR assessment of ischemic heart disease includes rapid first-pass contrast agent enhanced myocardial perfusion CMR.[119] Numerous saturation recovery-based perfusion techniques have been proposed to capture first-pass kinetics with one or two heartbeat temporal resolutions. Saturation methods established at lower fields are suboptimal for myocardial perfusion imaging at 7 T[32] because of their propensity for transmission field nonuniformities. To address this issue a novel saturation pulse train consisting of four hyperbolic-secant (HS8) RF pulses was proposed for effective saturation of myocardium at 7 T.[32] This approach facilitated an average saturation efficiency of 97.8% in native myocardium and afforded the first series of human first-pass myocardial perfusion images at 7 T.[32] The ability to produce exquisite in-plane spatial resolution at 7 T may offer greater diagnostic value for myocardial perfusion assessment and supports an extension of the perfusion assessment to the right ventricle. With sufficient acceleration and imaging speed, perfusion imaging is on the verge of 3D whole-heart coverage acquisitions[124] that might be furthered by the traits of UHF-MR.

Myocardial T2* Mapping

A growing number of reports refer to mapping the effective transverse relaxation time T2* in basic CMR research and clinical CMR applications. Myocardial T2* mapping provides means for noninvasive myocardial tissue characterization without the need for exogenous contrast agents. By making use of the blood-oxygen-level-dependent (BOLD) effect,[125] T2*-sensitized CMR has been proposed to probe changes in tissue oxygenation and perfusion, and has demonstrated the capability to reveal myocardial ischemia and perfusion deficits.[126–130] In clinical routine, T2* mapping has become the gold standard for myocardial iron assessment, an important parameter for diagnosis and therapy guiding in patients with myocardial iron overload.[131]

The linear relationship between magnetic field strength and microscopic susceptibility effects renders the move to $B_0 = 7$ T conceptually appealing for T2* mapping.[25,132–134] The enhanced susceptibility effects at 7 T may be useful to lower the detection level and to extend the dynamic range of the sensitivity for monitoring T2* changes. To avoid T2* quantification errors because of signal modulations induced by fat-water phase shift, echo times when fat and water are in phase are commonly used for T2* mapping.[135] Because of the reduction of the in-phase inter-echo time from 4.8 ms at 1.5 T to 1.02 ms at 7 T, UHF-MR enables rapid acquisition of multiple echoes.[17] Taking advantage of these properties, high spatial resolution and cardiac phase resolved T2* mapping has been demonstrated in the in vivo human heart at 7 T.[17] In contrast, studying temporal changes in T2* across the cardiac cycle at 1.5 T and 3 T is elusive because of scan time constraints which are prohibitive for CINE T2* mapping covering the cardiac cycle. The improved temporal resolution of T2* mapping at 7 T provides means for monitoring externally controlled variations of blood oxygenation, including short periods of hypoxia and hyperoxia test stimuli.[136,137]

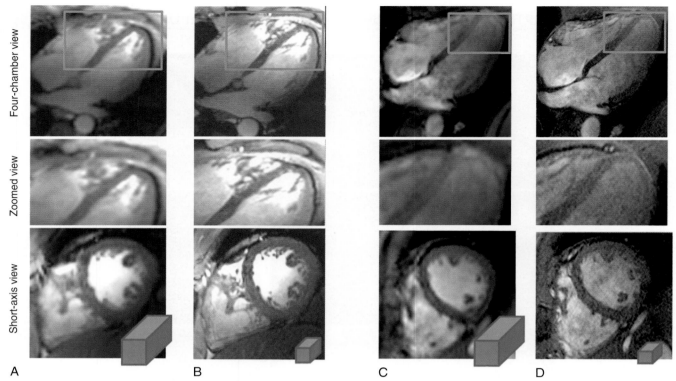

FIG. 13.11 Four-chamber views *(first row)* and short-axis views *(third row)* of the heart derived from two-dimensional CINE fast low angle shot acquisitions, generalized autocalibrating partial parallel acquisition reduction factor 2 using (A, B) a 32-channel modular transceiver (TX/RX) loop element array (see Fig. 13.1B and D) and (C, D) a 16-channel modular TX/RX bow-tie antenna array (see Fig. 13.1C and F). Different resolutions were employed: (A, C) standardized clinical protocol: spatial resolution $1.8 \times 1.8 \times 6$ mm³, (B) spatial resolution $1.1 \times 1.1 \times 2.5$ mm³ and (D) spatial resolution $0.8 \times 0.8 \times 2.5$ mm³. *Second row,* Magnified views of the ventricular trabeculae, demonstrating that spatial resolution enhancements by a factor of 6 or even 12 versus standardized protocols used in current clinical practice improve the delineation of subtle anatomical details of the heart. (From Niendorf T, Paul K, Oezerdem C, et al. W(h)ither human cardiac and body magnetic resonance at ultrahigh fields? Technical advances, practical considerations, applications, and clinical opportunities. *NMR Biomed.* 2016;29(9):1173–1197.)

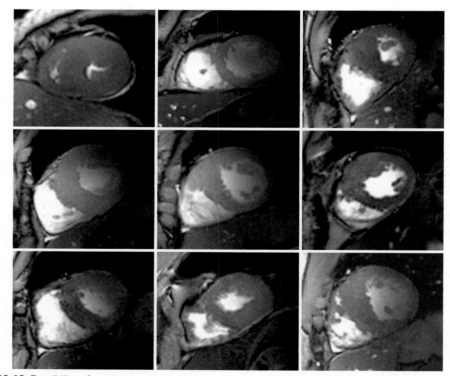

FIG. 13.12 Feasibility of cardiovascular magnetic resonance (CMR) in hypertrophic cardiomyopathy (HCM) patients at 7 T. High-resolution mid-ventricular short-axis CINE images obtained for nine HCM patients enrolled in an ultrahigh field CMR study demonstrating consistency in image quality. All images showed clinical diagnostic quality and were evaluable for cardiac chamber quantification. Spatial resolution is $1.4 \times 1.4 \times 4$ mm³.

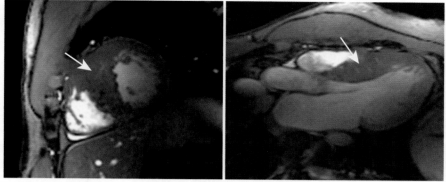

FIG. 13.13 Hypertrophic cardiomyopathy patient showing myocardial crypts detected with two-dimensional CINE fast low angle shot imaging at 7 T using a spatial resolution of 1.4 × 1.4 × 4 mm³. CINE images of a short-axis view *(left)* and a long-axis view *(right)* exhibit hyperintense signal in areas that were identified as myocardial crypts *(arrows)*. Fibrosis detected via late gadolinium enhancement at 3 T (not shown) and crypts do overlap.[40]

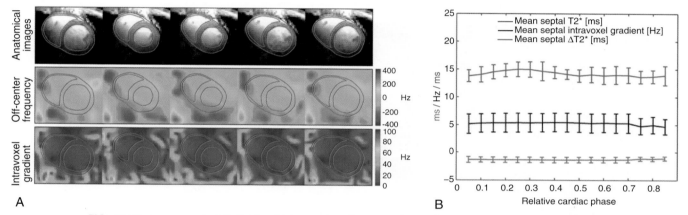

FIG. 13.14 Assessment of B_0 field and intravoxel gradient over the cardiac cycle derived from a short-axis view of the heart of a healthy subject obtained at 7 T. (A) *Top,* Anatomic magnitude images. *Middle,* Low pass filtered off-center frequency maps. *Bottom,* Intravoxel field gradient maps. (B) Plot of mean T2* *(blue)* and mean intravoxel B_0 gradient *(black)* in the intraventricular septum over the cardiac cycle for a cohort of healthy volunteers. An increase of T2* in systole can be observed. The estimated T2* shift caused by the B_0 variation assuming a common myocardial T2* value at 7 T of 15 ms is shown in *red.* Relative cardiac phase 0 indicates the beginning of systole. Macroscopic myocardial B_0 gradient variations over the cardiac cycle can be considered minor regarding their effects on T2*. Error bars indicate SD. (From Huelnhagen T, Hezel F, Serradas Duarte T, et al. Myocardial effective transverse relaxation time T2* correlates with left ventricular wall thickness: a 7 T MRI study. *Magn Reson Med.* 2017;77(6):2381–2389.)

For T2* mapping, a reasonable B_0 uniformity across the heart is essential such that susceptibility weighting is not dominated by macroscopic B_0 field inhomogeneities but rather by microscopic B_0 susceptibility gradients.[17] Because of increased susceptibility effects, this is of particular concern for UHF-CMR, but can be managed by dedicated B_0 shimming. Using local second-order shimming, a mean peak-to-peak B_0 difference of approximately 65 Hz was found across the left ventricle at 7 T,[17] which compares well with 3 T[138] and 1.5 T studies.[139] For myocardial anterior, anterolateral, and inferoseptal segments, a mean in-plane B_0 gradient of approximately 3 Hz/mm was observed. For CINE T2* mapping also, temporal changes of the macroscopic B_0 field across the cardiac cycle, induced by changes in cardiac macromorphology and the displacement of the diaphragm, need to be considered. Using cardiac-gated temporally resolved B_0 field mapping, it was demonstrated that such changes can be considered minor in the ventricular septum with respect to their influence on T2* even at 7 T (Fig. 13.14).[45] The mean absolute variation of the mean intravoxel

B_0 gradient in the interventricular septum over the cardiac cycle was approximately 0.4 ± 0.3 Hz/voxel. Regarding the mean observed septal T2* and intravoxel B_0 gradient over the cardiac cycle, the observed maximum intravoxel B_0 gradient variation translates into a T2* variation of approximately 0.7 ± 0.4 ms. With this B_0 uniformity across the heart and across the cardiac cycle, high spatial resolution and cardiac phase-resolved myocardial T2* mapping at 7 T is feasible,[17,25] as demonstrated in Fig. 13.15.[45]

For T2* mapping at 7 T, the longest mean T2* values were found for the anterior (T2* = 17.3 ms), anteroseptal (T2* = 16.8 ms), and inferoseptal (T2* = 16.3 ms) segments. Septal segments showed the lowest spatial variation in T2*, which is similar to that reported for 1.5 T and 3 T.[25] The inferior (T2* = 12 ms) and inferior lateral (T2* = 11.4 ms) wall yielded lowest T2* values with the spatial variation being significantly pronounced versus 1.5 T and 3 T.[25] The 7 T setup used facilitated a spatial resolution as good as 1.1 × 1.1 × 2.5 mm³, which helped to reduce intravoxel dephasing along the slice direction.[17]

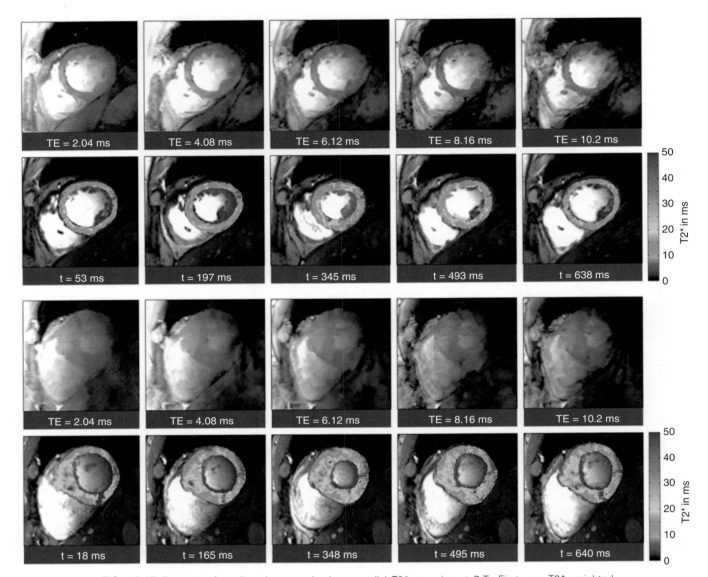

FIG. 13.15 Example of cardiac phase-resolved myocardial T2* mapping at 7 T. *First row,* T2*-weighted short-axis views of the heart for a mid-ventricular slice derived from multiecho gradient echo imaging at 7 T. Images were obtained at the echo times shown. A spatially adaptive nonlocal means denoising filter was applied.[177] *Second row,* Temporally resolved myocardial T2* maps of a short-axis view of the same volunteer derived from a series of T2*-sensitized two-dimensional (2D) CINE acquisitions covering the entire cardiac cycle (five cardiac phases out of a series of 20 cardiac phases are shown) overlaid onto conventional 2D CINE fast low angle shot images are displayed. *Third row,* T2*-weighted short-axis views and temporally resolved myocardial T2* maps of the heart for a mid-ventricular slice of a patient suffering from hypertrophic cardiomyopathy. An increase in septal T2* compared with healthy volunteers can be appreciated.

Myocardial T2* changes are commonly regarded to provide a surrogate for myocardial tissue oxygenation,[140] yet the factors influencing T2* are of multiple nature.[141] Further to blood oxygenation, blood volume fraction per tissue volume, hematocrit, the oxyhemoglobin dissociation curve, main magnetic field inhomogeneities, tissue susceptibility, and tissue microstructure or micromorphology were reported to govern T2*.[142–147] Cardiac macromorphology, including ventricular radius and ventricular wall thickness, constitutes another category of physiologic parameters that are substantially altered throughout the cardiac cycle. These alterations might affect blood volume fraction and the amount of deoxygenated hemoglobin (deoxyHb) per tissue volume, resulting in dynamic variation in myocardial T2* over the cardiac cycle. Detailing

T2* across the cardiac cycle using CINE T2* mapping revealed cyclic changes in septal T2* with a mean end-systolic T_2* increase of about 10% compared with end diastole (Fig. 13.16).[45] The periodic changes in interventricular septal myocardial T2* correlate well with changes in the septal wall thickness and with alterations in the LV radius throughout the cardiac cycle (see Fig. 13.16). The observed cyclic T2* variations were suggested to be dominated by changes in myocardial blood volume fraction rather than oxygenation, indicating that temporally resolved MR relaxation mapping could be beneficial for understanding cardiac (patho)physiology in vivo.[45]

The recent progress in in vivo histology and in fiber orientation tracking using T2*-weighted MR[143,144,148,149] suggests that the linear

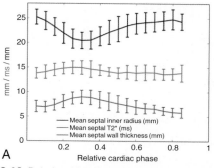
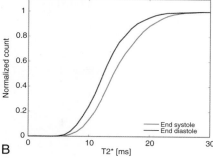

FIG. 13.16 Relationship of septal myocardial wall thickness, T2* and left ventricular (LV) inner radius in healthy volunteers at 7 T. (A) Time course of mean septal wall thickness, mean LV inner radius, and mean septal T2* plotted over the cardiac cycle averaged for 10 volunteers. Error bars indicate standard deviation. (B) Cumulative frequency plot of ventricular septal T2* in end systole and end diastole for all septal voxels of all volunteers. A clear shift to higher T2* in systole can be recognized. (From Huelnhagen T, Hezel F, Serradas Duarte T, et al. Myocardial effective transverse relaxation time T2* correlates with left ventricular wall thickness: a 7 T MRI study. *Magn Reson Med.* 2017;77(6):2381–2389.)

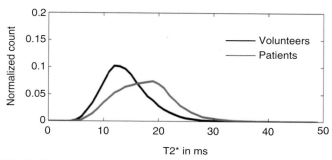

FIG. 13.17 Histogram showing the distribution of mid-ventricular septal T2* in healthy volunteers and patients suffering from hypertrophic cardiomyopathy (HCM). Data were derived from myocardial T2* mapping at 7 T. A clear shift toward higher T2* can be observed for HCM patients. The data were obtained and grouped for all cardiac phases for six HCM patients *(red line)* and 10 age-matched and body-mass-index–matched healthy volunteers *(black line)*.

relationship between T2* and B_0 might provide means to gain a better insight into the myocardial microstructure. Because the susceptibility effects depend on the orientation of blood-filled capillaries and microstructural arrangements with respect to the external magnetic field,[125,139,144,147,150] T2* mapping at 7 T might contribute to explorations into visualization of myocardial fibers, into the examination of helical angulation of myocardial fibers, or into the assessment of fibrotic tissue and other kinds of microstructural tissue changes. Results of the first cardiac patient study at 7 T investigating T2* in patients suffering from HCM demonstrated an increase of septal T2* compared with healthy controls[152] (Figs. 13.15 and 13.17). Mean septal T2* averaged over all subjects for all cardiac phases was found to be T2*$_{mean}$ = (17.5 ± 1.4) ms for HCM patients and T2*$_{mean}$ = (13.7 ± 1.1) ms for BMI-matched and age-matched healthy subjects. These findings provide encouragement that T2* mapping at UHF could provide an imaging-based biomarker that could support diagnosis and risk stratification in cardiomyopathies.

Myocardial T1 Mapping

Myocardial tissue characterization using T1-weighted LGE imaging is of proven clinical value for the assessment of ischemic heart diseases and also for nonischemic myocardial diseases.[119] T1-weighted imaging

is qualitative and subjective though, which spurs advancements toward myocardial T1 mapping.[153–155] At 7 T increased RF transmit power and improved B_0 shimming play complementary roles for myocardial T1 mapping which requires careful transmission field shaping and B_0 shimming. This requirement can be managed if quantification of and correction for imperfect inversion is applied.[23] For this purpose an adiabatic inversion pulse tailored for use in the heart in conjunction with a shortened modified Look-Locker inversion recovery (ShMOLLI) variant was employed.[23] Subject-averaged inversion efficiencies ranging from −0.79 to −0.83 (perfect inversion would provide −1) were accomplished across myocardial segments.[23] A T1 of normal myocardium has been reported to be 1925 ± 48 ms at 7 T[23] versus 1166 ± 60 ms at 3 T[156] and 721 ± 37 ms at 1.5 T.[155] Another method to address the challenge of imperfect inversion at UHF is to use saturation recovery methods instead of inversion recovery. Employing a saturation recovery single-shot acquisition (SASHA) technique with a saturation pulse train and saturation delays optimized for 7 T, T1 values comparable with an inversion recovery approach were obtained.[157] A T1 of 1939 ± 73 ms was reported in the intraventricular septum, employing a simple three-parameter fit model without the need for correction of imperfect inversion as required for ShMOLLI.

The prolonged T1 relaxation times at 7 T provide an enhanced blood/myocardium contrast superior to 1.5 T which afforded a revival of spoiled gradient echo imaging techniques at 7 T. Slice selective variable flip angle techniques provide an alternative for rapid parametric T1 mapping.[158] This approach obviates the need for inversion recovery preparation while being fast enough to meet the speed requirements of cardiac MR.

Fat-Water Imaging

Fat-water separated cardiac imaging provides a sensitive means of detecting intramyocardial fat, characterizing fibro-fatty infiltration, characterizing fatty tumors, and delineating epicardial and/or pericardial fat. The concept of fatty myocardium has also received attention because of its role in cardiomyopathy where the mismatch between myocardial fatty acid uptake and utilization leads to the accumulation of cardiotoxic lipid species.[159] Multiecho Dixon approaches using iterative decomposition have been shown to provide robust fat-water separation even in the presence of large field inhomogeneities.[160] Equipped with this technology, the feasibility of fat-water–separated cardiac imaging at 7 T has been demonstrated,[161] including its use for fat suppression in coronary artery imaging (Fig. 13.18). Yet, the Dixon approach constitutes a

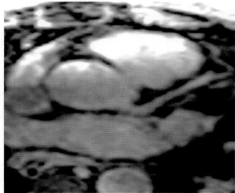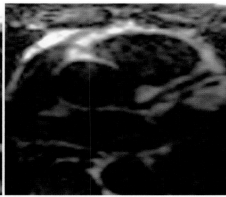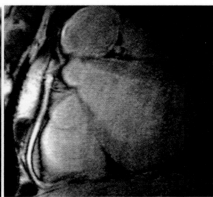

FIG. 13.18 Examples of early ultrahigh field cardiovascular magnetic resonance (UHF-CMR) application in healthy subjects: *Left, center,* Fat-water–separated (*left,* water image; *center,* fat image) coronary artery imaging showing the left main coronary artery using the Dixon approach at 7 T. *Right,* High-resolution image of the right coronary artery acquired with a spatial resolution of $0.45 \times 0.45 \times 1.2$ mm^3, which was facilitated by a navigator-gated free breathing three-dimensional gradient echo acquisition in conjunction with spectrally selective adiabatic inversion recovery at 7 T. (Courtesy Maurice Bizino and Hildo Lamb, Department of Radiology, Leiden University Medical Center, Leiden, The Netherlands.)

challenge for quantification of fat infiltration in myocardial disease. Chemical shift-resolved MR spectroscopy and imaging techniques provide a valuable alternative for fat quantification in the myocardium.

Coronary Artery Imaging

Coronary artery imaging (CAI) remains one of the most technically challenging applications in cardiovascular MRI because of small vessel size, vessel tortuosity, and physiologic motion.[162,163] UHF-CAI using noncontrast gradient echo imaging techniques suggested that image quality already approached that achieved for CAI at 3 T.[4,7,26] Coronary vessel sharpness at 7 T was found to be improved versus 3 T.[7] The early studies focused primarily on the right coronary. To afford appropriate coverage of all main coronary arteries, the capabilities of dynamic B_1^+ shimming were exploited.[86] The capabilities of UHF-CAI were furthered by employing high spatial resolution CAI (see Fig. 13.18).[26] For this approach, coronary vessel edge sharpness was found to be superior to the border sharpness accomplished in state-of-the-art CAI at 3 T. Visible vessel length and vessel diameter obtained at 7 T were competitive with 3 T.[26]

Traditional frequency selective fat saturation techniques used in CAI might suffer from large static field variations at 7 T, which may cause nonuniform and imperfect fat suppression over the target region, an effect which bears the risk of obscuring the delineation of coronary arteries. Here fat-water–separated imaging holds the promise of substituting conventional preparatory fat saturation techniques (see Fig. 13.18). This approach also promises to offset some of the RF power deposition constraints that come with conventional saturation recovery-based fat saturation that makes use of large flip angles.

Vascular Imaging

MR angiography (MRA) of the large vessels is a common CMR application. MRA stands to benefit from UHF-MR. The SNR gain can be used to counter the noise amplification caused by acceleration techniques employed to meet the high spatiotemporal resolution requirements of MRA. Potential applications include large-volume coverage, time-resolved phase velocity MRA (4D flow), which is an emerging technique for studying the flow pattern, or wall shear stress in large vessels. The feasibility of aortic 4D flow at 7 T was recently demonstrated.[35] For this purpose, a prospectively gated 4D flow sequence was applied. Another 4D flow MRA implementation at 7 T made good use of kt-generalized

autocalibrating partial parallel acquisition (GRAPPA) acceleration combined with dynamically applied B_1^+ shimming, toggling a setting tailored for the navigator used for respiratory gating and the imaging module.[44] Fig. 13.19 shows the blood velocity by path lines for different time points of the cardiac cycle within the human aorta derived from a 4D flow dataset acquired at 7 T with 1.2-mm isotropic spatial and 40.8 ms temporal resolution.

Perhaps UHF-MR forms another important enabling factor to transform the baseline SNR advantage into improved spatiotemporal resolution of contrast-enhanced MRA. To this end, an SNR gain for contrast-enhanced versus noncontrast-enhanced 4D flow MRA was reported to be approximately 1.4 at 7 T, which was found to be in accordance with 3 T and 1.5 T observations.[35]

Real-Time Imaging

Breath-held 2D CINE acquisitions segmented over regular 10 to 16 heartbeats are the clinical standard for LV morphology and function assessment. However, this approach is limited by physiologic (e.g., cardiac arrhythmias) constraints and the ability of the patients to hold their breath, which might cause inappropriate diagnostic information. Free-breathing real-time CMR achieves diagnostic quality in a single heartbeat[164] and bears the potential to change the landscape of cardiac diagnostics.[165–167] The SNR gain achieved by ultrahigh magnetic fields can help to counteract the loss of signal because of the undersampling needed for real-time acquisitions.

The accelerated imaging capabilities and the anatomic coverage of multichannel bow-tie antenna arrays (see Fig. 13.1E and F) supported free-breathing real-time imaging of the heart and of the aorta at 7 T (Fig. 13.20).[41] The spatial resolution of $1.2 \times 1.2 \times 6$ mm^3 and the frame rate of 30 frames per second fully meet if not excel the requirements of standardized LV structure and function assessment protocols used in today's CMR practice.[119] The real-time FLASH images of the aorta demonstrate the extended anatomic coverage of the 16-channel bow-tie antenna array along the head-feet direction, including details of the liver and the spine without B_1^+ signal voids (see Fig. 13.20).[41]

OPPORTUNITIES FOR DISCOVERIES

Exploiting the benefits of ultrahigh magnetic field strengths, X-nuclei imaging of the heart at 7 T moved into the spotlight of interest. In

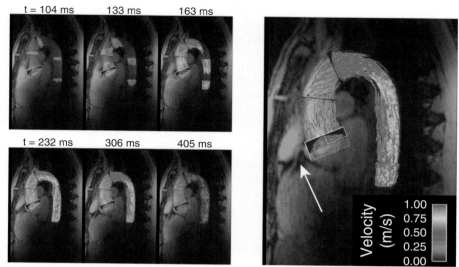

FIG. 13.19 Example of velocity data derived from four-dimensional flow measurements at 7 T using 1.2 mm isotropic spatial and 40.8 ms temporal resolution. *Left,* Pathline visualization of the blood velocity within the human aorta for different time points within the cardiac cycle relative to the R-wave of the electrocardiogram signal. *Right,* Enlarged view of time point 306 ms. The high spatial resolution allows for depicting the coronary artery in the magnitude image *(arrow).* (Courtesy Sebastian Schmitter, Center for Magnetic Resonance Research, University of Minnesota Medical School, Minneapolis, MN.)

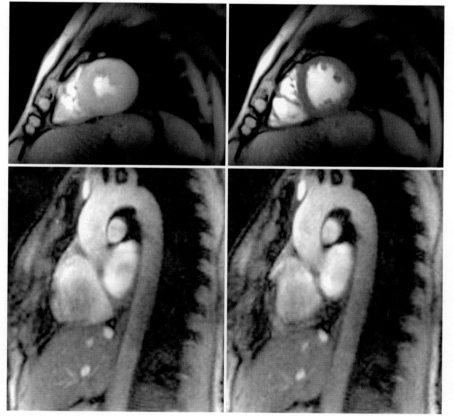

FIG. 13.20 Examples for free-breathing real-time imaging at 7 T. *Top,* Mid-ventricular short-axis view of the heart (*left,* systole; *right,* diastole) obtained with an 8-channel bow-tie antenna array (see Fig. 13.1E). *Bottom,* Coronal view of the aorta (*left,* systole; *right,* diastole) acquired with a 16-channel bow-tie antenna array (see Fig. 13.1F) demonstrating the 35 cm anatomic coverage of the 16-channel bow-tie antenna array along the head-feet direction, including details of the liver and the spine without transmission field–induced signal voids. Images were acquired at a rate of 30 frames per second using highly undersampled radial two-dimensional fast low angle shot with nonlinear inverse reconstruction at a spatial resolution of 1.2 × 1.2 × 6 mm³.

particular, sodium and phosphorus are two nuclei that promise to contribute to the understanding of physio-metabolic processes. This section describes pioneering work in the fields of [23]Na and ^{31}P cardiac imaging and spectroscopy at 7 T.

Sodium MRI

Sodium MRI ([23]Na MRI) is an emerging approach for gaining better insights into cellular metabolism, with a broad spectrum of biomedical imaging research applications.[168] Previous studies eloquently reported credible data on [23]Na MRI of the heart and demonstrated that [23]Na MRI is suitable for the detection and assessment of acute and chronic heart disease.[169] The rapidly decaying [23]Na signal and the low sensitivity of [23]Na MRI versus ^{1}H MR constitute a challenge for clinical [23]Na CMR. Once clinically feasible, sodium CMR holds the promise to become a valuable diagnostic tool for classifying viable from nonviable tissue in ischemic infarct patients. Recognizing the sensitivity gain and yet unimpaired transmission field homogeneity[19] because of the comparably low [23]Na resonance frequency, which is close to ^{1}H MRI at 1.5 T, it is conceptually appealing to pursue [23]Na CMR at 7 T at clinically acceptable acquisition times. To approach this goal, a local four-element transceiver RF surface coil customized for [23]Na CMR at 7 T was employed[37] to derive [23]Na images of the heart (Fig. 13.21) with a resolution of $6 \times 6 \times 6$ mm^3 using a density-adapted 3D radial acquisition technique.[170] These efforts also demonstrated that the sensitivity gain at 7 T enables CINE [23]Na imaging of the beating heart using a temporal resolution of 100 ms supported by retrospectively gated, density-adapted 3D projection reconstruction.[37,38]

Phosphorus Magnetic Resonance

Phosphorus MR affords in vivo insights into the energy metabolism and is an ideal candidate to benefit from the sensitivity gain and improved frequency dispersion at higher fields. To demonstrate the sensitivity gain, careful juxtaposition between cardiac ^{31}P MRS at 7 T and 3 T was conducted.[27] These pioneering studies revealed marked superiority of cardiac ^{31}P spectra at 7 T relative to 3 T (Fig. 13.22). SNR improvements of 2.8 for creatine phosphate (PCr)[27] together with a reduced standard deviation for the creatine phosphate/adenosine triphosphate (PCr/ATP) ratio were observed. This gain resulted in an enhanced quantification accuracy at 7 T. Myocardial [31]P T1 relaxation times are shorter at 7 T versus 3 T. These improvements could permit scan time reductions versus 3 T and might eventually allow metabolic probing of dynamic processes. For all these reasons it was concluded that 7 T will become the field strength of choice for cardiac ^{31}P MR spectroscopy tailored for probing myocardial energetics.[27] This manifests itself in a first 7 T ^{31}P MR spectroscopy study performed in a cohort of 25 patients with dilated cardiomyopathy (DCM),[42] where the PCr/ATP ratio was found to be significantly lower than that of healthy control subjects (see Fig. 13.22). These results are a precursor to a broader clinical study aiming at the assessment of the effects of energy-sparing drugs in patients with DCM.[42]

LOOKING AT THE HORIZON

Where do we stand? Although the lion's share of UHF-MR examinations today cover brain and neuroscience applications, cardiac imaging is another field that can benefit from UHF-MR. The eye-opening quality of recent anatomic, functional, and physiometabolic UHF-CMR insights into the heart have served as a driving force for application developments, which culminated in the breadth and detail outlined in this chapter. UHF-CMR helps to eliminate the main barriers standing in the way at low fields. Groundbreaking examples include the capability to detect subtle myocardial crypts which cannot be seen at lower fields, as well as unprecedented capacity and speed for real-time imaging. UHF-CMR opens new avenues into myocardial tissue characterization and will yield new insights by permitting phosphorus, sodium, and potassium MRI, which will reveal new dimensions of metabolism, bioenergetics, and tissue function of the heart and allow us to build many more bridges to molecular discovery. The pace of discovery is heartening and a powerful motivator to transfer the lessons learned from UHF-CMR research into broader clinical studies. These efforts are fueled by the quest for advancing the capabilities of cardiac imaging, with the implications feeding into MR physics, biomedical engineering,

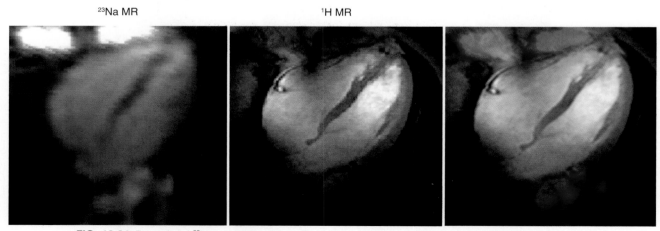

FIG. 13.21 Example of [23]Na magnetic resonance *(MR)* imaging of the heart at 7 T. *Left,* Sodium image of a four-chamber view of the heart acquired at 7 T. The [23]Na image of the heart was acquired using a density-adapted three-dimensional radial technique[139] with TE = 0.4 ms; TR = 11 ms; TRO = 7.1 ms; TX amplitude 115 V (~90% specific absorption rate), equivalent to a tip angle of 30 to 40 degrees; number of projections = 50,000; number of averages = 2; and a voxel size of $6 \times 6 \times 6$ mm^3. *Center,* Corresponding ^{1}H four-chamber view of the heart derived from two-dimensional CINE gradient echo imaging at 7 T. *Right,* Overlay of the sodium image *(color scale)* to the anatomical image *(gray scale)*. (Courtesy Dr. Helmar Waiczies, MRI.TOOLS GmbH, Berlin, Germany.)

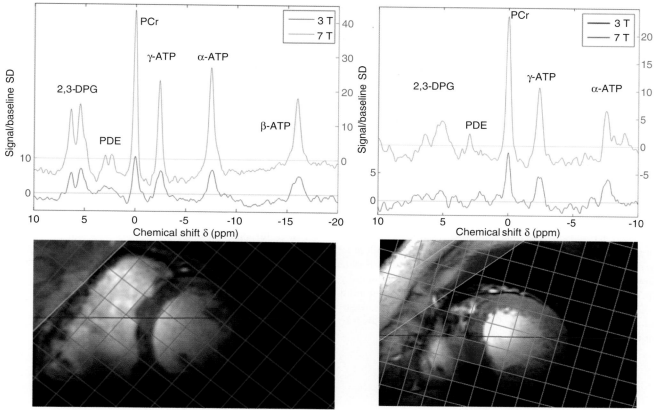

FIG. 13.22 Example of phosphorus spectroscopy in healthy subjects and patients with dilated cardiomyopathy at 7 T. *Top,* Comparison of single-voxel ^{31}P magnetic resonance (MR) spectra of the human heart obtained at 3 T *(blue)* and at 7 T *(red)* for a healthy volunteer *(left)* and for a patient with dilated cardiomyopathy *(right).* The voxel used for ^{31}P MR spectroscopy was placed in the middle of the interventricular septum, as illustrated in the short-axis views *(bottom)* of the heart obtained from a two-dimensional CINE fast low angle shot localizer scan at 7 T. [31]P MR spectroscopy at 7 T provided a signal-to-noise ratio advantage over ^{31}P MR spectroscopy at 3 T. (Courtesy Christopher Rodgers, Radcliffe Department of Medicine, University of Oxford, Oxford, UK.)

cardiology, internal medicine, and other related fields of basic research and clinical science.

How can clinical CMR at lower fields benefit from the progress in UHF-CMR? It is safe to state that the benefits of 7 T CMR innovations will be more seen at 3 T, where the suboptimal copy-and-paste approach to protocol migration from 1.5 T is being supplanted by the sort of application-targeted redesign which is essential for UHF-CMR. For example, whereas most of the effort on transmit-receive array structures for CMR is currently occurring at 7 T, recognition of the benefits of these structures may result in an eventual migration to 3 T ($\lambda_{\text{myocardium}}^{3T} \approx 30$ cm), where RF inhomogeneities and SAR limitations, although of less extent, remain significant in clinical CMR.[46,171,172] This is a powerful motivator to elucidate the performance of local multichannel surface RF coils versus large-volume body RF coil transmission for CMR at 3 T. A recent study demonstrated that CMR and cardiac chamber quantification at 3 T using local surface RF coil transmission is competitive when benchmarked against the today's 3 T CMR practice of large-volume body RF coil transmission.[173] CMR of patients equipped with passively conducting implants that constitute an SAR governed contraindication for cardiac MR in case of body RF coil transmission presents an application where local surface RF coil transmission provides a vital alternative over RF body coil excitation. Another example is interventional CMR employing imaging-guided navigation of conducting catheters. It was also shown that the B_1^+ efficiency benefits of a local transmission coil array versus

body coil transmission can be translated into a reduction in the TR. This 1/TR enhancement is conceptually appealing for the reduction of banding and off-resonance artifacts frequently encountered for 2D CINE SSFP imaging at 3 T. TR shortening also benefits rapid imaging that supports real-time assessment of the heart rather than relying on the interpolation of data acquired during multiple synchronized heartbeats commonly used in today's segmented CINE acquisitions.

What will the foreseeable future bring? It is no surprise that the future of UHF-CMR will not end at 7 T and that the field is moving apace to even higher fields. Physicists, engineers, and pioneers from related disciplines have already taken a further step into the future, in their minds, with something they are calling extreme field MR (EF-MR).[174] This envisions human MR at 20 T[103,110,174–176] and it is an important leap of the imagination because it aims to fill a crucial "resolution gap" in our understanding of human biology. Although discoveries are pouring in on the molecular and cellular level every day, it is extremely difficult to integrate these findings into a coherent picture of the functions of tissues and pathologic processes at a mesoscopic level above that of the cell. There is a wide gap between the view of biologists and clinicians that is begging to be filled. Extreme field MR is probably an ideal technology that will reach between these levels in vivo by bridging a crucial gap in resolution in space and time. Arguably, ^{1}H CMR at 20 T might be challenging in the first run, because of electrodynamic constraints. Yet, the frequencies of X-nuclei at 20 T are below the ^{1}H resonance frequency at 7 T, with the exception of ^{31}P and ^{19}F. This makes technologies established for ^{1}H MR at 7 T ideal candidates to be perfected and fine-tuned for heteronuclear CMR at 20 T. For example, the sensitivity gain at 20 T is expected to reduce scan times for ^{31}P and ^{23}Na by a factor of 8 versus today's 7 T capabilities. This promises ^{23}Na MR with a sub-millimeter spatial resolution in 5- to 10-minute scan time and offers the potential for probing the myocardial energetics with ^{31}P spectroscopy MRS in clinically acceptable scan times.

Do we need extra resources and a willingness to invest? Yes. Exploring new territory requires extra resources—and the will to go there. Obviously for a while the most high-end instruments will be costly and only accessible to a few; ideally through National Research Infrastructure Facilities. That cannot be an argument, however, against making the leap forward. Although the first 20 T class MR instruments will probably be devoted to discovery and to proof of principle, the findings will be crucial guides to making the best use of lower-resolution imaging techniques at 3 T and 7 T. The only thing that could keep the dream of human MR at 20 T from becoming reality would be a failure to follow the path and see what develops. Will the clinic eventually be able to follow us to even higher fields? It always does, if a whole community of experts devotes their creative efforts to the task. With this in mind UHF-CMR remains in a state of creative flux and productive engagement in this area continues to drive further developments for the sake of cardiac imaging.

ACKNOWLEDGMENTS

The authors wish to acknowledge the members of the Berlin Ultrahigh Field Facility (BUFF), Berlin, Germany; the working group for Cardiac Magnetic Resonance, Charité, Berlin, Germany; Maurice M. Bizino and Hildo Lamb, Department of Radiology, Leiden University Medical Center, Leiden, the Netherlands; Thea Marie Niendorf, Aachen, Germany and Anna Tabea Niendorf, Aachen, Germany; Christopher Rodgers, Radcliffe Department of Medicine, University of Oxford, Oxford, UK; Sebastian Schmitter, University of Minneapolis, Minnesota, USA; and Helmar Waiczies, MRI.TOOLS GmbH, Berlin, Germany who kindly contributed examples of their pioneering work or other valuable assistance. This work was supported (in part, TN) by the DZHK (German Centre for Cardiovascular Research) and by the BMBF (Federal Ministry of Education and Research). This work was funded (in part, TN) by the Helmholtz Alliance ICEMED—Imaging and Curing Environmental Metabolic Diseases, through the Initiative and Network Fund of the Helmholtz Association (ICEMED-Project 1210251). LW received support from the BMBF (Federal Ministry of Education and Research, "KMU-innovativ": Medizintechnik MED-373-046).

REFERENCES

A full reference list is available online at ExpertConsult.com

14

Clinical Cardiovascular Magnetic Resonance Imaging Techniques

David C. Wendell, Wolfgang G. Rehwald, John D. Grizzard, Raymond J. Kim, and Robert M. Judd

The first dedicated cardiovascular magnetic resonance (CMR) clinical services opened in the United States in mid-1990s. Since that time, CMR imaging has become routine at most academic medical centers, with a number of centers now running multiple CMR scanners dedicated to cardiovascular imaging studies. Although different centers still differ somewhat with regard to the exact clinical CMR imaging protocols employed, in recent years cross-institutional CMR protocols have become much more consistent. In this chapter we focus on the clinical CMR imaging techniques that we routinely use at our institution, and we believe these are now representative of most high-volume dedicated CMR clinical services.

The dedicated CMR clinical service at the Duke Cardiovascular Magnetic Resonance Center (DCRMC) first opened in July 2002. Since that time, we have experimented with and evaluated many approaches to CMR and have directly observed their effects on overall clinical volume. As shown in Fig. 14.1, clinical volume at the DCRMC has grown steadily since our service first opened and currently consists of approximately 4000 billed CMR imaging procedures per year.

From 2002 to 2010 the percentage of each type of CMR test we performed varied somewhat as the types of patients referred to us evolved, and as we ourselves modified the tests we offered. From 2010 to 2015 (the latest year data are available), however, the tests we offer and perform have remained relatively constant.

Fig. 14.2 summarizes the indications for CMR scans, as well as the corresponding current procedural terminology (CPT) codes used for billing. These data were pooled across four US hospitals with dedicated CMR clinical services and, as such, portray an arguably representative picture of clinical practice patterns in the United States. The largest referral indication for CMR was heart failure, followed by ischemia evaluation and vascular disease. The most common CPT codes were 75561 (morphology and function with/without contrast), 75565 (velocity flow), and 71555 (magnetic resonance angiography [MRA]). About 20% of all CMR scans involved stress testing (CPT code 75563). Unlike the four-hospital data of Fig. 14.2, however, at our institution roughly 50% of our CMR scans involve stress testing. The DCMRC definition of a "CMR Stress Test" can briefly be described as a group of three individual scans:

1. Cines (to examine biventricular contractile function).
2. Adenosine stress/rest perfusion (to examine regional myocardial perfusion).
3. Late gadolinium enhancement (LGE; to examine viability/infarction).

The DCMRC CMR Stress Test is described in more detail in a paper by Klem et al.,[1] and has arguably become the bread and butter of our clinical service.

Through the years our philosophy about how to perform CMR has evolved into the concept of a CMR "exam menu" which has not only allowed us to streamline our clinical service but has also made it considerably easier for us to teach CMR to cardiology fellows and level 2 trainees. The underlying idea of the examination menu (Fig. 14.3) is that most if not all routine clinical CMR can be performed simply by combining one or more items from a predetermined menu and performing these scan protocols/pulse sequences in a single consistent manner. As can be seen from Fig. 14.3, the CMR Stress Test is simply one combination of items from the examination menu. Virtually every patient we examine simply undergoes one or more of the items shown in the menu and, perhaps more importantly, only rarely do we find it necessary to perform a scan not listed there.

Accordingly, the remainder of this chapter focuses on providing more detail about each of the items on the examination menu, with an emphasis on providing practical information typically not provided in other CMR textbooks. In the Conclusion section of this chapter we present typical examples of how the items on the examination menu can be combined to answer common diagnostic questions in cardiology, such as the detection of coronary artery disease (CAD) and the evaluation of aortic disease.

SCOUTING ("SCAN" = "SCOUT")

The thoracic scout examination is the simplest and most commonly used CMR procedure performed during the CMR examination. The goal of the scout examination is to establish the anatomic position of the heart and the short-axis and long-axis views of the heart. Anatomic variations from patient to patient cause both the short-axis and long-axis cardiac views to lie at arbitrary angles with respect to scanner coordinates. These views are then obtained using "double oblique" planes.

The first step in determining the proper double-oblique views is to acquire images along the axes of the scanner: that is, axial, sagittal, and coronal planes passing through the thoracic cavity. Fig. 14.4 shows typical examples of scout images. These scout images are used to prescribe single-oblique images: that is, perpendicular to the axial image of Fig. 14.4, going through the left ventricle (LV) parallel to the septum *(dashed yellow line)*. The single-oblique images (pseudo two-chamber and pseudo four-chamber views) are used to determine the true short axis of the heart (doubly oblique). Therefore the goal of the scout is to acquire a series of images similar to that of Fig. 14.4 which define the short and long axis of the heart.

The pulse sequence we use for the scout images is based on balanced steady-state free precession (bSSFP). The underlying concept of bSSFP

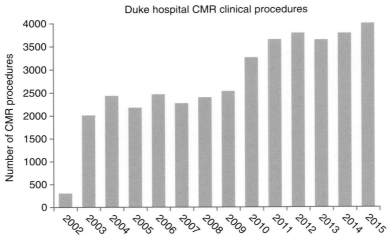

FIG. 14.1 Annual Duke Cardiovascular Magnetic Resonance *(CMR)* Center clinical volume. A "Procedure" corresponds to a current procedural terminology code.

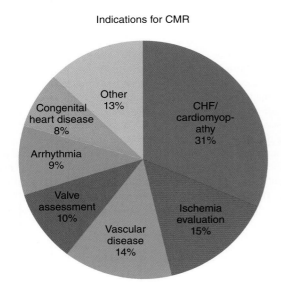

Indications for CMR

CPT CODE	CPT DESCRIPTION	# Reports	%
75561	MORPHOLOGY & FUNCTION W/ WO CONTRAST	4,723	66%
75565	VELOCITY FLOW MAPPINGS	3,714	51%
71555	CHEST MRA	3,312	46%
75563	STRESS MORPHOLOGY & FUNCTION W/WO CONTRAST	1,414	19%
75557	MORPHOLOGY & FUNCTION WITHOUT CONTRAST	270	3%
74185 72198 70549 73625	OTHER VASCULAR: Abdomen, pelvis, neck, lower extremity	761	10%

CMR clinical procedures (8,242 scans across four US hospitals)

FIG. 14.2 Recent (2010–2014) makeup of cardiovascular magnetic resonance *(CMR)* clinical referral indications across four US hospitals. *CHF,* Congestive heart failure; *CPT,* current procedural terminology; *MRA,* magnetic resonance angiography.

1 — Scout
2 — Left ventricular/right ventricular cine
3 — Stress–rest myocardial perfusion
4 — Late gadolinium enhancement
5 — Morphology
6 — Angiography
7 — Flow/velocity

FIG. 14.3 The Duke Cardiovascular Magnetic Resonance Center "exam menu." See text for details.

was described in the mid-1980s[2] but only since the late 1990s has CMR scanner hardware been capable of achieving the bSSFP magnetization state. Fig. 14.5 shows the bSSFP pulse sequence timing diagram characterized by its elegant simplicity, with symmetry around the data acquisition window on all three gradient axes. The axis labeled "slice" serves to select the slice to be imaged. The waveforms on the "read" axis create the magnetic resonance (MR) signal as an echo (see "signal" axis on bottom). During the positive portion of the "read" waveform the MR signal is digitally sampled. The "phase" encoding axis imposes a different phase on each echo which allows spatial encoding of the

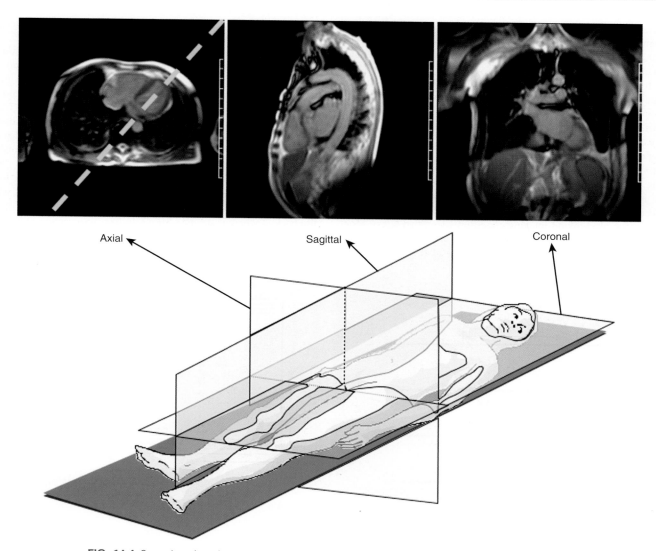

Axial   **Sagittal**   **Coronal**

FIG. 14.4 Scout imaging planes are typically obtained in the axial, coronal, and sagittal orientations.

second dimension called *y* in Fig. 14.6. In practice, the primary advantages of bSSFP imaging are: (1) fast imaging (i.e., short repetition time [TR]) and (2) very high signal-to-noise ratio (SNR) images. Accordingly, we use bSSFP not only for scouting but also for cine imaging (described in the Contractile Function section).

Acquiring any CMR image in essence involves filling the raw data space, often referred to as "*k*-space." Fig. 14.6 graphically depicts the process of filling *k*-space as a series of "lines" starting at the top and proceeding to the bottom. Each line is actually one echo (see zoomed-up box) acquired during the read event ("read" signal in Fig. 14.5). The echo runs in the *x*-direction. The *y*-dimension is the phase-encoding direction. For a bSSFP pulse sequence running on a typical modern CMR scanner the time needed to acquire each *k*-space line is approximately 3 ms. So, for the 100 *k*-space lines typical for scouting, the total image acquisition time is ~300 ms (100×3) or one-third of a second. This is fast enough to effectively freeze heart motion provided that the image data are acquired during diastole when the heart is relatively quiescent.

Acquiring the image data in diastole requires that the scanner hardware is "gated" to the cardiac cycle. This is typically achieved by having the scanner detect the R-wave of the electrocardiographic (ECG) signal and initiating the scan sequence at that time. In the following scouting

example we assume a heart rate of 60 beats per minute (RR duration = 1000 ms). The first "event" the scanner hardware must play out is a delay time of approximately 500 ms after the QRS (to get to diastole), followed by the 300 ms of image data acquisition. Fig. 14.7 graphically depicts cardiac gating for scout imaging.

MORPHOLOGY ("SCAN" = "MORPHOLOGY")

CMR scanning for cardiac morphology is used less often than cine imaging or even viability imaging, but the technical aspects of morphology, particularly as it relates to cardiac gating, are only modestly more complex than for scouting, so we present these next.

The "goal" of morphology scanning is essentially to create a series of parallel slices which "bread loaf" the thoracic cavity to examine vascular anatomy. Typically, three sets of black-blood and bright-blood images are acquired in the axial, coronal, and sagittal orientations. Once acquired, the scanner operator can then step through each series of image slices and understand the patient's vascular anatomy as well as plan additional scan planes.

It is often desirable to do this both with "black-blood" imaging (Fig. 14.8) and with "bright-blood" imaging (Fig. 14.9). The CMR pulse sequences used for black-blood and bright-blood morphology imaging are half-Fourier acquisition single-shot turbo spin echo (HASTE, Fig. 14.10A) and bSSFP (Fig. 14.5), respectively. Fig. 14.10A shows the pulse sequence timing diagram of the turbo spin echo sequence, and Fig. 14.10B shows the simplified spin echo sequence. HASTE is a special variant of the turbo spin echo sequence in which only 60% of k-space is sampled to reduce acquisition time.

Cardiac ECG gating for bSSFP morphology images is the same as that used for scouting, namely, by acquiring the entire image during a single diastolic phase (Fig. 14.11). For example, a set of 40 bSSFP images for morphology would require 40 consecutive heartbeats. ECG gating for HASTE imaging is also performed in diastole; however, these images are typically acquired every other heartbeat (e.g., 80 consecutive heartbeats). HASTE images require additional heartbeats to satisfy the black-blood imaging condition (described later). Morphology imaging typically takes 3 to 5 minutes and is performed with quiet respiration. For example, the acquisition of the 40 slices with

both bSSFP and HASTE slices would take 40 + 80 = 120 heartbeats (i.e., about 2 minutes).

Black-blood imaging is often advantageous for the examination of morphology because it allows clear differentiation of the inner portion of the vessel wall from the blood. Black-blood HASTE can be achieved by carefully combining CMR physics with the physiology of moving blood. The underlying reason that the blood appears black in HASTE images is caused by preparatory radiofrequency (RF) pulses before the HASTE readout (see Fig. 14.10). The basic concept is graphically depicted in Figs. 14.12 and 14.13. Soon after the R-wave, a brief (1–3 ms) RF pulse is played, which causes all of the magnetization in the body ("non-selective" or "hard" pulse) to flip upside down ("180 degrees" or "inversion" pulse). Immediately after this, a second RF pulse is played, which causes only the magnetization within the prescribed imaging slice to flip back to where it started ("slice-selective" re-inversion pulse). The net effect of these preparation pulses results in the magnetization outside the slice being inverted, whereas the magnetization within the prescribed

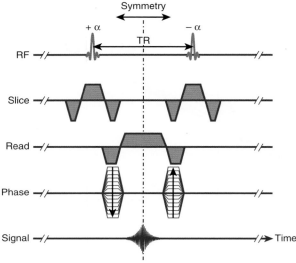

FIG. 14.5 Balanced steady-state free precession (bSSFP) pulse sequence timing diagram. In essence, bSSFP consists of rapid gradient echoes whose magnetization is preserved across multiple k-space lines, resulting in images with a high signal-to-noise ratio and short scan time. *RF*, Radiofrequency; *TR*, repetition time.

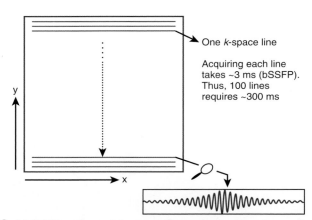

FIG. 14.6 Filling of raw data space. The raw data space for cardiovascular magnetic resonance is often referred to as "k-space" and must be filled line by line to generate an image. Each line contains one echo. Each echo is acquired after application of a different phase-encoding step (direction y) and thus contains different information. The k-space is filled using, for example, the pulse sequence of Fig. 14.5. Then this raw data undergoes a two-dimensional Fourier transform, resulting in an image of for example, Fig. 14.4. *bSSFP*, Balanced steady-state free precession.

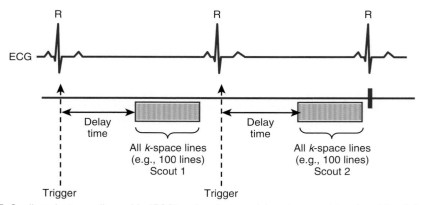

FIG. 14.7 Cardiac electrocardiographic (ECG) gating for scout imaging consists of a delay following the ECG R-wave and then rapid acquisition of the entire image in diastole. Imaging within a single heartbeat is made possible in part by the intrinsic speed of the balanced steady-state free precession pulse sequence. *ECG*, Electrocardiogram.

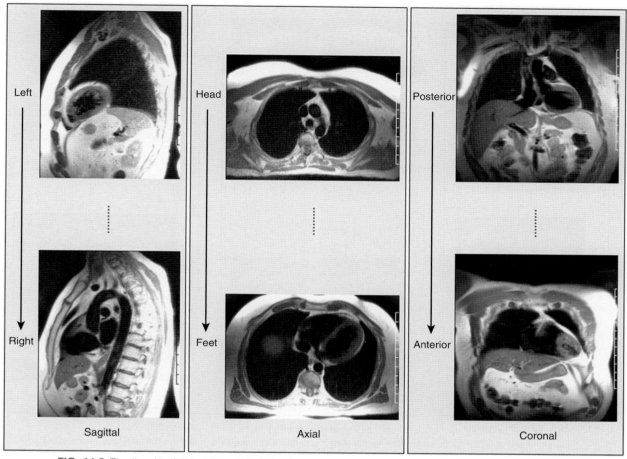

FIG. 14.8 The "goal" of "black-blood" half-Fourier acquisition single-shot turbo spin echo imaging. Shown are a series of parallel images across the entire thoracic cavity which can then be inspected to determine vascular anatomy. Usually, sagittal, axial, and coronal stacks are acquired.

imaging slice is restored. During the interval between the preparatory pulses and the HASTE readout (see Fig. 14.13) the heart contracts and expels blood from the slice (see Fig. 14.12, *middle*), which is subsequently replaced by fresh blood from outside the slice (see Fig. 14.12, *right*), which was previously inverted. When the HASTE readout begins, the previously inverted blood is recovering with T1, and its curve crosses zero at the start of the HASTE readout. Consequently, the blood produces no signal and appears black. Thus black-blood HASTE is made possible by a clever combination of a "memory" effect related to CMR physics (T1 recovery) as well as to the physiology of moving blood (and therefore may have intermediate signal with stagnant blood flow). Such images are quite helpful in detecting abnormalities in large-vessel anatomy, especially when combined with bright-blood bSSFP images at the same location.

CONTRACTILE FUNCTION ("SCAN" = "CINE")

Contractile function is a fundamental part of the CMR examination. Contractile function imaging is used for global and regional wall motion assessment and has been demonstrated to be highly accurate and reproducible for LV and right ventricular (RV) volume, ejection fraction, and mass measurements.[3–5] In recent years, CMR has become widely accepted as the clinical gold standard for contractile function assessment. It has been used as an endpoint for the evaluation of

ventricular remodeling,[6–8] and as a reference method for other imaging techniques.[9–14]

The "goal" of cine imaging is to capture a movie of the beating heart to visualize its contractile function. Fig. 14.14 shows a representative example of a mid-ventricular short-axis slice during different time points within the cardiac cycle, from early systole to late diastole. Images are acquired with the same bSSFP sequence used in bright-blood and scout imaging (see Fig. 14.5). The advantage of bSSFP for cardiac function imaging is high SNR, high temporal resolution, and excellent blood–myocardium contrast, which helps identify the endocardial border. Typically, a stack of multiple short axis slices (5–6 mm thick) are acquired at 1-cm increments to provide full LV and RV coverage. Short-axis views can be planned perpendicular to the long-axis scout images described in the Scouting section. In addition, cine images can be obtained in multiple long-axis views such as the two-chamber, three-chamber, and four-chamber views.

A key consideration for cine imaging is the time required to acquire a movie of a single cardiac cycle. Current CMR scanners are unable to acquire high spatial and temporal resolution cine images in real time. For example, for a movie with 25 frames each with 96 lines, a total of $25 \times 96 = 2400$ lines need to be acquired. Considering that the acquisition time for one line is approximately 3 ms, the acquisition time to create a series of cine images would be 2400×3 ms $= 7200$ ms, which is considerably longer than the human cardiac cycle. Imaging speed

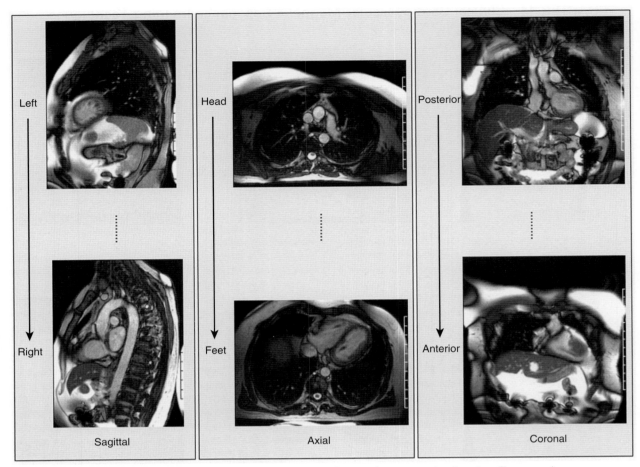

FIG. 14.9 The "goal" of "bright-blood" balanced steady-state free precession imaging. The same image planes used for half-Fourier acquisition single-shot turbo spin echo are acquired such that the two forms of images can be compared.

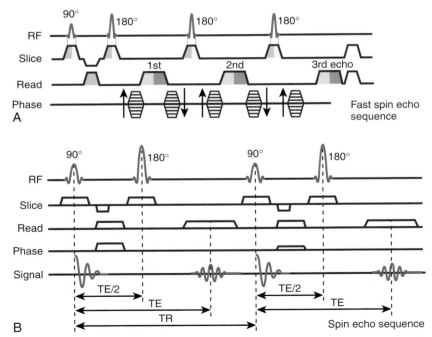

FIG. 14.10 Pulse sequence timing diagram for half-Fourier acquisition single-shot turbo spin echo (HASTE) (A) and for spin echo (B). In essence, HASTE consists of a series of spin echoes referred to as turbo spin echoes. Additional postprocessing steps are required to obtain the HASTE image. The spin echo sequence (B) is the predecessor of the turbo spin echo sequence (A). In HASTE, blood appears black in the resulting images because of the preparatory pulse described in Figs. 14.12 and 14.13. *RF,* Radiofrequency; *TE,* echo time; *TR,* repetition time.

could be reduced by acquiring fewer phase-encoding lines, but at the cost of spatial resolution (fewer lines per image) or temporal resolution (fewer movie frames). For cine imaging, image quality can be improved by using a segmented *k*-space acquisition assuming the beat-to-beat variation in heart rate is minimal.

The segmented *k*-space data acquisition collects only parts of each movie frame over 5 to 8 consecutive cardiac cycles and recombines the data to form a movie loop. Fig. 14.15 shows the scheme used for CMR in which only a fraction of *k*-space data is acquired for any given movie frame during any single heartbeat. This fraction is referred to as a "segment" (e.g., 16 *k*-space lines per segment in Fig. 14.15) and typically is adjusted by the scanner operator to produce an adequate number of movie frames (generally 16–20) given the patient's RR interval. Accordingly, the full *k*-space data for any one movie frame actually consists of multiple segments acquired during different cardiac cycles; the data are then reassembled during image reconstruction to form a movie depicting a single cardiac cycle (although compared with echocardiography, the data are not "real time"). For example, the scheme in Fig. 14.15 acquires 20 segments of 16 lines each in every cardiac cycle. Assuming that the scanner operator has chosen to obtain 96 *k*-space lines for each movie frame, the scan will acquire data across 96/16 = six heartbeats. In this example, the green segment is always acquired immediately after the R-wave and is used to reconstruct the first movie frame, the orange segment is acquired next and becomes the second movie frame, and so on. In practice, cine imaging is performed during breath-holding and takes 5 to 8 seconds for each cardiac view (e.g., one short-axis movie).

PERFUSION AT STRESS AND REST ("SCAN" = "PERFUSION")

Encouraged by a number of early clinical studies[1,15–19] adenosine stress–rest perfusion CMR has become more widespread in CMR centers. Perfusion CMR has been shown to accurately diagnose coronary artery disease with high sensitivity and specificity. Our center's approach of combining LGE CMR and rest–perfusion imaging with stress perfusion imaging is important for distinguishing true perfusion defects on stress images from artifacts.[1]

The "goal" of CMR perfusion imaging is to create a movie of the first passage of the CMR contrast media (typically gadolinium based) through the myocardium (e.g., first-pass perfusion). Fig. 14.16 gives an example of an adenosine stress perfusion scan as well as the corresponding rest perfusion scan in a patient with a stress-induced perfusion defect. The *blue slice* is shown at three representative time points: (1) before contrast arrival; (2) at the time of the contrast arrival in the RV; and (3) shortly after the time of the contrast arrival in the LV. During adenosine stress, two perfusion defects appear as dark regions in the anterior and inferolateral wall (hypoenhancement; see *arrows*) surrounded by bright contrast-enhanced normally perfused myocardium. In the corresponding

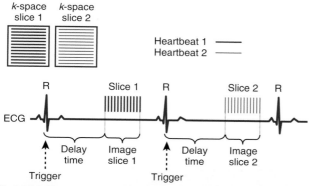

FIG. 14.11 Electrocardiogram *(ECG)* gating in half-Fourier acquisition single-shot turbo spin echo (HASTE) and balanced steady-state free precession (bSSFP) morphology imaging. Each HASTE and bSSFP morphologic image is acquired in a single diastolic image, similar to scout imaging. To skip systole, the wait period is inserted after electrocardiographic R-wave trigger detection.

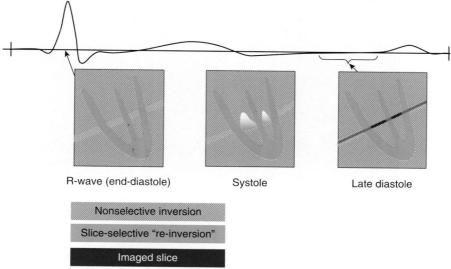

FIG. 14.12 Physiology of "black-blood" half-Fourier acquisition single-shot turbo spin echo imaging. Immediately after trigger detection a nonselective inversion *(green)* is played that is instantly followed by a slice-selective re-inversion *(orange)*. The so-prepared slice *(orange)* changes shape and position during cardiac contraction, but returns to its original geometry during diastole, when the blood is black and the heart has little motion. Nonblack re-inverted blood *(orange)* is expelled from the slice during systole. During diastole, an image is obtained from a slice *(blue)* that is thinner than and lies inside of the prepared slice *(orange)*.

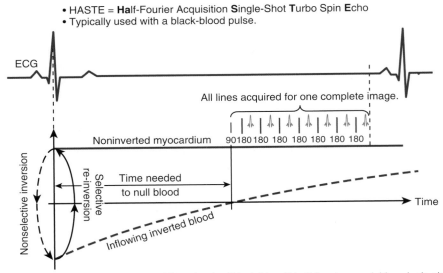

- HASTE = **Ha**lf-Fourier Acquisition **S**ingle-Shot **T**urbo Spin **E**cho
- Typically used with a black-blood pulse.

FIG. 14.13 Cardiac electrocardiogram *(ECG)* gating for "black-blood" half-Fourier acquisition single-shot turbo spin echo *(HASTE)* imaging; see text for details. Image acquisition starts when the magnetic relaxation curve of the inverted blood in the cavity is passing through zero/null signal: that is, when the blood is black. Note that in HASTE, the center lines of *k*-space are acquired first ("centric reordering"). Because these lines contain information of image brightness and contrast, they must be acquired while blood is "black": hence, at the beginning of the acquisition train.

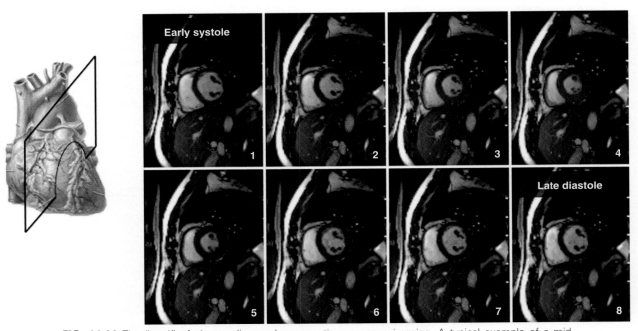

FIG. 14.14 The "goal" of cine cardiovascular magnetic resonance imaging. A typical example of a mid-ventricular series of short-axis cine images at the level of the papillary muscles, acquired with balanced steady-state free precession, is shown. Typically, the cine series contains about 20 image phases at each level, of which only eight are shown here because of space constraints.

rest perfusion images, conversely, perfusion appears normal in these regions, indicating normal resting perfusion with reduced coronary flow reserve, presumably because of the presence of hemodynamically significant coronary artery stenoses.

The sequences we use for perfusion imaging are based on a 90-degree saturation pulse followed by a gradient recalled echo readout (fast low angle shot [FLASH], Fig. 14.17).[20] Perfusion imaging data are acquired continuously rather than in the segmented manner previously described for cine imaging. A single image takes between 100 ms and 150 ms to acquire and, because of time constraints, imaging is typically performed throughout the entire cardiac cycle. All *k*-space lines for each of the 4 to 5 short-axis slice locations are acquired every cardiac cycle

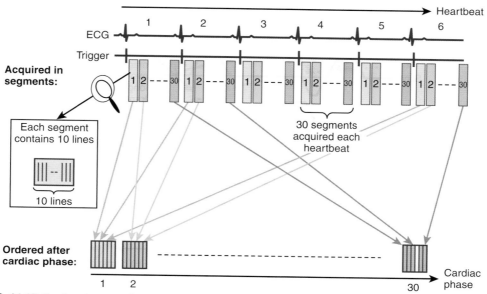

FIG. 14.15 Cardiac electrocardiogram *(ECG)* gating for cine imaging. Raw data lines are acquired in segments over the course of six successive heartbeats. The segments are then sorted in the *k*-space arrays for 20 movie frames/cardiac phases. Multiple lines form one segment, multiple segments form one *k*-space, and Fourier transform of one *k*-space yields one movie frame. See text for details.

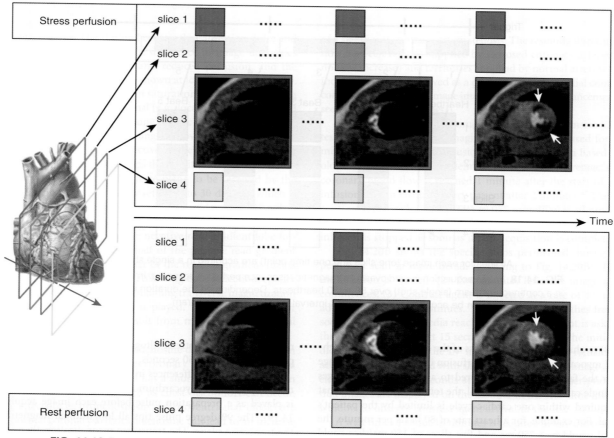

FIG. 14.16 The "goal" of cardiovascular magnetic resonance perfusion imaging. Stress and rest perfusion images are shown. In this example four slices *(basal red, green, blue, apical yellow)* are acquired with each heartbeat. An apical slice *(blue)* is shown at different time points throughout image acquisition (3 out of 50 time frames shown: before contrast arrival, at the time of the contrast arrival in the right ventricle, and shortly after the time of the contrast arrival in the left ventricle). Two stress perfusion defects appear as dark regions (hypoenhancement, *arrows*). They are surrounded by bright contrast-enhanced normally perfused myocardium. The defects are reversible as they are not present (no hypoenhancement, *arrows*) during rest perfusion.

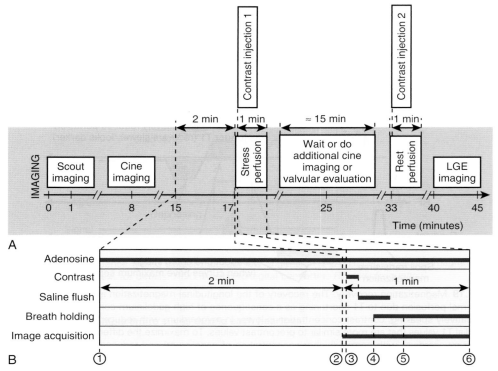

FIG. 14.20 (A) Timeline for a comprehensive cardiovascular magnetic resonance stress test. (B) The specific steps performed during the stress perfusion scan in more detail. Time points ❶–❻ are referenced in the text. Note that the time scale is not linear. See text for details. *LGE*, Late gadolinium enhancement.

VIABILITY AND INFARCTION ("SCAN" = "LATE GADOLINIUM ENHANCEMENT")

The clinical implications of viability imaging are steadily growing. Besides the assessment of acute and chronic myocardial infarction, LGE[24] has been used for the prediction of contractile improvement after revascularization,[25] for measuring the response to beta-blocker treatment,[26] for the differentiation of ischemic from nonischemic cardiomyopathies,[27] and for the diagnosis of various nonischemic cardiomyopathies.[28–30]

There is a large body of evidence that LGE can differentiate between nonviable and viable tissue.[24,31–34] Regions of irreversible injury exhibit high signal intensity (hyperenhancement) on T1-weighted images after administration of extracellular CMR contrast agent, such as Gd-DTPA. The underlying mechanism of hyperenhancement is that in acutely infarcted regions the ruptured myocyte membranes allow the extracellular contrast agent to passively diffuse into the intracellular space, resulting in an increased tissue-level contrast agent concentration, and therefore hyperenhancement. Chronic infarcts consist of dense scar with an increased interstitial space between collagen fibers (relative to normal myocardium) and therefore an increased distribution volume of the Gd-DTPA and, consequently, hyperenhancement.

The "goal" of LGE viability imaging is to create images with high contrast between the hyperenhanced nonviable tissue and normal myocardium for a clear delineation of these regions (Fig. 14.21). This is currently best achieved by using a segmented inversion recovery sequence.[34] So far, the best validated sequence for viability imaging is the segmented inversion recovery TurboFLASH sequence.[24,31–34] Fig. 14.22 displays the gating for a segmented inversion recovery sequence. The acquisition of multiple *k*-space lines in each cardiac cycle allows reductions in imaging times to the point where the entire image can be acquired during a single breath-hold of 6 to 10 seconds. The images

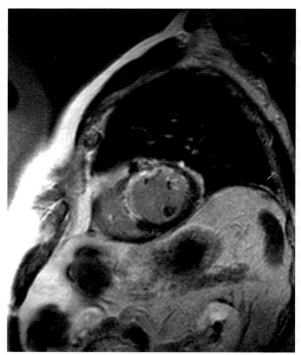

FIG. 14.21 The "goal" of late gadolinium enhancement viability imaging. The short-axis cardiovascular magnetic resonance image provides a clear delineation between nonviable (hyperenhanced) and viable (dark) myocardium.

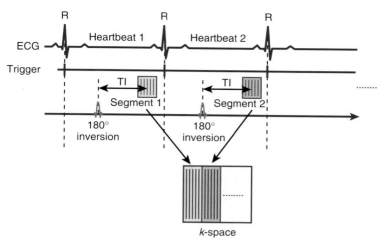

FIG. 14.22 Electrocardiogram *(ECG)* gating of the segmented inversion recovery sequence. See text for details.

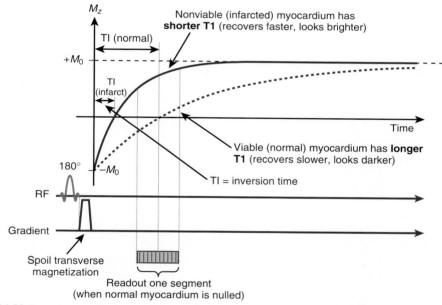

FIG. 14.23 Inversion recovery curve for viable and nonviable myocardium. See text for details. *RF,* Radiofrequency.

are acquired in mid-diastole by using a trigger delay to minimize the cardiac motion. The magnetization of the heart is prepared by a non-selective 180 degrees inversion pulse to create T1 weighting. The inversion time (TI) delay between inversion pulse and data collection (more precise, the center of *k*-space) is chosen such that the magnetization of viable (normal) myocardium is near its zero crossing, meaning that these regions appear dark (Fig. 14.23). Nonviable myocardium (acutely infarcted or scar), however, appears bright because of the shorter T1 (faster signal recovery curve in areas of Gd-DTPA; see Fig. 14.23). It is important to manually adjust the TI for each image to null normal myocardium to account for wash-out kinetics of the contrast agent.[35]

In recent years phase-sensitive inversion recovery (PSIR) sequences have been developed which relax the stringent constraint of selecting the appropriate TI on an LGE sequence.[36,37] The challenge with traditional LGE imaging is the selection of the correct null time for normal myocardium, which is continually changing as contrast is being cleared from the body. PSIR imaging uses an extra reference scan (acquired during the rest interval of a traditional IR image) to determine the polarity of the magnetization following an inversion pulse. Because normal myocardium has the longest T1 of the tissues normally imaged (normal myocardium, enhanced myocardium, and blood), the PSIR algorithm renders the normal myocardium black, regardless of the selected inversion time. A diagram of the pulse sequence and resulting images are shown in Fig. 14.24.

FLOW/VELOCITY IMAGING ("SCAN" = "FLOW/VELOCITY")

At the DCMRC, velocity-encoded (VENC) CMR imaging of blood flow is usually performed to measure velocities in arteries, veins, valves, and shunts. Typically, the overall goal is to evaluate the severity of an aortic valve stenosis or an intracardiac shunt (e.g., atria or ventricular septal defect). Furthermore, cardiac stroke volume can be calculated by summing up the area under the flow/velocity curve of the ascending aorta.

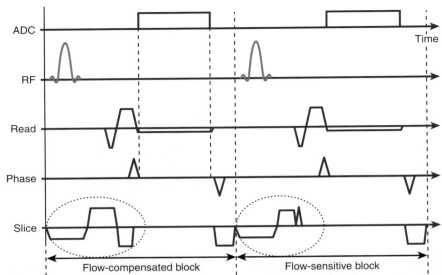

FIG. 14.26 Pulse sequence timing diagram of the velocity-encoded sequence. Gradients on the read axis are flow compensated. On the slice axis two gradient waveforms are shown inside the dotted ellipses; one that is insensitive to flow (flow-compensated block) and one that is sensitive toward flow (flow-sensitized block). The figure shows the sequence necessary to acquire one line of data. This is an example for assessment of through-plane flow, but in-plane flow can be imaged as well. *ADC,* Analog-to-digital converter; *RF,* radiofrequency.

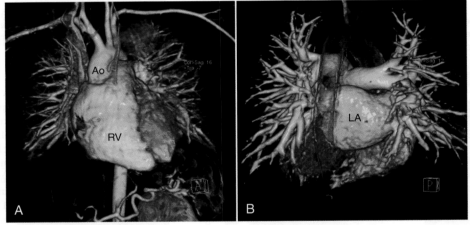

FIG. 14.27 Three-dimensional contrast-enhanced magnetic resonance angiography multiplanar reconstruction of the aortic root and thoracic aorta. This image was electrocardiogram-gated for high resolution of the aortic root in a young woman with a history of a bicuspid aortic valve and aortic root dilatation. (A) Anterior view showing the ventricles, aortic arch, and branch vessels. (B) Posterior view showing the pulmonary arteries and veins and the left atrium *(LA). Ao,* Aorta; *RV,* right ventricle.

affect image quality. In the case of highly dynamic structures such as the ascending aorta, we have also found it important to not only account for the systolic cycle length but also the period of time in early diastole when passive relaxation of the aorta occurs as a result of the elastic recoil of the vessel. This short period of "diastolic vessel relaxation" leads to appreciable vascular motion that can blur the edges of an angiogram and compromise its quality. These considerations were taken into account for obtaining the images of Fig. 14.27 because they would otherwise not be as crisp.

For contrast-enhanced MRA the most commonly used pulse sequence is a fast 3D spoiled gradient echo sequence. This is a variant of the FLASH technique that was discussed previously (see Fig. 14.17). The 3D data acquisition requires that an additional gradient be applied along the slice-encoding direction to encode the additional dimension. The data required for the 3D acquisition are much larger than the two-dimensional (2D) FLASH sequence and results in longer scan times (~15–20 seconds). Using parallel imaging techniques, more elegant *k*-space sampling, and faster gradient sets has decreased scan times significantly. Using state-of-the-art hardware and newer sequences, high-resolution ECG-gated contrast-enhanced MRA can be completed within a single breath-hold.

Contrast-enhanced 3D MRA is the most common type of angiography we use on the clinical service. We have found this scan to be easily incorporated into the clinical CMR examination without significantly changing the duration of the study or compromising the quality of the other components.

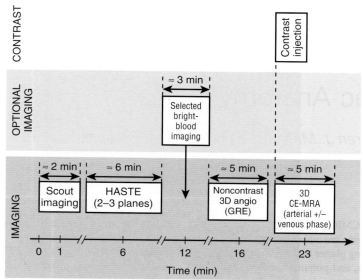

FIG. 14.28 Timeline of a typical contrast-enhanced magnetic resonance angiography *(CE-MRA)*. Note that the time scale is not linear. In addition to scouts, half-Fourier acquisition single-shot turbo spin echo *(HASTE)* and selected bright-blood balanced steady-state free precession images are obtained for analysis of extravascular structures and vascular structures which may not be in the angiographic field-of-view. A noncontrast three-dimensional *(3D)* angiogram is done before the contrast angiogram so that a subtraction image can be generated. A comprehensive study can be completed in 20 to 25 minutes. *GRE*, Gradient recalled echo.

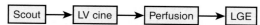

FIG. 14.29 Combination of menu items for the evaluation of a patient with coronary artery disease. This is the Duke cardiovascular magnetic resonance center (DCRMC) Cardiovascular Magnetic Resonance (CMR) Stress Test, which comprises approximately 50% of our 4000 annual procedures. The DCMRC CMR Viability Test (another 25% of our volume) is identical, except that perfusion imaging is not performed. *LGE*, Late gadolinium enhancement; *LV*, left ventricular.

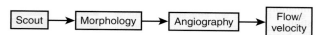

FIG. 14.30 Combination of menu items for evaluation of the aorta. Magnetic resonance angiography is the third-largest cardiovascular magnetic resonance procedure at our institution, after stress testing and viability.

CONCLUSION

The overall goal of this chapter was to describe an approach to routine clinical CMR that is based on selecting one or more scans from an examination menu and assembling these into a test. Fig. 14.29 shows how one would assemble a test for a patient referred for the evaluation of coronary artery disease. Specifically, one would perform scouting, cine imaging, perfusion imaging at stress and rest, and finally LGE imaging. The protocol of Fig. 14.29 is, in fact, identical to the CMR Stress Test[1] discussed in the introductory section of this chapter. Importantly, and as previously noted, this test now comprises approximately 50% of our 4000 annual CMR procedures. Similarly, Fig. 14.30 summarizes how one would approach CMR scanning of a patient referred for the evaluation of aortic disease. Additional information regarding the latest standards in CMR protocols is continually being updated through the Society for Cardiovascular Magnetic Resonance consensus document.[40]

In summary, although the definition of routine clinical CMR continues to evolve at our, and other, institutions, we have found it very useful to assemble a short list of predefined individual CMR scan protocols (the "exam menu"; see Fig. 14.3) from which one can create a "test package" specifically tailored to the diagnostic question. We have found that this approach substantially decreases the time needed to scan because the operator does not have to select amongst the literally hundreds of buttons on the scanner console while the patient waits idly inside the magnet (the buttons are predefined for each menu item). We have found that this approach significantly improves the throughput of our clinical CMR service. Perhaps more importantly, however, we have simultaneously found that this approach dramatically reduces the historically steep learning curve for new physicians interested in learning CMR.

REFERENCES

A full reference list is available online at ExpertConsult.com

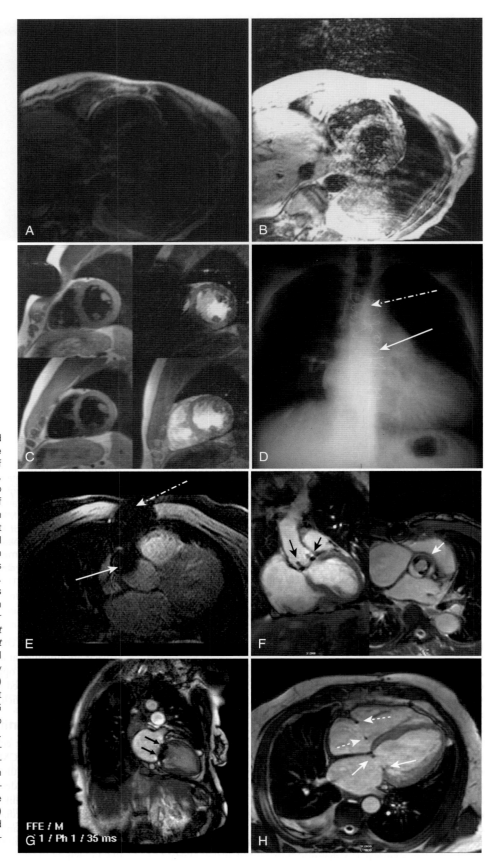

FIG. 15.4 (A) Artifacts due to respiration and poor gating. In this gated spin echo image there is mottling of the ventricular wall and loss of edge sharpness. (B) The same image as in A, but with the window and level adjusted to accentuate the artifact. There are ghosts of the chest wall related to respiratory motion and additional artifact over the heart as a result of poor electrocardiographic gating. (C) Metal artifact. The upper images were obtained with a safety pin present on the anterior subject's gown. The resultant signal void is very evident. The bottom row shows corresponding images after removal of the safety pin. Distortion from metal artifact is markedly more prominent/larger in the gradient recalled echo images *(right column)* than in the spin echo images *(left column)*. (D) Plain-film x-ray showing sternal wires *(dashed arrow)* and metallic coronary artery bypass graft (CABG) markers *(solid arrow)* in a patient with prior CABG surgery. (E) Artifact from sternal wires *(dashed arrow)* and CABG markers *(solid arrow)* on T1-weighted spin echo cardiovascular magnetic resonance imaging. (F) Signal voids *(arrows)* in two views of a bio-prosthetic aortic valve replacement by breath-hold cine balanced steady-state free precession imaging. The artifact results from the nonorganic struts. (G) Metal in bileaflet mitral valve prosthesis produces signal voids *(arrows)*. (H) There is minimal artifact from the tricuspid *(dashed arrow)* and mitral *(solid arrow)* annuloplasty rings.

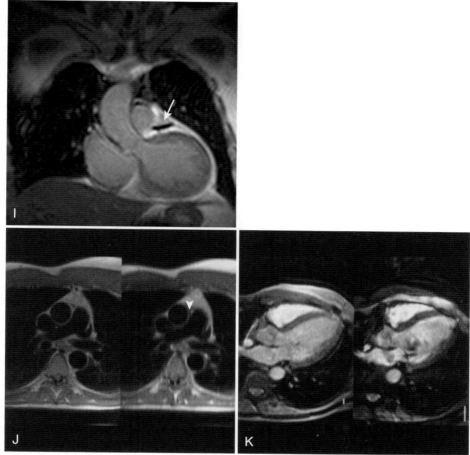

FIG. 15.4, cont'd (I) Metal artifact from a coronary artery stent in the left anterior descending coronary artery *(arrow)* seen on a scout image. (J) Chemical shift artifact. The image on the left is done with a relatively short signal acquisition time (wide bandwidth). The image on the right is done with a longer signal acquisition time (narrow bandwidth). This display accentuates the effect of the difference in chemical shift of water and fat, creating the artifactual space between the aortic wall at fat *(arrow)*. (K) Chemical shift artifact in echo planar imaging (EPI). In EPI, the chemical shift artifact occurs in the frequency-encoding direction (right to left in these images). The image on the left is obtained using a multishot EPI sequence with a relatively short EPI acquisition with each shot. The chemical shift artifact is indicated by the white line in the posterior chest wall. The image on the right is obtained using fewer shots with a longer EPI acquisition. The chemical shift is larger, as indicated by the longer white line posteriorly. The image is degraded by superimposition of anterior subcutaneous fat onto the heart. This problem can be addressed by adding fat saturation to the sequence.

systems provide arrhythmia rejection in an attempt to reduce these effects; however, use of these tools generally results in increased scan time because of rejection of cardiac cycles. Vectorcardiographic techniques, which exploit the difference between the normal vector and the vector of the artifact from the magnetohydrodynamic effect, have greatly facilitated reliable ECG gating.[12]

Respiratory Motion Artifacts (see Fig. 15.4A and B)

Respiration is associated with significant bulk cardiac motion. Motion in the craniocaudal direction is on the order of a centimeter in normal individuals.[13] This motion can result in significant image degradation with ghosting and blurring, particularly in those with inconsistent respiratory patterns. Strategies to reduce respiratory artifact include the use of breath-hold imaging, presaturation of the high-intensity signal from fat in the chest wall, and the use of respiratory gating. Respiratory gating may be accomplished using a thoracic bellows or by tracking the diaphragm position using a navigator echo (see Fig.

15.4).[14,15] These methods accept cardiac cycles only during some portion of the respiratory cycle. Respiratory gating can substantially improve image quality but increases total scan time. Real-time self-gating methods with continuous data acquisition are gaining increasing interest but are not yet in the clinical realm.[15a]

Metal Artifact (Fig. 15.4C to I)

Apart from safety considerations, pieces of metal outside or inside the body alter the local magnetic field and can result in artifacts. Patients must be screened carefully for the presence of metal, but despite vigilance, objects common in the hospital may still go with the patient into the scanner. Fig. 15.4C shows an artifact related to a safety pin on the patient's gown. Note that signal loss and distortion are present in both the fast spin echo and GRE images. However, the severity of artifact is worse in the GRE images, severely compromising interpretation of the RV and interventricular septum. Fig. 15.4D and E shows the artifacts related to sternal wires and coronary artery bypass graft markers. Fig.

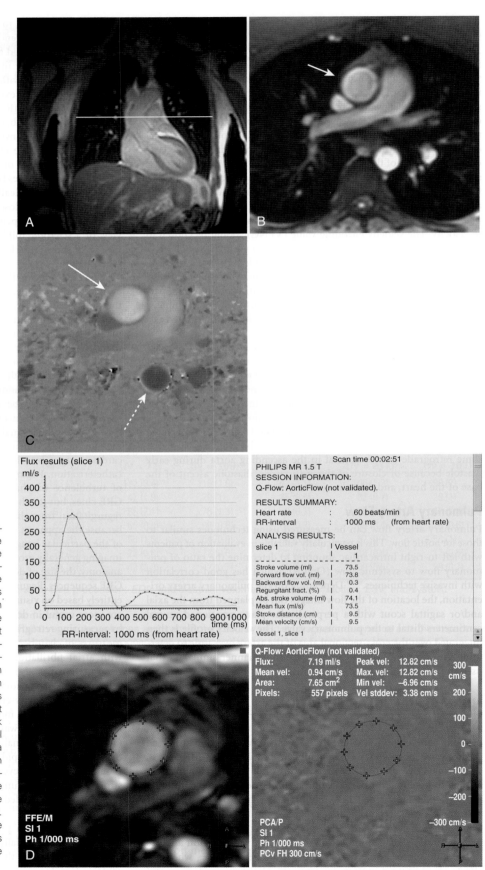

FIG. 15.6 (A) Coronal scout image for measuring aortic flow. The white line indicates the anatomic position of a flow sequence. The plane is positioned at the level of the bifurcation of the main pulmonary artery well above the aortic valve and perpendicular to the walls of the aorta. (B) Magnitude reconstruction from the flow sequence positioned in panel A. The imaging plane is transverse and positioned at the level of the bifurcation of the main pulmonary artery. The ascending aorta is seen anteriorly *(arrow)*. (C) Velocity map reconstruction from the same flow sequence as shown in panel B. The gray scale in this image indicates the velocity of motion toward the head as bright *(solid arrow, ascending aorta)* and away as dark *(dashed arrow, descending aorta)*. (D) Typical dataset for semiautomated analysis. The area of the ascending aorta is determined in each frame and the velocity over the area is integrated to calculate flow volume per frame. The top left subpanel shows a graph of flow volume over the cardiac cycle in the ascending aorta. The forward stroke volume, shown in the results listed in the upper right subpanel, is calculated by integrating the flow over the cardiac cycle.

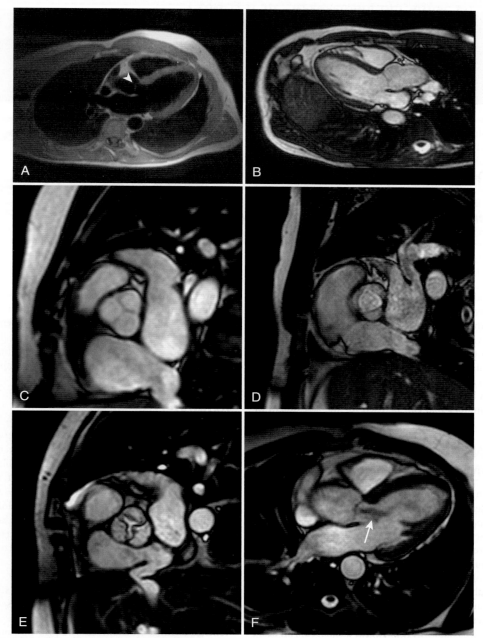

FIG. 15.7 (A) Double inversion recovery spin echo long-axis image. The aortic valve leaflets are demonstrated *(arrowhead)*. (B) A left ventricular outflow tract view acquired using breath-hold balanced steady-state free precession (bSSFP) imaging. (C) A normal trileaflet aortic valve depicted *en face* at end diastole (valve closed) by bSSFP imaging. (D) An open, normal trileaflet aortic valve seen during early systole. (E) An *en face* view of a sclerotic, mildly stenosed, trileaflet aortic valve also during early systole. Note the small opening and deformed leaflets as compared with panel D. (F) Aortic regurgitation is visualized qualitatively in the dephasing jet *(arrow)* in this bSSFP image.

CONCLUSION

CMR can be used to clearly delineate cardiac structure and assess function. As with any imaging technique, it is important to have a strategy for imaging and be familiar with the normal anatomy and potential artifacts. With this knowledge in hand, CMR can be a very effective tool in the noninvasive evaluation of nearly all cardiovascular diseases.

REFERENCES

A full reference list is available online at ExpertConsult.com

be easily and rapidly acquired to allow a visual, quantitative assessment of function, similar to that of echocardiography. The main advantage of CMR, however, lies in its quantitative accuracy and reproducibility.

of the LV; it is also subject to considerable partial volume effects, especially in the inferior wall. For this reason, more recently, short-axis slices were employed, and nearly all sites specializing in CMR have

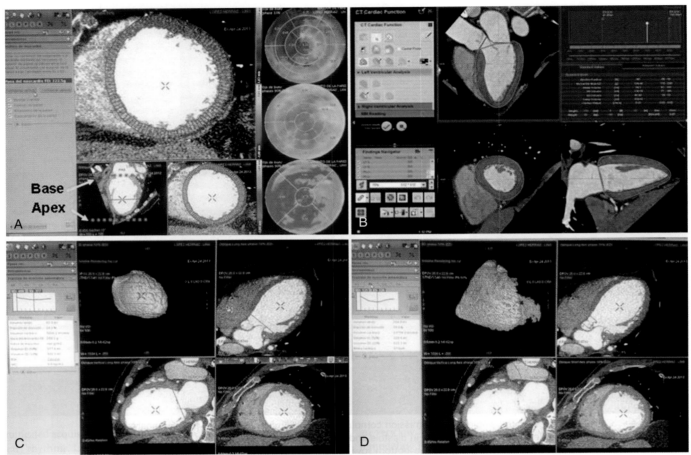

FIG. 16.5 Example of ventricular function analysis with computed tomography. A and B show, analogous to cardiovascular magnetic resonance, myocardial analysis for left ventricular (LV) function quantification both with ejection fraction and with wall thickening. C and D represent the ventricular threshold method for measurement of both LV (C) and right ventricular (D) volumes.

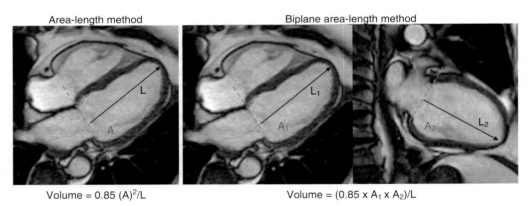

Area-length method Biplane area-length method

Volume = 0.85 (A)²/L   Volume = (0.85 x A₁ x A₂)/L

FIG. 16.6 Uniplane *(left)* and biplane *(right)* area-length method for measurement of left ventricular volumes and eventually function. Being a fast method, because only two planes are used, significant geometric assumptions are made that affect accuracy and reproducibility.

adopted this practice (Fig. 16.9). The question has been raised as to whether or not the right ventricular (RV) volumes should be measured in the axial orientation because this appears to have better interobserver and intraobserver reproducibility.[51,52] Yet the interstudy reproducibility of RV measurements in the short-axis orientation is good,[53] with differences not clinically significant and in practice, this orientation allows the LV and RV dimensions to be measured simultaneously. Rotational

long-axis views have also been proposed as an alternative to short-axis-derived methods because it has been suggested that they would have less partial-volume effects and would be less time consuming,[54] but this method has not gained wide acceptance so far.

In the past, to achieve full 3D coverage of the ventricle using conventional free-breathing gradient echo cine sequences, a total scanning time of 30 minutes or more was required, but on modern scanners with fast

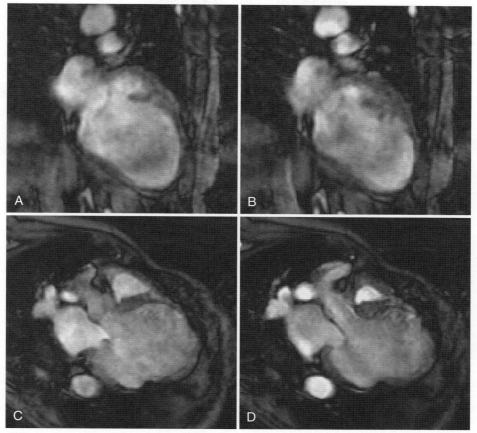

FIG. 16.7 A patient with ischemic heart disease in whom the left ventricle no longer conforms to geometric assumptions in either diastole (A, C) or systole (B, D) frames. Both the vertical long-axis (A, B) and the horizontal long-axis (C, D) views are illustrated.

imaging, a single cine can be acquired in just one breath-hold of about 8 to 10 seconds, with good spatial and temporal resolution, allowing the whole stack of images to be acquired in 5 to 8 minutes. This also has the considerable additional advantage of reducing breathing and movement artifacts. Moreover, real-time steady-state free precession (SSFP) imaging can acquire all the ventricular slices in just one breath-hold with acceptable accuracy and image quality. In patients who are unable to hold their breath consistently or who are orthopneic, solutions using the same sequence with more signal averages or combined with navigator echo imaging have been shown to be successful, during free breathing,[55] with a slight increase in the acquisition duration.

In addition to the left ventricle, it is important to remember the right ventricle, as its function is also known to be an important determinant of prognosis, both in coronary artery disease[56] and in heart failure,[57] congenital heart disease,[58] and pulmonary disease.[59,60] Global RV function is difficult to assess adequately by echocardiography, whereas radionuclide ventriculography suffers from assumptions concerning projection of overlapping structures unless research techniques such as first-pass techniques with ultra-short half-life isotopes are used. CMR does not experience such problems, and RV function and mass are well characterized. The right ventricle is discussed in greater detail in Chapter 39.

From Gradient Echo to Steady-State Free Precession Cine Sequences

Gradient recalled echo (GRE) cine sequences were the first ones to be implemented, but nowadays their use is limited to situations where

SSFP sequences are suboptimal, usually in patients with implanted devices that cause significant artifacts. SSFP sequences rephase the transverse magnetization that undergoes dephasing during phase encoding and readout between radiofrequency (RF) pulses; therefore imaging occurs when all transverse and longitudinal magnetization components are at steady state. SSFP cine imaging eliminates blood saturation artifacts and makes the cines independent of in-flow enhancement and based on the ratio of T2 to T1. This results, compared with GRE, in higher signal-to-noise ratio (SNR) and substantially improved blood-myocardium contrast,[61] which may allow easier delineation of the endocardial borders. At the epicardial border, fat-myocardium delineation is also improved.

The SSFP sequence runs at its best with ultrafast gradients because a very short repetition time (TR) is required to reduce the sensitivity of the sequence to movement artifact. Because of these characteristics, LV end-diastolic and end-systolic volumes are larger and LV mass is smaller with SSFP than with GRE.[62] In terms of reproducibility, only EF shows differences favoring SSFP, whereas SSFP and GRE are equal for volumes and mass reproducibility.

Nowadays, improved performance is no longer gained through improvements in gradient hardware. The introduction of parallel imaging, either image based such as sensitivity encoding (SENSE) or k-space-based such as generalized autocalibrating partially parallel acquisitions, provides alternative means for increasing acquisition speed. By using information from multiple receiver coils, images can be reconstructed from a sparsely sampled set of data, allowing for 2- to 3-fold acceleration of the imaging process. However, further increases in acquisition

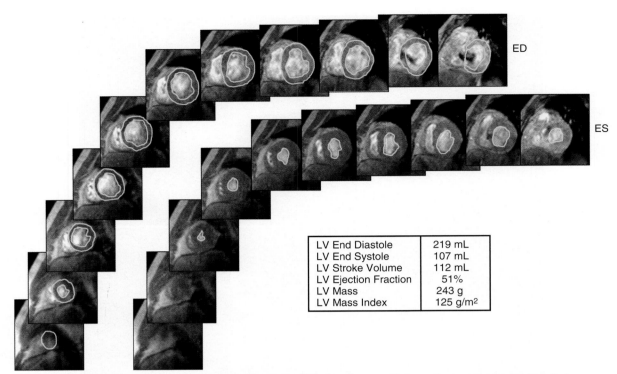

LV End Diastole	219 mL
LV End Systole	107 mL
LV Stroke Volume	112 mL
LV Ejection Fraction	51%
LV Mass	243 g
LV Mass Index	125 g/m²

FIG. 16.8 The end-diastolic *(ED)* and end-systolic *(ES)* slices from multiple contiguous short-axis cines that encompass the left ventricle *(LV)*, from base to apex, in a patient with ventricular dilatation and hypertrophy from chronic aortic regurgitation. The epicardial and endocardial borders are traced, and the summation values are shown. Note that there is one more image at end diastole[11] than at end systole,[10] reflecting the need to allow for the systolic descent of the atrioventricular ring, as described in the text. Note also the ingress of the LV outflow tract in the most basal end-diastolic image, where there is no ventricular mass, and the open ends of the LV myocardial horseshoe are joined together to form the appropriate volume.

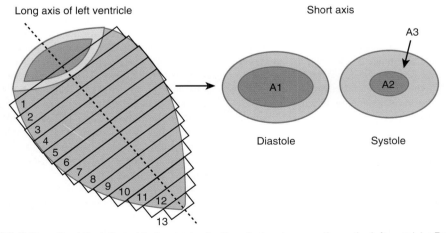

FIG. 16.9 Schematic of the left ventricular short-axis slices that encompass the entire left ventricle. Each slice is acquired as a cine. *A1,* End-diastolic endocardial area; *A2,* end-systolic endocardial area; *A3,* myocardium.

speed are difficult to achieve for current clinical field strengths and typical fields of view. More recently developed methods are based on temporal undersampling, *k-t* broad-use linear acquisition speed-up technique (BLAST) and *k-t* SENSE, have been proposed that significantly improve the performance of dynamic imaging, taking into account the similarity of image information at different time points during a dynamic series. These methods improve temporal resolution (5- to 8-fold acceleration) or spatial resolution for a given amount of acquisition, and they also enable the acquisition of 3D *k-t* BLAST SSFP cine sequences in one breath-hold that can be used for ventricular function assessment.[63] Another recently developed method is unaliasing by Fourier-encoding the overlaps using the temporal dimension (UNFOLD),[64] which works by forcing aliased signals to behave in specific ways through time, so unwanted signals are detected and removed, thus reducing the

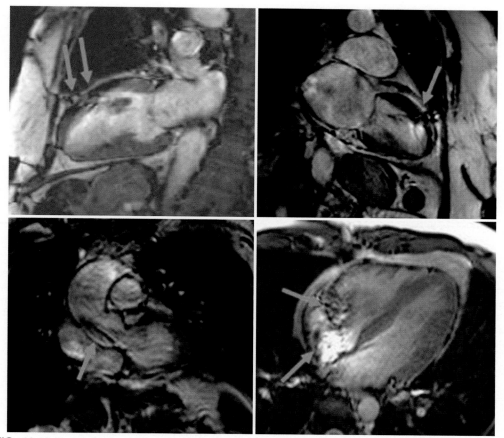

FIG. 16.10 The darkening artifact because of off-resonance effect *(top row, arrows)* and flow artifacts *(bottom row, arrows)* that are very frequent with cardiovascular magnetic resonance at 3 T.

amount of acquired data. This method can in theory be used with *k-t* SENSE and *k-t* BLAST to accelerate the acquisition and/or to suppress artifacts in free breathing.[65] All these techniques are very promising but still in development, and no specific data on their use in LV function assessment are available.

Steady-State Free Precession Cine Sequences at 1.5 T vs. 3 T Magnetic Fields

There is an overall quantitative improvement in SNR for myocardium and blood at 3 T, as well as variable increase of blood-to-myocardium contrast-to-noise ratio (CNR).[66] These SNR improvements can be translated into higher speed because they facilitate the use of parallel imaging, with higher acceleration factor and multichannel RF receiver coils, with less noise and almost identical parameters for SSFP imaging at both magnetic fields. However, accelerated acquisition results in the loss of SNR and in the introduction of noise nonuniformly, and there are some challenges that need to be addressed, including B_0 and RF inhomogeneity, limitation of flip angle and minimum achievable TR, longer T1, shortened T2* and off-resonance effects because of magnetic susceptibility gradients,[67] which together combine to offset the advantages from SSFP at 3 T, when a reproducible image quality for cine SSFP is important for the evaluation of ventricular function (Fig. 16.10). Comparative analyses of LV function indexes, mass, and volume using cine SSFP has shown no significant difference in values obtained at 3.0 T compared with 1.5 T.[68,69] Nonetheless, reference values for LV function parameters have been published.[70,71] Importantly, CNR

between blood and myocardium seems to be reduced in the RV at 3.0 T relative to LV, which may affect reproducibility of RV functional evaluation.

ACCURACY AND REPRODUCIBILITY OF CARDIOVASCULAR MAGNETIC RESONANCE

It is now widely accepted that CMR offers the reference standard for the noninvasive assessment of cardiac function, being both accurate[72,73] (Figs. 16.11 to 16.14) and reproducible in normal as well as abnormal ventricles, both with nonbreath-hold[74] and breath-hold techniques.[75,76] This is illustrated in Fig. 16.15, which shows the intraobserver, interobserver, and interstudy variability for volume and functional assessment by breath-hold CMR in dilated and normal ventricles, compared with conventional cine CMR.[75]

CMR has been shown to have higher reproducibility than 2DE for LV end-systolic volume (4.4% to 9.2% vs. 13.7% to 20.3%, $P < .001$), LVEF (2.4% to 7.3% vs. 8.6% to 19.4%, $P < .001$), and LV mass measurements (2.8% to 4.8% vs. 11.6% to 15.7%, $P < .001$), and this higher reproducibility allows for sample size reductions of 55% to 93%.[77] The excellent reproducibility of CMR versus 2DE can be illustrated by considering the sample size required for a drug trial designed to show a 10 g decrease in LV mass with antihypertensive treatment. A direct comparison of CMR with 2DE for reproducibility has shown that for an 80% power and a P value of .05, the sample size required would be 505 patients with 2DE but only 14 patients with CMR.[78] Equally, we have found that to show

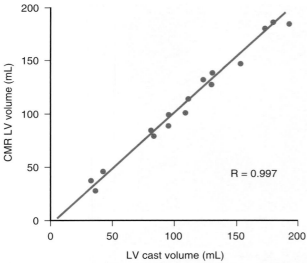

FIG. 16.11 Validation of left ventricular (LV) volume measurements by cardiovascular magnetic resonance (CMR). CMR-derived volume (vertical scale) is compared with the displacement volume of the LV casts from human postmortem hearts. There is excellent accuracy, and the regression line slope is close to identity. (From Rehr RB, Malloy CR, Filipchuk NG, et al. Left ventricular volumes measured by MR imaging. *Radiology*. 1985;156:717–719.)

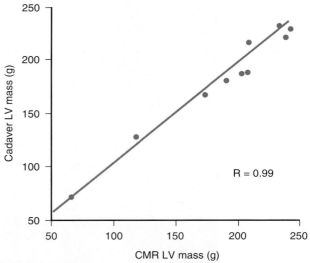

FIG. 16.13 Validation of left ventricular (LV) mass with comparison of cardiovascular magnetic resonance (CMR)-derived mass against human cadaver hearts. (From Katz J, Millikem MC, Stray-Gunderson J, et al. Estimation of human myocardial mass with MR imaging. *Radiology*. 1988;169:495–498.)

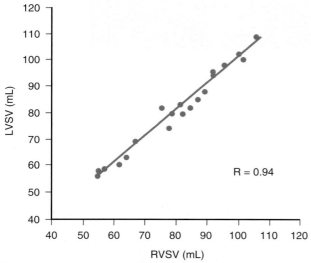

FIG. 16.12 Validation of right and left ventricular stroke volumes (RVSV and LVSV, respectively) in vivo using cardiovascular magnetic resonance (CMR) ventricular volume analysis. There is an excellent agreement between the stroke volumes of both ventricles, which is strong evidence that both measurements are accurate, because they are equivalent in vivo in the absence of valve regurgitation or shunting. (From Longmore DB, Klipstein RH, Underwood SR, et al. Dimensional accuracy of magnetic resonance in studies of the heart. *Lancet*. 1985;1:1360–1362.)

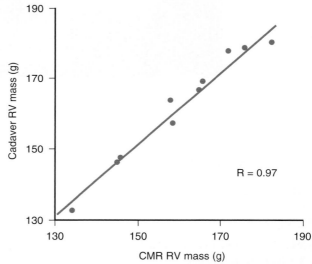

FIG. 16.14 Validation of right ventricular (RV) mass with comparison of cardiovascular magnetic resonance (CMR)-derived mass against postmortem bovine hearts. (From Katz J, Whang J, Boxt LM, Barst RJ. Estimation of right ventricular mass in normal subjects and in patients with primary pulmonary hypertension by nuclear magnetic resonance imaging. *J Am Coll Cardiol*. 1993;21:1475–1481.)

a 5% difference in EF with a 90% power and a *P* value of 0.05 would require only 7 normal subjects or 5 patients with dilated ventricles.[77] Similarly, CMR measurements of RV function parameters both in healthy subjects and in patients show good interstudy reproducibility (4.2% to 7.8% for RV end-diastolic volume, 8.1% to 18.1% for RV end-systolic volume, 4.3% to 10.4% for RV ejection fraction and 7.8% to 9.4% for RV mass), which was lower than that for the left ventricle for all

measures but only significantly for EF.[79] Three-dimensional echocardiography (3DE) and administration of contrast are claimed to improve accuracy and reproducibility. In a study[80] that compared 2DE, 3DE, and contrast-enhanced 3DE (CE3DE) with CMR in subjects with poor acoustic window, CE3DE showed the best agreement with CMR and was claimed to be the only acceptable alternative for CMR. In terms of reproducibility, another study[81] compared interreader variability for LV EF measurement with 2DE, 3DE, CE2DE, CE3DE, and CMR and obtained a variability of 14.3% for 2DE and 3DE, 8.0% for CE2DE, 7.4% for CE3DE and 7.9% for CMR, then showing that 3DE requires contrast application as much as 2DE to reduce interreader variability.

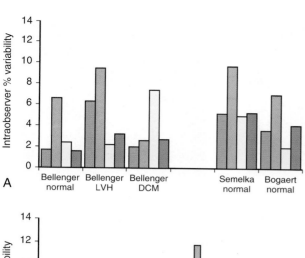

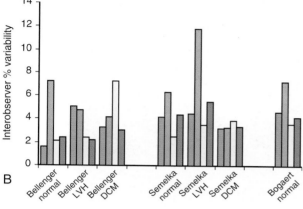

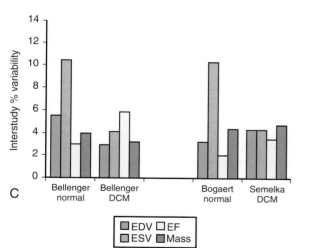

FIG. 16.15 The intraobserver (A), interobserver (B), and interstudy (C) percentage variability for end-diastolic volume (*EDV*), end-systolic volume (*ESV*), ejection fraction (*EF*), and left ventricular mass (*Mass*). Results using breath-hold gradient echo from our center in patients with heart failure and dilated ventricles (*DCM*) and left ventricular hypertrophy (*LVH*) are compared with breath-hold gradient echo in normals (Bogaert) and traditional, slower gradient echo cine imaging (Semelka).[65] Overall, the results are very similar (probably favoring the breath-hold imaging), both between techniques and between different population groups.

With respect to the right ventricle, a recent study has shown that 3DE underestimates RV volumes, with no significant differences in ejection fraction.[82] Reproducibility has significant implications for research and in particular for pharmaceutical companies, for which CMR offers a more cost-effective and time-effective research tool.

A PRACTICAL GUIDE TO FUNCTIONAL CARDIOVASCULAR MAGNETIC RESONANCE

In modern medicine, a balance must be struck between the information that can be gained from an investigation and the resources it demands. The following protocol is designed to be as efficient as possible in gaining the volumetric data from the ventricles of the heart[83] (see Chapter 15). Fig. 16.16 illustrates the sequence of pilot images used to achieve imaging in the long axis of the left ventricle and thereby the true short axis. A coronal pilot is first taken and used to acquire transverse pilots, which show both the mitral valve and the apex of the left ventricle. By taking a plane through the center of the mitral valve (halfway between the back end of the septum and the back end of the lateral wall) and the tip of the apex, the vertical long axis (VLA) is acquired. This VLA is used to plan the horizontal long axis (HLA), by again using a plane through the center of the mitral valve (halfway between the back of the anterior and inferior walls) and the tip of the apex. It should be noted that it is common to find centers describing planes that are parallel to the septum for the VLA and parallel to the inferior wall for the HLA, but these are not correct because they are likely to lead to the long-axis plane not passing through the center of the basal ring of the LV, and they may lead to an offset from the tip of the apex, which is also undesirable. This can lead to problems planning the short-axis cuts to adequately cover the full extent of left and right ventricles; in addition, it reduces the reproducibility of the short-axis plane positioning for repeated studies. Finally, the short-axis slices are placed on the HLA to encompass the heart. To achieve the most reliable results, which are the most reproducible, attention to detail is required. First, if the short-axis cuts are to be acquired by using a breath-hold cine sequence, then the VLA and HLA must also have been acquired by using a breath-hold and at end expiration. Second, in using breath-hold techniques, it is more reproducible to ask the patient to hold the breath at end expiration rather than elsewhere in the respiratory cycle; this applies to the pilots as well as to the cines.[84] Third, the first short-axis plane should be placed at the base of the heart, covering the most basal portion of the left and right ventricles just forward of the atrioventricular (AV) ring, and it should be placed on the end-diastolic HLA image. Finally, further short-axis planes should then be planned to move apically from this plane until the apex is encompassed. Although it is possible to acquire the VLA and HLA as single pilot images instead of cines, there is little practical merit in this because the time for two breath-hold cines is small, and the contraction pattern in these two planes is very useful during qualitative assessment of ventricular function. Nowadays, with the development of 3D postprocessing software solutions for analyzing the cines, these long-axis cines are mandatory. Also, full 3D analysis of atria as well as ventricles is simple and practical with automated analysis, in which case cines encompassing the entire heart should be acquired.

Following are some technical tips:

- Modern CMR scanners with faster gradients allow a shorter TR and echo time (TE), which improve the breath-hold length so this is no longer generally a problem for patients. If necessary, increasing the phase-encoded grouping (PEG) can reduce the breath-hold, but a compromise is reached because fewer phases will be captured with a higher PEG. The number of phases should be at least 15 to give adequate information on wall motion and cover end systole. Decreasing the field-of-view will also reduce the breath-hold time but may result in some wrap-around occurring at the edges of the image. If this remains remote from the heart, it may be considered an acceptable compromise. Typically, the best results are seen when the time between cine phases is <30 ms, and this yields a cine with approximately 25 to 40 frames in clinical practice.

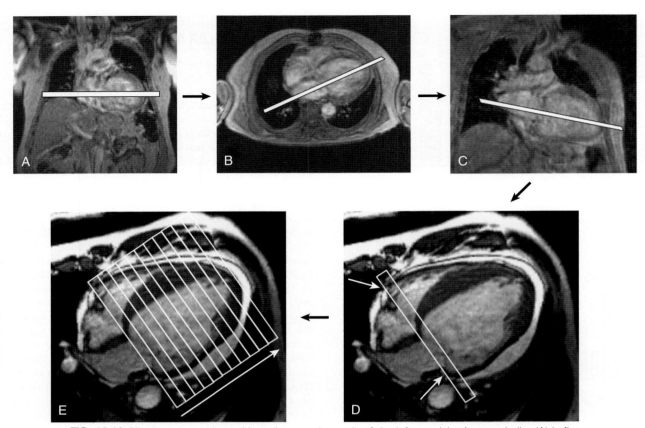

FIG. 16.16 Pilot images used to achieve the true short axis of the left ventricle. A coronal pilot (A) is first acquired and used to pilot the transverse image (B). The vertical long axis (C) is obtained from this and, subsequently, the horizontal long axis (D) is obtained, upon which a stack of short-axis cines are placed (E).

- The ECG gating can be prospective or retrospective. In prospective gating, images are acquired during systole and the beginning of diastole, whereas with retrospective gating, images from the whole cardiac cycle are obtained. Although the breath-hold with prospective gating is shorter, it is advisable to use retrospective gating, which allows diastolic function to be assessed. In patients with arrhythmia, retrospective gating may sometimes yield better image quality, but when ventricular ectopics are present, a good strategy is to use prospective gating with an acquisition window shorter than the coupling interval, so the acquisition is not disturbed by the ectopics.

- A slice thickness of 8 mm at 1.5 T provides adequate spatial resolution without overly increasing the number of slices and thereby the analysis time. It also limits partial volume effects. A 2 mm slice gap is commonly used to allow easy calculation of volumes because the center of each slice is then 1 cm apart. There are no formal studies to aid in the choice of slice thickness, but 8 mm is a reasonable consensus. Some centers prefer thinner slices, but it is important to maintain acceptable SNR and image quality. Three-dimensional imaging may eventually allow more partitions with thinner slices.

- Analysis of the short-axis slices is relatively straightforward, provided that the quality of the images is reasonable (mainly depending on accurate ECG gating and good breath-holding). The main source of error is in separating the ventricles from the atria. Identifying this basal slice is made more difficult by the through-plane descent of the AV ring in systole, which is usually about 1 cm. This makes the placement of the first, most basal short-axis slice very important. By ensuring that this basal slice is carefully positioned on the

end-diastolic, end-expiratory breath-hold HLA image just forward of the AV ring, the first short-axis cine will, by definition, contain end-diastolic volume and mass within both ventricles. However, at end systole, the basal slice will include only atrium, owing to descent of the AV ring, and, mostly, the systolic area in the basal cine is not included in the analysis of the systolic volume. In general, the next slice down contains both end-diastolic and end-systolic volume. An alternative to this rigorous approach is to oversample with short-axis slices into the atrium and attempt to retrospectively differentiate ventricle from atrium on the basis of the degree of descent of the AV ring in the long-axis images and whether the chamber dilates or contracts in systole. In general, we prefer not to oversample but to ensure that the first basal slice is acquired correctly because this leads to a reproducible approach and is more time efficient for both acquisition and analysis and because oversampling relies more heavily on good image quality to differentiate atrium from ventricle. Also, although at some point it has been suggested that a binary cutoff should be used for analysis of the basal slice, it has been shown[85] that fully inclusive quantification, rather than binary cutoffs that omit basal LV myocardium, yields smallest CMR discrepancy with echocardiography-measured LV mass and nonsignificant differences with necropsy-measured LV weight.

- Papillary muscles and endocardial trabeculae should be excluded from the LV volume and included in the LV mass. Although there is no clear consensus at present, LV mass is usually taken from the end-diastolic images. LV mass by CMR varies by a small amount from end diastole to end systole, and this may be due to expulsion of intramyocardial blood into the venous system, or to partial volume effects. The reproducibility of LV diastolic volumes is in general better than at end systole because the volumes are larger and delineation of trabeculae is easier, and this is probably as good a reason as any for working from the end-diastolic images to determine mass, but in addition, if the routine above is followed, there may be doubt as to whether LV mass is present in the most basal LV slice at end systole if its quality is less than ideal, but by definition, LV mass is always present at end diastole in the most basal slice.

- Normal reference ranges have been reported for LV[86,87] and RV[88] dimensions and systolic function. This is important because most LV and RV parameters are dependent on gender, age, and body surface area. The reference data are shown in Tables 16.1 (LV) and 16.2 (RV) and Fig. 16.17 (LV).
- For the very best interstudy reproducibility for follow-up studies and drug trials, it is necessary to go the extra mile in the analysis and always have the first set of cines with the regions of interest (ROIs) on screen alongside the follow-up cines during the analysis. At least a printout on paper of the first study and the ROIs used for analysis is required for comparison. For this reason, we routinely print out the diastolic and systolic ROIs in a systematic way for every patient on whom volumes are analyzed.
- Currently, a number of analysis softwares for automated postprocessing of the cines with a 3D analytical approach are available that take into account the motion in systole of the AV ring, by incorporating

VLA and HLA cines to define accurately the mitral valve position at each phase in the cardiac cycle. These softwares provide a fast analysis of ventricular dimensions in most patients, leaving manual analysis limited to studies with poor image quality because of arrhythmia or difficulty in breath-holding.

OTHER CARDIOVASCULAR MAGNETIC RESONANCE MEASURES OF GLOBAL FUNCTION: BRIEF SYNOPSIS

Systolic Function

There are other ways to derive important functional information from the heart besides volumetry alone. For example, flow in the major vessels is easily measured with great accuracy by using velocity mapping.[89] If the aortic flow is measured over a complete cardiac cycle, this represents the LV stroke volume. The RV stroke volume can likewise be found from flow in the pulmonary artery. Cardiac output can be easily derived by using the following formula: cardiac output = stroke volume × heart rate. The measurement of stroke volume, which is useful in valve disease[90,91] and for determining the need for surgery in cardiovascular shunting, is noninvasive and quantitative. The peak flow velocity and acceleration, which are derived from the flow curves, have been used to determine the burden of ventricular ischemia during dobutamine stress (see Chapter 17). Recently, tissue tracking technologies such as speckle tracking echocardiography and feature tracking CMR (CMR-FT)

TABLE 16.1 Normal SSFP LV Volumes, Systolic Function, and Mass (Absolute and Indexed to BSA) by Age Decile (Mean, 95% CI) in Males and Females

	20–29 Years	30–39 Years	40–49 Years	50–59 Years	60–69 Years	70–79 Years
Males	ABSOLUTE VALUES					
EDV (mL), SD 21	167 (126–208)	163 (121–204)	159 (117–200)	154 (113–196)	150 (109–191)	146 (105–187)
ESV (mL), SD 11	58 (35–80)	56 (33–78)	54 (31–76)	51 (29–74)	49 (27–72)	47 (25–70)
SV (mL), SD 14	109 (81–137)	107 (79–135)	105 (77–133)	103 (75–131)	101 (73–129)	99 (71–127)
EF (%), SD 4.5	65 (57–74)	66 (57–75)	66 (58–75)	67 (58–76)	67 (58–76)	68 (59–77)
Mass (g), SD 20	148 (109–186)	147 (109–185)	146 (108–185)	146 (107–184)	145 (107–183)	144 (106–183)
	INDEXED TO BSA					
EDV/BSA (mL/m²), SD 9.0	86 (68–103)	83 (66–101)	81 (64–99)	79 (62–97)	77 (60–95)	75 (58–93)
ESV/BSA (mL/m²), SD 5.5	30 (19–41)	29 (18–39)	27 (17–38)	26 (15–37)	25 (14–36)	24 (13–35)
SV/BSA (mL/m²), SD 6.1	56 (44–68)	55 (43–67)	54 (42–66)	53 (41–65)	52 (40–64)	51 (39–63)
EF/BSA (%/m²), SD 3.3	34 (28–40)	34 (28–40)	34 (28–40)	34 (28–41)	34 (28–41)	34 (28–41)
Mass/BSA (g/m²), SD 8.5	76 (59–93)	75 (59–92)	75 (58–91)	74 (57–91)	73 (57–90)	73 (56–89)
Females	ABSOLUTE VALUES					
EDV (mL), SD 21	139 (99–179)	135 (94–175)	130 (90–171)	126 (86–166)	122 (82–162)	118 (77–158)
ESV (mL), SD 9.5	48 (29–66)	45 (27–64)	43 (25–62)	41 (22–59)	39 (20–57)	36 (18–55)
SV (mL), SD 14	91 (63–119)	89 (61–117)	87 (59–115)	85 (57–113)	83 (56–111)	81 (54–109)
EF (%), SD 4.6	66 (56–75)	66 (57–75)	67 (58–76)	68 (59–77)	69 (60–78)	69 (60–78)
Mass (g), SD 18	105 (69–141)	106 (70–142)	107 (71–143)	108 (72–144)	109 (73–145)	110 (74–146)
	INDEXED TO BSA					
EDV/BSA (mL/m²), SD 8.7	82 (65–99)	79 (62–96)	76 (59–93)	73 (56–90)	70 (53–87)	67 (50–84)
ESV/BSA (mL/m²), SD 4.7	28 (19–37)	27 (17–36)	25 (16–34)	24 (14–33)	22 (13–31)	21 (12–30)
SV/BSA (mL/m²), SD 6.2	54 (42–66)	53 (40–65)	51 (39–63)	50 (37–62)	48 (36–60)	47 (34–59)
EF/BSA (%/m²), SD 4.7	39 (30–48)	39 (30–49)	40 (30–49)	40 (31–49)	40 (31–49)	40 (31–49)
Mass/BSA (g/m²), SD 7.5	62 (47–77)	62 (47–77)	63 (48–77)	63 (48–78)	63 (48–78)	63 (49–78)

BSA, Body surface area; *CI,* confidence interval; *EDV,* end-diastolic volume; *EF,* ejection fraction; *ESV,* end-systolic volume; *LV,* left ventricular; *SD,* standard deviation; *SSFP,* steady-state free precession; *SV,* stroke volume.

TABLE 16.2 Normal SSFP RV Volumes, Systolic Function, and Mass (Absolute and Indexed to BSA) by Age Decile (Mean, 95% CI) in Males and Females

	20–29 Years	30–39 Years	40–49 Years	50–59 Years	60–69 Years	70–79 Years
Males			ABSOLUTE VALUES			
EDV (mL), SD 25.4	177 (127–227)	171 (121–221)	166 (116–216)	160 (111–210)	155 (105–205)	150 (100–200)
ESV (mL), SD 15.2	68 (38–98)	64 (34–94)	59 (29–89)	55 (25–85)	50 (20–80)	46 (16–76)
SV (mL), SD 17.4	108 (74–143)	108 (74–142)	107 (73–141)	106 (72–140)	105 (71–139)	104 (70–138)
EF (%), SD 6.5	61 (48–74)	63 (50–76)	65 (52–77)	66 (53–79)	68 (55–81)	70 (57–83)
Mass (g), SD 14.4	70 (42–99)	69 (40–97)	67 (39–95)	65 (37–94)	63 (35–92)	62 (33–90)
			INDEXED TO BSA			
EDV/BSA (mL/m²), SD 11.7	91 (68–114)	88 (65–111)	85 (62–108)	82 (59–105)	79 (56–101)	75 (52–98)
ESV/BSA (mL/m²), SD 7.4	35 (21–50)	33 (18–47)	30 (16–45)	28 (13–42)	25 (11–40)	23 (8–37)
SV/BSA (mL/m²), SD 8.2	56 (40–72)	55 (39–71)	55 (39–71)	54 (38–70)	53 (37–69)	52 (36–69)
EF/BSA (%/m²), SD 4	32 (24–40)	32 (25–40)	33 (25–41)	34 (26–42)	35 (27–42)	35 (27–43)
Mass/BSA, (g/m²), SD 6.8	36 (23–50)	35 (22–49)	34 (21–48)	33 (20–46)	32 (19–45)	31 (18–44)
Females			ABSOLUTE VALUES			
EDV (mL), SD 21.6	142 (100–184)	136 (94–178)	130 (87–172)	124 (81–166)	117 (75–160)	111 (69–153)
ESV (mL), SD 13.3	55 (29–82)	51 (25–77)	46 (20–72)	42 (15–68)	37 (11–63)	32 (6–58)
SV (mL), SD 13.1	87 (61–112)	85 (59–111)	84 (58–109)	82 (56–108)	80 (55–106)	79 (53–105)
EF (%), SD 6	61 (49–73)	63 (51–75)	65 (53–77)	67 (55–79)	69 (57–81)	71 (59–83)
Mass (g), SD 10.6	54 (33–74)	51 (31–72)	49 (28–70)	47 (26–68)	45 (24–66)	43 (22–63)
			INDEXED TO BSA			
EDV/BSA (mL/m²), SD 9.4	84 (65–102)	80 (61–98)	76 (57–94)	72 (53–90)	68 (49–86)	64 (45–82)
ESV/BSA (mL/m²), SD 6.6	32 (20–45)	30 (17–43)	27 (14–40)	24 (11–37)	21 (8–34)	19 (6–32)
SV/BSA (mL/m²), SD 6.1	51 (39–63)	50 (38–62)	49 (37–61)	48 (36–60)	46 (34–58)	45 (33–57)
EF/BSA (%/m²), SD 5.2	37 (27–47)	38 (27–48)	38 (28–49)	39 (29–49)	40 (30–50)	41 (31–51)
Mass/BSA (g/m²), SD 5.2	32 (22–42)	30 (20–40)	29 (19–39)	27 (17–37)	26 (16–36)	24 (14–35)

BSA, Body surface area; *CI*, confidence interval; *EDV*, end-diastolic volume; *EF*, ejection fraction; *ESV*, end-systolic volume; *RV*, right ventricular; *SD*, standard deviation; *SSFP*, steady-state free precession; *SV*, stroke volume.

have enhanced the noninvasive assessment of myocardial deformation in research and clinical practice. CMR-FT has emerged as a useful tool for the quantitative evaluation of global and regional cardiac function, through quantification of biventricular mechanics from measures of myocardial deformation. The technology is common to both modalities, and derived parameters to describe myocardial mechanics are similar but with different accuracies and reproducibilities.[92] CMR-FT provides a fast assessment of longitudinal strain,[93] which is an independent predictor of survival in several cardiomyopathies,[94] as well as circumferential and radial strain. Also, normal values of references have been published.[95] CMR-FT has a reasonable agreement with myocardial tagging[96] and a there is a high correlation with 2DE and 3DE.[97] Although CMR-FT is a promising technique for evaluation of systolic and diastolic, global, and regional function, at present more work is needed to accelerate analysis, which is still time consuming, to assess differences in results obtained with different software packages, and, more importantly, on standardization of acquisition and analysis, applicability, and reference values. This is discussed in more detail in Chapter 22.

Diastolic Function

For diastolic function, phase-contrast CMR can be applied to measure, analogous to 2DE, both mitral inflow at the tip of the mitral valve leaflets and tissue velocity at the annulus. This technique is fast and reproducible, with good agreement with Doppler echocardiography.[98] Still, a mitral valve tracking technique should be implemented to overcome the limitation of not measuring velocities at the same level throughout the cardiac cycle. The same approach could be applied to the analysis of the pulmonary venous flow, but the lack of a dedicated postprocessing tool makes routine use of the PVF difficult. Cine CMR also allows direct visualization of the abnormal diastolic filling in dilated ventricles with inflow directed not toward the apex but toward the free wall, giving rise to a well-developed circular flow pattern turning back toward the septum and outflow tract, persisting through diastole.[99] With the current analysis softwares it is possible to measure volumes over a complete cardiac cycle, obtaining a volume curve whose first derivative is the flow curve; normal values of LV diastolic function with this method have been described and are shown in Fig. 16.18.[86] With the same approach, RV diastolic function curves have been produced and are shown in Chapter 39.[88] Left atrial dilatation is also a good marker of diastolic dysfunction; atrial volumes are easy to obtain with CMR.[100] Studies of myocardial velocity in diastole with tissue phase contrast allow evaluation of myocardial velocities during diastole and systole, in the same way as Doppler tissue imaging does in echocardiography.[101] Other techniques such as tagging, spectroscopy, or elastography have been used to assess myocardial relaxation and/or stiffness but more experience is needed before these techniques can be promoted. More details of the assessment of diastolic function can be found in Chapter 39.

Regional Function

Cine CMR sequence allows a qualitative assessment of regional cardiac function in the same way as with echocardiography, but with improved

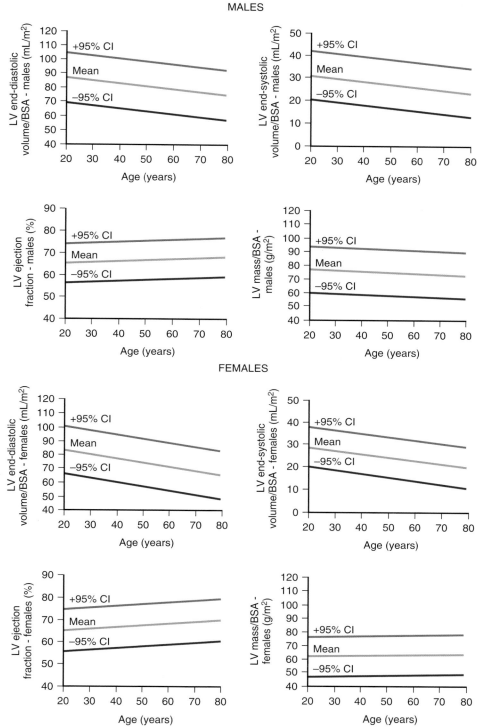

FIG. 16.17 Left ventricular *(LV)* volumes, mass, and function in systole normalized to age and body surface area *(BSA)* for males and females. *CI,* Confidence interval.

image quality and a lower loss of nonvisualized segments. In addition, it is possible to image routinely in the true long and short axis of the heart without compromises that result from restricted angulation caused by awkward acoustic windows. This wall motion analysis can be performed at rest, with low-dose dobutamine for detection of viable myocardium[102,103] and high-dose dobutamine for detection of ischemia.[104,105]

Studies using real-time CMR are now being published; these too show that CMR is superior to dobutamine stress echocardiography in patients with limited acoustic access.[106,107]

Several methods based on cine CMR have been suggested to provide quantitative assessment of wall motion and wall thickening.[108] In reality, however, myocardial dynamics are more complicated than simple

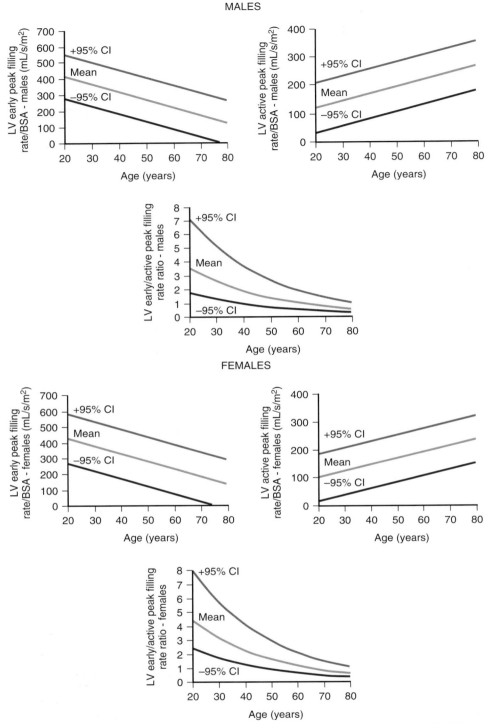

FIG. 16.18 Left ventricular *(LV)* function in diastole normalized to age and body surface area *(BSA)* for males and females. *CI,* Confidence interval.

thickening and 2D motion because of a complex interaction of contraction, expansion, twisting, and through-plane motion. This is best measured by the process of tagging,[109,110] which quantifies local deformation parameters and accurately measures several determinants of local loading conditions, such as wall thickness and curvature. These factors, combined with systolic blood pressure, give a measure of local loading, and by using the relation between local loading and deformation, a measure of local performance is produced. Tagging is discussed in more detail in Chapter 22. Also, as discussed earlier, myocardial phase contrast and CMR-FT may allow for quantification of local myocardial deformation in systole and diastole, with potential applicability in studies for detection of ischaemia and viability (Fig. 16.19).

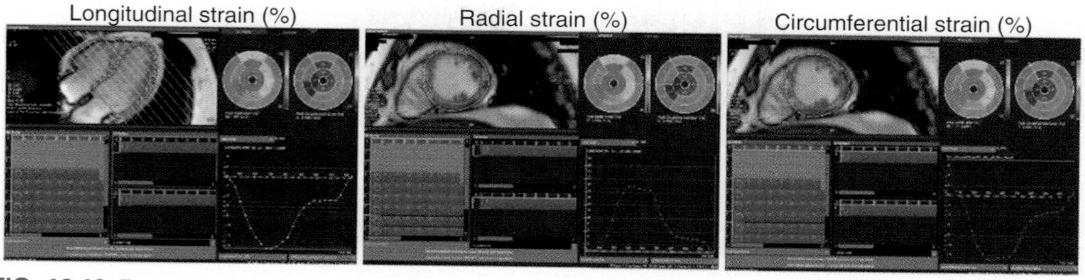

FIG. 16.19 Example of strain quantification with cardiovascular magnetic resonance feature tracking. Longitudinal, radial, and circumferential strain can be measured with this technique. Although longitudinal strain is usually given as a global value for the whole left ventricle, circumferential and, especially, radial strain can be provided on a segmental basis. The same approach can be used for the right ventricle and the left atrium. *BSA*, Body surface area; *CI*, confidence interval; *LV*, left ventricular.

THE FUTURE

CMR offers a rapid, accurate, and reproducible assessment of cardiac function that is free of geometric assumptions and is truly noninvasive. At present, CMR analysis of cardiac function is reasonably fast. Automated analysis softwares are already in use which allow for a fast 3D approach to ventricular measurement. Strategies to further decrease breath-hold time and implementation of 3D volume cine acquisitions should be achievable. Generalization of quantification of myocardial mechanics either with CMR-FT or other approaches is expected. As CMR becomes faster, acquisition protocols will become shorter and this will make the technique more cost effective for assessment of cardiovascular disease.

REFERENCES

A full reference list is available online at ExpertConsult.com

Stress Cardiovascular Magnetic Resonance: Wall Motion

R. Brandon Stacey and W. Gregory Hundley

Master and Oppenheimer described the first stress test in 1929.[1] Several methods of assessing myocardial ischemia have subsequently been developed, including those that incorporate electrocardiograms (ECGs), echocardiography, myocardial scintigraphy, and, most recently, cardiovascular magnetic resonance (CMR). Since 1987,[2] stress CMR has been used to identify inducible ischemia,[3] measure contractile reserve,[4] and identify those at risk of future myocardial infarction (MI) and cardiac death.[5,6] In this chapter, we review the utility of CMR wall motion stress testing, including the pharmacologic agents used during the procedure, the evolution of the procedure from dobutamine stress echocardiography (DSE), the performance and safety of a dobutamine stress CMR (DCMR) examination, and the efficacy of DCMR in identifying inducible ischemia, myocardial viability, and cardiac prognosis.

INTRAVENOUS DOBUTAMINE AND ATROPINE

Developed in 1975 by Tuttle and Mills,[7] dobutamine is a synthetic beta-1-selective catecholamine agonist that binds to myocyte beta-1-receptors and increases intracellular calcium concentrations and myocardial contraction.[8] Dobutamine was first employed as a stress-testing agent in 1984.[9] In addition to enhancing myocardial contractility, it increases the heart rate by promoting peripheral vasodilation and a reflex tachycardia.[8]

Because of rapid metabolism by catechol-*O*-methyltransferase, dobutamine's onset of action and half-life are both approximately 2 minutes; inactive metabolites are readily excreted by the kidneys and liver.[10] At low doses, <10 µg/kg/min, myocardial contractility is augmented and minor peripheral vasodilation occurs.[11] As the dose increases (20–40 µg/kg/min), heart rate and myocardial oxygen demand are increased along with myocardial work.[12] In study participants with flow-limiting epicardial stenoses, intravenous dobutamine promotes an oxygen supply/demand mismatch that induces left ventricular (LV) wall motion abnormalities.[13,14]

Intravenous dobutamine increases myocardial oxygen demand in a fashion similar to exercise, and thus is useful for stress testing in study participants whose exercise ability is limited as a result of peripheral vascular disease, physical incapacitation, or chronic deconditioning.[15] Other benefits of dobutamine include its tolerance for peripheral vein infusion and its effectiveness in both perfusion and wall motion imaging.[16]

The common side effects associated with dobutamine administration for stress include chest pain, ventricular ectopy, dyspnea, nausea, hypertension, and arrhythmias. Despite its relative safety, dobutamine is specifically contraindicated in study participants with hypertrophic obstructive cardiomyopathy, epicardial luminal narrowings of >50% in the left main coronary arterial segment, severe aortic stenosis, second- and third-degree atrioventricular block, sudden death syndrome, supraventricular tachycardia, and previous episodes of dobutamine hypersensitivity.

Although dobutamine exhibits positive inotropic activity, its chronotropic response can be suboptimal. Studies using changes in LV wall motion to identify inducible ischemia exhibit heightened sensitivity in appreciating flow-limiting epicardial luminal narrowing when the heart rate response during testing exceeds 85% of the age-predicted maximum heart rate (APMHR) response (220 − age in years).[17] For this reason, intravenous atropine may be needed to achieve an adequate peak heart rate response during testing. Atropine is a naturally occurring alkaloid that is a competitive antagonist of muscarinic cholinergic receptors; it increases heart rate by inhibiting vagal tone.[18] It is particularly useful in study participants taking beta-blockers, rate-limiting calcium antagonists, or those possessing a high parasympathetic drive. Atropine may be administered in increments of 0.1 to 0.3 mg, up to a total of 2 mg, to facilitate the achievement of >85% the APMHR during testing. Common side effects of atropine include dry mouth, tachycardia, and hallucinations.[10] Abnormally high heart rates after atropine administration are best treated with intravenous beta-blockers or rate-limiting calcium channel antagonists.

SAFETY PROFILE OF DOBUTAMINE AND ATROPINE STRESS TESTING

Safety is a primary concern for physicians and health care providers who administer dobutamine/atropine stress examinations.[16,19,20] The safety profile of dobutamine/atropine stress has been reported in 6 large studies, 3 using DSE and 3 using DCMR (Table 17.1). Garcia et al.,[23] Picano et al.,[24] and Geleijnse et al.[25] reported on the adverse events associated with DSE. These were classified into major and minor complications. Major complications included death, ventricular fibrillation, sustained ventricular tachycardia, complete atrioventricular block, acute MI, rupture of the LV free wall or ventricular septal defect, transient ischemic attack, and severe hypotension. Minor complications included nausea, anxiety, and atropine poisoning with hallucinations lasting up to several hours in the absence of either myocardial ischemia or hypotension.

Across the 3 DSE studies, the rates of major and minor complications ranged from 0.1% to 4%, and 38% to 71%, respectively. Wahl et al.,[26] Kuijpers et al.,[27] and Hamilton et al.[28] have reported on the incidence of major and minor side effects associated with DCMR. In Wahl's study of 1000 participants, 54% received atropine; in Kuijpers' study of 400 participants, none received atropine; and in Hamilton's study of 469 participants, 27% received atropine. There were no episodes of ventricular fibrillation, MI, or death during DCMR (see Table 17.1). The number of study participants sustaining other major events was

TABLE 17.1	Safety Profile of Select DSE and DCMR Studies				
Study	Modality	No. of Patients	Minor Events	Major Events	Deaths
Picano[24]	DSE	2799	78%	5%	0
Geleijnse[25]	DSE	2246	71%	5%	0
Garcia[23]	DSE	325	57%	21%	1
Hamilton[28]	DCMR	469	67%	0%	0
Kuijpers[27]	DCMR	400	71%	3%	0
Wahl[26]	DCMR	1000	64%	6%	0

Major complications included death, ventricular fibrillation, supraventricular tachycardia, atrioventricular block, acute myocardial infarction, rupture of the left ventricular free wall or ventricular septal defects, transient ischemic attacks, or severe symptomatic hypotension. Minor complications included nausea/vomiting, anxiety, hypotension, and atropine poisoning with hallucinations lasting several hours in the absence of myocardial ischemia.

DCMR, Dobutamine stress cardiovascular magnetic resonance; *DSE,* dobutamine stress echocardiography.

From Mandapaka S, Hundley WG. Dobutamine cardiovascular resonance: a review. *J Magn Reson Imag.* 2006;24(3):499–512.

0.6%, 0.2%, and 0% respectively. The percentage of participants sustaining minor events in all three studies combined was 54%. In these studies, the rates of major and minor events observed during DCMR are similar to those reported with DSE and would be expected as the dose administration is similar.

It is important to recognize that the major events are usually associated with continued administration of pharmacologic stress in the setting of concurrent myocardial ischemia. For this reason, it is important to identify ischemia promptly, and to discontinue the DCMR protocol when ischemia is recognized.[29] In the studies reported above, many of the study participants (56%) who developed side effects had known coronary atherosclerosis and a diminished resting LV ejection fraction (LVEF).[30] For this reason, a high level of scrutiny is used when reviewing image or ST-segment data for ischemia in the setting of reduced LVEF. Because of the risk of major adverse events, certain study participants should not receive intravenous dobutamine and atropine. Medications used for testing and emergency medications (Table 17.2) for treatment of potential cardiac complications need to be readily available to improve the probability of a successful outcome should complications occur during DSE.

DOBUTAMINE STRESS ECHOCARDIOGRAPHY

Since 1977, transthoracic echocardiography (TTE) has been used to acquire images before, during, and after treadmill or bicycle exercise stress, or pharmacologically induced stress.[31] During DSE, images are acquired in four standard imaging planes: parasternal short-axis (PSAX), parasternal long-axis (PLAX), apical four-chamber (A4C), and apical two-chamber (A2C) views.[32,33] The most common dobutamine infusion protocol used involves initiating dobutamine at 5 to 7.5 µg/kg/min for a period of 3 minutes, followed by 10 µg/kg/min for 3 minutes and subsequent increments of 10 µg/kg/min in 3-minute increments to a maximal dose of 50 µg/kg/min. If the patient does not achieve 85% of their APMHR, supplemental atropine is administered in 0.1 mg to 0.3 mg increments per minute (up to 2.0 mg total) until the target heart rate is reached.[34]

Throughout the test, the four echocardiographic planes are reviewed to monitor for ischemia. During testing, LV myocardial wall motion is defined as 1 = normal, 2 = hypokinesis, 3 = akinesis, and 4 = dyskinesis. Myocardial ischemia is defined as an increase in wall motion score during testing, or the persistence of severe hypokinesis during testing.[35,36] The scoring system is determined using a 17-segment model defined by the American Heart Association and American College of Cardiology.[37,38] A DSE is interrupted when there is evidence of ischemia in at least two adjacent segments, severe hypertension or

hypotension, dysrhythmias, unstable angina, or unexpected neurologic findings.[21]

DSE is useful for assessing risk of future MI, death, and the need for coronary intervention.[39,40] For many years, it was the modality of choice for risk stratification of cardiovascular events for patients being considered for noncardiac surgery.[41,42] However, DSE is of minimal value in study participants with poor acoustic windows, often because of a large body habitus, prior cardiothoracic surgery, or pulmonary disease.[17,43,44] In addition, there is a high interobserver variability for image interpretation; consequently, the accuracy of the test depends heavily on the proficiency of both the sonographer (acquisition) and physician (interpretation).[29,45]

DOBUTAMINE STRESS CARDIOVASCULAR MAGNETIC RESONANCE

CMR is well suited to overcome the acquisition and interpretative limitations encountered during DSE. It has no acoustic window limitations and thus can obtain comprehensive visualization of the LV myocardium regardless of body habitus.[46–48] In addition, image acquisition can be standardized and there is less reliance on an individual technologist's technique for acquiring high-quality images.

DCMR is commonly performed on short, 1.5 tesla (1.5 T) closed-bore systems, with bore diameters ranging from 55 to 70 cm. At the initiation of the DCMR examination, a 12-lead ECG is performed outside of the magnet. After intravenous access is established, study participants are told to lay flat on the CMR scanning table with a phased-array surface coil, brachial blood pressure cuff, pulse oximetry monitor, and respiratory gating belt attached (Fig. 17.1).[49] A physician and nurse are present throughout testing to continuously monitor the heart rate and rhythm, respiratory rate, oxygen saturation, and blood pressure. The protocol is similar to that described for DSE in that dobutamine infusions are started at 5 to 7.5 µg/kg/min, followed by 10, 20, 30, 40, and 50 µg/kg/min infusions in 3-minute stages. If study participants do not achieve 85% of their APMHR, atropine is added in 0.1 mg to 0.2 mg/min increments (up to 2 mg total) to augment the heart rate response (Fig. 17.2).

Breath-hold cine balanced steady-state free precession (bSSFP) images are obtained in three apical views (horizontal, vertical, and apical long axis) and in at least three short-axis LV planes (base, middle, and apex) at each level of pharmacologic stress (Fig. 17.3). If Simpson's rule is used to calculate LV volumes, short slices spanning the entire LV from base to apex can be acquired.[50] These views are also obtained after 10 minutes of recovery to confirm that LV wall motion has returned to baseline. After the patient is removed from the magnet, the 12-lead

End diastole   End systole   End systole

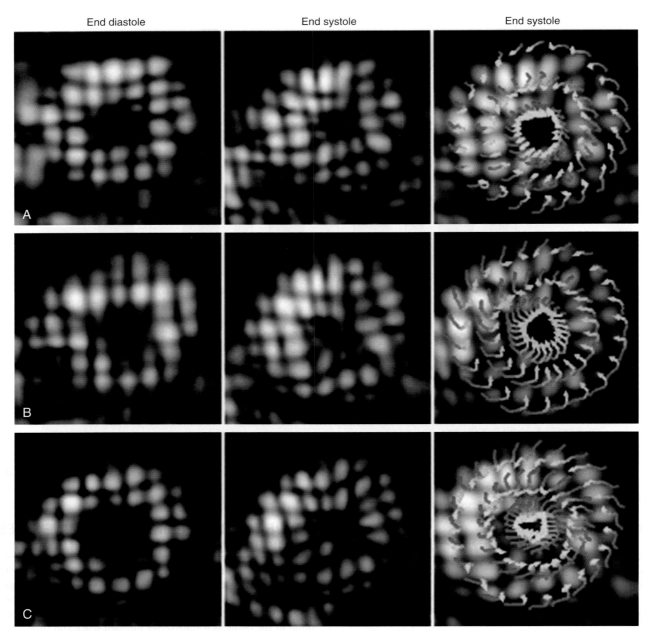

FIG. 17.13 Representative tagging end-diastolic and end-systolic apical cardiovascular magnetic resonance images of a patient without significant coronary artery disease. (A) Rest. (B) Low-dose dobutamine stress. (C) High-dose dobutamine stress. Note the increase in systolic rotation and endocardial motion from rest to low-dose stress. (From Paetsch I, Foll D, Kaluza A, et al. Magnetic resonance stress tagging in ischemic heart disease. *Am J Physiol Heart Circ Physiol.* 2005;288:H2708–H2714.)

tagging helps in a quantitative analysis of systolic and diastolic function during both low- and high-dose dobutamine stress.

Another potential development for the use of tissue tagging during DCMR is the use of automated analyses of the images with harmonic phase magnetic resonance (HARP). Image inspection with HARP enables substantial reduction of tag analysis times. Developed by Osman et al.,[82,83] this technique concentrates on the Fourier transformation of tagged images, which is directly related to the motion of the tag lines. The HARP technique can be used with any tagging strategy provided the tag pattern is planar and tag lines are placed a uniform distance from one another. In addition to wall motion and thickening, myocardial strain can be analyzed. Selecting tag filter specifications for the images requires

up to 20 minutes, but once the filter is set, a full quantitative analysis of the data typically takes less than 3 minutes. This represents a substantial time savings over manual analysis, which can take up to 8 hours. Further research is proceeding in this area to provide users with a mechanism to obtain quantitative tag data in near real time. By standardizing acquisitions of tagged images, one can preset the filter and provide very efficient myocardial strain mapping. By extracting HARP images directly from the raw data using faster microprocessors, the possibility of on-line detailed quantitative assessment of two-dimensional (2D) myocardial strains for use during stress testing may become a reality in the near future.

Pan et al.[84] have proposed a potentially fast and semiautomatic method for tracking three-dimensional (3D) cardiac images. Using a

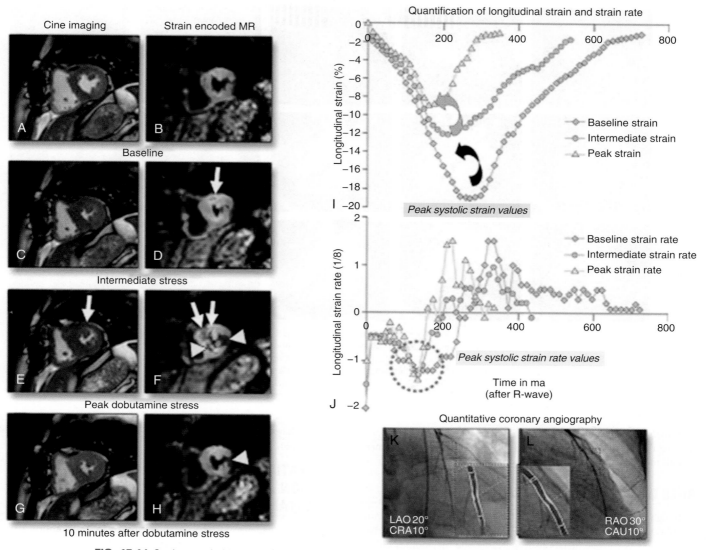

FIG. 17.14 Strain-encoded images (SENC) in a patient with coronary artery disease: mid–short-axis SENC and cine images are shown (A–H). With cine images, inducible ischemia is detected only during peak stress in the mid-anterior left ventricular wall (E, *arrow*). Conversely, with SENC, a strain defect is already observed during intermediate stages (D, *arrow*). The arrowheads indicate signal voids on SENC images due to low signal-to-noise ratio (F and H). Peak systolic strain values decrease as stress increases (I), but peak systolic strain rate remains unchanged (J). These findings were further investigated by coronary angiography, which confirmed a 68% stenosis of the left anterior descending artery (K and L). *MR,* Magnetic resonance. (From Korosoglou G, Lehrke S, Wochele A, et al. Strain-encoded CMR for the detection of inducible ischemia during intermediate stress. *JACC Cardiovasc Imaging.* 2010;3(4):361–371.)

material mesh model that is built to represent a collection of material points inside the LV wall, the phase time-invariance property of material points is then used to track mesh points. With a series of 9 timeframe CMR images, researchers were able to initialize settings, build the mesh, and track the 3D images in approximately 10 minutes. Eventually, more complex mesh algorithms will be developed that will allow 3D calculation of regional and global wall motion in real time.

Another technique used to assess myocardial strain is strain-encoded (SENC) imaging. This technique is a modified SPAMM tagging sequence.[85] In contrast to other tagging methods, the SENC gradient is applied orthogonal to the imaging plane. The magnitude of SENC images at both a high-tuning frequency and a low-tuning frequency are computed and placed over the anatomic slice image, which produces the strain map.[85] This can be done for long- or short-axis images (Fig. 17.14). In the setting of a DCMR, images are obtained at baseline and at rest. It has been studied at both 1.5 T and 3 T.[86] Initial analyses are promising and have demonstrated that SENC is as robust as other techniques and may improve the identification of myocardial ischemia and contractile reserve during both intermediate and full-dose dobutamine stress testing.[87,88]

Feature-tracking analysis may be used to measure LV thickening during DCMR. This technique uses standard bSSFP images to calculate both longitudinal and radial strain.[89] Both LV and right ventricular (RV) longitudinal strain are calculated from the four-chamber view (Fig. 17.15), and the LV radial strain is obtained from the short-axis view. Initial studies demonstrated the feasibility of feature-tracking analysis and, subsequently, demonstrated a reduced interobserver variability in

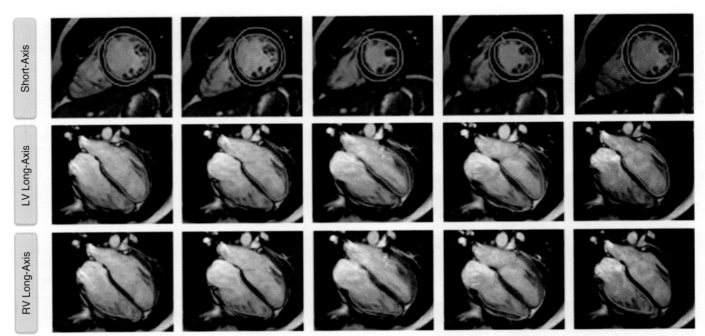

FIG. 17.15 Tracking in the short-axis and long-axis orientation. The figure shows a representative example of the tracking in short-axis and long-axis orientation of the left ventricle *(LV)* and right ventricle *(RV)*.[30] (From Schuster A, Kutty S, Padiyath A, et al. Cardiovascular magnetic resonance myocardial feature tracking detects quantitative wall motion during dobutamine stress. *J Cardiovasc Magn Reson.* 2011;13:58.)

identifying wall motion abnormalities.[90] Even at less than peak doses of dobutamine, feature tracking has been able to identify the development of wall motion abnormalities.[91]

ROLE OF DOBUTAMINE PERFUSION IMAGING

Although much of the focus during DCMR is on the increase in contractility and heart rate, dobutamine also indirectly increases coronary blood flow. As cardiac metabolism increases, the metabolites induce coronary arteriolar vasodilation, resulting in increased coronary blood flow. Initial studies comparing wall motion and perfusion during DCMR showed that perfusion defects had the potential to differentiate LV wall motion abnormalities because of true myocardial ischemia from heart rate–related bundle branch blocks.[92] Subsequently, myocardial perfusion during DCMR has been found to enhance the utility of DCMR for detecting myocardial ischemia. In a series of 42 study participants, Falcao et al.[93] found that by adding perfusion imaging to standard wall motion analysis in DCMR, the sensitivity to detect obstructive CAD went from 80% to 92%. In a larger series of 455 study participants, Gebker et al.[94] found that by adding perfusion imaging during DCMR, the sensitivity for detecting obstructive CAD increased from 85% to 91%, but they also found that the specificity was reduced because of artifacts and nonspecific perfusion abnormalities.

Dobutamine-related perfusion assessments may have clinical utility in other disease states. For those participants with concentric LV hypertrophy, the addition of perfusion imaging improves the sensitivity of DCMR for obstructive CAD. In a series of 187 participants who underwent DCMR before invasive x-ray coronary angiography, Gebker et al.[95] found that the addition of perfusion imaging to wall motion analysis improved the accuracy in identifying obstructive CAD from 71% to 82% in those with concentric LV remodeling. When interpreting dobutamine perfusion imaging from CMR, it is critical to interpret any perfusion defects identified with findings obtained

from LGE because prior infarcts also have associated perfusion defects (Fig. 17.16).

LIMITATIONS TO LEFT VENTRICULAR WALL MOTION ASSESSMENTS DURING DOBUTAMINE STRESS

A frequent challenge for the interpretation of LV wall motion stress testing relates to predobutamine and postdobutamine wall motion analyses in individuals with resting LV hypokinesis (e.g., those with LV wall motion abnormalities because of prior MI).[96] In these circumstances, it can be difficult to ascertain whether a segment that is persistently hypokinetic (rest and stress) exhibits myocardial ischemia or whether residual functioning myocytes within and around a previously scarred infarct cannot mount a contractile response that overcomes the stationary forces related to the scar.[97–99]

Those patients with resting LV concentric hypertrophy may not develop an inducible LV wall motion abnormality in the setting of epicardial coronary artery stenoses.[100] In a large DSE series, Smart et al.[100] showed that there were fewer recognized stress-induced LV wall motion abnormalities among individuals with CAD and LV concentric remodeling. Interobserver agreement of the LV wall motion assessment was high when LV systolic function was normal or significantly reduced, but agreement was reduced as the LV systolic function became impaired or significant hypertrophy was present.[97] In study participants with LV concentric remodeling, it should be recognized that it may be difficult to fully appreciate the functional changes associated with ischemia. By lowering wall stress, a significant determinant of myocardial oxygen demand, LV hypertrophy may make it more difficult to reach the ischemic threshold needed to produce wall motion abnormalities.[101,102]

Finally, when interpreting LV wall motion during intravenous dobutamine, one assumes that cardiac workload will increase to a sufficient degree during dobutamine stress such that a wall motion abnormality will occur because of reduced oxygen supply delivered through a stenosis epicardial coronary artery. Interestingly, in a prospective series of 278 older adults who underwent DCMR, Vasu et al.[101] demonstrated that nearly 60% of dobutamine-induced perfusion defects were not associated with corresponding LV wall motion abnormalities during dobutamine.

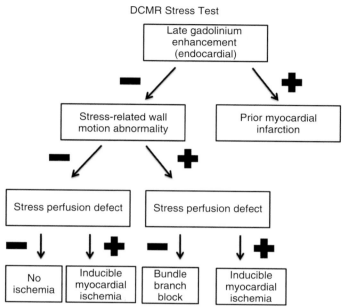

DCMR Stress Test

FIG. 17.16 Algorithm to interpret left ventricular wall motion abnormalities provoked during dobutamine stress cardiovascular magnetic resonance *(DCMR)*.

The stress discordance may have resulted from an inadequate stress load because older individuals are often more sensitive to the vascular effects of dobutamine. In the elderly, dobutamine may reduce both LV preload (by reducing the end-diastolic volume) and LV afterload manifest as a lower blood pressure with dobutamine. Both effects decrease their LV wall stress during dobutamine. This situation can occur more frequently when LV hypertrophy is present, causing further reductions in LV end-diastolic volume because of the relatively small LV cavity size. This finding is demonstrated in Fig. 17.17 in which a 64-year-old male who underwent DCMR demonstrated a hyperdynamic LV wall response to dobutamine, but displayed an associated apical perfusion defect at peak stress. X-ray coronary angiography revealed multivessel disease, including a 90% proximal left main stenosis. If one did not assess myocardial perfusion during the test and only focused on LV wall motion, inducible myocardial ischemia may have been missed.

ADENOSINE AND DIPYRIDAMOLE AS WALL MOTION STRESS AGENTS DURING CARDIOVASCULAR MAGNETIC RESONANCE

Dipyridamole, adenosine, and regadenoson exert their effect through coronary vasodilation, producing up to 5-fold increase in coronary artery blood flow. The safety profile of dipyridamole is favorable, with a well-known and low complication rate. Side effects include chest pain, shortness of breath, flushing, and dizziness, all of which can be reversed with aminophylline administration.[103] Pennell et al.[104] were the first to report the use of vasodilator dipyridamole with CMR in the assessment of LV wall motion. In 40 study participants, dipyridamole was infused at a dose 0.56 mg/kg, along with a 10-mg bolus after 10 minutes. Compared with thallium tomography, the sensitivity for detecting new wall motion abnormalities and identifying perfusion defects associated with ischemia was 67%.[105] After review of the data, however, there was an

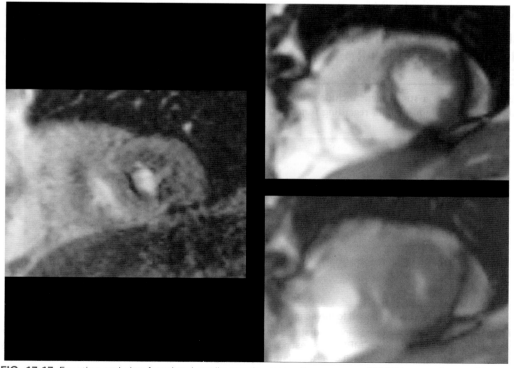

FIG. 17.17 Function and cine functional cardiovascular magnetic resonance (CMR) images from a 64-year-old man obtained during a dobutamine CMR. On the left, an apical perfusion defect is demonstrated. On the right, still short-axis images of end diastole and end systole demonstrate no left ventricular wall motion abnormality.

TABLE 18.1   **Assessment of Coronary Artery Disease: Characteristics of Stress-Only Protocol and Stress-Rest Protocol**

		Stress-Only Perfusion Protocol	Stress-Rest Perfusion Protocol
Acquisitions		Hyperemic data only	Hyperemic and rest data waiting time between acquisitions
Oxygen demand–perfusion relation			
• For resting perfusion		Not applicable	Determined by "confounding factors"
			• Heart rate
			• Contractility
			• Loading condition
• For hyperemic perfusion		Oxygen demand–supply uncoupled	Oxygen demand–supply uncoupled
Analysis		Only hyperemic data	Two analyses (stress and rest) matching anatomy for rest/stress condition "late enhancement effect" for second acquisition
"Ideal" MR parameter–perfusion relation		Linear for low perfusion range (no perfusion increase during hyperemia in myocardium supplied by significantly stenosed vessel)	Linear for both resting and hyperemic perfusion, because CFR is calculated as hyperemic data/rest data
Normal/abnormal discrimination		With normal database for regional hyperemic perfusion	With normal database for regional CFR
Viability assessment		With late enhancement acquisition advantage: acquisition window: minutes	Low resting perfusion indicates scar disadvantage: acquisition window: seconds (first pass)
Assessment of perfusion and viability			
• CMR:	• Perfusion	Hyperemic perfusion	With resting perfusion yielding CFR
	• Viability	Late enhancement	Resting perfusion
• SPECT:	• Perfusion	Hyperemic perfusion (tracer injection at stress)	—
	• Viability	Rest-tracer redistribution (tracer injection at rest)	—
• PET:	• Perfusion	Perfusion (flow tracer injection at stress)	With resting perfusion yielding CFR
	• Viability	Rest FDG uptake (metabolic tracer injection at rest)	—

"Stress" indicates hyperemic condition induced by adenosine or dipyridamole.
CFR, Coronary flow reserve; *CMR,* cardiovascular magnetic resonance; *FDG,* fluorodeoxyglucose; *MR,* magnetic resonance; *PET,* positron emission tomography; *SPECT,* single-photon emission computed tomography.

degranulation. Despite this profile, it is a very safe stressor as was shown in the EuroCMR registry with only two severe reactions in 18,840 patients.[44] In clinical routine, an insufficient hemodynamic response to adenosine can occur. Karamitsos and colleagues[45] proposed a high-dose regimen for adenosine (by increasing the standard dose of 140 µg/kg/min for 3 minutes to 210 µg/kg/min for 7 minutes), which was safely applied in patients with suspected CAD, increasing the proportion of adequate hemodynamic response (heart rate increase >10 beats per minute or systolic blood pressure decrease >10 mm Hg) from 82% to 98%. Conversely, dipyridamole induces hyperemia by blocking adenosine re-uptake. Finally, regadenoson represents a more selective adenosine 2A receptor, which is administered as a single intravenous (IV) bolus. This compound was shown to induce hyperemia at a similar degree to adenosine[46] and it was also successfully used in studies on prognosis (see later).[47,48]

ENDOGENOUS VERSUS EXOGENOUS CONTRAST MEDIA

Endogenous Contrast Media

Arterial spin labeling exploits the fact that unsaturated protons entering saturated tissue shorten the tissue T1.[49–52] Using appropriate electrocardiogram (ECG)-triggered pulse sequences, T1 measurements are performed after global and slice-selective spin preparation. Absolute tissue perfusion is then calculated by assuming a two-compartment model. It should be kept in mind that this approach assumes that the direction of flowing blood in intramural vessels is orthogonal to the slice orientation, which is not the case for all myocardial layers. Furthermore,

fiber orientations change during contraction and relaxation, making this approach problematic in the beating heart.

In blood-oxygen-level-dependent (BOLD) imaging, deoxygenated and thus paramagnetic hemoglobin shortens T2 relaxation time and therefore can be used as an endogenous contrast media (CM) (although oxygenated hemoglobin is slightly diamagnetic, causing less T2 shortening). A T2- or T2*-weighted pulse sequence allows for an estimation of an increased content of oxygenated blood. During pharmacologically induced hyperemia, oxygen content will increase in well-perfused myocardium but not in myocardium supplied by a stenosed vessel (which is associated with a higher O_2 extraction). However, signal differences in normally perfused regions versus hyperemic regions (with a 4-fold increase in flow) were reported to be as low as 32% in an experimental study.[53] These BOLD data correlated closely with microsphere data, but the slope of the correlation was as low as 0.08. This limitation in signal difference might be problematic, because CM first-pass studies suggested several hundred percent of signal change being required for a reliable stenosis detection.[54] In another study applying BOLD, $\Delta R2$ measurements yielded an adequate slope of 0.94.[55] But again, the sensitivity to absolute flow changes was low, because a 100% increase in flow yielded a signal increase of only 5% (i.e., a change in myocardial R2 of 0.94/s) in that study.[55] Accordingly, in a recent study in patients, R2 increased by only 16% during adenosine stress in nonstenotic areas (although adenosine is typically increasing flow 300%–500%).[56] The BOLD approach is also sensitive to magnetic field inhomogeneities, predominantly occurring in the posterior wall close the coronary sinus draining deoxygenated blood. Considering these aspects, the robustness of the method is not yet fully explored.[57,58]

Exogenous Contrast Media for Perfusion Cardiovascular Magnetic Resonance

These CM are typically injected into a peripheral vein, and the signal change in the myocardium occurring during the first-pass of the CM is measured by a fast CMR acquisition. All CM first-pass techniques either under development or in clinical routine are designed to meet the following requirements: (1) provide high spatial resolution to permit detection of small subendocardial perfusion deficits, (2) provide adequate cardiac coverage to allow for assessment of the extent of perfusion deficits, (3) feature high CM sensitivity to generate optimum contrast between normally and abnormally perfused myocardium during CM first pass, and (4) allow acquisition of perfusion data every one to two heartbeats to yield signal intensity–time curves of adequate temporal resolution that allow for extraction of various perfusion parameters (see later). To reach these goals, high-speed data acquisition and time-efficient magnetization schemes are most important. Because the first pass of CM during hyperemia lasts only 5 to 10 seconds, breathing motion is minimized by a breath-hold maneuver, although cardiac motion is eliminated by ECG triggering. This control of cardiac and breathing motion in perfusion CMR preserves its high spatial resolution of data acquisition: on the order of 1 to 2 mm × 1 to 2 mm. This is not the case for scintigraphic techniques with acquisition windows of several minutes, which preclude breath-holding for elimination of respiratory motion, and ECG triggering during single-photon emission computed tomography (SPECT) studies requires higher tracer amounts to improve counts statistics.

Extravascular Contrast Media

For perfusion CMR techniques, the relationship between myocardial CM concentration and myocardial signal depends on a variety of factors. Normal perfusion can cause a signal increase during first pass of a gadolinium (Gd) chelate when combined with a T1-weighted pulse sequence, although a T2-weighted sequence with a higher dose of a Gd chelate can even cause a signal drop during first pass.[59,60] This is fundamentally different from ischemia detection based on the assessment of wall motion, where new onset of dysfunction unambiguously indicates the presence of ischemia.[61]

Today, extravascular Gd chelates are most commonly used for first-pass perfusion CMR in combination with heavily T1-weighted pulse sequences. These CM are excluded from the intracellular compartment (i.e., from viable cells with intact cell membranes); therefore a perfusion deficit during the first pass reflects either hypoperfused viable myocardium (which would become ischemic during inotropic stress) and/or scar tissue (with severe reduction of perfusion even at rest). To differentiate hypoperfused tissue further, it is recommended to inject another dose of CM and to wait for the establishment of a dynamic equilibrium of CM concentrations in the various compartments (blood, viable myocardium, scar tissue), to obtain conditions where tissue CM concentrations are governed by distribution volumes (and no longer by perfusion).[62] During this condition, which typically occurs within 10 to 20 minutes after CM injection in humans, late enhancement imaging (with the inversion time set to null normal myocardium) is ideal to discriminate hypoperfused but viable myocardium as dark tissue from scar, which appears bright.[63,64] For viability assessment, scintigraphic techniques also exploit the equilibrium distribution of tracers, which is observed after rest injection or rest reinjections. However, the radioactive tracers are not taken up by scar tissue, which consequently appears as a cold spot, whereas viable tissue appears as a hot spot (see Table 18.1).

Several multicenter studies were performed for the assessment of the optimal CM dose for perfusion imaging. This is important because higher CM doses can cause susceptibility artifacts at the subendocardium, where differences in CM concentrations between blood and myocardium are high during first pass. Strongly T1-weighted sequences showed an absence of a susceptibility-induced signal drop in the subendocardial layer up to doses of 0.15 mmol/kg of an extravascular Gd chelate, which resulted in superior diagnostic performance of doses of 0.1 and 0.15 mmol/kg versus 0.05 mmol/kg for semiautomatic analysis of the upslope parameter[4] (Fig. 18.3).

Intravascular Contrast Media

For albumin-targeted MS-325[65] and polylysine-Gd compounds[66,67] differences between normally perfused and stenosis-dependent hypoperfused myocardium were reported in animals. However, these intravascular Gd-based CM have not advanced into clinics. Ultrasmall superparamagnetic particles of iron oxide (USPIO) nanoparticles were used for perfusion studies in humans (however, this CM is no longer under investigation because its iron accumulation in the liver).[68] For T2*-enhancing CM, not only the concentration of CM in the voxel but also its intravoxel distribution (homogeneous vs. inhomogeneous) determines its T2*-shortening effect, rendering such a T2*-approach susceptible to vessel architecture (vessel orientation, intervessel distance), which also may compromise quantitative approaches.

Hyperpolarized Contrast Media

Conventional Gd chelates modulate the magnetic resonance (MR) signal by accelerating the relaxation rates of surrounding water protons. However, at a field strength of 1.5 T, the polarization level of the spin population of the MR active nuclei at the thermal equilibrium is low (several parts per million), and only the vast abundance of water molecules in the human body enables generation of a measurable signal. Because the polarization level of water protons increases with magnetic flux density, a higher signal is achieved at higher field strength. Alternatively, however, the polarization level of the spin population of specific nuclei (such as liquid ^{13}C in various compounds) could be increased by a factor of up to 100,000 (compared with polarization of water protons at the thermal equilibrium) by dynamic nuclear polarization[69] or parahydrogen-induced polarization.[70] With these hyperpolarized CM, signal is received only from the ^{13}C-nuclei; therefore no signal from background tissue is obtained. This feature appears ideal for absolute quantification of perfusion because signal is directly proportional to the amount of ^{13}C molecules similar to radioactive tracers, where radioactivity is directly proportional to tracer concentration. Similarly to radioactive tracers, the signal from hyperpolarized ^{13}C-nuclei also decays (with specific time constants depending on the type of the ^{13}C-compound), because the spin population of the ^{13}C-molecules is far away from thermal equilibrium. In addition, repetitive radiofrequency pulsing further destroys longitudinal magnetization depending on the pulse sequence type and the imaging parameters. Johansson and colleagues showed that depolarization can be approximated by a monoexponential function with a time constant T_D and successfully applied this concept for cerebral perfusion quantification.[71] Recently, sophisticated spiral pulse sequences became available, which allowed for myocardial perfusion and metabolism quantification in small animals[72] and for the first time in humans.[73]

PERFUSION CARDIOVASCULAR MAGNETIC RESONANCE: WHAT IS ESTABLISHED AND WHAT IS NOT

Cardiovascular Magnetic Resonance Data Readout

Echo planar readout strategies are well suited to speed up data acquisition,[74,75] particularly when segmented to reduce the echo time and

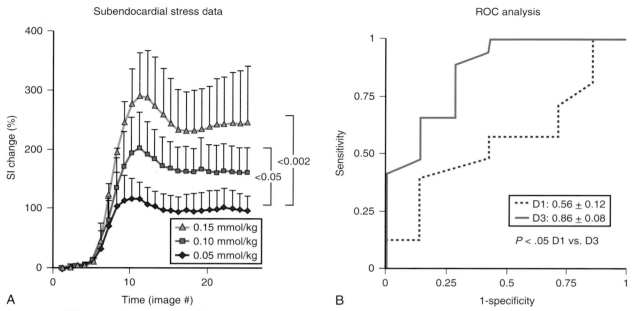

FIG. 18.3 (A) Increasing doses of the extravascular contrast medium gadolinium diethylenetriamine penta-acetic acid from 0.05 to 0.10 and 0.15 mmol/kg administered intravenously induce an increasing myocardial signal in the subendocardium (inner half of myocardial wall) during first pass.[4] (B) Even a dose as high as 0.15 mmol/kg did not cause measurable susceptibility-induced signal loss in the subendocardial layer using a hybrid echo planar pulse sequence (echo time: 1.3–2.2 ms). Accordingly, the highest dose *(D3)* detected stenoses with ≥50% diameter reduction significantly better than the 0.05 mmol/kg dose *(D1)*. *ROC*, Receiver operator characteristics; *SI*, signal intensity.

consequently to render the pulse sequence less prone to susceptibility artifacts (hybrid echo planar pulse sequences).[1,54,65,76,77] With these accelerated pulse sequences, several *k*-lines are acquired following a single radiofrequency excitation, reducing the repetition time (TR) per *k*-line down to less than 2 ms and consequently reducing the total acquisition window per slice substantially. This enables the acquisition of a stack of slices every one to two heartbeats, allowing for multislice acquisitions. Conventional nonsegmented fast gradient echo (FGE; or Turbo fast low angle shot [TurboFLASH]) pulse sequences were also used for perfusion imaging, however, resulting in relatively long readout windows.[61,78–84] Alternatively, FGE can be combined with parallel imaging techniques[85] or strategies that exploit the spatiotemporal correlations of image data to considerably speed up the data acquisition.[86] Improving cardiac coverage without the need to reduce spatial and/or temporal resolution would be beneficial because the extent of CAD correlates with outcome. In a recent study in human volunteers, the loss in signal-to-noise ratio (SNR) given by $g * \sqrt{R}$ (with g being the so-called geometry factor and R the accelerating factor) was compensated for by a longer TR (due to the implementation of temporal sensitivity encoding, a modification of sensitivity encoding [SENSE][85]) and increasing the readout flip angle from 20 to 30 degrees. This accelerated hybrid echo planar saturation recovery technique yielded twice as many slices as that obtained with the nonparallel approach whereas SNR improved by approximately 20%.[87]

Readout strategies during steady-state conditions of magnetization (steady-state free precession [SSFP] sequences) appear promising because they preserve magnetization and, thus a high SNR. In a human volunteer study, however, banding artifacts (probably because of longer readout periods or off-resonance) were problematic and myocardial signal increase was rather low (approximately 40% of baseline signal).[88] Recently, Jogiya et al.[89] compared an FGE with a SSFP readout in a three-dimensional (3D) acquisition at 3 T. To optimize the radiofrequency

(RF) deposition homogeneity, a dual-source parallel RF transmission approach was applied. To allow for 3D undersampling with acquisition windows of 191 ms and 211 ms for FGE and SSFP, respectively, *k-t* (*k*-space) BLAST (broad linear speed-up technique) and *k-t* PCA (principal component analysis) reconstructions were used. In 15 volunteers, overall image quality was good, but more susceptibility, that is, dark-rim artifacts, were observed in the SSFP acquisitions compared with FGE.[89] Currently, SSFP-based techniques are not recommended for clinical use because of a relatively high level of artifacts compared with (hybrid) FGE readouts.

Magnetization Preparation

Although 180-degree preparation was used in the past,[61,78–84,90] a 90-degree magnetization preparation is now generally accepted as the most efficient way to achieve T1 weighting because it shortens the delay time to 100 to 150 ms[1,54] and, additionally, it renders the sequence heart rate independent. Partial preparation flip angles (e.g., of 45–60 degrees) were suggested, which allow for shorter delay times.[65,76] However, this limited the dynamic range of signal response[54] and it is no longer recommended (Fig. 18.4).

The relationship between CM concentration and MR signal is not only dependent on the flip angle of the preparation pulse but also on the readout flip angle, as shown in Fig. 18.4. To shorten the delay time, it is also important to place the readout of the data into phases of minimal cardiac motion, into late systole and mid-diastole, which is achieved with a delay time of about 120 ms. Because length of systole varies relatively little with a changing heart rate (as occurs during pharmacologically induced hyperemia), these delay times are robust to place the data collection into stable heart phases irrespective of heart rate. To further accelerate data collection, it was proposed to play out one single nonslice-selective 90-degree saturation pulse,

Effect of imaging parameters:
α_{prep}, delay time, $\alpha_{read-out}$

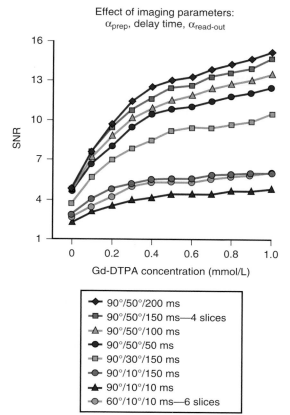

- ◆ 90°/50°/200 ms
- ■ 90°/50°/150 ms—4 slices
- △ 90°/50°/100 ms
- ● 90°/50°/50 ms
- ■ 90°/30°/150 ms
- ● 90°/10°/150 ms
- ▲ 90°/10°/10 ms
- ● 60°/10°/10 ms—6 slices

FIG. 18.4 These phantom measurements demonstrate that optimization of a hybrid echo planar pulse sequence[76] with respect to the delay time between magnetization preparation and readout, readout flip angle, and preparation flip angle can improve signal response of gadolinium diethylenetriamine penta-acetic acid *(Gd-DTPA)*-doped phantoms from 80% (of nondoped phantoms) to 250%, which ultimately increased diagnostic performance in patients.[54] *SNR,* Signal-to-noise ratio.

and to acquire the entire stack of slices thereafter.[2] With this scheme, however, the delay time varies from slice to slice, and consequently, CM sensitivity becomes dependent upon slice position and acquisition order, which is likely to affect data analysis. In a modified version of a saturation recovery preparation, the entire myocardium is prepared by a 90-degree saturation pulse except the slice which is immediately imaged after preparation ("notch technique").[91] With this scheme, the readout time for slice$_n$ equals the preparation time for the next slice, that is, slice$_{n+1}$, and so on. This approach allows acquisitions of up to 7 slices every 2 heartbeats (at a heart rate up to 115 beats per minute). Currently, identical saturation recovery preparation of each acquired slice is recommended to allow for consistent signal response and easy data analysis.

Field Strength: 1.5 T Versus 3 T

Systematic data comparing the diagnostic performance of perfusion CMR at 1.5 T and 3 T are still sparse. Increasing the field strength from 1.5 T to 3 T increases the available magnetization, as was demonstrated in a study in volunteers, in which myocardial signal during the first pass (at 0.1 mmol/kg Gd-diethylenetriamine penta-acetic acid [DTPA] IV) was 2.6 times higher at 3 T than at 1.5 T (relative to baseline signal).[92] However, this increase was observed in the anterior wall, whereas signal increased by only 1.7 times in the posterior wall. This inhomogeneous signal increase might be disadvantageous, and larger clinical trials would

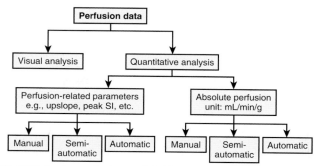

FIG. 18.5 A scheme for better definition of possible analysis strategies. In this scheme, "quantitative" results are given in numbers, which allow for an objective comparison of studies both longitudinally (e.g., monitoring disease activity) as well as from patient to patient (e.g., patient data vs. normal database). Such quantitative results are obtained either manually (and thus are associated with some observer dependence), in a semiautomatic fashion—that is, with some observer interaction—or automatically, thus eliminating any observer interaction with the data and thereby completely eliminating analysis variability. *SI,* Signal intensity.

be required to demonstrate a potential advantage of perfusion imaging at 3 T. In a recent study, a novel spatiotemporal correlation approach was implemented (5× *kt*-SENSE) on a 1.5 T and a 3 T machine.[93] In patients with suspected CAD, the 1.5 T and 3 T machines yielded spatial resolutions of 1.5 × 1.5 mm^2 and 1.3 × 1.3 mm^2 (with otherwise identical temporal resolution and coverage). The areas under the receiver operator characteristics (ROC) are under the curve (AUC) for CAD detection (defined as >50% diameter reduction on coronary angiography) were not different with 0.80 and 0.89, respectively ($P = .21$), despite slightly higher SNR on 3 T, indicating that the high diagnostic performance of perfusion CMR at 1.5 T is hard to improve.[93] Accordingly, in the EuroCMR registry, out of 27,781 examinations, only 5.9% were performed on 3 T machines, whereas 29.3% of all examinations were adenosine stress studies.[9]

ANALYSIS OF PERFUSION DATA

With increasing experience, an observer will be able to visually differentiate hypoperfused regions from artifacts, both typically causing lower signal during first-pass conditions.[5,84,90,94] However, the advantage of experience is traded for subjectivity, that is, reduced interreader reproducibility. Therefore a computer-assisted or automatic analysis of perfusion data would be highly desirable and could potentially render CMR perfusion analyses fully reproducible. Because many different analysis procedures are currently in use, some common definitions for analysis characteristics are proposed in Fig. 18.5.

Visual Assessment

Although visual reading can provide accurate diagnoses, adequate reproducibility should not rely on individual experience but on standardized criteria that in particular would differentiate signal loss due to hypoperfusion from artifacts. This indicates that reading criteria should also assess image quality, which in turn depends on the pulse sequence, the CM type and dose, and, importantly, the experience and care in data acquisition. Signal loss in the subendocardium, which is most sensitive for perfusion abnormalities, can be caused by susceptibility artifacts occurring during the time window when CM concentration differs most between the blood pool and the myocardial tissue. Thus long persistence of signal loss during first pass is suggestive of the presence of true hypoperfusion in the subendocardium. However, these timing criteria also depend on the dose of CM injected, the injection rate and site, and the dispersion of the bolus within the pulmonary circulation. Currently, CM doses of 0.075 to 0.10 mmol/kg of a Gd chelate (with injection rates of 4–8 mL/s intravenously [IV]) are recommended and typically used in clinical routine. With such a setting, a reduced signal increase in the subendocardium lasting for ≥3 frames (i.e., during ≥3–6 heartbeats) during hyperemic first pass is highly suggestive for ischemia as established in trials on diagnostic performance.[3,4,6–8] Most trials on outcome[10–15,47,48,95,96,153] use this or similar criteria demonstrating an excellent prognostic power (for more details, see also Table 18.4 later). A signal reduction consistent with a territory supplied by an individual coronary artery is also supporting the diagnosis of CAD, whereas artifacts predominantly distribute along the phase direction (because spatial resolution is often reduced along phase) or may occur in regions with inhomogeneous magnetic field characteristics as observed in the inferior wall (where air is extending between diaphragm and inferior wall of the left ventricle).[97] Criteria for quality assessment of perfusion data were derived from multicenter studies[4,5] and validated for interobserver reproducibility in multicenter registry data,[98] as given in Table 18.2.

Quantitative Approach

Dedicated algorithms for perfusion data analysis would allow comparison of signal responses in an individual patient with a normal database, rendering the technique less observer dependent. Because myocardial signal response is strongly dependent on imaging parameters, a normal database should be updated in case the pulse sequence and/or the imaging parameters would be modified (e.g., by a hardware or software upgrade). On the basis of such a normal database, perfusion studies can be compared between patients, and even more importantly, the perfusion situation; that is, the activity or progression of CAD can be monitored by serial perfusion CMR studies in the same patient. To allow for better comparisons between various analysis strategies, it appears reasonable to clarify some confusion that may exist with expressions such as semiquantitative and semiautomatic. In Fig. 18.5 quantitative relates to the analysis output obtained as numbers (which may be related to perfusion or may represent perfusion itself). These aspects should be separated from the issue of how the data are extracted from the imaging set, which may occur manually (with considerable observer interaction with the data and corresponding time requirements), semiautomatically (with some observer interaction), or fully automatically. A fully automatic approach is time saving (no labor needed for analysis) and eliminates any observer variability, although it is anticipated that high-quality data would be required for an automatic approach. A quantitative approach is also ideal to generate ROC, which are the adequate means for assessment of test performance. Once a ROC curve has been determined (for a given acquisition and analysis protocol), the optimum cost-effectiveness of the protocol can be calculated (optimum point on the ROC), because cost-effectiveness changes with changing portions of false and true negatives and positives.

Quantitative Approach: Perfusion-Related Parameters

First-pass perfusion studies are typically performed during breath-holding, and therefore any type of quantitative analysis should start with a registration of the first-pass data over time: that is, motion in the data

---

TABLE 18.2 Perfusion Cardiovascular Magnetic Resonance: Acquisition—Data Quality—Reading/Interpretation

Acquisition	Quality	Reading

• Saturation recovery preparation
• Myocardial SI increase during FP >250%–300% of precontrast baseline SI
• CM dose: (0.075)—0.10 mmol/kg IV
• Acquisition window (readout): ≤150 ms in mid-late systole and/or mid-diastole
• Spatial resolution: ≤1.5–2 × ≤1.5–2 mm
• Slice thickness: ≤10 mm
• Acquisition of ≥3 slices every 1–2 RR
• No breathing during FP
• Reliable ECG triggering
• Adequate vasodilation
	• Severe artifacts (3 points each)
	  • Abrupt breathing motion during first pass
	  • >2 mistriggers and/or ES during FP or AF
	  • Wrap-around artifacts, ghosts, blurring, and metallic artifacts in ≥3 slices
	• Intermediate artifacts (2 points)
	  • Wrap-around artifacts, ghosts, blurring, and metallic artifacts in 2 slices
	• Minor artifacts (1 point each)
	  • Respiratory drift (small respiratory excursions) during FP
	  • 1–2 mistriggers and/or ES during FP
	  • Wrap-around artifacts, ghosts, blurring, and metallic artifacts in 1 slice
		The perfusion deficit is:
		• clearly visible (minimal SI increase during FP) during ≥3 phases (i.e., ≥3 heartbeats and ≥6 heartbeats, respectively, in 1–2 RR acquisitions)
		• extends to ≥50% of wall thickness
		• encompasses ≥50% of segment
		• matches a coronary artery territory (except CABG patients)
		• resides within viable tissue (LGE-negative tissue)

Comments The recommended acquisition parameters were derived from single-center[3] and multicenter trials,[4,6–8] which confirmed their high diagnostic performance	These quality criteria were derived from multicenter studies[4,5] and were validated with multicenter registry data.[98] Criteria are modified from Klinke et al.[98] The maximum score is 9, which would indicate severe artifacts in 3 slices or more. A score <4 indicates good quality, scores 4–6 indicate intermediate quality (and AUC for CAD detection decreases by ~10% vs. good quality), scores >6 indicate inadequate quality	Visual reading criteria are derived from large single-center[1,153] and multicenter trials[4,6–8] and most studies on the prognostic power of perfusion CMR (as given in Table 18.4) use these or similar reading criteria. Perfusion deficits are typically assessed in the 17-segment AHA model (not including the LV apex)[157]

AF, Atrial fibrillation; *AHA,* American heart Association; *AUC,* area under the curve; *CABG,* coronary artery bypass grafting; *CAD,* coronary artery disease; *CMR,* cardiovascular magnetic resonance; *ECG,* electrocardiogram; *ES,* extra-systoles; *FP,* first pass; *LGE,* late gadolinium enhancement; *LV,* left ventricular; *SI,* signal intensity.

caused by breathing and/or diaphragmatic drift should be eliminated either by a manual procedure or by (semi-)automatic algorithms.[99,100]

To improve SNR, cardiac perfusion studies are performed with phased-array coils. Therefore analyses of signal intensity–time curves have to correct for inhomogeneous coil sensitivities. For this purpose, it has been suggested to subtract precontrast signal from the first-pass signal intensities.[2] However, signal reception by a phased array coil does not cause a constant offset of signal over the field of view; therefore a division of first-pass signal by precontrast signal for correction is required.[1,4]

From the resulting signal intensity–time curves calculated for various transmural or subendocardial segments covering ideally the entire left ventricular myocardium, many parameters can be extracted. The applicability was demonstrated for the peak signal intensity,[61,65,78,101] signal change over time (upslope),[1,54,81–83,101–104] arrival time, time to peak signal, mean transit time,[101,102,105,106] area under the signal intensity–time curve,[107] and others. For the upslope of the signal intensity–time curve, a relatively close correlation with perfusion data is reported in both animal[102,108] and human studies,[1] at least for the low-flow range. Its robustness could also be demonstrated in a multicenter trial.[4] This upslope parameter is relatively insensitive to CM recirculation because it uses the initial portion of the signal intensity–time curve only, which also reduces its sensitivity for motion (most patients are able hold their breath for this short time period). The upslope parameter is also proposed to correct for differences in arterial input by dividing myocardial upslope data by the blood-pool signal upslope.[1,54,82,83,103,104] This approach is suboptimal for input correction because the upslope–CM concentration relationship is flat at higher CM concentrations, which occur in the blood pool during first pass and which are even higher during hyperemic condition. An experimental study demonstrated linearity between the upslope parameter and perfusion measured by microspheres for low perfusion values only (below approximately 1.5 mL/min/g) (Fig. 18.6A).[108] A similar limitation for upslope estimates was described for humans using PET perfusion measurements as the standard of reference (Fig. 18.6B).[1]

Quantitative Approach: Absolute Tissue Perfusion

For blood-pool CM, which do not mix homogeneously in the tissue compartment but are restricted to the intravascular compartment, the so-called bolus tracking approach can be applied, which is based on the central volume principle given by

$$V_B = F \times MTT \qquad \text{Eq. 18.1}$$

where MTT is the mean transit time (expected distribution of transit times for the blood through the tissue volume) and V_B is blood volume.

Because the conventional extravascular Gd chelates do not cross the intact blood-brain barrier, this model is generally used for cerebral perfusion measurements. Also, hyperpolarized ^{13}C-CM (see later) can

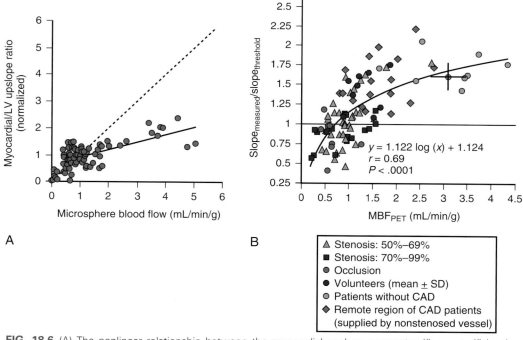

FIG. 18.6 (A) The nonlinear relationship between the myocardial upslope parameter ("corrected" by the signal upslope in the left ventricular [LV] blood pool) and the microsphere blood-flow measurements in canine experiments.[108] Linearity exists for low-flow situations only (up to approximately 1.5 mL/min/g). (B) Similar nonlinearity between the myocardial upslope parameter (normalized by the threshold upslope value) and the myocardial blood flow measured by positron emission tomography (PET) in patients with and without coronary artery stenoses. Normalization of the myocardial upslope by the threshold upslope value (which discriminates between stenotic and nonstenotic flow) results in a ratio of ≥1 for flow in nonstenosed vessels.[1] CAD, Coronary artery disease; MBF, myocardial blood flow; SD, standard deviation. (Reproduced with permission from Christian TF, Rettmann DW, Aletras AH, et al. Absolute myocardial perfusion in canines measured by using dual-bolus first-pass MR imaging. Radiology. 2004;232:677–684; Schwitter J, Nanz D, Kneifel S, et al. Assessment of myocardial perfusion in coronary artery disease by magnetic resonance: a comparison with positron emission tomography and coronary angiography. Circulation. 2001;103:2230–2235.)

act as an intravascular tracer[71]; hence, this model could be applied for cardiac studies using these CM.

In the myocardial tissue, however, the conventional Gd chelates behave as extravascular CM. Therefore the CM first-pass techniques with residue detection will be discussed next. It is assumed that CM diluted in blood enters the tissue via the artery, transits the capillaries, and leaves the tissue through the venous system. Then the Fick principle relates the CM concentration in the tissue to the arterial input and venous outflow by a convolution integral. This model takes both CM inflow and outflow into account and assumes a freely diffusible CM that is homogeneously mixed within a single tissue compartment.[109] It is given by

$$C_T(t) = F \cdot \int_0^t C_A \cdot (\tau) \cdot e^{-F/\lambda(t-\tau)d\tau} = C_A(t) \otimes F \cdot e^{-F/\lambda \cdot t} \qquad \text{Eq. 18.2}$$

where C_T is the tissue CM concentration at time t, C_A is the CM concentration in blood, F is tissue perfusion (in milliliters per minute per gram), λ is the tissue-blood partition coefficient, and $\otimes$ denotes convolution. If C_T and C_A are known, a two-parameter fit yields F and λ (by application of a three-parameter fit, blood volume V_B can be incorporated into the model as well). Several deconvolution procedures have been used to obtain F.[108,110–113] For nonfreely diffusible CM, the extraction fraction E must also be taken into account,[114–116] where E is related to F by

$$K_i = E \times F = F(1 - e^{-PS/F}) \qquad \text{Eq. 18.3}$$

where PS is the permeability-surface-area product (in milliliters per gram per second) and K_i is the unidirectional influx constant (in milliliters per gram per second). For all these models, knowledge about the arterial input function (i.e., the measurement of the arterial CM concentration over time) is mandatory. Consequently, the signal intensity–CM concentration relationship over the full range of CM concentrations occurring in the blood pool during first-pass conditions must be known.[66,111,117,118] Although higher CM doses yield an appropriate CNR level for the signal response in the myocardium, such high doses are likely to cause a clipping of the signal intensity–time curve in blood from which a conversion of signal intensities into CM concentration is problematic. To solve this problem, a dual-bolus approach was presented,[108] in which a small CM bolus is injected first for determination of an arterial input function, followed by a larger CM bolus to achieve an adequate signal response in the myocardium. In dogs, this approach yielded absolute values of tissue perfusion in close agreement with microsphere measurements. Alternatively, Gatehouse and colleagues[119] proposed a dual T1 sensitivity method. This elegant approach uses a single high-dose CM bolus injection, which provides a high signal response in the myocardium although preventing clipping of the blood pool signal at peak effect of the bolus. To measure blood signal (with low T1 sensitivity for very short T1), a short saturation recovery time is applied, although it is longer for measurement of myocardial signal (high T1 sensitivity for longer myocardial T1). Furthermore, the low T1-sensitive blood-pool measurements are performed at a low spatial resolution to accelerate acquisition. With this dual T1 sensitivity single-bolus approach, CFR estimates in volunteers closely matched those from dual bolus measurements. Although this dual T1 sensitivity single-bolus technique is available as work-in-progress packages for clinical application, to our knowledge, no larger clinical studies evaluated its performance for CAD detection in comparison to nonquantitative "visual" approaches.

Once a reliable arterial input function has been obtained, diffusion of water molecules between the intravascular and extravascular compartments must be taken into account, because conventional Gd chelates exert their effect indirectly through water proton relaxation, which modifies the MR signal during first pass.[120–123] An extravascular CM mixed homogeneously in the extravascular space by diffusion would generate a maximum signal during first pass of 20% of fully relaxed magnetization (assuming an extracellular compartment of 20% and the absence of water exchange between compartments). For an intravascular CM, the maximum achievable signal during first pass would further decline to approximately 10% of fully relaxed magnetization (assuming a blood volume in tissue of 10% and no water exchange between compartments). In rat experiments, however, extravascular and intravascular CM yielded approximately 70% and 50%, respectively, of fully relaxed magnetization during first pass, indicating that water exchange across both capillary vessel wall and cell membranes strongly affects signal.[120] Water exchange conditions can be categorized into fast, intermediate, and slow. If tissue $1/T_1$ ($= r_1$) increases linearly with intravascular r_1 and hence myocardial signal response in the presence of a CM would be unaffected by water exchange, the water exchange regimen is called fast. Studies by Larsson and colleagues[124] and others[121–123] demonstrated that intravascular–extravascular water exchange is the rate-limiting step for signal behavior in tissue (slow exchange regime). Similar to radioactive tracers, E of extravascular CM varied with increasing myocardial perfusion.[116,125,126] By assuming rather small changes in E for resting and hyperemic conditions and therefore using E as a constant, K_i at rest and during hyperemia was calculated, from which a perfusion index or CFR was derived.[127,128] In asymptomatic patients, myocardial perfusion was quantitatively assessed by first-pass perfusion CMR and a relation was found for hyperemic perfusion impairment and reduced segmental contractile function at rest, demonstrating the feasibility to quantify myocardial perfusion by first-pass techniques; however, no attempt was undertaken to use these perfusion data to detect CAD in this population.[129] In a subgroup of the CE-MARC (Clinical Evaluation of Magnetic Resonance Imaging in Coronary heart disease) population, myocardial first-pass perfusion data were subject to four different models to quantitate stress mean blood flow and myocardial perfusion reserve and to evaluate the potential to detect CAD.[130] In a cohort of 50 patients, CAD was defined as an ischemia-positive SPECT result and a ≥70% diameter stenosis in quantitative coronary angiography, and absence of CAD was defined as an ischemia-negative SPECT and no diameter stenosis >50% in quantitative coronary angiography. Thus patients with severe ischemia were compared with normals, whereas "intermediate" ischemia patients were excluded from the study. In this highly preselected patient population, quantitative stress mean blood flow yielded high sensitivities and specificities to discriminate the ischemic from nonischemic patients and the four methods (Fermi model, uptake model, one-compartment model, and model-independent deconvolution) yielded no difference in performance with AUCs of 0.86, 0.85, 0.85, and 0.87, respectively. To our knowledge, no larger clinical studies are available that tested a quantitative approach in a suspected CAD population at intermediate risk and, therefore, a quantitative approach cannot (yet) be recommended for clinical application.

Besides precision, the variability of parameter estimates is another important aspect of perfusion measurements. On the basis of simulations for the determination of regional blood volume, intravascular CM[131,132] were less sensitive for noise than were extravascular CM.[114] Despite a large body of computer simulations[114,131] and experimental data,[66,111] the clinical value of absolute quantitative measures of perfusion for the detection of CAD in patients remains unproven. A 95% confidence interval (CI) of −45% to −82% to +45% to +82% for absolute perfusion quantification[66,110] suggests that the sensitivity of these techniques to detect changes in perfusion might be limited. Also, short periods of ischemia can cause endothelial leakage,[133,134] which would complicate absolute perfusion assessment by intravascular CM in patients. For intravascular CM based on hyperpolarization (hyperpolarized ^{13}C-CM), water exchange does not affect the MR signal; consequently, perfusion quantification models could become easier. However, for these compounds, the time course of depolarization has to enter the formula for perfusion models (see later).[71] Similar to the approach used by Klocke et al., that is, to use the area under the signal intensity time curve during first pass as a measure of perfusion,[107] Lau and co-workers applied this concept successfully to measure myocardial perfusion in rats after co-injection of hyperpolarized ^{13}C-pyruvate and ^{13}C-urea to simultaneously quantify myocardial metabolism and perfusion, respectively.[72] Because the hyperpolarized ^{13}C-technique is applicable in patients, this perfusion approach may be considered as an alternative to conventional Gd-based techniques. However, to our knowledge, this technique has not yet been tested in humans.

CLINICAL PERFORMANCE OF PERFUSION CARDIOVASCULAR MAGNETIC RESONANCE

Single-Center Studies: Visual Interpretation

Visual discrimination of normal from severely abnormal findings is certainly feasible; however, it should be kept in mind that development of CAD is a progressive process that passes from mild to moderate to severe lesions (most likely by repetitive plaque ruptures). It might be in this intermediate range of lesions where visual assessment becomes difficult, and relating the patient data to a normal database might be particularly advantageous for this population advancing from nonobstructive to mildly obstructive CAD. Results of several studies applying a visual reading are given in Table 18.3.[3,90,94,135–142] In a recent study, first-pass perfusion CMR was compared with SPECT.[135] A visual

assessment of MR stress and rest dynamic data of 69 patients yielded a sensitivity and specificity of 90% and 85%, respectively, for the detection of stenoses with 70% or more diameter reduction on quantitative coronary angiography (QCA) at 0.075 mmol/kg of Gd-DTPA (injected at 4 mL/s into a peripheral vein). CMR performed significantly better with areas under the ROC curves (AUC) of 0.89 to 0.91 for two observers versus AUC of 0.71 to 0.75 for SPECT.[135] In the large single-center CE-MARC study, 647 patients were investigated with first-pass perfusion CMR, SPECT, and invasive x-ray coronary angiography (see Table 18.3).[3] An excellent diagnostic performance to detect CAD (defined as ≥50% diameter stenosis) was observed with an AUC of 0.84. Furthermore, this CE-MARC trial also confirmed the superiority of perfusion CMR over SPECT to detect CAD as demonstrated in the multicenter MR-IMPACT trial (see later and Fig. 18.7B).[6] Recently, perfusion CMR was also evaluated at 3 T. Plein et al.[93] reported an excellent sensitivity and specificity to detect CAD of 90% and 83%, respectively, which was, however, not superior to that obtained at 1.5 T. This might be explained among other factors by the lower field homogeneities typically encountered at higher fields strengths that can cause irregular RF deposition and, consequently, segmental signal variabilities during first pass. However, the higher field strength yields better SNR, which could be "invested" in 3D techniques. Accordingly, three studies demonstrated high sensitivities and specificities to detect CAD ranging from 88% to 94% and from 74% to 81%, respectively, in comparison to anatomy (see Table 18.3).[140–142] Particularly high sensitivity and specificity of 3D perfusion CMR was achieved versus fractional flow reserve (FFR).[141] One of these 3D perfusion CMR studies also compared CMR versus SPECT to detect CAD, but no superiority of CMR versus SPECT was found in that small population of 33 patients.[142]

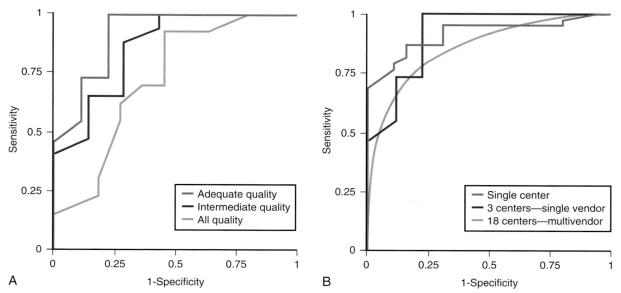

FIG. 18.7 (A) The important influence of data quality on test performance given by the area under the receiver operating characteristic curve (AUC).[4] If all categories of data quality are entered in the analysis, AUC is rather low. Applying a blinded read to eliminate data with low quality (most of them caused by breathing motion) resulted in 86% of data *(intermediate category)*, and AUC improves. In this study, a hybrid echo planar pulse sequence was applied and yielded five to seven slices every two RR intervals (with triggering on every other R-wave only). Thus only some slices are acquired during cardiac phases with minimal motion (end-systolic and mid-diastolic phase), whereas other slices fall within rapid motion phases. Eliminating these slices degraded by motion further increased test performance, yielding an AUC of 0.91 *(adequate quality)*. (B) A similar trend is demonstrated for quality reduction in studies with increasing numbers of participating sites,[1,3] which is most evident for multivendor data.[4,6,7]

TABLE 18.3 Clinical Performance of Perfusion Cardiovascular Magnetic Resonance: Detection of Coronary Artery Disease in Patients

Authors	N and Centers	Vendor[a]	Prep/ Slices[b]	CM	Dose	Rest[c]	Stress	Analysis	Reference Standard	Sens	Spec	AUC
Single-Center Studies												
Hartnell et al.[94]	14/1	S −	IR-2D/1	Gd-DTPA	0.04	+	Dip	Visual	QCA (≥70%)	83%[d]	100%	—
Eichenberger et al.[82]	8/1	S −	2D/3	Gd-DOTA	0.05	+	Dip	Upslope	QCA (≥80%)	65%[e]	76%[e]	—
Walsh et al.[90]	46/1	S −	IR-2D/3	Gadoteridol	0.10	+	Dip	Visual	^{201}Th/^{99m}Tc scinti	89%	44%	—
Bertschinger et al.[54]	24/1	S −	SR-2D/4	Gd-DTPA-BMA	0.10	−	Dip	Upslope$_{trans}$	QCA (≥50%)	82%	73%	0.76
Al-Saadi et al.[83]	34/1	S −	IR-2D/1	Gd-DTPA	0.025	+	Dip	Upslope CFR	QCA (≥75%)[f]	90%	83%	—
Schwitter et al.[1]	57/1	S −	SR-2D/4	Gd-DTPA-BMA	0.10	−	Dip	Upslope$_{subendo}$	QCA (≥50%)	87%	85%	0.91
Schwitter et al.[1]	43/1	S −	SR-2D/4	Gd-DTPA-BMA	0.10	−	Dip	Upslope$_{subendo}$	^{13}NH$_3$-PET (CFR)	91%	94%	0.93
Nagel et al.[2]	84/1	S −	SR-2D/5	Gd-DTPA	0.025	+	Ado	Upslope CFR	QCA (≥75%)[f]	88%	90%	0.93
Ishida et al.[135,g]	104/1	S −	SR-multi	Gd-DTPA	0.075	+	Ado	Visual	QCA (≥70%)	90%	85%	0.90[h]
Doyle et al.[104]	138/1	S −	SR-multi	Gd-BOPTA	0.04	+	Dip	Upslope CFR	QCA (≥70%)	57%	85%	—
Plein et al.[136]												
1.5 T	37/1	S −	SR-2D/4	Gd-Butrol	0.10	−	Ado	Visual	QCA (≥50%)	90%	83%	0.80
3 T	37/1	S −	SR-2D/4	Gd-Butrol	0.10	−	Ado	Visual	QCA (≥50%)	90%	83%	0.89
Rieber et al.[144]	43/1	S −	SR-2D/3	Gd-DTPA-BMA	0.05	+	Ado	Upslope CFR	FFR (≤0.75)	88%	90%	0.93
Costa et al.[158]	11/1	S −	SR-2D/3	Gd-DTPA	0.10	+	Ado	Fermi CFR	FFR (≤0.75)	86%[i]	60%[i]	—
Lockie et al.[137]												
3 T	42/1	S −	SR-2D/3	Gd-DTPA	0.05	+	Ado	Visual	FFR (<0.75)	82%	94%	0.92
Per segment	38/1							Fermi CFR		80%	89%	0.89
Watkins et al.[138]	101/1	S −	SR-2D/3	Gd-DTPA-BMA	0.10	+	Ado	Visual	QCA (≥70%)	97%	78%	—
									FFR (<0.75)	91%	94%	—
Greenwood et al.[3]	647/1	S −	SR-2D/3	Gd-DTPA	0.05	+	Ado	Visual	QCA (≥50%)	—	—	0.84
Greenwood et al.[139]	235♀/1	S −	SR-2D/3	Gd-DTPA	0.05	+	Ado	Visual	QCA (≥50%)	82%	89%	0.90
Manka et al.[140] 3T	146/1	S −	SR-3D	Gd-DTPA	0.10	+LGE	Ado	Visual 3D	QCA (≥50%)	92%	74%	—
								Visual 3 slices		88%	74%	—
Jogiya et al.[141] 3T	53/1	S −	SR-3D	Gd-Butrol	0.075	+LGE	Ado	Visual 3D	FFR (<0.75)	91%	90%	0.89
								Visual 3 slices	FFR (<0.75)	85%	84%	0.85
								Visual 3D	QCA (≥50%)	88%	80%	—
Jogiya et al.[142] 3T	33/1	S −	SR-3D	Gd-Butrol	0.075	+LGE	Ado	Visual	QCA (≥50%)	94%	81%	—
Multicenter Studies[j]												
Wolff et al.[5]	99/3	S +	SR-2D/7	Gd-DTPA	0.05	+	Ado	Visual	QCA (≥50%)	93%	75%	0.90
Giang et al.[4]	99/3	S +	SR-2D/7	Gd-DTPA	0.10	−	Ado	Upslope$_{subendo}$	QCA (≥50%)	91%	78%	0.91
Schwitter et al.[6]	241/18	M +	SR-2D/3	Gd-DTPA-BMA	0.10	+	Ado	Visual	QCA (≥50%)	90%	73%	0.87
Schwitter et al.[7]	425/33	M +	SR-2D/3	Gd-DTPA-BMA	0.075	+	Ado	Visual	QCA (≥50%)	—	—	0.75
	112♀/33	M +	SR-2D/3	Gd-DTPA-BMA	0.075	−	Ado	Visual	QCA (≥50%)	—	—	0.76
Manka et al.[146]	120/2	S −	SR-3D	Gd-DTPA	0.10	+LGE	Ado	%Vol$_{hypo\ at\ peak}$	FFR (<0.75)	86%	86%	0.90
Manka et al.[147] 3T	150/5	S −	SR-3D	Gd-Butrol	0.075	+	Ado	Visual	FFR (<0.80)	85%	91%	0.91

[a]Single vendor (S) vs. multivendor (M): − indicates *without* and + indicates *with* external supervision by European Medicines Agency and/or US Food and Drug Administration.

[b]Prep slices: magnetization preparation by saturation recovery (SR) and inversion recovery (IR), respectively. Single and multi, single-slice, and multislice acquisition, respectively. Multislice acquisitions indicated as 4 or 7 slices refer to 4 or 7 slices acquired every 2-RR interval.

[c]+ indicates rest perfusion performed; − indicates rest perfusion not performed.

[d]Comparison on a regional basis (5 segments/heart evaluated).

[e]Comparison on a regional basis (48 segments/heart evaluated).

[f]Vessel area reduction (in all other studies: vessel diameter reduction).

[g]Patients with history of myocardial infarction and/or resting wall motion abnormalities excluded.

[h]AUC (mean of two readers) for subset of 69 patients who also had a single-photon emission computed tomography (SPECT) study (AUC for SPECT: 0.73; $P < .001$ versus magnetic resonance).

[i]Per segment analysis (44 segments in 11 patients)

[j]Multicenter studies, diagnostic performance is given for best CM dose (for dose ranges tested, see text).

AUC, Area under the curve; *CM*, contrast media (all gadolinium chelates); *Fermi CFR*, calculation of coronary flow reserve by quantitation based on Fermi-constrained deconvolution using cutoffs between 1.6–2; *FFR*, fractional flow reserve; *LGE*, late gadolinium enhancement; *QCA*, quantitative coronary angiography (diameter reduction); *PET-CFR*, positron emission tomography coronary flow reserve; *scinti*, scintigraphy; *Upslope$_{trans}$*, upslope data derived from full wall thickness; *Upslope$_{subendo}$*, upslope data derived from subendocardial layer; *Upslope CFR*, coronary flow reserve calculated from upslope data (ratio of slope:rest/hyperemia).

All studies performed on 1.5 T, if not mentioned otherwise. Studies with $N \geq 7$ included.

Single-Center Studies: Quantitative Semiautomatic Analysis

The rate of myocardial signal change (upslope) during CM first pass is most widely used to quantitatively assess perfusion data.[1,2,54,80-83,101,143,144] From a rest-stress protocol, a CFR index ($slope_{hyperemia}/slope_{rest}$) was derived and yielded a sensitivity and specificity of 90% and 83%, respectively, for the detection of stenoses with 75% or more area reduction on QCA (at a CFR threshold of 1.5).[83] For an arterial input correction, the upslope of signal in the left ventricular blood pool was used; furthermore, the dose of the extravascular CM Gd-DTPA was kept at 0.025 mmol/kg body weight to minimize clipping of the blood-pool signal intensity–time curve. The same CFR index derived from multislice perfusion data (with peripheral administration of the same CM dose) yielded a similar performance with a sensitivity and specificity of 88% and 90%, respectively, for the detection of stenoses with 75% or more area reduction on QCA,[2] and it also correlated well with FFR.[144] When CFR was determined by perfusion CMR in women, a specificity of 85% for the detection of CAD (defined as ≥70% diameter reduction on QCA) was achieved, although sensitivity was only 57%.[104] This test performance at 0.04 mmol/kg of Gd-BOPTA compares well with the results of a recent dose-finding study for the dose of 0.05 mmol/kg of Gd-DTPA (see Fig. 18.3B).[4]

A stress-only protocol provided a comparable performance of the hyperemic upslope parameter when thresholds were derived from a normal database, resulting in a sensitivity and specificity of 87% and 85%, respectively, for the detection of stenoses of ≥50% diameter reduction on QCA.[1] This stress-only protocol avoids the need for matching myocardial regions for rest and stress condition and therefore offers easy analysis of the subendocardial layer, where perfusion abnormalities are most severe (Fig. 18.8).[1,143] In a comparison of the subendocardial CMR upslope data with PET perfusion data, a sensitivity and specificity of 91% and 94%, respectively, were reported.[1]

Multicenter Studies

Perfusion CMR appears to represent the most accurate method currently available for the noninvasive assessment of myocardial perfusion in humans, as evidenced in multicenter trials.

In a multicenter single-vendor trial, a stress-only protocol combined with a semiautomatic data analysis (upslope) performed best with CM doses as high as 0.10 to 0.15 mmol/kg Gd-DTPA, yielding an AUC of 0.91 ± 0.07 and 0.86 ± 0.08, respectively, with corresponding sensitivity/specificity of 91%/78% and 94%/71%, respectively.[4] Thus this multicenter trial confirmed the high diagnostic performance of the stress-only approach proposed in an earlier single-center study.[1] However, in this multicenter study, the high diagnostic performance was achieved in data with adequate quality only. For this purpose, a blinded quality reading was performed first, which eliminated 14% of all studies (see Fig. 18.7A). An example from a study at the dose of 0.15 mmol/kg is shown in Fig. 18.9. With adequate data quality, a κ-value of 0.73 was obtained for interobserver agreement,[4] which compares favorably with κ-values of 0.80 for multicenter SPECT data.[145] As expected with an increasing number of participating sites, homogeneity of data quality, and hence test performance, is likely to deteriorate, as demonstrated in a comparison between single-center and multicenter perfusion CMR studies (see Fig. 18.7B).

Recently, the diagnostic performance of a 3D perfusion approach was evaluated at 1.5 T in two centers[146] and at 3 T at five centers[147] in a single-vendor design. Interestingly, in the two-center study at 1.5 T, high sensitivity and specificity of 86% each were achieved versus FFR of ≤0.75 by quantifying the ischemic myocardium with a threshold <2 SD of remote myocardium measured at the peak myocardium signal.

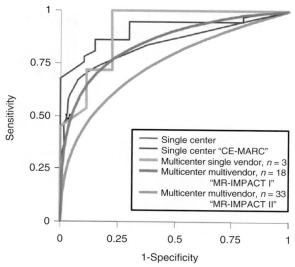

FIG. 18.8 These receiver operating characteristic curves demonstrate superiority of subendocardial first-pass perfusion data over transmural perfusion data for detection of stenoses with ≥50% diameter reduction on quantitative coronary angiography,[1,54] supporting the general knowledge of the subendocardium being most sensitive for hypoperfusion. In these two studies, perfusion data of patients were compared with a normal database. If susceptibility artifacts were to reduce signal response in the subendocardium, this approach would correct, to a certain extent, because the normal database would also contain lower threshold values (provided that both patient data and normal data are acquired and analyzed with the identical protocol and software).

Because this analysis is technically easy to accomplish, this approach warrants further testing in a multivendor setting.

As discussed previously, perfusion CMR has advantages over SPECT with respect to spatial resolution, motion suppression, and lack of attenuation artifacts. This suggests superiority of perfusion CMR over SPECT.[135] In the MR-IMPACT multicenter program (MR-Imaging for Myocardial Perfusion Assessment in Coronary Artery Disease Trial),[6] 241 patients underwent both invasive coronary angiography and SPECT within ± 4 weeks of a perfusion CMR study (see Fig. 18.7B).[6] In this trial, monitored by official authorities (US Food and Drug Administration [FDA], European Medicines Agency [EMA]), no serious adverse events occurred in the 234 patients dosed with Gd-DTPA-BMA. MR-IMPACT confirmed the high diagnostic performance of the MR first-pass perfusion approach at a dose of 0.1 mmol/kg Gd-DTPA-BMA with an AUC of 0.86 for the detection of CAD (defined as ≥50% diameter reduction on QCA, see Fig. 18.7B). Most importantly, it also showed superiority of perfusion CMR over nongated SPECT imaging for the detection of CAD.[6] From this MR-IMPACT trial, detailed reading and quality criteria were derived and tested in the MR-IMPACT II trial. To compare perfusion CMR with gated SPECT the MR-IMPACT II was launched in 33 centers in the United States and Europe (see Fig. 18.7B). The MR-IMPACT II also tested the "minimal effective" CM dose of 0.075 mmol/kg to detect CAD (in comparison to 0.1 mmol/kg in MR-IMPACT I), and it is also the largest multicenter SPECT trial using ^{99m}Tc-tracers available so far.[8] This trial (monitored by the regulatory authorities FDA and EMA) analyzed 425 patients all undergoing perfusion CMR, SPECT, and invasive x-ray coronary angiography. The MR-IMPACT II confirmed the superiority of perfusion CMR versus gated SPECT with significantly larger AUCs for the detection of CAD.[7] Perfusion CMR also performed better than gated SPECT in the multivessel disease group, in men, in women, as well as in the subgroup without infarction.[7] Because

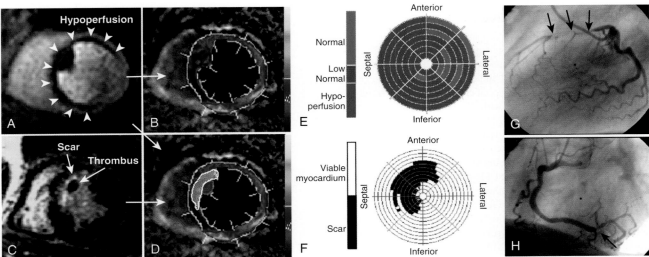

FIG. 18.9 In this example of a 59-year-old patient, a first-pass perfusion deficit is shown in panel A (at the peak effect of the bolus), encompassing approximately two-thirds of the left ventricular circumference. From the time series of first-pass data, an upslope map is generated and compared with a normal database, allowing the color coding of pixels with reduced and normal wash-in kinetics in shades of blue and red, respectively (B). Late enhancement imaging for detection of scar tissue is shown in panel C. Combining perfusion (A) and viability (C) data into a single map (D) allows discrimination of hypoperfused viable (jeopardized) tissue (blue area in panel D) from hypoperfused scarred tissue (*white area* overlaid in panel D). Perfusion and viability are also demonstrated in polar map format of the subendocardial layer (inner half of the myocardial wall) in panels E and F, respectively. (G) Coronary angiography reveals an occlusion of the left anterior descending coronary artery in this patient *(arrows)*, with collateral vessels that protected the anterior and septal wall from transmural infarction. The large circumflex artery is not stenosed, explaining the normal perfusion pattern in the lateral wall in the polar map (E), whereas a stenosis at the crux of the right coronary artery *(arrow* in H) causes hypoperfusion of the inferior wall. With this stress-only perfusion approach combined with a late enhancement approach, the various tissue components (normal viable, ischemic, and scar) can be defined within various myocardial layers with a single magnetic resonance one-stop-shop examination. Owing to the extensive areas of hypoperfusion in viable myocardium, the patient was revascularized.

these results were obtained from a large network of 33 participating centers, representing data quality currently achievable over a substantial spectrum of centers and MR machines, these data together with MR-IMPACT I data[6] and large single-center data[3] were important to integrate the perfusion CMR techniques into international guidelines for the work-up of CAD.[148–152]

Perfusion Cardiovascular Magnetic Resonance and Prediction of Outcome

To recommend perfusion CMR for the management of patients with known or suspected CAD, it is crucial to demonstrate that the technique is able to reliably detect CAD: that is, to detect relevant coronary artery stenoses in patients. This goal was undoubtedly achieved with the many positive studies performed during the last decades, as summarized in Table 18.3. Nevertheless, a method is of most value if it can discriminate patients with good prognosis from those with an increased risk for cardiovascular complications; that is, if it can identify patients in need for a specific treatment as, for example, revascularizations. In all studies listed in Table 18.4,[10–13,15,16,47,48,95,153] the annual event rate for cardiac death and nonfatal myocardial infarction (MI) was below 0.9%, with the exception of two studies with a percentage of known CAD of at least 43%[14,96] and one study performed early (in 2009).[154] Fig. 18.10 shows a very low event rate in ischemia-negative patients in terms of cardiac death and nonfatal MI (bars to the right), although the event rate is high in all studies for ischemia-positive patients (bars to the left), providing clear evidence for the prognostic power of perfusion

CMR. Interestingly, there is a trend toward higher complication rates in CMR-positive patients in the earlier studies compared with more recent ones (inlet in Fig. 18.10), which might reflect the clinical situation that, nowadays, patients with ischemia proven by CMR have better chances to get revascularized than in the beginnings of perfusion CMR when this method was not yet accepted to guide treatment. This view is supported by the low event rate observed in the EuroCMR registry population for both ischemia-negative and ischemia-positive patients, clearly indicating that the use of CMR in patients with suspected CAD can yield a high event-free survival rate.[16] In this context, it is also noteworthy to mention that CMR-guided management of suspected CAD can reduce costs in comparison to invasive strategies, even when FFR is used to guide interventions by ischemia testing.[16]

PERSPECTIVES

A main feature of CAD is its chronic course over several decades. CAD may become clinically overt by symptoms in an early stage of disease, but it may also remain silent for many years, becoming symptomatic suddenly by an acute MI. Because symptoms are not always present heralding an imminent infarction or symptoms may be atypical and therefore may be misinterpreted, up to 60% of cardiac deaths occurred in the United States outside the hospital or before the patients reached the catheterization laboratory for rescue intervention in the year 2004.[155] It can be concluded that such a reactive strategy (i.e., evaluating a patient primarily when the patient is exhibiting symptoms) is often inadequate.

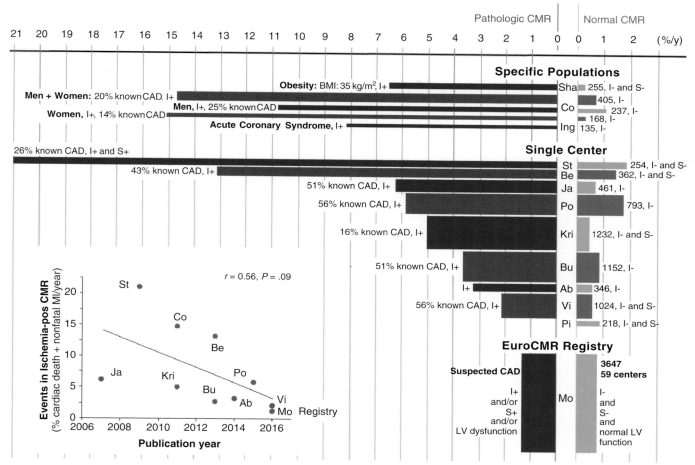

FIG. 18.10 Event rates are shown for patients with ischemia-positive cardiovascular magnetic resonance (*CMR; bars to the left*) and ischemia-negative CMR (*bars to the right*). Bar thickness is proportional to the sample size. Smaller studies (*thinner bars*) tend to yield larger differences in outcome between ischemia-positive and ischemia-negative patients than large studies (*thicker bars*). Irrespective of study size, the outcome is excellent for ischemia-negative patients. *Insert,* Studies performed earlier tend to yield a worse outcome in ischemia-positive patients than studies performed recently. This may be explained by the fact that, nowadays, treating physicians are aware of the prognostic power of perfusion CMR and therefore they revascularize CMR-positive patients regularly. In the EuroCMR registry, 20.4% of the patients were ischemia positive in at least 1 segment and 17.4% of these patients underwent revascularization (typically with 2 or more ischemic segments). These excellent EuroCMR registry outcome data of 3647 patients demonstrate the value of CMR to manage patients with suspected coronary artery disease (*CAD*). In this registry, the CMR approach also reduced costs versus an invasive strategy.[16] Abbreviations between bars and in the inset refer to the first author's name (as used in Table 18.4). *I+* and *S+* indicate patients positive for ischemia and scar (by late gadolinium enhancement), respectively. Numbers to the right of bars indicate size of study population. For details on imaging parameters, contrast media dose, stress agent, etc., see Table 18.4. *BMI,* Body mass index; *LV,* left ventricular; *MI* myocardial infarction.

A more successful strategy would focus on an earlier detection of CAD (i.e., a noninvasive detection of severe and, thus dangerous coronary lesions by CMR) and treating these lesions before they rupture, thereby preventing acute myocardial infarctions. Such an active strategy would monitor the disease process over many years and would indicate the need for action in case of a significant lesion. Because the factors triggering the progression of CAD are not yet well known, a repetitive evaluation of the coronary circulation is required. Perfusion CMR is an ideal tool

to monitor CAD over time because it can be repeated when needed, owing to a lack of radiation. It yields a high sensitivity and specificity for the detection of obstructing lesions and, as a short examination, it is well tolerated by patients. An active strategy could potentially reduce the high number of "prehospital" cardiac deaths significantly, which would represent a major success in cardiac care. Large single-center and registry data indicate that perfusion CMR can reduce costs substantially in comparison with invasive strategies in a population of

TABLE 18.4 **Prognosis**

Study	Year	Tesla	Sequence	Stress	CM	Dose	Analysis	Follow-Up (Median Months)	Known CAD	N
Steel (St)	2009	1.5	SR-7 (2RR) Hybrid FGE	Ado	Gd-DTPA	0.1	Visual S+r+LGE	17	26%	254
Bertaso (Be)	2013	1.5	SR-3	Ado	Gd-DTPA	0.1	Visual S+r+LGE	22	43%	362
Jahnke (Ja)	2007	1.5	SR-3 (FGE/SSFP)	Ado	Gd-DTPA	0.05	Visual S+r	27	51%	461
Pontone (Po)	2015	1.5	SR-3	Dip	Gd-BOPTA	0.1	Visual S	27	56%	793
Krittayaphong (Kri)	2011	1.5	InvR-3	Ado	Gd-DTPA	0.05	Visual S+LGE	35	16%	1232
Buckert (Bu)	2013	1.5	SR-3	Ado	Gd-DTPA	0.1	Visual S+r+LGE	50	51%	1229
Abbasi (Ab)	2014	3	SR-3	Rega	Gd-DTPA	0.1	Visual S+LGE	23	—	346
Vincenti (Vi)	2016	1.5/3	SR-4 (2RR)	Ado	Gadobutrol	0.1	Visual S+LGE	30	45%	1024
Pilz (Pi)	2008	1.5	SR-5 (2RR) hybridFGE	Ado	Gd-DTPA-BMA	0.1	Visual S+LGE	12	—	218
Specific Patient Populations										
Shah (Sha)	2014	1.5 3	SR-3	Ado Rega	Gd-DTPA	0.1	Visual S+LGE	25	BMI 35 kg/m²	255
Coelho-Filho (Co)	2011	1.5 3	SR-5 (2RR) SR-5 (1RR)	Ado Dip	Gd-DTPA	0.075–0.1	Visual S+LGE	30	20% Men: 25% Women: 14%	405 237 168
Ingkanisorn (Ing)	2006	1.5	SR-9 (2RR) Hybrid FGE	Ado	Gd-DTPA-BMA	0.1	Visual Fn+S+LGE	15	ACS	135
Registry										
Moschetti (Mo)	2016	1.5 or 3	SR-3–5 (1–2 RR)	Ado Dip	Gd chelates	—	Visual S+LGE or S+r+LGE	12	Suspected CAD	3647

For abbreviations of first authors refer to Fig. 18.3.

2RR, Acquisition on every other heartbeat; *ACS,* acute coronary syndrome; *Ado,* adenosine (at standard dose of 140); *Analysis,* S+r+LGE: all datasets, that is, stress perfusion, rest perfusion, and *LGE* (late gadolinium enhancement) are used for analysis; *BMI,* body mass index; *CAD,* coronary artery disease; *Dip,* dipyridamole (at standard dose of 0.84); *Fn,* left ventricular systolic function; *Gd-DTPA* (Magnevist); *Gd-BOPTA* (Multihance); *Gd-DTPA-BMA* (Omniscan); *hybridFGE,* hybrid fast-gradient echo echo-planar pulse sequence; *InvR,* inversion recovery; *Rega,* regadenoson; *SR,* saturation recovery; *SR-3,* the number indicates the number of slices acquired per R-R interval; *SSFP,* steady-state free precession.

low[16] to intermediate risk[18] (i.e., in a suspected CAD population), while an excellent outcome is achieved.[16] This is of paramount importance because costs for cardiovascular disease management are expected to increase from $315 billion in 2010 (direct and indirect costs in the United States) to $918 billion in 2030.[155] To determine the cost effectiveness of perfusion CMR in various disease populations, future prospective randomized trials on economics are warranted. From a technical point of view, (semi-)automatic analyses of perfusion CMR data would be desirable to replace visual approaches to increase reproducibility and reduce costs through reduction of reading time.

REFERENCES

A full reference list is available online at ExpertConsult.com

19

Acute Myocardial Infarction: Cardiovascular Magnetic Resonance Detection and Characterization

Andrew Arai

Cardiovascular magnetic resonance (CMR) can characterize acute myocardial infarction (AMI) in unique ways and with high quality. Cine CMR can assess left ventricular (LV) volumes, ejection fraction (LVEF), and regional wall motion in ways comparable to a high-quality transthoracic echocardiogram. Late gadolinium enhancement (LGE) is generally considered the reference standard in imaging chronic myocardial infarction and the method works well for AMI as well. CMR stress testing is capable of detecting residual myocardial ischemia. Various important complications of myocardial infarction can be imaged, such as LV dysfunction, thrombus, ventricular septal defect, aneurysm, pseudoaneurysm, and valvular complications. Newer CMR methods for quantifying myocardial T1, T2, T2*, and extracellular volume fraction (ECV) are providing quantitative insights into the pathophysiology and characterize AMI in ways that are not currently possible with alternative modalities. Thus CMR is highly relevant and a powerful diagnostic tool for complex problems in AMI patients.

CARDIOVASCULAR MAGNETIC RESONANCE FOR DETECTING ACUTE CORONARY SYNDROME AND ACUTE MYOCARDIAL INFARCTION

Balanced steady-state free precession (bSSFP) cine CMR[1] has been accepted as a reference standard for assessing LV mass, volumes, and LVEF.[2,3] Cine CMR is a powerful method for detecting regional wall motion abnormalities, as is evidenced by the diagnostic accuracy of dobutamine stress tests.[4–6] This is an important set of validations because dobutamine stress testing poses some of the most extreme challenges for assessing regional wall motion (see Chapter 17). The diagnostic information must be acquired quickly (usually within about 2 minutes) at a time when the heart rate is 85% of age-predicted maximum and patients may be experiencing angina.

Cine CMR can assess regional wall motion with high image quality, allowing diagnosis of small wall-motion abnormalities with confidence that might be missed by other methods. For example, Fig. 19.1 illustrates a case in which a presumptive diagnosis of clinically unrecognized myocardial infarction could be made based on a focal anteroseptal wall-motion abnormality that was missed on a good-quality noncontrast enhanced transthoracic echocardiogram.

Cine CMR also performed well in detecting acute coronary syndrome (ACS) in patients presenting to an emergency department with at least 30 minutes of chest pain. Both qualitatively and quantitatively, regional wall-motion abnormalities by cine CMR had an accuracy of 82% for ACS, 89% for non–ST elevation myocardial infarction (NSTEMI), and 98% for ischemic heart disease.[7] One important reason cine CMR performed so well may have related to how early patients were imaged after presentation to the emergency department. Specifically, 87% of subjects were scanned before the 4-hour troponin was available. By studying patients within 6 hours of presentation to the emergency department, stunned myocardium offers an additional mechanism that is capable of detecting infarction or unstable angina. When combined with LGE, the sensitivity for AMI increased to 100%. An example of a rest perfusion abnormality in a patient with a normal initial electrocardiogram (ECG) and normal initial troponin is shown in Fig. 19.2.

However, a single CMR scan of regional wall motion does not differentiate acute from chronic conditions. In patients with no history of myocardial infarction, a definite regional wall-motion abnormality is reasonably specific for coronary artery disease (CAD) even though there are other conditions that can cause regional wall-motion abnormalities, such as myocarditis. However, using T2-weighted imaging to characterize the acuity of regional wall-motion abnormalities, Cury et al.[8] replicated the primary findings of Kwong et al.[7] but improved the specificity for diagnosing ACS.

Plein et al. formally studied the additive value of each available CMR method for diagnosing ACS. In that study, an LV wall motion by cine CMR had lower sensitivity (68%), perhaps as a result of the later timing of the CMR scan during the index hospitalization. In that setting, stress perfusion and CMR coronary angiography were the most sensitive components, and the comprehensive analysis of all methods used had 96% sensitivity.[9] Ingkanisorn et al. also found that stress perfusion CMR had high diagnostic accuracy for detecting patients with possible ACS presenting to the emergency department.[10] An example of a patient with a stress-induced perfusion defect that extends beyond the myocardial infarction is shown in Fig. 19.3. In that study, CMR did not miss any patients with major adverse cardiac events over about 1 year of follow-up.

A series of studies from Wake Forest University examined the diagnostic accuracy and cost effectiveness of CMR to detect CAD in patients presenting to the emergency department with chest pain. Miller et al. found that use of adenosine stress CMR to assess patients with acute chest pain who were triaged to a chest pain observation unit had lower short-term[11] and 1-year costs[12] than those managed with standard inpatient care. In lower risk patients presenting to the emergency department with chest pain, provider-selected evaluation reduced costs compared with mandated stress CMR.[13] That study was interesting because the primary stress test modality used was transthoracic echocardiography in 62% of patients. The primary provider used stress CMR in 32%, single proton emission computed tomography (SPECT) in only 2%, and computed

End diastole　　　　　　End systole

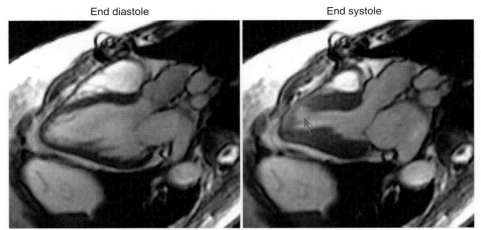

FIG. 19.1 A small dyskinetic wall motion abnormality associated with myocardial infarction was not seen on transthoracic echocardiography. The cine cardiovascular magnetic resonance is shown at end diastole and end systole. The red arrow points to the wall-motion abnormality.

Cine

Rest perfusion

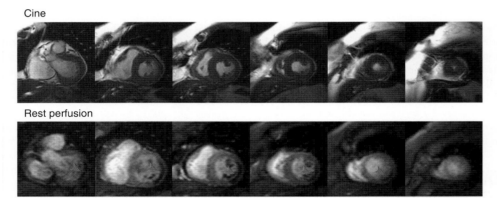

FIG. 19.2 Perfusion defect *(red arrowheads)* associated with acute myocardial infarction in a patient with no prior coronary disease. This patient presented to the emergency department within the 1st hour after onset of chest pain. Cardiovascular magnetic resonance (CMR) was performed within 1 hour after arrival in the hospital, and the initial electrocardiogram and troponin-I were normal. The diagnosis of acute myocardial infarction was subsequently confirmed by troponin-I assays 8 hours after presentation (6 hours after CMR) and by coronary angiography. Multiple parallel short axis images allow determination of the amount of myocardium at risk.

Cine　　　Late gadolinium enhancement　　　Adenosine perfusion

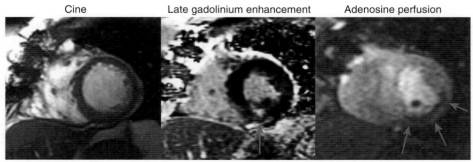

FIG. 19.3 Adenosine stress perfusion defect *(three red arrows)* clearly extends beyond the edges of the very small inferior myocardial infarction on the late gadolinium enhancement image.

tomography (CT) in 2%. In the setting of intermediate-risk patients with chest pain in an observation unit with a negative initial ECG and negative initial troponin, CMR was again a cost-effective modality.[14]

Although CMR is not commonly used to evaluate patients with chest pain in the emergency department, these studies demonstrated several important concepts. Cine CMR is a powerful method of assessing global and regional LV systolic function and is useful in patients with acute presentations of possible CAD. However, the multiple ways that CMR can characterize the heart, including stress perfusion, LGE of myocardial infarction, and other methods create an even more powerful diagnostic tool. Despite the relatively high costs of CMR, the modality has high diagnostic accuracy and can be cost effective in the management of patients with possible ACS when applied to appropriate risk categories.

LATE GADOLINIUM ENHANCEMENT OF ACUTE MYOCARDIAL INFARCTION

LGE-CMR is accepted as a reference standard method for imaging myocardial scar. Before discussing applications of LGE, it is important to understand the different mechanisms leading to hyperenhancement of AMI versus the fibrotic or collagen scar associated with chronic myocardial infarction. As summarized in Fig. 19.4, after intravenous injection, gadolinium (Gd)-based contrast agents rapidly enter the interstitial space, as represented by the yellow between cardiomyocytes. Thus contrast-enhanced normal or viable myocardium has a T1 that is shorter than native T1. The intact cell membranes of viable cells exclude Gd-based contrast agents from the intracellular space; hence the dark intracellular space in the diagram. Using inversion recovery methods,[15] the inversion time is adjusted to null normal myocardium, making it appear dark on the LGE images.

Acutely infarcted myocardium enhances more strongly with Gd-based contrast agents than viable myocardium because damage to cell membranes allows Gd into what used to be the intracellular space. This is represented by yellow in both the intracellular and extracellular spaces in Fig. 19.4. Finally, chronically infarcted myocardium also enhances strongly with Gd-based contrast agents because collagen scar has relatively little cellular volume and thus a large volume of distribution as represented by extensive yellow patches in Fig. 19.4.

VALIDATION OF LATE GADOLINIUM ENHANCEMENT IN ACUTE MYOCARDIAL INFARCTION

LGE-CMR is currently the highest-resolution method for detecting AMI and provides an exquisitely sensitive diagnostic test. In animal studies in which histopathology was used as a reference standard for determining what is normal or infarcted myocardium, the bright zones on LGE CMR correlate closely in size and location to the infarct delineated by triphenoltetrazolium chloride (TTC) histopathology.[16] These experiments examined acutely infarcted canine hearts and some experiments included a transient coronary occlusion in a different coronary territory to document that stunned myocardium did not enhance whereas infarcted myocardium did enhance. The bright myocardium on LGE-CMR corresponded closely to the infarcted myocardium in reperfused and nonreperfused canine infarction at 4 hours, 1 day, 3 days, 10 days, 4 weeks, and 8 weeks postinfarction.[17] That study also found no difference in signal intensity between viable myocardium in the area at risk (AAR) versus remote myocardium.[17] In another study using electron probe x-ray microanalysis, Gd concentration was high in the infarcted myocardium but not statistically different between viable

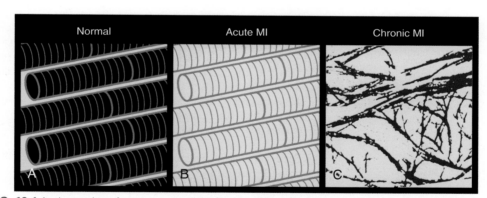

FIG. 19.4 In the setting of acute myocardial infarction (MI), different types of myocardium have distinctive appearances on late gadolinium enhancement (LGE) images. (A) Normal: The myocardium outside the ischemic area at risk is characterized by healthy cardiomyocytes (striped cylinders) with intact cell membranes. Extracellular gadolinium contrast agents arrive via the bloodstream and rapidly enter the interstitial space (yellow regions) but are excluded from the intracellular space (black regions). Thus normal myocardium has a shorter T1 after contrast administration, but the amount of enhancement is modest, and the inversion recovery time can be adjusted to make normal myocardium appear uniformly dark (nulled). Viable or salvaged myocardium within the area at risk has intact cell membranes and therefore excludes gadolinium contrast agents from the intracellular space. However, some aspect of the ischemic period reversibly damaged this part of the heart enough to raise the water content and thus lengthen the T2 of the tissue. Therefore the area at risk is brighter than normal myocardium on T2-weighted images. The salvaged myocardium appears essentially normal on LGE cardiovascular magnetic resonance (CMR). (B) Acute MI: The myocardium is characterized by loss of cell membrane integrity. As long as there has been adequate reperfusion, gadolinium contrast agents rapidly enter not only the interstitial space but also what used to be the intracellular space. As indicated by the extensive yellow in the diagram, acutely infarcted myocardium enhances significantly more than normal myocardium and appears bright on LGE CMR. Acutely infarcted myocardium also appears bright on T2-weighted images, owing to the tissue swelling. (C) Chronic MI: Chronically infarcted myocardium enhances strongly as a result of the relatively small number of viable cells and extensive interstitial space within the collagen scar.

myocardium in the AAR versus remote myocardium.[18] The elevations in Gd concentration were 2 to 3 times higher still in the chronically infarcted myocardium than in acutely infarcted myocardium. Failing to find an elevation in Gd concentration in the viable portion of the AAR is likely related to the detection limit of the assay and underpowered statistics owing to small sample size. This concept becomes important when one considers newer data finding CMR abnormalities in the salvaged myocardium[19]; techniques that detect abnormalities in the viable AAR are described later in this chapter. Beyond this subtlety, there is general agreement that the hyperenhanced myocardium on LGE images corresponds closely to infarcted myocardium by pathological standards in animals.

Clinical trials helped validate that LGE imaging of AMI is a clinically validated measurement of infarct size (Table 19.1). The infarct size visualized by LGE-CMR correlated with the degree of elevations of creatine kinase-MB (CKMB) or troponin.[20–22] Several studies demonstrated that the recovery of function could be predicted by the transmural extent of LGE-CMR in AMI patients.[20,21,23–25] The relationship between transmural extent of infarction and recovery of function was used by Kim et al.[26] and Selvanayagam et al.[22] to validate CMR viability

imaging in patients with chronic CAD undergoing revascularization. Bullock et al.[27] recommend using a higher transmural extent of hyperenhancement in the context of AMI than recommended for chronic infarction.

With a slightly different interpretation of the LGE findings, Ichikawa et al.[28] found that the amount of viable-appearing myocardium was a better predictor of functional recovery postinfarction than the transmural extent of hyperenhanced myocardium. In a study of patients with AMI, Baks et al.[29] found that LGE could predict recovery of function distal to a totally occluded coronary artery, but the effect was modulated by the presence or absence of microvascular obstruction.

LGE-CMR imaging for AMI appears to be more sensitive than SPECT imaging. This concept was already known for chronic infarction.[30] In the setting of AMI, three studies showed that LGE-CMR was more sensitive than SPECT for detecting the infarct.[31–33] These studies showed that CMR was more likely to detect small infarcts, as evidenced by lower troponin elevations, NSTEMI, and infarcts in the circumflex territory.

As further evidence of the benefits of high-resolution CMR imaging of AMI, Ricciardi et al.[34] helped prove the sensitivity of LGE-CMR

TABLE 19.1 **Clinical Validations of Late Gadolinium Enhancement Cardiovascular Magnetic Resonance in Myocardial Infarction**

Reference	N	Acute ± Chronic	Major Findings
Ricciardi et al.[34]	14	Acute	Microinfarcts were detected in patients who had PCI-related elevations in CKMB. Two patterns of
	6	Chronic	MI were observed: small side branch occlusion and distal embolization.
Choi et al.[20]	24	Acute	Within 7 days of AMI, infarct size correlates with peak CKMB. There is an inverse relationship
		Chronic	between the transmural extent of infarct and the likelihood of regional recovery of function.
Gerber et al.[25]	20	Acute	In patients 4 days after AMI, LGE predicted recovery of regional function better than did perfusion
		Chronic	images, which significantly underestimated the amount of irreversible injury.
Beek et al.[24]	30	Acute	In patients 1 week after AMI, there was an inverse relationship between the transmural extent of
		Chronic	infarction and the likelihood of regional recovery of function.
Ingkanisorn et al.[21]	33	Acute	In patients 2 days after acute PCI, MI size correlated with peak troponin. AMI size predicted chronic
	20	Chronic	LVEF and regional function. Infarct size decreased from 16%–11% of the LV.
Lund et al.[33]	60	Acute	SPECT and CMR infarct size correlated, but SPECT had 80% sensitivity and CMR had 100%
			sensitivity. SPECT missed 6 of 30 inferior AMI.
Ibrahim et al.[32]	33	Acute	LGE-CMR was superior to SPECT in detecting myocardial necrosis after reperfused AMI because
			CMR detects small infarcts missed by SPECT.
Baks et al.[23]	22	Acute	LGE predicted recovery of function after AMI better than perfusion imaging.
		Chronic	
Selvanayagam et al.[35]	50	Acute	All patients with a troponin elevation (as low as 3.7 mg/L) associated with PCI exhibited new
	24	Chronic	abnormal LGE. Troponin level correlated with AMI size.
Ichikawa et al.[28]	18	Acute	Thickness of nonenhanced myocardium had better diagnostic accuracy than percent transmural
		Chronic	enhancement for predicting improvement in systolic wall thickening.
Baks et al.[29]	22	Acute	Segments without MVO had early increased wall thickness and late partial functional recovery.
		Chronic	Segments with MVO showed late wall thinning and no functional recovery at five months.
Gerber et al.[99]	16	Acute	Infarct size by CT and CMR correlated well (r = 0.89), although the two standard deviation limits of
	21	Chronic	agreement were about 35 g. Interobserver agreement and interstudy agreement were good.
Kumar et al.[100]	37	Acute	In patients with inferior AMI, LGE CMR detected right ventricular infarction more frequently than
		Chronic	echocardiography or electrocardiography.
Ibrahim et al.[31]	78	Acute	AMI was detected more often by CMR than by SPECT, specifically for non–Q-wave AMI and for the
			left circumflex territory.
Plein et al.[101]	25	Acute	LGE mass is highest in Q-wave AMI, intermediate in non–Q ST elevation AMI, and lowest in non-ST
			elevation AMI.
Kim et al.[36]	282	Acute	Multicenter validation of LGE imaging of both acute and chronic infarction.
	284	Chronic	
Total	764	Acute	

AMI, Acute myocardial infarction; *CKMB*, creatine kinase-MB; *CMR*, cardiovascular magnetic resonance; *CT*, computed tomography; *LGE*, late gadolinium enhancement; *LV*, left ventricle; *LVEF*, left ventricular ejection fraction; *MI*, myocardial infarction; *MVO*, microvascular obstruction; *PCI*, percutaneous coronary intervention; *SPECT*, single photon emission computed tomography.

imaging by detecting two types of embolic infarction in patients undergoing percutaneous coronary intervention (PCI) who had mild elevations in creatine kinase-MB. The microinfarcts ranged in size from 0.7 to 12.2 g. Selvanayagam et al.[35] also found new abnormalities by LGE-CMR in patients with post-PCI elevations in troponin and could detect abnormities in all patients, including troponin levels as low as 3.7 μg/L. Before those studies, there had been debate over whether the post-PCI biomarker elevations truly represented infarction because older imaging methods generally could not reliably detect abnormalities in <10% of the myocardium.

The culmination of validation studies of LGE as an imaging marker of infarction was a multicenter clinical trial led by Kim et al.[36] As a study intended to get US Food and Drug Administration approval for the contrast agent gadoversetamide, participants were randomized to one of four doses of: 0.05, 0.1, 0.2, or 0.3 mmol/kg. The sensitivity of CMR for detecting infarction increased with rising dose of gadoversetamide reaching 99% for AMI and 94% chronic infarction. Likewise, the accuracy of LGE-CMR for identifying infarction location also increased with rising dose of gadoversetamide and was 99% for AMI and 91% for chronic infarction.

Overall, the transmural extent of infarction predicts recovery of function in patients with either acute and chronic infarction although the relationship is tighter for chronic infarction.

MICROVASCULAR OBSTRUCTION AFTER ACUTE MYOCARDIAL INFARCTION

LGE is dependent on enough perfusion to get Gd to the myocardium. In a nonreperfused AMI, there will be a severe perfusion defect (see Fig. 19.2) unless there is significant collateral circulation. In the setting of successfully opening the epicardial coronary artery, microvascular obstruction (MVO) and related "no-reflow" phenomena can prevent reperfusion in the core of the MI[37] as shown in Fig. 19.5. CMR is generally accepted as the best noninvasive imaging test for detecting MVO.

There are four interrelated mechanisms that can lead to MVO or no reflow: ischemic injury, reperfusion injury, distal embolization, and individual susceptibility.[38,39] Although vascular tissue has lower energetic requirements than cardiomyocytes, if the duration and severity of ischemia is severe enough, then severe ischemic capillary damage may occur. Endothelial protrusions, swelling of endothelial cells, and endothelial blebs may block the capillary lumen. Gaps in the endothelial

may open and allow red blood cells into the extravascular space, a situation that will lead to abnormal iron in the interstitial space of the myocardium. Ischemic injury to cardiomyocytes can lead to edema and increased pressure in the tissue. When tissue pressures exceed capillary perfusion pressure, edema can further decrease perfusion through the myocardium. Reperfusion injury is accompanied by white blood cells, platelets, and accompanying vasoconstrictors such as endothelin and thromboxane-A2. Reperfusion injury to the myocardium may exacerbate tissue edema and may cause release of oxygen free radicals that cause further damage to cardiomyocytes and the vasculature. Distal embolization of thrombus and cholesterol plaque can compromise microvascular reperfusion despite effective epicardial PCI. Finally, some patients may have genetic or other susceptibilities to microvascular injury that modulate the likelihood of this complication of AMI.

Judd et al.[40] reported that the hypoenhanced regions within an otherwise contrast-enhanced AMI corresponded to regions of no reflow in a 2-day reperfused canine model. That same year, Lima et al.[41] published that similar findings were observed in patients after AMI when imaged by contrast-enhanced CMR. Shortly thereafter, Wu et al.[42] published one of the first CMR prognosis studies. They found that patients with AMI characterized by having MVO had higher adverse cardiovascular event rates than patients without MVO.

The relative prognostic significance of different CMR imaging characteristics will be addressed more completely later in this chapter.

T1, T2, T2*, AND ECV AS QUANTITATIVE CMR CHARACTERISTICS OF AMI

Signal intensity on CMR depends on the T1, T2, T2*, and proton density characteristics of different tissues and fluids in the body. In the last several years, it has become possible to produce quantitative maps of myocardial T1, T2, and T2* and ECV.[43] The application of these methods to characterization of AMI has led to interesting and objective observations that indicate CMR can image and differentiate infarcted myocardium, salvaged myocardium, and remote myocardium.

Using LGE imaging alone to estimate the AAR in AMI, Hillenbrand et al.[44] reported that one can infer the presence of salvaged myocardium based on a transmural extent of AMI that is less than the full wall thickness. The concept behind this method is based on the wavefront theory of AMI[45] where the infarction starts at the endocardium and progresses toward the epicardium with longer durations of coronary

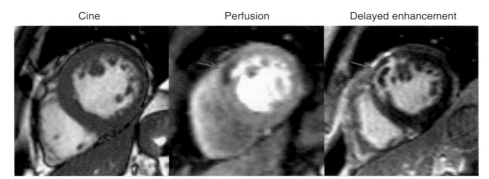

| Cine | Perfusion | Delayed enhancement |

FIG. 19.5 Appearance of acute myocardial infarction complicated by severe microvascular obstruction. The signal intensity of myocardium appears relatively uniform on the cine image in this acute anteroseptal myocardial infarction. A first pass perfusion cardiovascular magnetic resonance (CMR) image reveals a dark zone consistent with low perfusion (red arrow). Severe microvascular obstruction is present, because the perfusion defect is still present on late gadolinium enhancement CMR 10 minutes after the injection of contrast. As is often seen, the dark patch of microvascular obstruction is surrounded by a rim of bright infarcted myocardium. One can also see that the resolution of the late gadolinium enhancement image and overall image quality is better than the perfusion image.

TABLE 19.3 **Indications for Cardiovascular Magnetic Resonance in the Guidelines Published by the European Society of Cardiology That May Be Applicable to Patients After Myocardial Infarction[a]**

	Class	Level
Recommendations for CMR in Patients With STEMI		
If echocardiography is not feasible, CMR may be used as an alternative for assessment of infarct size and resting LV function.	IIb	C
For patients with multivessel disease, or in whom revascularization of other vessels is considered, stress testing or imaging (e.g., using stress myocardial perfusion scintigraphy, stress echocardiography, positron emission tomography, or CMR) for ischemia and viability is indicated before or after discharge.	I	A
CMR in Patients With Suspected Non–ST-Elevation Acute Coronary Syndromes		
In patients with no recurrence of chest pain, normal ECG findings and normal levels of cardiac troponin (preferably high sensitivity), but suspected acute coronary syndrome, a noninvasive stress test (preferably with imaging) for inducible ischemia is recommended before deciding on an invasive strategy.	I	A
CMR in the Context of Myocardial Revascularization		
Stress CMR, stress-echo, SPECT or PET are recommended in subjects with intermediate pretest probability for suspected coronary artery disease and stable symptoms.	I	A
To achieve a prognostic benefit by revascularization in patients with coronary artery disease, ischemia has to be documented by noninvasive imaging.	I	A–C
Recommendations for CMR in Acute and Chronic Heart Failure		
CMR imaging is recommended to evaluate cardiac structure and function, to measure LVEF, and to characterize cardiac tissue, especially in subjects with inadequate echocardiographic images or where the echocardiographic findings are inconclusive or incomplete (but taking account of cautions/contraindications to CMR).	I	C
Myocardial perfusion/ischemia imaging (echocardiography, CMR, SPECT, or PET) should be considered in patients thought to have coronary artery disease, and who are considered suitable for coronary revascularization, to determine whether there is reversible myocardial ischemia and viable myocardium.	IIa	C

[a]The guidelines were abstracted by von Knobelsdorff-Brenkenhoff and Schulz-Menger.[98] Note that there are other potential indications such as evaluating for intracardiac thrombus that are not currently mentioned in European Society of Cardiology guidelines.
CMR, Cardiovascular magnetic resonance; *LV*, left ventricle; *PET*, positron emission tomography scan; *SPECT*, single proton emission computed tomography; *STEMI*, ST-elevation myocardial infarction.

CONCLUSION

CMR offers a wide range of imaging methods suitable for detecting AMI and assessing many clinically important questions. The combination of cine, perfusion, and LGE-CMR is a powerful and useful test. Some patients may benefit from more detailed imaging with velocity-encoded CMR or T2-weighted images. Table 19.3 provides a summary of reasonable clinical indications for CMR after AMI, which are a subset of recently published appropriateness criteria.[98] Note that postinfarct patients must be imaged efficiently and quickly.

REFERENCES

A full reference list is available online at ExpertConsult.com

20

Acute Myocardial Infarction: Ventricular Remodeling

David Lopez and Christopher M. Kramer

Approximately 550,000 Americans will suffer an acute myocardial infarction (AMI) each year.[1] Despite major advances in AMI therapies, mortality and incident heart failure (HF) remain significant problems. Five-year mortality is estimated at 36% in men and 47% in women.[1] The five-year incidence of HF ranges from 16% in men to 22% in women.[1] These adverse outcomes have been unequivocally linked to the development of significant left ventricular (LV) dilation and reduced systolic function after AMI, otherwise known as post-MI negative LV remodeling.

LV remodeling refers to structural and functional myocardial changes that can occur in response to physiologic stress such as exercise or because of a pathologic insult such as AMI. Postinfarction LV remodeling is an intricate cascade of biologic events set forth by the release of intracellular chemokines from necrotic myocytes and increased wall stress due to infarct region contractile and diastolic impairment.[2] Remodeling is a healing and compensatory process that restricts myocardial damage while maintaining cardiac output.

Multiple studies have demonstrated different patterns of post-MI remodeling with varying degrees of LV dilation. LV dilation may be transient, limited or progressive.[3–5] Differences in the onset of dilation have been observed. It can occur acutely (within 10 days) and/or later during the healing process.[4,5] Progressive dilation has been observed even years after MI.[6] Controlled ventricular remodeling is ultimately achieved by the formation of a strong collagen scar and remote myocardium hypertrophy which counteract intracavitary forces, thereby limiting progressive ventricular dilation.[2] In this case, ventricular remodeling is compensatory. However, in many instances, particularly with large transmural infarcts, the remodeling process is overwhelmed by the increased LV wall stress.[7] Ongoing dilation and remote contractile impairment ensues[8,9] (Fig. 20.1) in a process known as negative postinfarction LV remodeling, which increases risk of HF and mortality.

The prognostic significance of negative post-MI remodeling has been demonstrated with the use of various imaging modalities, including chest radiographs,[3] invasive x-ray left ventriculography,[10] radionuclide ventriculography,[9] and echocardiography.[6,11–13] In 1973 Kostuk and colleagues showed various patterns of LV remodeling and the association between the extent of negative remodeling and clinical outcomes by measuring serial left heart dimensions using calibrated chest radiographs.[3] Subsequent investigations established LV ejection fraction (EF) as a strong predictor of survival after AMI.[11,14] By 1987 White and colleagues found that LV end-systolic volume (ESV) measured by x-ray left ventriculography 1 to 2 months after MI was a more powerful predictor of survival than end-diastolic volume (EDV) and LVEF.[10]

Although these modalities have laid the foundation of our understanding of post-MI LV remodeling, their utility has been hindered by technical and safety limitations. Chest radiographs are insensitive to RV and LV volumes and systolic function. Invasive x-ray left ventriculography and radionuclide techniques expose patients to potentially harmful ionizing radiation, making their routine repeated use in humans less desirable. Echocardiography is limited in a subset of patients by the availability of acoustic windows for proper endocardial definition. Finally, two-dimensional (2D) modalities, such as x-ray left ventriculography and echocardiography, rely on geometric assumptions to calculate ventricular volumes that may not apply in hearts regionally deformed by MI.

Cardiovascular magnetic resonance (CMR) is a technique that can overcome many of the limitations mentioned above. As a result it has emerged as a valuable noninvasive modality for the assessment of cardiac disease. CMR provides a comprehensive, volumetric, accurate, and reproducible cardiovascular evaluation beyond ventricular volumes. With the use of CMR it is possible to characterize the myocardial tissue for the localization and quantification of myocardial edema, microvascular obstruction (MVO), intramyocardial hemorrhage, and infarct burden. Hence, CMR is particularly well suited for the evaluation of post-MI remodeling. In this chapter we will review the research and clinical utility of CMR in the evaluation of post-MI ventricular remodeling,

VENTRICULAR VOLUMES, EJECTION FRACTION, AND MASS

LV cavity dilation and systolic dysfunction are the hallmarks of postinfarct remodeling and can be accurately quantified with high spatial and temporal resolution using cine CMR. Early breath-hold cine imaging used fast low-angle shot (FLASH), a spoiled gradient recalled echo (GRE) sequence. Currently, balanced steady-state free precession (bSSFP) is the most commonly used pulse sequence because of faster acquisition times, improved temporal resolution, and optimal contrast between the myocardium and the blood pool.[15,16] The use of bSSFP facilitates qualitative and quantitative assessment of cardiac anatomy and function mainly by improving endocardial border definition.

Unlike echocardiography, acoustic windows do not limit CMR; therefore images can be acquired in any desired orientation to accurately depict LV morphology and function. A carefully prescribed stack of short-axis slices extending from the cardiac base to the apex provides a three-dimensional (3D) dataset that can be used to make accurate ventricular morphologic measurements at end diastole (ED) and end systole (ES) without the need for geometric assumptions, as is the case with 2D modalities (Fig. 20.2). Ventricular volumes are calculated using the summation of disks method.

CMR derived LV volumes and mass have been validated with phantom, animal and human studies[17–19] and currently considered the clinical reference standard for other imaging modalities.[20] Although accuracy is important, reliability may be even more important because it dictates the validity of differences between serial examinations.

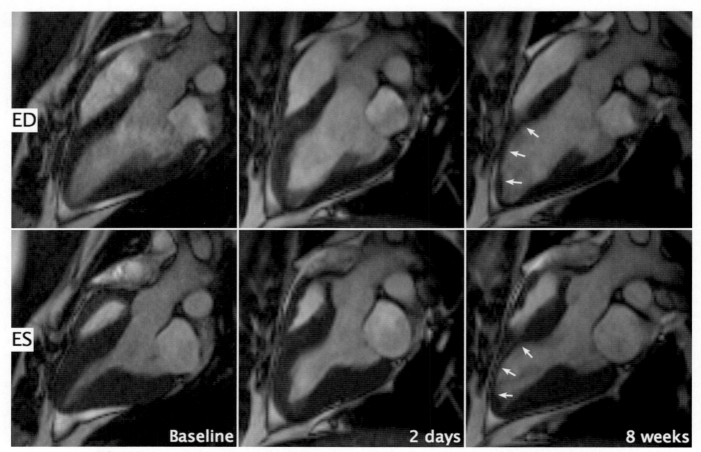

FIG. 20.1 Representative cine images from a swine model of percutaneous left anterior descending artery 90-minute occlusion followed by reperfusion illustrate negative ventricular remodeling 8 weeks after infarction. Note the anterior infarct region wall thinning and akinesis *(arrows). ED,* End diastole; *ES,* end systole.

Volumetric measurements by CMR provide high-interstudy, interscan, and interobserver reproducibility in normal hearts and those deformed by prior MI.[21–23] Interstudy, interobserver, and intraobserver reproducibility of CMR-derived RV volumes is also excellent in healthy controls, patients with HF, ventricular hypertrophy, and congenital heart disease.[24,25] Because of improved reproducibility compared with echocardiography, CMR facilitates the identification of clinically significant ventricular changes in serial examinations after AMI. The reduced variability of the measurement significantly reduces the sample size needed to detect differences between treatment arms in clinical trials.[26]

Cine CMR has been successfully used to evaluate post-MI remodeling in animal models and humans. Konermann and colleagues[27] studied the reliability of CMR in the evaluation of LV morphology and function in post-MI patients. They compared cine CMR LV volumes and LVEF with 2D echocardiography (2DE), radionuclide, and x-ray left ventriculography in a group of 65 patients who suffered a transmural MI and did not undergo thrombolysis or angioplasty. Good correlation was found between x-ray and radionuclide ventriculography. However, correlation with 2D echocardiography was limited because of inconsistent 2DE image quality. In this study, the investigators also demonstrated good correlation between creatine kinase (CK)-derived infarct size and CMR infarct mass determined from cine images.

In a follow-up publication, Konermann et al.[7] reported the natural history of LV remodeling in the same group of 65 patients at 1, 4, and 26 weeks post-MI. Medical therapy was limited to nitrates, beta-blockers, aspirin, and diuretics. Only those patients with first transmural infarcts were included in the study. Infarct transmurality and size were defined by clinical, electrocardiographic, and enzymatic criteria. The extent of negative remodeling was not only dependent on the enzymatic size but also on the location of the infarct. Small infarcts caused modest but concordant ED and ES dilation, so that LVEF remained stable. Individuals with large anterior infarcts developed an unbalanced, progressive diastolic and systolic dilation that resulted in a marked reduction in LVEF. Infarct region thinning was almost always observed at 6 months except for small posterior infarcts. LV stroke volume index (SVI) was smaller in large anterior MI, but there was no statistically significant difference in LV SVI between 1 and 26 weeks post-MI. Despite a significant LVEF reduction in those with large infarcts, stroke volume was maintained at the expense of ventricular dilation. No clinical difference between the groups was observed when analyzing New York Heart Association (NYHA) symptom classification. Four patients died before the completion of the study and all had large anterior MI.

In a cohort of 26 patients with reperfused anterior AMI, Kramer et al.[28] used cine tissue tagging to evaluate morphologic changes, LVEF, and regional intramyocardial function of myocardium adjacent and remote to the infarct. All patients received either angiotensin-converting enzyme inhibitor (ACEI) or beta-blocker. Most patients received ACEI and about half received both agents. Imaging was done on day 5 ± 2 and week 8 ± 1 after MI. There was a significant increase in LV end-diastolic volume index (EDVI) with stable end-systolic volume index (ESVI). Therefore there was an improvement in global LVEF 8 weeks post-MI. The increased LVEF was mediated by contractile improvement

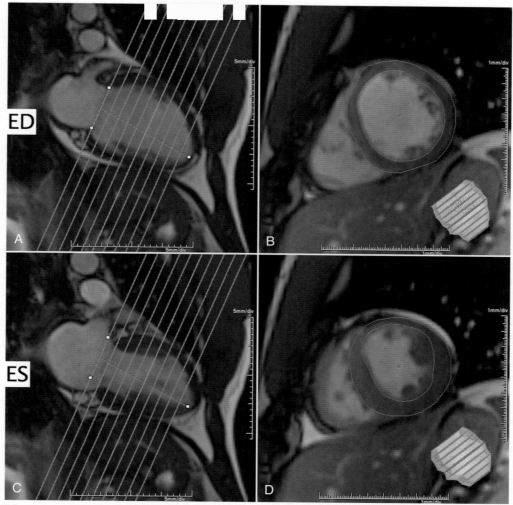

FIG. 20.2 A carefully prescribed stack of short-axis slices extending from the cardiac base to the apex (A) provides a three-dimensional dataset (B and D) that can be used to make accurate left ventricular (LV) morphologic measurements at end diastole *(ED)* and end systole *(ES)* without the need for geometric assumptions. It is important to account for in-plane motion of the mitral annulus (C) to avoid overestimation of the end-systolic volume and underestimation of the LV ejection fraction.

and normalization in the adjacent and remote regions, respectively. Enzymatic infarct size correlated with the degree of diastolic dilation.

REGIONAL CONTRACTILITY

Although LVEF is the most commonly used global metric of LV systolic function, it does not provide information regarding regional performance. In fact, segmental systolic abnormalities because of AMI may sometimes be concealed by a normal global LVEF. Accordingly, to understand the contributing factors to global functional alterations during the remodeling process, it is important to characterize regional contractile performance in the adjacent and remote noninfarcted myocardium. In clinical practice this is usually done by subjective visual scoring of segmental endocardial motion and thickening using cine CMR images. However, visual assessment can be insensitive to subtle abnormalities and is subject to greater interobserver variability. Thus objective methods to quantify contractile function have been developed. Wall thickening and endocardial motion can be measured from cine CMR images. A more accurate[29] assessment of intramyocardial contractility in the infarcted

heart can be determined by measuring strain with the use of myocardial tissue tagging sequences such as spatial modulation of magnetization (SPAMM)[30] and phase-based sequences such as displacement encoding with stimulated echoes (DENSE).[31] More recently, feature tracking analysis has allowed the measurement of circumferential and longitudinal strain from bSSFP cine images.[32,33]

Wall Thickening and Endocardial Displacement: Cine Cardiovascular Magnetic Resonance

In their chronicle of nonreperfused AMI, Konermann et al.[7] assessed regional LV contractility by measuring wall thickening and the endocardial motion toward the center of the LV cavity using cine CMR. Progressive changes in endocardial motion were identified in the infarct and remote regions during the 6-month follow-up period. The extent of regional LV dysfunction correlated with infarct size and location. The infarct region of large anterior AMI had the greatest reduction in endocardial motion, which progressed to dyskinesis (displacement away from the cavity center) at 6 months. Changes in wall thickening were not observed in the viable myocardium. It is worth noting that the authors averaged the adjacent and remote myocardium wall thickness in their analysis. Hence, regional differences could not be identified between these segments.

Holman et al.[34] investigated the regional contractility of 25 patients 3 weeks after anterior MI. An optimized 3D analysis of the myocardium centerline was implemented to improve accuracy of wall thickness measurement. Some 100 equidistant chords were constructed between the endocardial and epicardial contours of short-axis cine images. The starting point was defined as the inferior RV insertion site, which was labeled for ED and ES, allowing to correct for rotational motion. Wall thickening was reduced in the left anterior descending (LAD) artery territory compared with a normal database. The dysfunctional LV myocardial mass 3 weeks after MI, when any myocardial stunning should have resolved, correlated with enzymatic infarct size.

Strain Imaging
Tissue Tagging

CMR strain imaging in animal and human studies has contributed greatly to our understanding of regional myocardial function during the post-MI remodeling process. In an ovine model of surgical LAD ligation,[35] SPAMM myocardial tissue tagging was used to measure circumferential and longitudinal myocardial shortening at baseline, 1 week, 8 weeks, and 6 months after AMI. Shortening within infarcted regions was reduced throughout the study period. A persistent difference in intramyocardial shortening was found between noninfarcted regions adjacent to and remote from the infarct border. Function in adjacent noninfarcted regions fell markedly at 1 week after AMI and partially improved by 8 weeks, but remained depressed relative to baseline and to remote regions at 6 months. These findings were reproduced by Moulton et al.[36] using a similar ovine model and DANTE (delays alternating with nutations for tailored excitation) myocardial tagging. In addition to systolic strain, Moulton et al. evaluated diastolic and isovolemic strains. They found abnormal, positive strain during isovolemic contraction in the border zone, suggesting that isovolemic myocardial fiber stretching contributes to LV systolic dysfunction in these segments.

Epstein et al.[37] used myocardial tissue tagging to characterize acute regional function in a murine model of LAD occlusion and reperfusion. The percent circumferential shortening was measured for the infarct, adjacent and remote regions. A gradient of contractile dysfunction was found from the infarct to the remote region 1 day post-AMI compared with baseline. Thomas et al.[37a] used tissue tagging to characterize regional contractile changes in a rat model of LAD ligation at 1 to 2, 3 to 4, 6 to 8, and 9 to 12 weeks post-AMI. In this study, changes in the maximum and minimum principal stretches and strains, and the orientation of the principal stretch angle were measured. At 1 to 2 weeks post-AMI, significant changes were found in a gradient fashion from the infarct to the remote region. These abnormalities persisted relatively unchanged up to 12 weeks post-MI. The principal strain direction became more circumferentially oriented during the study period.

Using CMR tissue tagging in a cohort of patients within the first week after reperfused LAD AMI without significant disease in other coronary territories and with an EF of <50%, Kramer et al.[38] found a significant reduction in remote region intramyocardial shortening compared with controls. Once again, there was a decrease in contractile function in all myocardial segments in a gradient fashion similar to the findings in animal studies. When this patient group was re-imaged at 8 weeks after AMI, there was improvement in regional function in all segments, including normalization of contractile function in the remote myocardium.[28] The impact of early reperfusion is evident by the improvement in infarct region strain.

CMR myocardial tagging was used to assess the correlation between regional function and loading conditions in 16 patients after successful reperfusion of a first anterior MI compared with 31 age-matched controls.[39] All patients had received optimal medical therapy with beta-blockers and ACEIs. Imaging was performed 1 and 12 weeks postinfarction. The LV myocardium was divided into 32 cuboid segments, defined by 4 endocardial and 4 epicardial node points derived from short- and long-axis tagged images. Regional LVEF was calculated using a pie-shaped volume defined by the endocardium and the center of the LV. This parameter was viewed as a composite marker of regional deformation. A relative metric of regional load was defined as the product of the systolic blood pressure and the mean radius of curvature in the short and long axes divided by the segment wall thickness. In healthy controls, an inverse relationship between regional LVEF and load was demonstrated. In contrast for the MI patients, the average load values significantly increased in a graded fashion from remote to infarct segments between the acute and chronic time points. At 12 weeks, remote regional LVEF decreased with a similar correlation coefficient to changes in load as controls; therefore the change in LVEF was because of an increase in loading conditions and a worsening of myocardial function. No change in regional LVEF was observed in the adjacent segments, indicating some improvement in myocardial function. The infarct segments demonstrated an average increase in regional LVEF even with significant increases in load representing an even greater true improvement in myocardial function. This study demonstrated that CMR could be used to assess LV function post-MI and differentiate improvement in intrinsic myocyte function from changes in deformation that occur as a response to alterations in Frank-Starling conditions.

Phase-Based Strain Imaging

In 1999 advanced, phase-based, strain imaging techniques were introduced to facilitate and optimize strain analysis compared with tissue tagging methods. These included harmonic phase magnetic resonance (HARP)[40] and DENSE.[31] These methods were validated with traditional tagging sequences in animal and human studies.[41–45]

Azevedo et al.[46] used tissue tagging with HARP analysis in combination with contrast-enhanced (CE)-CMR and radioactive microspheres to evaluate the relationship between strain properties and myocardial injury in a canine model of 90-minute LAD or left circumflex (LCX) occlusion followed by 24 hours of reperfusion. In this early period the areas at risk as defined by radioactive microspheres with preserved systolic strain and strain rate demonstrated significantly reduced diastolic strain rate compared with the remote regions. Similar to the findings of Gerber et al.,[47] infarct segments with MVO demonstrated even greater reduction in systolic and diastolic strain than those without.

In a canine model of reperfused LAD, Ashikaga et al.[48] used DENSE to generate 3D-displacement maps, CE CMR imaging to generate infarct maps, and epicardial electrical recordings to generate electrical activation maps. CMR examinations were completed between 3 and 8 weeks post-AMI. Electrical activation times were significantly delayed in the infarct zone, but preserved in the border and remote areas. Conversely, all strain parameters were impaired in the border zone, which was not different from the infarct region. Hence, contractile abnormalities in the border segments were not mediated by impaired electrical activation. In the remote segments there was a typical[42] transmural strain gradient from subendocardium to subepicardium, which was not observed in the infarct or border zone regions. Positive circumferential and longitudinal strains were observed in the border zone indicative of abnormal systolic stretch.

In a canine model that typically created subendocardial infarcts with large areas at risk, recovery of systolic function was evaluated with DENSE imaging and correlated to T2-weighted (T2W) imaging representing the area at risk.[49] T2W area at risk was validated with microsphere measurements. At 2 months post-AMI there was resolution of the T2W abnormalities representing the area at risk. This correlated with a significant improvement in radial and circumferential strain compared with the acute post-MI setting. However, contractile function in the area at risk remained significantly depressed compared with remote sectors.

Feature Tracking

More recently anatomical feature tracking of cine bSSFP images or feature tracking CMR has been introduced as a practical solution for strain analysis.[32] Although the information obtained via this method is mostly limited to the endocardium and epicardium, it still provides relevant and comparable information when compared with traditional tissue tagging.[33] Its application to post-MI remodeling has been limited[33a]; however, given its ease of use, it is likely to rapidly gain popularity as it has in many other disease states.

MYOCARDIAL FIBER STRUCTURE: DIFFUSION TENSOR MAGNETIC RESONANCE IMAGING

An evolving technique to study post-MI remodeling is diffusion-weighted magnetic resonance imaging (MRI). The ability to visualize and characterize the myocardial fiber structure is important to better understanding cardiomyopathies, including post-MI remodeling. Diffusion tensor imaging (DTI) is a form of diffusion-weighted CMR which has been validated against histology as a rapid and nondestructive method to depict the myocardial fibers' architecture.[50,51] Early animal and human studies have consistently shown that early after MI, the infarct region is characterized by increased diffusivity and decreased fractional anisotropy.[52–54] Investigators have also shown a difference in the distribution of right- and left-handed helix fibers between the infarct and remote regions. In a study of 37 patients imaged about 4 weeks after their first MI, a transmural gradient of left- and right-handed helical fibers was observed between the infarct and remote regions.[52] In the infarct region the percent of right-handed fibers was lowest in association with a greater percent of left-handed fibers. Using 3D DTI tractography, Sosnovik et al.[53] performed in vivo imaging of mouse hearts 24 hours and 3 weeks after mid-LAD infarct or ischemia-reperfusion injury. DTI imaging findings were compared with CMR and histologically determined infarct and area at risk regions. Areas of increased T2, representing tissue edema, demonstrated increased diffusivity and decreased fractional anisotropy as well as loss of fiber tracts. The loss of tract coherence was uniform across the area at risk and included infarct and viable fibers when compared with late gadolinium enhancement (LGE) and histopathology. In the infarct group there was persistent loss of fiber tracts 3 weeks post-MI. Therefore presence of collagen fibers did not restrict diffusion adequately to resolve tracts by DTI. In the ischemia-reperfusion group, diffusivity and fractional anisotropy returned to baseline 3 weeks after the injury; however, fiber architecture remained abnormal, albeit relatively preserved compared with infarcted hearts.

TISSUE CHARACTERIZATION

To thoroughly understand post-MI remodeling, it is crucial to precisely characterize the location, size, transmural extent, and type of ischemic injury. In the event of epicardial vessel occlusion, the myocardium subtended by the vessel segments distal to the occlusion is at risk of infarction. This territory is known as the area at risk. A sufficiently prolonged occlusion leads to irreversible injury, or infarction, of the entire area at risk. If a vessel is opened before the occurrence of permanent injury, a percentage of the area at risk is salvaged. The salvaged myocardium exhibits reversible contractile dysfunction, or stunning. A more deleterious form of injury can occur within the infarct core because of persistent ischemia or "no-reflow" caused by MVO. In a number of infarcts with MVO, intramyocardial hemorrhage may also occur. CMR stands out from other imaging modalities because of its superior tissue characterization capability. With the use of various noncontrast and contrast-enhanced CMR sequences, we can identify and quantify the area at risk, areas of irreversible infarction, salvaged myocardium, MVO, and intramyocardial hemorrhage, which are all important parameters that influence post-MI remodeling.

Infarct Characterization and Predictors of Left Ventricular Remodeling

Infarcted myocardium can be identified by various CMR pulse sequences, including cine, CE-CMR, and, more recently, T1 mapping. Today, CE-CMR, specifically LGE, is considered the reference standard for acute and chronic infarct characterization.

Late Gadolinium Enhancement

LGE images are acquired at least 10 minutes after gadolinium (Gd) administration using an inversion-recovery T1-weighted (T1W) pulse sequence. Gd shortens the T1 relaxation of the surrounding protons; therefore areas of increased Gd appear hyperintense on T1W imaging. Although Gd-based contrast media are extracellular, the loss of cell membrane integrity and altered Gd wash-in and wash-out kinetics lead to increased Gd in acute infarcts.[55,56] In chronic MI, Gd is increased because of an increase in extracellular space, with formation of a collagenous scar as well as alterations in contrast kinetics. Consequently, both AMI and chronic MI will appear as bright myocardial regions on LGE imaging (Fig. 20.3).

LGE imaging precisely and reproducibly demonstrates acute and chronic infarcts in comparison to histology.[55,57] This was best demonstrated in an elegant canine study by Kim et al.[55] in which acute infarcts

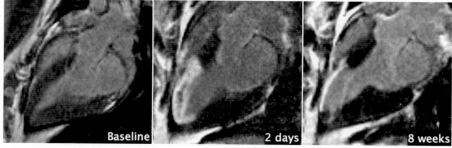

FIG. 20.3 Representative late gadolinium enhancement images from a swine model of left anterior descending artery occlusion and reperfusion. Note the increased wall thickness and hypoenhanced core 2 days postinfarction, followed by infarct resorption/wall thinning at 8 weeks.

were created by coronary ligation. A second artery was instrumented to create reversible ischemic injury. CMR examinations were performed at 1 day, 3 days, and 8 weeks postischemic injury. LGE images were acquired 30 minutes after Gd administration. Compared with histology, the extent of LGE by ex vivo imaging was the same as the extent of myocardial necrosis in the acute phase and the extent of collagenous scar at 8 weeks after reperfused and nonreperfused ischemic injury. Therefore areas of LGE specifically represent permanent myocardial injury and not stunned or salvaged myocardium. It should be noted that the accuracy of in vivo LGE is influenced by multiple factors, including imaging delay after contrast injection,[56,58] spatial resolution,[57] and postprocessing methodology.[59] When a standardized approach is applied, LGE imaging reproducibly quantifies acute and chronic infarcts with excellent interscan, intraobserver and interobserver agreement.[60,61]

This technique has been useful to define the evolution of infarct size in vivo. Rochitte et al.[62] demonstrated an increase in infarct size from 2 to 48 hours after reperfused 90-minute LAD occlusion in a canine model. However, the investigators did not report the changes in wall thickness or circumferential expansion index to further characterize the pattern of infarct size growth in this very early phase after ischemic injury. They also observed up to 3-fold increase in the size of MVO in the infarct core, which correlated with thioflavin-S myocardial blood flow assessment. Fieno et al.[63] assessed chronic infarct remodeling in canines after 45-minute, 90-minute, or permanent LAD occlusion. Imaging was performed on day 3, 4 weeks, and 8 weeks after MI. The infarct size at 8 weeks post-AMI decreased on average by 75% of the size on day 3, but as much as 90% in the case of small infarcts caused by the 45-minute occlusion. True infarct expansion was not observed. Although the overall myocardial mass decreased, the non-infarcted myocardium mass increased on average by 15%. The infarct involution findings were consistent with those of Richard et al.,[64] who measured infarct size on pathologic specimens 4 days, 2 weeks, and 6 weeks after 6 hours of reperfused or permanent circumflex occlusion in an open chest canine model. In both experiments, reperfusion appeared to accelerate infarct healing, but did not impact the final infarct size. Early infarct expansion and cardiac rupture were not observed in these studies.

Infarct involution has been demonstrated in humans as well. Ingkanisorn et al.[65] evaluated infarct size within 5 days of an AMI in 33 patients, 20 of whom returned for follow-up imaging more than 8 weeks after MI. Acute infarct size correlated well with troponin-I. At follow-up, infarct size decreased from 16% to 11% of the LV mass. Choi et al.[66] also reported a significant decrease in infarct size between week 1 and week 8 post-MI in 25 patients after reperfused AMI. The involution of MI size tended to be greater in those with MVO.

LGE CMR has been recognized as a powerful predictor of LV remodeling, regional and global functional recovery, and major adverse cardiac events (MACE) following AMI. Choi et al.[67] performed LGE on 24 patients within 7 days of revascularization post-MI. Scans were repeated at 8 to 12 weeks to assess functional recovery. There was an inverse relationship between transmural extent of LGE and segmental recovery. Interestingly, the extent of dysfunctional myocardium with zero or <25% transmural enhancement was a better predictor of global functional recovery than peak cardiac enzyme level or total infarct size by LGE. Ingkanisorn et al.[65] found a better correlation between acute LGE infarct size and follow-up LVEF than between acute LVEF and follow-up LVEF. This is probably caused by the presence of stunned, yet viable, myocardium in the setting of early reperfusion. Lund et al.[67a] imaged 55 patients within 1 week of reperfused MI and approximately 8 months later. LGE infarct size of 24% of the LV area predicted LV remodeling, as defined by an increase in EDV index of ≥20%, with a sensitivity and specificity of 92% and 93%, respectively. In a cohort of 231 patients

with prior MI (at least 3 months), Di Bella et al.[68] found that LGE >12.7% of LV mass, EDV >105 mL/m², and a wall motion score index >1.7 were independently associated with cardiac death or appropriate intracardiac defibrillator shocks. Patients with all three factors had a 4-year event rate of 29.6%, whereas those with none of these factors had an event rate of 3.5%.

No-Reflow Phenomenon: Microvascular Obstruction and Intramyocardial Hemorrhage

It has been shown in animal and clinical studies that opening an occluded epicardial artery does not always result in homogeneous reperfusion of the area at risk.[69] This is known as the "no-reflow" phenomenon. Areas of no-reflow can be detected in vivo by various modalities, including angiography, single-photon emission computed tomography (SPECT), positron emission tomography (PET), and contrast echocardiography, but are best evaluated by CE-CMR. In the CMR literature, no-reflow zones have been referred to as areas of MVO. Areas of MVO are detected by CE-CMR as hypoenhanced regions within the infarct core on dynamic first-pass perfusion imaging during Gd administration or on LGE imaging after Gd administration (Fig. 20.4). LGE imaging 2 to 5 minutes after contrast injection reveals so-called *early* MVO and imaging after 10 minutes reveals *late* MVO. It has been demonstrated that areas of early MVO tend to be larger than late MVO, which suggests that early MVO illustrates a penumbra of slow collateral flow in addition to true no-reflow regions. Therefore early MVO is more sensitive, whereas late MVO is more specific for no-reflow. A recent systematic review shows that the prevalence of early MVO is greater than that of late MVO (65% vs. 54%, respectively).[70]

The mechanisms of the no-reflow phenomenon are incompletely understood but may include vasoconstriction mediated by inflammatory cells, external compression from surrounding edema, and microembolization of atherosclerotic cellular debris leading to small vessel plugging.[69] Regardless of the exact mechanism, studies have demonstrated that this phenomenon is mediated by reperfusion injury. Rochitte et al.[62] and Wu et al.[71] showed that MVO size, as detected by in vivo CE-CMR and validated with thioflavin-S, peaks 48 hours after reperfusion and plateaus from 2 to 9 days after reperfusion. Areas of MVO involute thereafter and are rarely seen on follow-up CMR 1 month or later after AMI.

The presence of any MVO has been repeatedly associated with worse myocardial remodeling and clinical outcomes. This was first demonstrated by Wu et al.,[72] who found that early MVO predicts infarct transmurality, LV function, and remodeling after 16 months, and was also a powerful independent prognostic indicator of MACE even after controlling for infarct size. Gerber el al.[47] studied the effect of MVO on myocardial strain and reported that the extent of MVO correlates with significant decreases in infarct region stretch and reduced radial strain in the adjacent regions. Nijveldt et al.[73] evaluated the impact of early, mid, and late MVO in 63 patients who received percutaneous coronary intervention (PCI) and optimal medical management. They found that MVO was a better predictor of adverse remodeling at the 4-month follow-up CMR. Cochet et al.[74] compared the prognostic significance of MVO as detected by first-pass perfusion to late MVO in 187 patients and showed that by multivariate analysis both methods are predictors of 1-year MACE. However, late MVO had an odds ratio (OR) over 3 times that of first-pass perfusion (8.7 vs. 2.5). These results are summarized in a recent systematic review by Hamirani et al.,[70] showing that both early MVO and late MVO are associated with lower LVEF, increased ventricular volumes and larger infarct size, and predict worse adverse remodeling. However, late MVO appears to portend greater risk of MACE compared with early MVO (OR 4.3 vs. 2.6), which may be a function of its improved specificity for true no-reflow zones. Furthermore, late MVO is more likely to contain

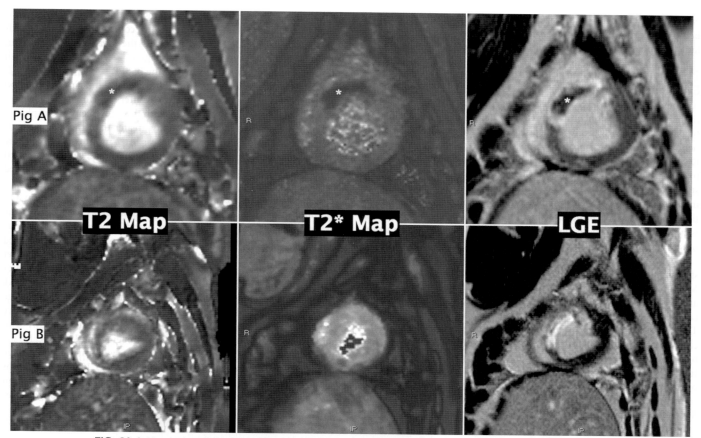

FIG. 20.4 Hypoenhanced infarct core may represent intramyocardial hemorrhage or microvascular obstruction (MVO). Intramyocardial hemorrhage *(* on Pig A panels)* can be seen with T2 mapping, but is best demonstrated on T2* mapping. Areas of MVO are not seen with T2 or T2* mapping *(Pig B). LGE,* Late gadolinium enhancement.

intramyocardial hemorrhage,[70] which may represent a more severe ischemic injury.

Intramyocardial Hemorrhage

Intramyocardial hemorrhage occurs as the result of capillary endothelial necrosis.[75] In the early era of reperfusion therapy, intramyocardial hemorrhage was considered a deleterious effect of reperfusion.[76,77] This idea was later challenged by Fishbein et al.,[78] who demonstrated that intramyocardial hemorrhage only occurs in areas with existing microvascular damage before epicardial reperfusion. Therefore intramyocardial hemorrhage is probably a manifestation of preexisting capillary injury and not caused by reperfusion. It is worth noting that whether intramyocardial hemorrhage is a consequence of reperfusion or a manifestation of underlying injury, it is always dependent on the duration of ischemia.[76–78]

Intramyocardial hemorrhage is mostly observed in areas of no-reflow and cannot be differentiated from nonhemorrhagic MVO by CE-CMR. However, CMR is the only modality that allows in vivo visualization of intramyocardial hemorrhage with the use of T2-weighted or T2*-weighted imaging (see Fig. 20.4). T2*W imaging has been validated in animals and is considered the preferred method because of improved sensitivity compared with T2W imaging.[79–81]

An increasing body of literature indicates that the presence of intramyocardial hemorrhage may represent a more severe form of injury in the ischemic spectrum. However, its clinical prognostic value is not well defined. In their systematic review Hamirani et al.[70] identified 9 studies comprising 1106 patients that evaluated the impact of intramyocardial

hemorrhage on LV remodeling, and the pooled analysis demonstrates that intramyocardial hemorrhage is associated with larger ventricular volumes, infarct size, and lower LVEF. In a recent study of 151 patients, Kandler et al.[81] also report that intramyocardial hemorrhage, as detected by T2*, was independently associated with larger infarct size, larger LV volumes, smaller salvage index, and lower LVEF. In a study of 346 patients with reperfused ST elevation MI (STEMI) within 12 hours of symptom onset, Eitel et al.[82] evaluated the prognostic significance of intramyocardial hemorrhage, as defined by hypointense core on T2W imaging. Intramyocardial hemorrhage was observed in 35% of the patients and it was associated with larger acute infarct size, MVO size, less myocardial salvage, and lower LVEF. Using stepwise multiple Cox-regression analysis, the presence of intramyocardial hemorrhage was an independent predictor of MACE 6 months after AMI (hazard ratio 2.04), whereas late MVO alone was not. The addition of intramyocardial hemorrhage to a predictive model that included clinical history, LV function, and infarct size increased the c-statistic (area under the curve [AUC]) from 0.76 to 0.8 ($P = .046$). The results of this study require confirmation in larger multicenter studies.

Bulluck et al.[83] reported a new insight regarding the fate of intramyocardial hemorrhage in a cohort of STEMI patients who had CMR within the first week post-MI and a follow-up examination 5 months later. Review of T2 and T2* maps at both time points indicated that about 87% of those with intramyocardial hemorrhage had evidence of residual iron deposits in the infarct zone. The T2 relaxation times were higher in infarcts with residual iron deposits. Adverse remodeling was

nitric oxide synthase knockout mice compared with wild-type mice. Furthermore, the circumferential extent of wall thinning was reduced in inducible nitric oxide synthase knockout mice. This effect was evident by day 7 post-MI and persisted at the final CMR scan on day 28 post-MI.

Pharmacologic agents that may limit reperfusion injury and MVO might also be useful in limiting LV remodeling post-MI. Nicorandil is an adenosine triphosphate-sensitive potassium channel agonist which has been used as an antianginal agent in Asia and Europe because of its nitrate-like effect.[113] Krombach et al.[114] demonstrated that nicorandil treatment in rats after coronary artery ligation before reperfusion reduced infarct size assessed by CMR LGE. Subsequently, they fed nicorandil to rats before coronary ligation and reperfusion and for 8 weeks post-MI. At 8 weeks post-MI the nicorandil-treated groups had improved LVEF, EDV, ESV, and wall thickening in remote infarct regions and periinfarct regions relative to controls that experienced initial infarcts of the same size.[115]

Nahrendorf et al.[116] studied the role of 3-hydroxy-3-methylglutaryl-coenzyme A (HMG-CoA) reductase inhibition in LV remodeling to determine whether the mechanism of any positive effect on remodeling was nitric oxide synthase dependent. Adult rats underwent left coronary ligation followed by treatment with placebo, cerivastatin, or cerivastatin plus N-methyl-L-arginine methyl ester (L-NAME), a nitric oxide synthase inhibitor. Rats fed cerivastatin had a significantly lower LV mass at 4 and 12 weeks post-MI. However, LV volume was similar among all three groups. L-NAME abolished the effects of cerivastatin. The authors concluded that HMG-CoA reductase inhibitors diminished LV hypertrophy and helped to preserve function but not LV dilatation in a mechanism that appears to involve nitric oxide synthase.

The same group also tested the effect of testosterone on LV remodeling based on data demonstrating a higher 2-year mortality post-MI in women than in men. Rats were treated with placebo, testosterone, or orchiectomy, starting 2 weeks before sham procedure or LAD occlusion.[117] CMR was performed 2 weeks and 8 weeks after LAD ligation. Hemodynamic measurements including LV end-diastolic pressure (LVEDP) and mean arterial pressure (MAP) were recorded. At 8 weeks, testosterone therapy augmented LV hypertrophy with associated reduction in LVEDP. No difference in LVEF, cardiac output, or MAP was observed between the groups.

CMR has also been used to study the role of mechanical restraint devices to limit LV remodeling after acute MI. Blom et al.[118] used an ovine model of LAD occlusion to create an anterior MI in 10 animals. Five sheep received the Acorn device 1 week after acute MI. At 12 weeks after MI animals treated with the Acorn device had a significantly smaller LV epicardial surface area compared with controls. Furthermore, border zone systolic regional radial strain was improved at 12 weeks in sheep that were treated with the Acorn device.

In the past decade multiple investigators have used CMR techniques to evaluate the effects of stem cell transplantation in small- and large-animal models.[119–123] CMR has been useful to assess changes in volumes, contractile function, infarct size, energetics,[122] and cell engraftment with the use of iron-oxide labeling.[120,123]

Human Studies

Numerous studies have used CMR to assess the effects of post-MI antiremodeling therapies and many more are underway. Schulman et al.[124] randomized 43 patients with a Q-wave AMI within 24 hours of symptom onset to intravenous enalaprilat and then oral ACEI therapy or placebo for 1-month post-MI. Twenty-three of the patients underwent CMR at 1 month post-MI for evaluation of infarct expansion. The infarct expansion index was defined as the ratio of the infarct to noninfarct endocardial segment length. Other parameters measured included infarct segment length and wall thickness. ACEI therapy was associated with a reduced infarct segment length (7.9 ± 1.0 cm vs. 10.6 ± 0.9 cm in controls) and a lower infarct expansion index (1.1 ± 0.3 vs. 1.8 ± 0.3 in controls). The greatest impact of ACEI therapy on infarct expansion was found in the subgroup with anterior infarcts. Johnson et al.[125] used CMR to assess ACEI therapy post-MI in a study of 35 patients who had an LVEF >40% after their first acute Q-wave MI. Studies were performed at 1 week and 3 months post-MI. Volumetric cine CMR was used to quantify LV EDVI, ESVI, and mass. Therapy with the ACEI ramipril contributed to a fall in LV mass index (LVMI; from 82 ± 18 to 79 ± 23 g/m^2), whereas there was no significant change in control patients (77 ± 15 to 79 ± 23 g/m^2). No significant change in LV EDVI was noted in either the treatment group or controls in these patients with mild LV dysfunction at baseline.

CMR was used to evaluate the effects of beta-blockade administered before revascularization in those presenting with Killip Class II or less anterior STEMI in the METOCARD-CNIC (Effect of Metoprolol in Cardioprotection During an Acute Myocardial Infarction) trial.[126] Infarct size was smaller and ejection fraction higher in the treatment arm without a difference in 24-hour outcomes. Groenning et al.[127] performed CMR three times over 6 months on 41 patients enrolled in the MERIT-HF (Metoprolol CR/XL Randomized Intervention Trial in Congestive Heart Failure) study. These were patients with chronic stable HF who had been randomized to metoprolol succinate or placebo. At 6 months the metoprolol group experienced a significant decrease in LVEDVI (150 mL/m^2 at baseline to 126 mL/m^2 at 6 months, $P = .007$) and LVESVI (107 mL/m^2 at baseline to 81 mL/m^2 at 6 months, $P = .001$), with a concomitant increase in LVEF (29% at baseline to 37% at 6 months, $P = .005$). There was no change among these variables in the placebo group. Dubach et al.[128] performed CMR on 26 patients with a mean LVEF of $26 \pm 6\%$ who were randomized to bisoprolol fumarate or placebo. After 1 year, the treatment group experienced an increase in LVEF (25.0 ± 7 vs. $36.2 \pm 9\%$; $P < .05$) and a trend toward smaller LVEDV and LVESV. The control group experienced no change. More recently, Bellenger et al.[129] performed CMR on 34 patients with chronic stable HF who were participating in the CHRISTMAS (Carvedilol Hibernation Reversible Ischaemia Trial, Marker of Success) trial. This is a double-blind study comparing carvedilol and placebo. The patients underwent CMR at baseline and at 6 months. The carvedilol group experienced a decrease in LVESVI (-9 vs. $+3$ mL/m^2, $P = .0004$) and in LVEDVI (-8 vs. 0 mL/m^2, $P = .05$) with a concomitant increase in LVEF ($+3$ vs. -2%, $P = .003$) relative to control. These studies demonstrate that differences in LV structure because of pharmacologic therapy of acute MI can be demonstrated with CMR in relatively small-sized patient cohorts. Studies using echocardiography post-MI have required a much larger group of patients (on the order of several hundreds) to demonstrate quantifiable differences between treatment and control groups.[130]

It is well established that early revascularization minimizes infarct size and reduces MACE. On the other hand, the benefits of late infarct artery revascularization in clinical practice is less evident. A CMR pilot study of 16 patients showed that reperfusion within 2 weeks of MI mitigated ventricular remodeling compared with delayed intervention 3 months post-MI. Subsequently, Silva et al.[131] published a study in which 36 patients with an occluded infarct related artery were randomized to PCI or optimal medical management. At 6 months there was no difference in LV volumes or regional contractility. However, global LVEF improved in the PCI group and became worse in the conservative management group. Bellenger et al.[132] used CMR to assess whether the presence of infarct zone viability would affect LV remodeling after late recanalization of an infarct related artery. Twenty-six patients were randomized to PCI (14 patients) or medical management (12 patients) after an anterior MI. PCI was performed on an average of 26 days post-MI. The initial CMR study, which included a dobutamine stress protocol to assess myocardial viability, occurred at an average of 7.7 weeks post-MI. The follow-up CMR study occurred at an average of 10.8 months post-MI. In the PCI group, there was a significant correlation between the number of viable segments and improvement in LVEF and ESV. No significant relationship existed between EDV and viable segments in the PCI group. No correlation between viability and any of the aforementioned metrics of remodeling was noted in the conservatively treated group. Despite these findings, the Occluded Artery Trial (OAT), which randomized 2166 stable patients to PCI versus medical therapy 3 to 28 days post-MI, found no difference in MACE between the groups.[133]

CMR has become an important tool to assess the effect of stem cell transplantation. Following a series of animal studies, multiple clinical trials have been conducted to assess stem cell therapy after MI. Unfortunately the results of stem cell therapy, particularly with bone marrow-derived mononuclear cells, have been disappointing. A meta-analysis by de Jong et al.[134] comprised 22 randomized controlled trials between 2002 and 2013 and found that stem cell treatment increased LVEF by 2.1% in the treatment arm as a result of the preservation of ESV. However, no beneficial effect was observed in trials that used CMR to assess ventricular remodeling. Furthermore, no reduction in MACE was observed after a median follow-up of 6 months.

CMR has also been used in studies assessing nontraditional therapies of LV remodeling postinfarction. Dubach et al.[135] studied 25 patients with LV dysfunction after MI (EF 32 ± 6%) and randomized them to

2 months of exercise in a rehabilitation program or control. Cine CMR was performed and LV volumes, mass, and EF measured. At the end of the training period, no differences were noted between groups in any of the aforementioned parameters. In addition, no differences were noted within groups over time. Exercise capacity increased in the treated group, but no deleterious effects on global parameters of LV remodeling were found, contrary to previously published data.[136]

Finally, Heydari and colleagues examined high-dose omega-3 fatty acids in a double blind, placebo-controlled study of 358 patients with AMI.[137] By intention-to-treat analysis, those randomized to omega-3 fatty acids had a significant reduction in LV systolic volume index and noninfarct myocardial fibrosis.

CONCLUSION

With the use of CMR it is possible to accurately and reproducibly measure post-MI remodeling, including ventricular volumes, mass, EF, regional contractile function, and infarct size. CMR has proved instrumental in the understanding of the mechanism of remodeling and plays an important role in the development of therapeutic interventions intended to minimize remodeling. CMR will undoubtedly be used with increasing frequency as surrogate endpoints for clinical trials to prevent post-MI remodeling.

REFERENCES

A full reference list is available online at ExpertConsult.com

21

Myocardial Viability

Udo P. Sechtem and Heiko Mahrholdt

The detection of residual myocardial viability in a patient with regional or global severe left ventricular (LV) dysfunction is of clinical importance to plan the therapeutic strategy because revascularization of dysfunctional but viable myocardium may improve LV function.[1] Several imaging techniques have been shown to be successful in detecting myocardial viability; these include LV angiography using appropriate interventions,[2] perfusion scintigraphy,[3] positron emission tomography (PET),[4] and echocardiography.[5] More recently, cardiovascular magnetic resonance (CMR) has gained widespread acceptance as a technique to identify viable myocardium and distinguish it from myocardial necrosis and scar.[6–9] This chapter reviews the current knowledge of how these techniques can be used in humans to guide clinical decision making and predict recovery of function after revascularization of dysfunctional myocardium.

All scientific papers on the value of imaging techniques for detecting myocardial viability use the well-known statistical terms of sensitivity, specificity, and the predictive values. The sensitivity of a test is commonly defined as the number of true positives divided by the sum of true positives and false negatives. In other words, the sensitivity of a test is the number of diseased persons with a positive test divided by the total number of diseased persons. Common sense might suggest that scar tissue and, hence, absence of viability might indicate the presence of disease. The total number of diseased people or segments would thus be the number of people with scar or segments without recovery of function. The presence of viability would be synonymous with a healthy state (relatively speaking), and the total number of viable, healthy people or segments would appear as the denominator in the formula for calculating specificity. In the viability literature, however, sensitivity indicates the ability of a test to identify viable myocardium, and specificity is an indicator of how well the test performs when it comes to detecting scar. Positive and negative predictive values are used accordingly. This needs to be borne in mind when it comes to the interpretation of test results reported later in this chapter.

FEATURES OF VIABLE MYOCARDIUM DETECTABLE BY CARDIOVASCULAR MAGNETIC RESONANCE

Scar Formation and Left Ventricular Wall Thickness

Myocardium is commonly defined as viable if it shows severe dysfunction at baseline but recovers function with time either spontaneously (myocardial stunning) or following revascularization (hibernating myocardium).[10,11] Clinically, stunned myocardium may be found in patients with early reperfusion of an infarct-related artery. If there is no residual high-grade stenosis, blood flow at rest will be normal and the myocardium will recover spontaneously after a few days. Patients with hibernating myocardium often present with severe triple vessel disease, globally depressed LV function, and prominent dyspnea but

often surprisingly little angina. This type of dysfunction is often more chronic, and previous myocardial infarction may or may not be reported in the history. Pathology may reveal regions of transmural scar, regions with predominantly subendocardial scar, and regions with mixtures of scar and viable myocardium.

Severe wall thinning is the hallmark of transmural chronic myocardial infarction. However, wall thinning is the end result of infarct healing, and it may take up to 4 months before the remodeling process is completed. In contrast to the severe thinning of chronic transmural scar, the best example for which is the thin-walled anterior LV aneurysm, acute and subacute transmural infarcts may not yet have reached the stage of thinning because local infarct remodeling is incomplete.[12] In contrast with transmural myocardial infarction, which may or may not appear thinned, depending on infarct age, healed nontransmural infarcts usually do not develop severe thinning. Some thinning may be observed, however, depending on the degree to which the endocardially located infarct extends throughout the wall. Therefore the finding of preserved myocardial wall thickness in diastole in a patient with a known chronic infarct that is more than 4 months old will likely represent nontransmural infarction with a substantial rim of viable myocardium surrounding the endocardial scar. If the infarct is more recent than approximately 4 months, preserved end-diastolic wall thickness cannot be used to distinguish between viable and nonviable myocardium.

Patients with small subendocardial infarcts may, however, also present with regional wall thinning despite the presence of substantial amounts (>50% of wall thickness) of viable myocardium.[13,14] In a case described by Kim and Shah,[13] diastolic thickness of the anterior wall on a long-axis late gadolinium enhancement (LGE) CMR image measured only 5 mm. However, the subendocardial rim of scar was only 1.5 mm of total wall thickness, indicating the presence of substantial amounts of viable myocardium. Indeed, recovery of the myocardium occurred following revascularization. Shah et al.[14] systematically looked at more than 1000 consecutive patients who had LGE CMR for viability assessment and found that 19% of them had regional wall thinning. Within these regions, the extent of scarring was 72%. However, 18% of thinned regions had only limited scar burden (≤50% of total extent). Among patients with thinning undergoing revascularization and follow-up cine CMR (*n* = 42), scar extent within the thinned region was inversely related to regional and global contractile improvement. End-diastolic wall thickness in thinned regions with limited scar burden increased from 4.4 mm to 7.5 mm after revascularization (*P* < .001) with resolution of wall thinning (Fig. 21.1). Thus regional wall thinning may be possible in myocardium that has only little subendocardial scarring probably because of ventricular remodeling, and full recovery of function may occur following revascularization. The ratio of viable to total myocardium (viable plus nonviable) irrespective of wall thickness in the dysfunctional region may therefore be more

Before revascularization CMR

After revascularization

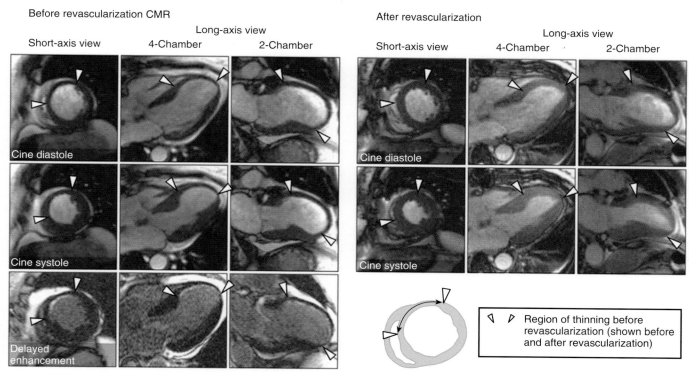

FIG. 21.1 A patient with subendocardial scar and regional akinesia and wall thinning. *Left*, Before revascularization, cine-cardiovascular magnetic resonance *(CMR)* still frames in systole and diastole demonstrate akinesis and thinning of the anteroseptal, anterior, and apical walls. Delayed-enhancement images demonstrate limited scar burden (≤50%) within the thinned region. *Right*, After revascularization, cine-CMR still frames demonstrate improvement in myocardial contractility along with reversal of thinning in the previously thinned region. End-diastolic wall thickness changed from 4.5 to 9.5 mm after revascularization. (Modified from Shah DJ, Kim HW, James O, et al. Prevalence of regional myocardial thinning and relationship with myocardial scarring in patients with coronary artery disease. *JAMA.* 2013;309:909–918.)

accurate than end-diastolic wall thickness in predicting functional improvement.

Contractile Reserve of Viable Myocardium

A well-known feature of viable myocardium is augmented contractility in response to a suitable stimulus.[11] Such stimuli include sympathomimetic agents[5] or postextrasystolic potentiation.[2] In contrast, necrotic or scarred tissue will not respond to such stimulation. Today, the most widely used mode of stimulation is to infuse low doses of dobutamine up to 10 µg/kg/min. If a contractile reserve can be elicited, the responsive myocardium will usually recover function after appropriate revascularization.[15] However, it appears that there is also some spontaneous improvement in the response to dobutamine over the course of infarct healing after reperfused myocardial infarction, which may affect the accuracy of this viability marker after myocardial infarction.[12]

Noninvasive Observation of Tissue Edema

Irreversible myocardial damage occurs after approximately 30 to 120 minutes of ischemia. Very early changes can be observed by electron microscopy; these changes include intracellular edema and swelling of the entire cell, including the mitochondria. The sarcolemma ruptures, and there is free exchange between the extracellular and intracellular compartments. In some infarcts, light microscopy reveals changes just a few hours after the onset of ischemia; these changes are most pronounced at the periphery of the infarct. After 8 hours, there is edema of the interstitium, and infiltration of the infarct zone by neutrophils

and red blood cells becomes evident. Small blood vessels undergo necrosis, and karyolysis of muscle cell nuclei can be observed. Plugging of capillaries by erythrocytes is most pronounced in the center of the infarct. If reperfusion can be achieved at an early stage, the resulting infarcts contain a mixture of necrosis and hemorrhage within zones of irreversibly injured myocytes.

Myocardial edema is associated with prolonged magnetic resonance (MR) relaxation times, and this leads to characteristically increased signal intensity on MR images, which are sensitive to such changes.[16] By using modern T2-weighted pulse sequences, the edema associated with acute infarcts can be depicted, and this can be used to differentiate between acute and chronic infarcts.[17]

No-Reflow Phenomenon and Early Hypoenhancement With Gadolinium

A feature of the central necrotic region within a myocardial infarct is intracapillary red blood cell stasis.[18] Plugging of the capillaries leads to tissue hypoperfusion. This hypoperfusion is primarily related to the resulting reduced functional capillary density rather than reduced microvascular flow rates.[19] This decrease in functional capillary density results in a prolonged washin time constant. This lack of reperfusion despite restoration of flow in the epicardial vessel is known as the *no-reflow phenomenon*. When the myocardium is imaged by CMR early after injection with gadolinium (early gadolinium enhancement), no-reflow zones appear dark in comparison with the surrounding rim regions of the infarct.[20]

Late Gadolinium Enhancement in Infarcted Tissue

Gadolinium chelates are commonly used as CMR contrast agents. These metabolically inert molecules are distributed extracellularly, and they shorten both T1 and T2 relaxation times. Rupture of myocyte membranes leads to an increased volume of distribution of CMR contrast agents with a corresponding increase in the effective voxel concentration of such agents.[21,22] Thus a higher concentration of gadolinium contrast agents leads to a more pronounced shortening of relaxation times. CMR images are usually T1 weighted (because the RR interval is approximately 800 ms, which corresponds to the T1 value of myocardium), and this will result in a higher signal intensity of infarcted as compared with normal tissue once the contrast material has fully penetrated the infarct region. The time–concentration curve of MR contrast agents in infarct tissue does not correspond to that in blood or normal tissue kinetics. Thus, while early hypoenhancement of infarcted regions after injection of contrast material is caused by delayed contrast penetration,[19] late enhancement in infarction is due to both increased volume of distribution and slow contrast washout. The enhancement pattern that is seen will depend on regional differences in tissue washin/washout kinetics, as well as the time after injection of contrast when the image is acquired. LGE has now been extensively validated in animal and human studies, and with improved imaging sequences (notably the use of inversion recovery to null signal from normal myocardium), the signal-to-noise ratio of enhanced to unenhanced tissue is dramatically higher than with previous sequences, at approximately 500%. This has led to greatly improved image quality and a substantial increase in use of the technique. In animal experiments, the area of LGE has been shown to correlate closely with areas of infarction,[23] and for the first time in vivo, high-quality imaging of the distribution of scar is possible.

High-Energy Phosphates and Viability

The primary energy reserve in living myocardial cells is stored in the form of creatine phosphate and adenosine triphosphate (ATP). Depletion of total myocardial creatine, creatine phosphate, and ATP follows severe ischemic injury, as shown in biopsy samples obtained from patients during cardiac surgery or necropsy. Using ^{31}P magnetic resonance spectroscopy (MRS), it is possible to measure the myocardial content of phosphocreatine and ATP.[24] ^1H-MRS has a higher sensitivity than ^{31}P-MRS and has the ability to detect the total pool of phosphorylated plus unphosphorylated creatine in skeletal and cardiac muscle.[25] MRS is currently not used clinically and is not discussed further in this chapter.

CARDIOVASCULAR MAGNETIC RESONANCE TO DETECT VIABLE MYOCARDIUM IN ACUTE MYOCARDIAL INFARCTION

Signal Intensity Changes on T2-Weighted Images

Myocardial edema accompanies acute myocardial necrosis. On T2-weighted spin echo images, the increased water content leads to an increase in signal intensity.[26] T2-weighted spin echo images acquired early after myocardial infarction (within 10 days) demonstrate that the infarct site is a region of high signal intensity in comparison with normal myocardium.[27] The advent of modern rapid pulse sequences, which produce a higher contrast between edematous and normal myocardium, has led to some revival of T2-weighted CMR.[28]

However, it is important to keep in mind that there are several potential pitfalls to the acquisition and interpretation of T2-weighted images, including the necessity to differentiate the signal from slowly flowing blood in the ventricle from increased signal intensity from a region of infarction and to recognize artifactual variation of signal intensity in the myocardium because of respiratory motion or residual cardiac motion. Thus careful optimization of all imaging parameters is required for achieving interpretable results during T2-weighted image acquisition (Fig. 21.2).

Late Enhancement With Gadolinium in Acute Infarction

In the mid and late 1990s, Kim and Judd developed late enhancement imaging.[19,23] Within a short time, LGE CMR became widely used because of its high image quality, simplicity, and high resolution allowing clear demarcation of the transmural extent of necrosis and scar. The T1-weighted segmented inversion recovery pulse sequence that is employed in most centers acquires images in mid diastole when cardiac motion is minimal (Fig. 21.3).[29] Segmentation of k-space makes it possible to acquire images during a breath-hold, which reduces motion artifacts as compared with the older T1-weighted techniques. With the appropriate choice of the inversion time and imaging 10 to 20 minutes after the intravenous application of contrast material, the signal intensity of normal myocardium is nulled but the infarcted tissue becomes very bright (Fig. 21.4). Kim and colleagues[23] clearly demonstrated that this technique provides precise images of acute and subacute infarcts irrespective of transmurality and reperfusion status (Fig. 21.5).

The time between contrast injection and starting the imaging process is important, as contrast concentration and hence enhancement of a region vary over time. Normal regions with normal contrast washin and washout reach a constant enhancement within 2 to 3 minutes.[19] The border zones of an infarct, however, have longer time constants for washin and washout as compared with normal, and these time constants are even longer in the center of the infarct (see later). Consequently, both core and border zone of the infarct appear dark during the early phase of contrast washin (Fig. 21.6). Later, core and normal myocardium have similar signal intensities, but the border zone begins showing some enhancement. When contrast washout begins in normal myocardium at about 10 minutes after injection, core and border zones of the infarct are enhanced, and this persists in the core of the infarct at late stages of contrast washout. At this time, the border zones have already returned to near-normal signal intensities.

There has been debate about whether LGE occurs exclusively in regions with myocardial necrosis or also in edematous viable border zones around infarcted areas. However, the observation by Saeed and colleagues[30] that the Gd-DTPA-enhanced region overestimates true infarct size by approximately 8% was not supported by other animal studies.[31] Fieno and colleagues[32] compared ex vivo CMR with triphenyltetrazolium chloride–stained sections and confirmed that the spatial extent of enhancement was the same as the spatial extent of infarction at every stage of healing from day 1 to 8 weeks. The ischemic area at risk was defined by fluorescent microparticles injected into the left atrium with the infarct-related artery occluded. Enhanced regions were smaller than the ischemic area at risk at every stage of healing (Fig. 21.7). Image intensities of viable myocardium within the risk region were the same as those of remote, normal myocardium. A possible explanation for the discrepant findings of Saeed and colleagues and the group of Kim and Judd is that Saeed and colleagues used a different pulse sequence than that found to be highly and reproducibly accurate for infarct sizing.

It is important to note that accurate infarct imaging requires constant adjustment of the TI if imaging cannot be completed within 5 minutes. This is necessary because the null point of normal myocardium depends on the concentration of the contrast agent at any given point in time. As contrast washout from normal myocardium occurs at a comparatively rapid pace, TI increases continuously, necessitating corresponding increases of TI to achieve perfect nulling of normal myocardium. Typical TI values range from 310 ms at 10 minutes to 385 ms at 30 minutes

Black-Blood T2-Weighted MRI: Procedure for Optimizing Image Timing

Step 1: At the same short-axis location, acquire multiple images in 50 ms increments throughout diastole.

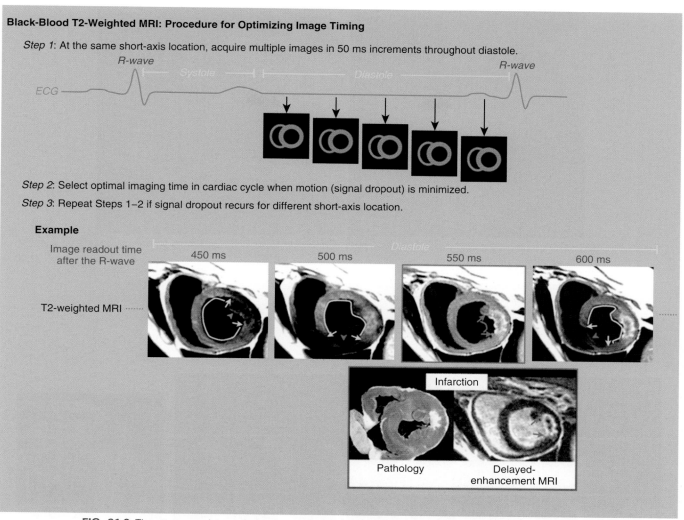

Step 2: Select optimal imaging time in cardiac cycle when motion (signal dropout) is minimized.

Step 3: Repeat Steps 1–2 if signal dropout recurs for different short-axis location.

FIG. 21.2 The steps used to optimize image timing for black-blood T2-weighted cardiovascular magnetic resonance (CMR). This involved choosing a midventricular short-axis slice, obtaining test images throughout diastole, and inspecting the images to determine the best timing of readout based on the absence of signal loss (dropout) artifact. Signal loss was determined visually and defined as a myocardial region with obviously reduced signal on one but no other test images. Example images from one subject demonstrate that small changes in timing (≈50 ms) can affect the presence and location of dropout artifact *(green arrowhead)*. Note that when dropout artifact is present, the remaining myocardium appears hyperintense *(yellow arc)*, which could confound interpretation. This usually leads to overestimation of T2-abnormality size because dropout typically affects only a fraction (<50%) of the myocardium in the slice. The image with optimal timing *(red box)* demonstrates no region with dropout and an obvious area of hyperintensity *(red arc)* in the region of acute infarction as demonstrated by pathology and in vivo late enhancement CMR *(red arrows)*. ECG, Electrocardiogram; *MRI*, magnetic resonance imaging. (From Kim HW, Van Assche L, Jennings RB, et al. Relationship of T2-weighted MRI myocardial hyperintensity and the ischemic area-at-risk. *Circ Res.* 2015;117:254–265.)

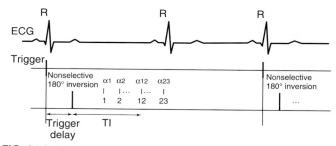

FIG. 21.3 Segmented inversion recovery fast gradient echo sequence with TI set to null normal myocardium after contrast agent administration. *ECG,* Electrocardiogram. (From Simonetti OP, Kim RJ, Fieno DS, et al. An improved MR imaging technique for the visualization of myocardial infarction. *Radiology.* 2001;218:215–223.)

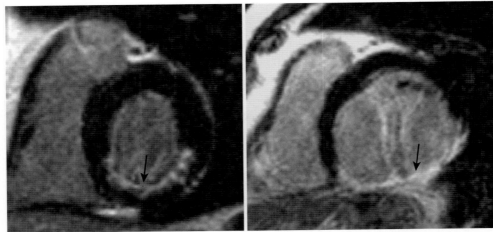

FIG. 21.4 Nontransmural inferior myocardial infarct *(left panel)*. This patient presented with acute onset of ST-elevation myocardial infarction and was revascularized by catheterization approximately 120 minutes after first onset of symptoms. Note the preserved wall thickness *(arrow)* in the region with subendocardial late gadolinium enhancement. The transmural inferolateral myocardial infarct displayed in the right panel is several months old. Note the thinning *(arrow)* of the infarcted area, which is considered to be a hallmark of transmural infarcts.

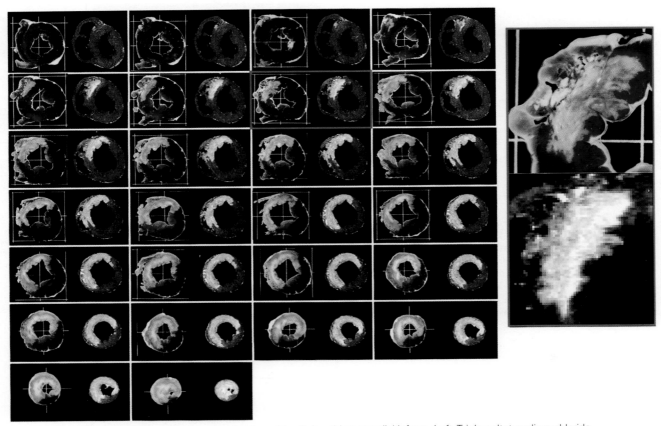

FIG. 21.5 Postmortem images of a dog with a 3-day-old myocardial infarct. *Left,* Triphenyltetrazolium chloride (TTC)-stained slices of the left ventricle showing the infarct as nonstained white areas, whereas normal myocardial cells stain red. Slices are arranged from base to apex, starting in the upper left and advancing from left to right and then from top to bottom. *Right,* Insert showing a magnification. There is excellent matching of the enhanced areas in the ex vivo magnetic resonance images with the necrotic zones in the necropsy slices. (From Kim RJ, Fieno DS, Parrish TB, et al. Relationship of MRI delayed contrast enhancement to irreversible injury, infarct age, and contractile function. *Circulation.* 1999;100[19]:1992–2002.)

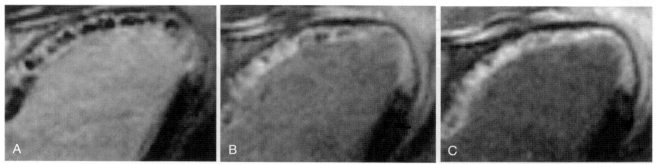

FIG. 21.6 Temporal changes in signal intensity after 0.2 mmol/kg gadolinium-diethylenetriaminepentaacetic acid was administered intravenously in a patient after primary percutaneous transluminal coronary angioplasty plus stenting of the left anterior descending coronary artery for anterior myocardial infarction. Magnified three-chamber view at 2 minutes (A), 15 minutes (B), and 30 minutes (C). (From Beek AM, Kühl HP, Bondarenko O, et al. Delayed contrast-enhanced magnetic resonance imaging for the prediction of regional functional improvement after acute myocardial infarction. *J Am Coll Cardiol.* 2003;42[5]:895–901.)

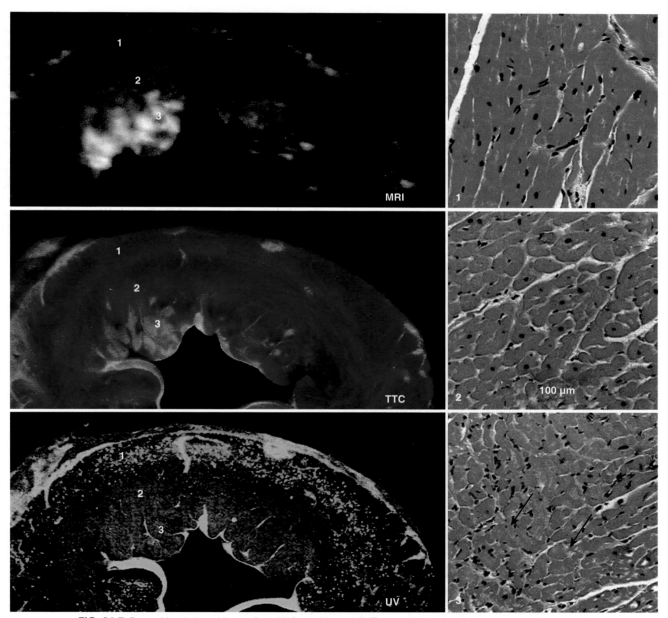

FIG. 21.7 Dog with a 1-day-old reperfused infarct. *Upper left,* The ex vivo magnetic resonance enhancement image. *Middle left,* The matching triphenyltetrazolium chloride *(TTC)*-stained myocardial slice. *Bottom left,* The myocardium at risk as the blue-appearing region without fluorescent microparticles. *Right,* Light microscopy views of region 1 (not at risk, not infarcted), region 2 (at risk but not infarcted), and region 3 (infarcted). Arrows point to contraction bands. *MRI,* Magnetic resonance imaging; *UV,* ultraviolet. (From Fieno DS, Kim RJ, Chen EL, et al. Contrast-enhanced magnetic resonance imaging of myocardium at risk: distinction between reversible and irreversible injury throughout infarct healing. *J Am Coll Cardiol.* 2000;36[6]:1985–1991.)

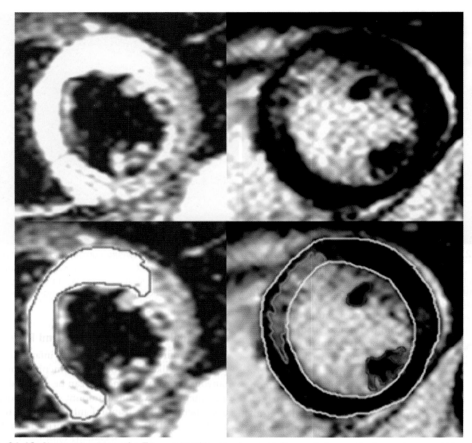

FIG. 21.12 Short-axis slices of a T2-weighted image *(upper left panel)* demonstrating edema contours *(red, lower left panel)*, which are speculated to represent the ischemic area risk, and the corresponding late enhancement image *(upper right panel)* with endocardial *(green)*, epicardial *(yellow)*, papillary *(dark blue)*, and infarcted *(red)* contours *(lower right panel)* in a patient with anterior myocardial infarction. The suspected myocardial salvage was calculated from the ischemic area at risk on T2-weighted images minus infarct area on late enhancement images. (From Eitel I, Desch S, Fuernau G, et al. Prognostic significance and determinants of myocardial salvage assessed by cardiovascular magnetic resonance in acute reperfused myocardial infarction. *J Am Coll Cardiol.* 2010;55:2470–2479.)

intensity zone on T2-weighted images is related to the ischemic area at risk measured by microspheres in an animal model as the gold standard. Whalen et al.[47] reported that there is an increase in tissue water of about 88% in myocardial regions that are completely infarcted (postmortem data). In contrast, Jennings et al.[48] found an increase of tissue water of only 9% in reversibly injured myocardium which persisted for less than 24 hours after reperfusion.

Based on the data from Whalen and Jennings, there is at least a 9-fold difference in tissue water content between reversibly and irreversibly injured myocardium, casting serious doubt that there is any pathophysiologic basis for the quantification of the area at risk, or the salvaged area using T2-weighted imaging. These doubts are supported by experimental data from the Duke group,[49] who recently studied 21 canines and 24 patients to determine whether T2-weighted images delineate the area at risk. Matching the pathophysiology described by Whalen and Jennings, they found no relationship between the transmural extent of T2-intense regions and that of the ischemic area at risk ($P = .97$) because the tissue water content of reversibly injured myocardium is only increased by 9% for less than 24 hours after the acute event. Instead, there was a strong correlation with that of infarction ($P < .0001$) because tissue water content in infarcted myocardium is increased by 88%. There was a fingerprint match of T2-intense regions with the intricate contour of infarcted regions by late enhancement and pathology (Fig. 21.13).

Thus based on the pathophysiology and the recent results from the Duke group, T2-weighted imaging should not be used to measure myocardial salvage, either to inform patient management decisions, or to evaluate novel therapies for acute myocardial infarction. The earlier reports of other groups[45,46] (see also Fig. 21.12), which are not in line with the pathophysiology and the recent gold standard animal data from Duke described above, are most likely explained by the frequent pitfalls in the acquisition and interpretation of T2-weighted images (see also Fig. 21.2). In the future new T2-weighted mapping techniques may overcome the limitations of conventional T2-weighted imaging described earlier.[50]

Wall Thickness and Wall Thickening Measurements

After an acute ischemic event, structural changes occur within the infarct zone, and infarct healing with scar formation is completed by approximately 3 to 4 months.[51] Thinning of the infarct region may occur early, especially in large anterior myocardial infarcts, but transient thickening of the infarcted segment because of edema[52] has also been observed. The consequence of infarct thinning is an increase in the size of the infarcted segment, known as infarct expansion.[53] However, even in transmural infarcts, infarct expansion may not occur in patients with open infarct-related arteries. Such patients are encountered more often today with the widespread use of thrombolysis and

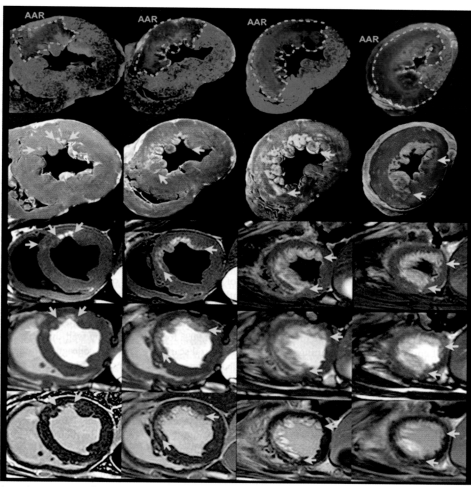

FIG. 21.13 A comparison between cardiovascular magnetic resonance (CMR) and pathology at multiple short-axis level in one subject with substantial salvage. The area at risk *(AAR)* by histopathology *(top row, orange outline)* is nearly 100% transmural at every short-axis location, whereas T2 intense *(third and fourth rows)* and infarcted regions *(second and bottom row)* are clearly nontransmural *(yellow arrows)*. The most basal slice shows a particularly large discrepancy between the full-thickness AAR and the region of infarction, which is tiny and subendocardial. For all slices, T2 intense regions closely resemble the shape of infarction, not the AAR. *MI,* Myocardial infarction; *MRI,* magnetic resonance imaging; *TTC,* triphenyltetrazolium chloride. (From Kim HW et al. Relationship of T2-weighted MRI myocardial hyperintensity and the ischemic area-at-risk. *Circ Res.* 2015;117:254–265.)

angioplasty of the infarct artery.[54] Therefore transmural necrosis and nontransmural necrosis may have the same wall thickness early after myocardial infarction. Both conditions may also be associated with complete absence of resting function early after the acute event. However, it should be remembered that even a small amount of wall thickening in a region of interest indicates the presence of residual contracting cells and hence of viable myocardium.

CARDIOVASCULAR MAGNETIC RESONANCE IN CHRONIC MYOCARDIAL INFARCTION

As previously discussed, chronic myocardial infarcts are structurally different from acute myocardial infarcts. The most obvious difference is that chronic transmural infarcts may be very thin, owing to infarct expansion and remodeling.[55] Consequently, this feature can be detected by CMR and can be used to distinguish between chronic transmural scar and residual viable myocardium in the infarct area. However, caution must be used when observing a small area of pronounced wall thinning

in order to not assume that the entire region perfused by an occluded coronary artery is completely scarred. Frequently, myocardial cells in the border zone survive, and ischemia of this border zone alone may cause substantial symptoms in a patient. Moreover, wall thinning may also occur in some patients who only have thin subendocardial scar yet show substantial end-diastolic wall thinning in a region of severely reduced wall motion. Therefore in a patient with single-vessel disease, previous myocardial infarction, and anginal symptoms, restoration of blood flow by re-establishing patency of the occluded artery may be justified in the presence of ischemia to improve symptoms, despite evidence of substantial wall thinning of the infarct zone.

Myocardial Wall Thickness as a Feature of Viable Myocardium

The hypothesis that thinned and akinetic myocardium usually[14] represents chronic scar has been tested by comparing CMR findings with those obtained by PET and single-photon emission computed tomography (SPECT) in identical myocardial regions.[56,57] Comparison of CMR

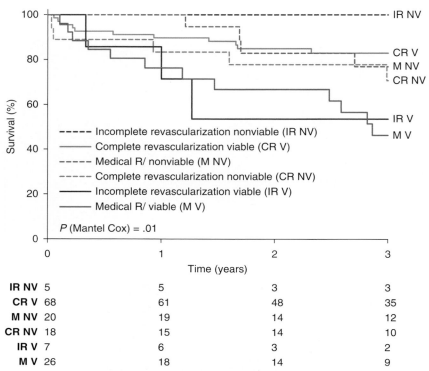

IR NV 5	5	3	3
CR V 68	61	48	35
M NV 20	19	14	12
CR NV 18	15	14	10
IR V 7	6	3	2
M V 26	18	14	9

FIG. 21.18 Kaplan-Meier survival curves comparing overall 3-year survival in subgroups of patients according to treatment and presence of myocardial viability in dysfunctional myocardium. Survival was significantly worse in patients with dysfunctional viable myocardium remaining under medical treatment or undergoing incomplete revascularization not including dysfunctional myocardium than in other subgroups. *CR,* Complete revascularization; *IR,* incomplete revascularization not including dysfunctional region; *M,* medical treatment; *NV,* nonviable myocardium; *R/,* remaining under medical treatment; *V,* viable myocardium. (From Gerber B, Rousseau MF, Ahn SA, et al. Prognostic value of myocardial viability by delayed-enhanced magnetic resonance in patients with coronary artery disease and low ejection fraction—impact of revascularization therapy. *J Am Coll Cardiol.* 2012;59:825–835, with permission of the publisher.)

Klein and colleagues[75] found that the area of LGE measured by CMR correlated closely with myocardial infarcts defined by PET in patients with ischemic cardiomyopathy, but CMR showed the extent of infarct transmurality more clearly (Fig. 21.21).

Comparison of Different Cardiovascular Magnetic Resonance Techniques for the Diagnosis of Viability

Wellnhofer and colleagues[76] compared LGE CMR with dobutamine CMR (5 and 10 μg/kg/min) for assessment of myocardial viability. Both techniques were performed in 29 patients with chronic CAD and resting LV dysfunction (mean LVEF, 32% ± 8%). Cine CMR imaging at rest was repeated 3 months after revascularization to determine wall motion improvement. The transmurality of LGE was assessed visually, using a five-grade scale. Similarly, wall motion was assessed visually. Using a cutoff value of 25% transmurality of LGE, the authors found that contrast-enhanced CMR correctly identified 73% of hibernating segments, but dobutamine CMR was better and identified 85% correctly. The results for sensitivity and specificity of Wellnhofer and colleagues for dobutamine CMR are slightly worse that those reported by Baer and associates,[57] whose patient group had a higher EF (42 ± 16%). However, the sensitivity found by Wellnhofer and colleagues for scar transmurality less than 50% is much better than the 50% found by Gunning and colleagues,[77] who studied a patient group with more severely depressed LV function (mean LVEF, 24% ± 8%). In contrast, the sensitivity of dobutamine CMR in the Wellnhofer study dropped sharply to values below 60% in segments with a scar transmurality of

50% or more. Thus in severely impaired ventricles, low-dose dobutamine CMR has a suboptimal sensitivity but a preserved high specificity at around 90%. This has been known from studies using dobutamine echocardiography in which similar low sensitivity values of 50% or less were reported. The lower sensitivity of dobutamine echocardiography in detecting viable myocardium in regions with reduced function and perfusion may indicate that some regions of hibernating myocardium have such delicately balanced reductions in flow and function, with exhausted coronary flow reserve, that any catecholamine stimulation to increase oxygen demands will merely result in ischemia and inability to elicit enhanced contractile function.[78] However, it is just the patients with global severe depression of function in whom viability testing is clinically most meaningful. In such patients, it has been demonstrated that LGE CMR predicts improvement in severely dysfunctional segments.[79] In an editorial accompanying the paper by Wellnhofer and colleagues, Kim and Manning[80] comment that contractile reserve has a reduced predictive accuracy if more severe dysfunction is present at rest. In this most important subgroup of patients, LGE CMR appears to have a higher accuracy than dobutamine CMR. From a practical point of view, LGE CMR has the additional advantage in that it does not require pharmacologic stress and thus involves less risk and subsequently less monitoring of the patient. Furthermore, it is likely easier and less observer dependent for interpretation.

Dobutamine and LGE CMR can also be used as complementary techniques to make the diagnosis of viability. Kaandorp and associates[81] studied 48 patients with chronic coronary artery disease and a mean

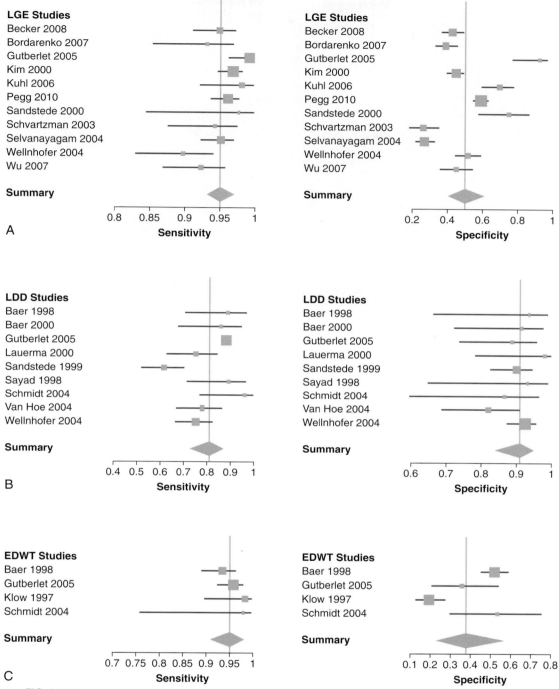

FIG. 21.19 Forest plots of sensitivity and specificity from 24 prospective cardiovascular magnetic resonance studies evaluating myocardial viability. Eleven studies used late gadolinium enhancement *(LGE)* (A), nine studies used low-dose dobutamine *(LDD)* (B), and four studies used end-diastolic wall thickness *(EDWT)* (C) as viability parameters. The size of the square plotting symbol is proportional to the same size for each study. Horizontal lines are the 95% confidence intervals, and the summary sensitivity and specificity are calculated based on the bivariate approach. (From Romero J, Xue X, Gonzalez W, Garcia MJ. CMR imaging assessing viability in patients with chronic ventricular dysfunction due to coronary artery disease. *JACC Cardiovasc Imaging.* 2012;5:494–508, with permission.)

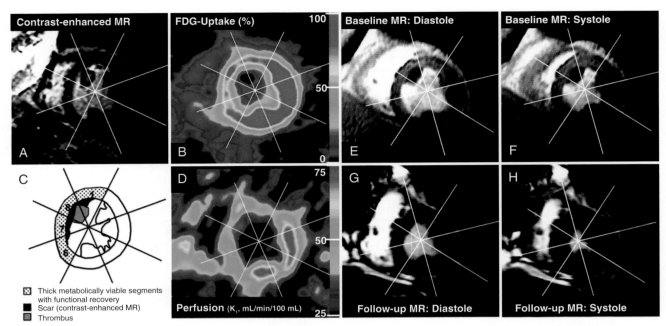

FIG. 21.20 A 59-year-old patient 5 months after an anteroseptal myocardial infarction. Contrast-enhanced magnetic resonance *(MR)* (A) shows a small subendocardial zone of scar *(bright)* with adjacent thrombus *(black,* segment 8). A thick rim of viable tissue is observed (segments 1 and 6 through 8 in A) that corresponds to segments with preserved ^{18}F-fluorodeoxyglucose *(FDG)* uptake (B), whereas perfusion in these segments is reduced (D). A schematic in C illustrates this situation, with segments 1 and 6 through 8 consisting of metabolically viable segments with a thick rim of viable tissue on MR. Contractile function is severely reduced in these segments before revascularization (E and F), but has normalized 9 months after coronary artery graft bypass surgery (G and H). (From Knuesel PR, Nanz D, Wyss C, et al. Characterization of dysfunctional myocardium by positron emission tomography and magnetic resonance: relation to functional outcome after revascularization. *Circulation.* 2003;108[9]:1095–1100.)

ejection fraction of 37% ± 10%. Regional dysfunction was present in 41% of segments, and 61% of those had contractile reserve. The likelihood of a contractile improvement with dobutamine was highest (75%) in segments with small amounts of subendocardial scar, lowest (17%) in those with transmural scar, but intermediate (42%) in segments with intermediate infarct transmurality. The authors suggest an approach where LGE CMR is sufficient at both extreme ends but dobutamine CMR should be added to optimally predict outcome in segments with intermediate amounts of scar transmurality.

Viability Testing After Surgical Treatment for Ischemic Heart Failure Trial

Despite promising data pointing to substantial value of LGE CMR for predicting recovery of chronically dysfunctional myocardium, the recent STICH trial employed only SPECT imaging or dobutamine echocardiography for preoperative viability assessment. The STICH study randomized 1212 patients with an ejection fraction of less than 35% and coronary artery disease suitable for CABG to receive optimal medical therapy for heart failure and coronary artery disease (602 patients) or optimal medical therapy plus CABG (610 patients). Only 601 of the 1212 patients underwent assessment of myocardial viability.[82] Of these, 298 received medical therapy plus CABG and 303 received medical therapy alone—yet the decision to perform viability testing was not randomized and treatment was not assigned in a randomized fashion based on viability status. Over a median follow-up of 5.1 years, 178 of 487 (37%) patients with viable myocardium and 58 of 140 patients without viable myocardium (41%) died. The hazard ratio for death

among patients with viable myocardium was 0.64 (*P* = .003) (Fig. 21.22). However, after adjustment for other baseline variables, this significant association with mortality was no longer significant. Hence there was no significant interaction between viability status and treatment assignment with respect to mortality (Fig. 21.23).

The viability substudy of STICH has been criticized for several methodologic problems.[83] First, there were significant baseline differences between the patient groups that did and did not undergo viability testing. Second, 81% of patients undergoing viability testing showed viability, which is much higher than in previous studies where only about 50% of patients demonstrated significant myocardial viability. Thus it is conceivable that the patients enrolled in the STICH trial represented a different population from previous viability studies and that this fact may have influenced the results, which contradicted the results of these earlier studies. Third, unusual viability criteria were employed in the STICH trial. These criteria were rather conservative, which makes it more surprising that such a high percentage of patients demonstrated significant viability. For dobutamine echocardiography, ≥5 dysfunctional segments with evidence of contractile reserve were required. For SPECT, ≥11 viable segments (irrespective of baseline contractility) had to be present. Using two different imaging methods that had different definitions of viability further disturbs the homogeneity of the two groups of patients defined as having viable myocardium or absence of viability. Thus one would expect to find different patients in groups defined by these criteria than in groups defined by traditional viability criteria. Again, this may have influenced the surprising results. However, when the data of the STICH viability substudy were separately

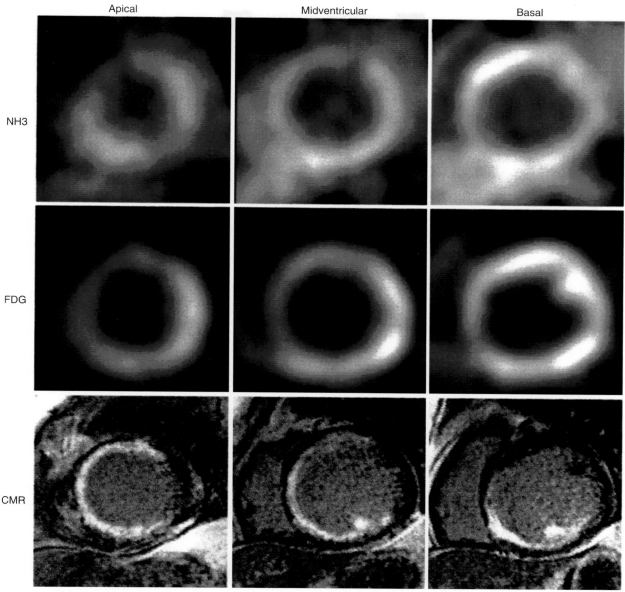

FIG. 21.21 Three short-axis views (apical, equatorial, and basal) of a positron emission tomography viability study with assessment of rest perfusion *(NH3; top)* and glucose metabolism *(FDG; middle)*. *Bottom,* Cardiovascular magnetic resonance *(CMR)* images in corresponding slices show enhancement. Note that in segments with reduced perfusion and metabolism, there is an increased CMR signal. Because of better spatial resolution in CMR, distinction between transmural, subendocardial, and papillary defects can be made. The border between enhanced and normal areas is distinct. (From Klein C, Nekolla SG, Bengel FM, et al. Assessment of myocardial viability with contrast-enhanced magnetic resonance imaging: comparison with positron emission tomography. *Circulation.* 2002;105[2]:162–167.)

analyzed for the dobutamine echocardiography and SPECT cohorts, the results remained the same.[84] Fourth, almost 20% of patients had LVEF >35% when images were reanalyzed at the core laboratory. A higher LVEF would reduce the potential for improvement with revascularization. However, EFs in most previous studies were higher than in STICH.[70,85] Fifth, there was a large imbalance in clinical variables in each of the viability groups, which led to equalization of results after statistical correction for these imbalances. Sixth, it is unclear whether patients receiving revascularization had complete revascularization of viable tissue.

It has been debated whether different imaging techniques with higher sensitivities and specificities such as PET or CMR could have altered the results.[83,86] For practical reasons, these techniques could not be employed in such a large multicenter study, which was performed in 127 sites in 26 countries. Moreover, it is likely that the definitions employed and the advances of medical therapy since the time of the early viability studies influenced the unexpected results more than the choice of the imaging techniques. This is reflected in the considerably lower mortality rates of patients with viable myocardium treated medically in the STICH trial than in a previous metaanalysis.[70] Thus the

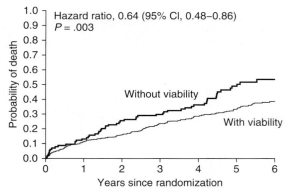

No. at risk

Without viability	114	99	85	80	63	36	16
With viability	487	432	409	371	294	188	102

FIG. 21.22 Kaplan-Meier analysis of the probability of death, according to myocardial viability status. The comparison that is shown has not been adjusted for other prognostic baseline variables. After adjustment for such variables on multivariable analysis, the between-group difference was not significant (*P* = .21). *CI*, Confidence interval. (From Bonow RO, Maurer G, Lee KL, et al. Myocardial viability and survival in ischemic left ventricular dysfunction. *N Engl J Med.* 2011;364:1617–1625, with permission of the publisher.)

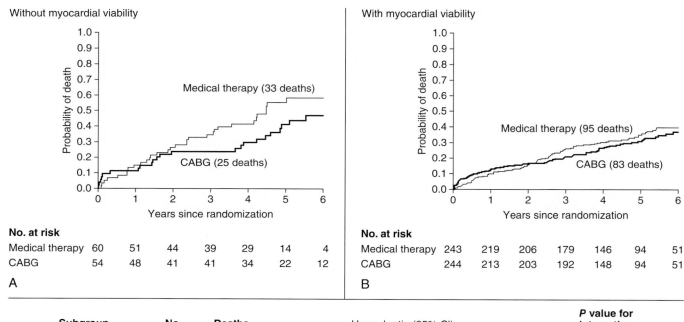

No. at risk (A)

Medical therapy	60	51	44	39	29	14	4
CABG	54	48	41	41	34	22	12

No. at risk (B)

Medical therapy	243	219	206	179	146	94	51
CABG	244	213	203	192	148	94	51

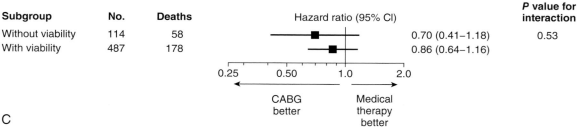

Subgroup	No.	Deaths	Hazard ratio (95% CI)		P value for interaction
Without viability	114	58		0.70 (0.41–1.18)	0.53
With viability	487	178		0.86 (0.64–1.16)	

CABG better — Medical therapy better

FIG. 21.23 Kaplan-Meier analysis of the probability of death according to myocardial viability status and treatment. At 5 years in the intention-to-treat analysis, the rates of death for patients without myocardial viability were 41.5% in the group assigned to undergo coronary artery bypass grafting *(CABG)* and 55.8% in the group assigned to receive medical therapy (A). Among patients with myocardial viability, the respective rates were 31.2% and 35.4% (B). There was no significant interaction between viability status and treatment assignment with respect to mortality (*P* = .53) (C). *CI*, Confidence interval. (From Bonow RO, Maurer G, Lee KL, et al. Myocardial viability and survival in ischemic left ventricular dysfunction. *N Engl J Med.* 2011;364:1617–1625, with permission of the publisher.)

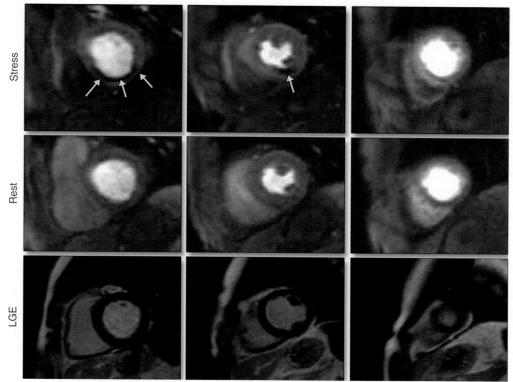

FIG. 21.24 Adenosine stress perfusion images *(top)* show the presence of a subendocardial inducible defect in the basal and mid-cavity inferior wall *(arrows)*, not present at rest *(middle)*. Late gadolinium enhancement *(LGE)* images demonstrate a viable inferior wall with absent myocardial enhancement (no infarction) *(bottom)*. (From Bucciarelli-Ducci C, Auger D, Di Mario C, et al. CMR guidance for recanalization of coronary chronic total occlusion. *JACC Cardiovasc Imaging.* 2016;9:547–556.)

results of STICH suggest that viability testing is not a prerequisite for decisions regarding medical versus surgical management in patients with severely reduced EFs. Imaging should be reserved for those patients in whom management decisions are difficult in view of age, comorbidities, or complex coronary anatomy, and in whom the demonstration of substantial viability might tilt the scale toward revascularization.[84]

In contrast with the difficult clinical scenario of identifying viable myocardium in patients with severely reduced EFs, identification of myocardial ischemia and viability is a "must" in patients with chronically occluded coronary arteries.[87–89] Recently, Bucciarelli-Ducci et al.[90] demonstrated in 50 consecutive patients with chronic total occlusions (CTOs) that most patients with inducible perfusion deficits and myocardial viability (infarct transmurality <50% by LGE CMR) within the CTO arterial territory before percutaneous coronary intervention had complete or near-complete resolution of CTO-related perfusion defects (Fig. 21.24). Moreover, these patients selected on the basis of ischemia and viability in the CTO-related myocardium as demonstrated by CMR had favorable reverse remodeling and improvements in the quality of life.

CONCLUSION

CMR provides a variety of methods of obtaining information on residual viability after myocardial infarction. Indirect signs of viability that can be observed by CMR are any sign of wall thickening at rest (which is detectable with high accuracy by cine CMR), wall thickening after stimulation by low-dose dobutamine, preserved wall thickness, and a preserved viable epicardial rim. On the other hand, myocardial necrosis is characterized by LGE (possibly with a low-intensity core region because of no reflow) of the infarct area after injection of gadolinium, reduced wall thickness (in chronic infarcts) without a substantial viable rim, and the absence of a contractile reserve during dobutamine stimulation.

Evaluation of viable myocardium is most important in patients with severe LV dysfunction because these patients can gain most from revascularization if substantial amounts of myocardium are present. Recent data from the STICH trial questioned the value of viability imaging for improving outcome in these patients. Unfortunately, the information available about the value of CMR techniques in identifying patients with global LV dysfunction who have a high likelihood of profiting from a coronary revascularization is still scarce. Low-dose dobutamine CMR may be less accurate than LGE CMR in this patient group. In patients with regional LV dysfunction, however, in whom the need for revascularization needs to be established, both dobutamine CMR and LGE CMR are well validated and can be used clinically. Depiction of zones of acute necrosis by observing enhancement after gadolinium carries substantial promise for detailed studies of the effects of different treatment strategies for acute myocardial infarction, as well as for treatment in the early and late postinfarction phase. In contrast, CMR may not be able to hold its initial promise for identifying the area at risk and distinguishing it from the area of infarction.

REFERENCES

A full reference list is available online at ExpertConsult.com

22

Cardiovascular Magnetic Resonance Tagging for Assessment of Left Ventricular Diastolic Function

El-Sayed H. Ibrahim and Matthias Stuber

Left ventricular (LV) diastolic function has been recognized as an important factor in the pathophysiology of many common cardiovascular diseases. Dilated and hypertrophic cardiomyopathy (HCM), coronary artery disease (CAD), and systemic hypertension are all associated with abnormal LV filling dynamics. Diastolic dysfunction has also been increasingly appreciated as a major cause of heart failure (HF), especially in the elderly. Although invasive hemodynamic measures/assessment of diastole are considered the gold standard, echocardiographic methods, including tissue Doppler imaging, have gained greater use in the clinical assessment of LV diastolic function because of their noninvasive acquisition, which greatly facilitates serial assessments. In cardiovascular magnetic resonance (CMR) imaging, with the advent of parallel imaging, three-dimensional (3D) data collection, spiral and balanced steady-state free precession (bSSFP) imaging, and higher magnetic field strength, the prolonged tag persistence permits easier access to diastole. Together with rapid state-of-the-art software analysis tools, quantification of LV diastolic wall motion can now easily be performed using CMR.

CARDIAC MOTION

Systolic and Diastolic Heart Motion

During systole, the heart performs a complex motion analogous to "wringing" a towel, and as a result, the base and apex rotate in opposite directions. There is counterclockwise rotation at the apex and clockwise rotation at the base.[1] In parallel, the atrioventricular valvular plane (basal left ventricle and right ventricle) descends toward the apex. The lateral free wall of the right ventricle performs a more pronounced long-axis contraction than the lateral wall of the left ventricle.[2] During isovolumic relaxation, the myofibrils return to their resting state from the contracted state. This process is accompanied by a rapid untwisting at the apex, whereas the volume and cavity shape of the heart remain nearly unchanged. This rapid untwisting typically lasts less than 75 ms and precedes the early passive filling phase of the ventricles. During this filling phase, practically no rotational components can be seen at the apex of the healthy heart.[3]

Understanding different diastolic strain components and their intrinsic mechanisms during different pathologic conditions allows for better understanding of diastolic dysfunction.[4] Isovolumic relaxation is associated with changes in principal strains and untwisting, which are all related to an apparent increase in the LV volume, likely reflecting expansion of the LV myocardium.[5] The diastolic shear strain rates are linearly related to the corresponding preceding systolic shear strain components. Nevertheless, the torsional recoil is uncoupled

from end-systolic volume or associated strains.[6] In normal subjects, the circumferential-longitudinal shear strain decreases before the axial strain.[7] Furthermore, the early-diastolic filling efficiency can be augmented during exercise stress in an effort to maintain stroke volume despite shortened diastole.[8] Studying early-diastolic strain patterns through myocardial strain analysis allows for comparing normal subjects with those with diastolic dysfunction. Therefore clinicians would be able to identify patients with regional diastolic dysfunction that places them at the risk of HF and sudden cardiac death following pathologic conditions such as myocardial infarction (MI), and aortic stenosis (AS).

Assessment of Cardiac Rotation/Motion: Noncardiovascular Magnetic Resonance Methods

With echocardiographic imaging, the myocardium has relatively poor internal structure because of the absence of structural landmarks, making limited quantification of parameters, such as rotation, stress, and strain.[9,10] Several invasive methods have been reported during diastole to examine cardiac motion. One approach is the surgical/invasive implantation of tantalum markers into the midwall of the myocardium.[11] In combination with x-ray angiography, the motion of these markers can then be recorded with high temporal and spatial resolution. Using such an approach, alterations in diastolic untwisting have been observed in patients who have undergone heart transplantation shortly before rejection.[12] Although this method is very powerful, it is invasive, requires ionizing radiation, and is inappropriate for routine and repeated clinical use. Alternative angiographic "markers," such as tracking of the bifurcations of the coronary arteries,[13] suffer from the limited number of landmarks and their irregular geometric distribution. Furthermore, they only provide motion information about the epicardial layers of the myocardium.

Assessment of Cardiac Rotation/Motion: Cardiovascular Magnetic Resonance Methods

Similar to echocardiography, conventional cine CMR images do not provide information about the internal structure of the myocardium. However, a CMR myocardial tagging technique, spatial modulation of magnetization (SPAMM), originally proposed by Axel[15] and further developed and refined by others, offers the opportunity to assess strain noninvasively. With these methods, the magnetization of the muscle tissue is spatially modulated, or "tagged," by the application of a specific time series of radiofrequency (RF) pulses and magnetic field gradients. The tagging is typically applied immediately after the R-wave of the electrocardiogram (ECG). Images are then acquired during successive heart phases in which the tags may be identified as dark lines or grids. Because these tags are spatially fixed with respect to the muscle tissue at the time of the tag's application, local myocardial motion can be derived from the translation, rotation, and distortion of the tags on the myocardium. However, because of the relaxation effects, the tags fade rapidly and cannot be reliably detected after end systole (approximately 300 ms after tag application). This is a serious drawback for the quantification of systolic and diastolic dynamics of the heart wall. Another limitation is that this approach does not compensate for through-plane motion. These limitations have been resolved through the development of the complementary SPAMM (CSPAMM) technique,[3,16] on which we will focus in the remainder of the chapter.

COMPLEMENTARY SPATIAL MODULATION OF MAGNETIZATION: TECHNICAL DEVELOPMENTS

Complementary Spatial Modulation of Magnetization Tagging[17]

One limitation of SPAMM tagging is the fading of the tagging pattern through the cardiac cycle as a result of longitudinal magnetization relaxation. The loss of tagging contrast toward the end of the cardiac cycle results in unrecognizable tagging pattern, which precludes the analysis of diastolic heart phases. It was not until 1993 when Fischer et al.[16] introduced the CSPAMM sequence to resolve this problem (Fig. 22.1). To grasp the idea behind CSPAMM, it is necessary to understand the magnetization evolution with time in a tagging sequence. Immediately after applying the tagging module of the pule sequence, the whole magnetization is tagged or modulated (90-degree RF pulses are assumed here) and stored in the longitudinal position. With time, the magnetization experiences longitudinal relaxation, trying to reach the equilibrium state. This has two effects on the stored tagging pattern: (1) introducing a growing nontagged magnetization offset (we call it here the DC component, borrowing the term *direct current* [DC] from electrical engineering); and (2) reducing the magnitude of the tagged component (the peak-to-peak difference of the sinusoidal tagged magnetization). Thus, during the imaging stage, the excited magnetization has two components: tagged and DC, with the DC overhead impairing the visibility of the (already fading) tagged component. It should be noted that the multiple applications of RF pulses during the imaging (data acquisition) part of the sequence also contributes to reducing the tagged magnetization component (each RF pulse consumes part of the tagged magnetization stored in the longitudinal direction). The solution provided by CSPAMM consisted of two parts: eliminating the nontagged (DC) magnetization and enhancing the fading tagged magnetization. To eliminate the nontagged magnetization, two consecutive SPAMM scans are acquired with exactly the same parameters, except for the polarity of one of the tagging RF pulses. The 90-degree/90-degree tagging RF pulses in the first scan modulate the magnetization with a positive sinusoidal pattern, whereas the 90-degree/−90-degree RF pulses in the second scan result in a negative sinusoidal pattern. Note that the DC magnetization component is the same in both scans at corresponding time points. Therefore, the overhead DC magnetization can be simply eliminated by subtracting the images in the first scan from the corresponding images (at the same heart phases) in the second scan. This subtraction has also the effect of improving the image's signal-to-noise ratio (SNR) by 40% as two acquisitions with independent noise terms are added together. To resolve the second problem of fading tagging contrast, the concept of "ramped flip angle" was introduced. Basically, during the imaging stage, the flip angles of the RF pulses determine how much magnetization is tipped into the transverse plane for data acquisition. Thus increasing the flip angles through the cardiac cycle compensates for the fading tagging contrast as a larger percentage of the available longitudinal magnetization is used at later heart phases.

Complementary Spatial Modulation of Magnetization With Slice-Following

Because of through-plane cardiac motion, two-dimensional (2D) cine imaging of the heart may not show the same myocardial tissue throughout the cardiac cycle; rather, the imaging plane shows whatever tissue lies inside it at the time of data acquisition. This could lead to inaccurate assessment of myocardial motion; for example, an apparent myocardial thickening in a basal short-axis slice could be in fact caused by myocardial basal displacement toward the apex. Slice-following CSPAMM[3] was developed as an improvement of the original CSPAMM technique to resolve the through-plane motion problem. The technique is based on implementing slice-selective tagging instead of the nonselective tagging used in conventional CSPAMM. A thin slice of interest is tagged by switching one (or both) of the tagging RF pulses with a slice-selective pulse, which has the effect of confining the tagging pattern inside the slice of interest (whose slice thickness = Δz, as shown in Fig. 22.2). Later, during the data acquisition part of the sequence, a thicker slice (whose slice thickness of Δs encompasses the thin tagged slice) is excited. The excited slice should be thick enough to accommodate the thin tagged slice despite its displacement in the through-plane (z) direction. Because nontagged magnetization is eliminated in CSPAMM, the only source of signal in the resulting image comes from the initially tagged slice, regardless of its displacement in the through-plane direction. This ensures that the same myocardial tissue is imaged during the whole cardiac cycle, and that apparent motion illusions are eliminated. The choice of the imaging slice thickness has to be carefully considered to ensure inclusion of the tagged slice throughout the cardiac cycle, and at the same time to avoid unnecessary thickness that would only add noise to the image.

Typically, double oblique short-axis sections of the myocardium are tagged with a slice thickness of 6 to 8 mm. Subsequently, 16 to 20 sequential heart phase images are acquired with a temporal resolution (Δt) of about 35 ms. With this high temporal resolution, rapid motion components, such as diastolic untwisting, can be identified readily. Because the ratio of wanted to unwanted signal components must be optimized, the thickness of the imaged volume (Δs; see Fig. 22.2) must be reduced to a minimum. Therefore it depends on the level of the tagged slice with respect to its level on the long axis. For basal LV images, where a long-axis contraction of more than 20 mm may be expected for the lateral right ventricular (RV) free wall,[2] a slice thickness of 30 mm is typically chosen. For midventricle slices, a slice thickness of 25 mm is appropriate, and at the apex, a slice thickness of 20 mm is used because of reduced through-plane motion. For suppression of breathing-induced motion artifacts, a repetitive breath-holding scheme[3,16] or single breath-hold techniques[18] can be applied. Furthermore, for high-resolution CSPAMM tagging, the two SPAMM acquisitions could be acquired with a 90-degree phase shift between them before constructing the CSPAMM images.[19]

Considering the location of the relevant tagging information in *k*-space, a reduced *k*-space acquisition scheme can be applied.[3,16] Hereby, two sets of orthogonally line tagged images are acquired. Subsequent combination of these acquisitions results in grid-tagged images (Figs. 22.3 and 22.4). With this method, acquisition time is significantly reduced and image resolution perpendicular to the line tags is not affected. Fig. 22.3 shows 20 heart phase images with a temporal resolution of 37 ms acquired at an apical slice of a healthy subject.[18] The grid structure remains visible, with a high contrast up to the last acquisition in late diastole (>700 ms). No fading of the tags is seen in the images. Therefore the method is well suited for the quantification of diastolic heart wall motion.

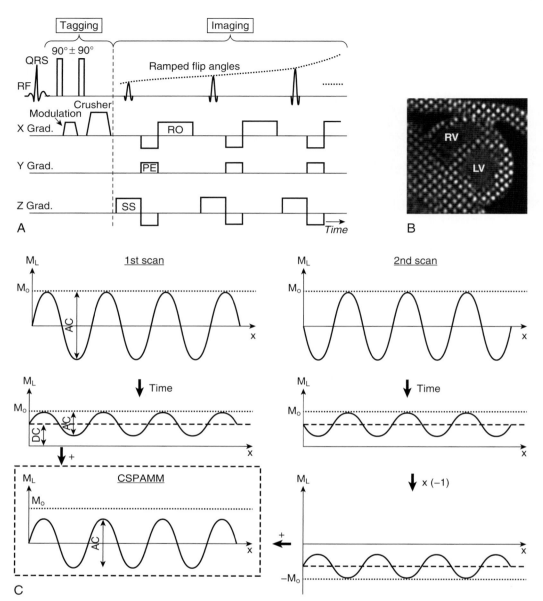

FIG. 22.1 (A) Complementary spatial modulation of magnetization *(CSPAMM)* pulse sequence. The sequence runs two SPAMM sequences, with the polarity of the second tagging radiofrequency *(RF)* pulse changed in the second SPAMM acquisition. Notice also the ramped flip angles of the imaging RF pulses to compensate for fading tagging. (B) Example of a grid-tagged CSPAMM image. Notice that nontagged tissues appear black because of the elimination of the offset DC signal. (C) The concept of magnetization subtraction in CSPAMM. Two scans are acquired as shown in the pulse sequence, which results in positive and negative sinusoidal tagging patterns from the first and second scans, respectively. With time, the tagging patterns experience longitudinal relaxation, trying to reach equilibrium magnetization *(M$_o$)*. Magnetization relaxation has two effects on the tagging pattern: the peak-to-peak *(AC)* magnitude is decreased and the tagging pattern has nonzero average *(DC)* value. However, the DC component is the same in both scans. Thus, at any time point, when two corresponding images (obtained from the first and second acquisitions at the same time point) are subtracted, the DC component cancels out and the peak-to-peak tagging magnitude doubles. *Grad,* Gradient; *LV,* left ventricular; *RV,* right ventricular. (From Ibrahim el-SH. Myocardial tagging by cardiovascular magnetic resonance: evolution of techniques—pulse sequences, analysis algorithms, and applications. *J Cardiovasc Magn Reson.* 2011;13:36.)

Data Acquisition Trajectory in Complementary Spatial Modulation of Magnetization

Although traditionally segmented *k*-space gradient recalled echo (GRE) techniques are used for signal readout, both T1 relaxation and serial RF excitations for imaging are responsible for the fading of the tags.

T1 can only be increased by going to a higher magnetic field strength, and the number of RF excitations can be reduced by using alternative imaging sequences with fewer RF excitations. Hereby, echo planar imaging (EPI)[18,20] (see Fig. 22.3) and, more recently, spiral imaging[21] proved to be very valuable alternatives (see Fig. 22.4).

Spiral imaging provides a time-efficient *k*-space coverage, which makes it a very powerful alternative to EPI for signal readout of the tagged myocardium. Because a small number of excitation RF pulses is needed in spiral imaging, the tagging pattern persists longer, leading to improved tagging contrast.[22] Furthermore, spiral imaging allows for efficient coverage of the *k*-space in a short amount of time, leading to

imaging at a very high temporal resolution. Finally, the short echo time (TE) of spiral acquisition allows for minimizing flow and motion artifacts.[23] Ryf et al.[21] combined CSPAMM with interleaved spiral imaging, which allowed for acquiring high spatial resolution (4-mm tag separation) or high temporal resolution (77 frames per second) grid-tagged images in a single breath-hold (see Fig. 22.4).

Together with EPI and spiral readouts, the use of bSSFP was exploited by Herzka et al.,[24] who found that bSSFP leads to an improved tagging contrast compared with the more conventional GRE imaging. In another study, Zwanenburg et al.[25] combined CSPAMM with bSSFP imaging for a single breath-hold scan. In this approach, the steady-state magnetization is stored in the longitudinal direction using an $\alpha/2$ flip-back RF pulse immediately before tagging preparation. Imaging proceeds normally, although excitation is achieved using a series of the linearly increasing start-up angles (LISA) technique to minimize off-resonance artifacts. Ibrahim et al.[26] developed a technique for improving the CSPAMM tagging contrast in bSSFP cine images by optimizing the RF excitation angles to compensate for tags fading during the cardiac cycle, similar to Fischer's approach for the gradient echo CSPAMM-tagged cine images.[16]

With the advent of parallel and 3D imaging, 3D assessment of myocardial motion based on 3D CSPAMM lattice tagging was reported by Ryf et al.[27] Fig. 22.5 shows an isosurface-rendered image based on 3D

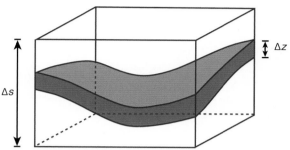

FIG. 22.2 Slice-following principle. An initially tagged planar slice of the thickness d*z* translates and distorts during the cardiac cycle. A volume of the thickness d*s* is imaged multiple times during the cardiac cycle. This volume must encompass the potential extent of the motion of the tagged, thin slice.

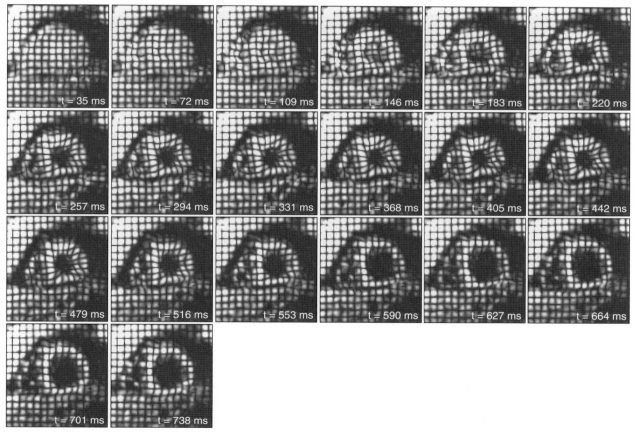

FIG. 22.3 Twenty apical left ventricular short-axis images in a healthy adult subject acquired with complementary spatial modulation of magnetization tagging. The systolic images include frames 1 to 9 (331 ms after the R-wave of the electrocardiogram), and the diastolic images are shown in frames 10 to 20 (368 to 738 ms). The temporal resolution in these images is 37 ms, and two line-tagged acquisitions were combined to create a grid-tagged image off-line. During systole, a counterclockwise apical rotation is seen, followed by a rapid clockwise untwisting in frames 10 to 15 (368 to 553 ms) during early diastole. This precedes the filling phase (frames 16 to 20; 590 to 738 ms) of the ventricles.

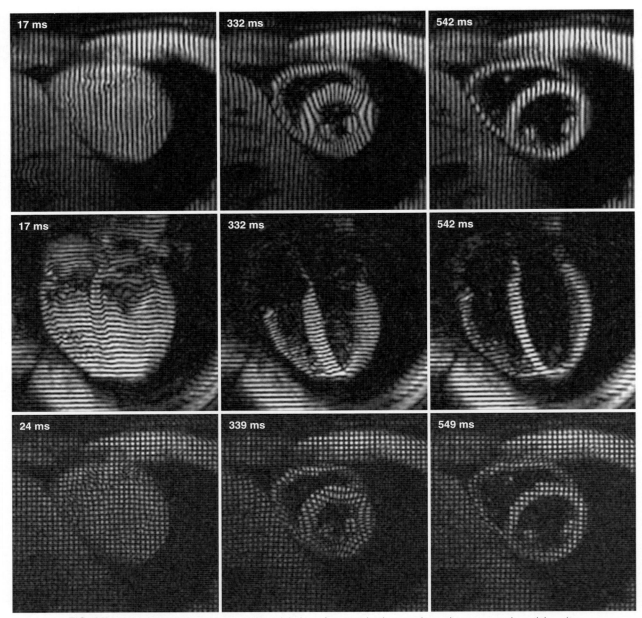

FIG. 22.4 Spiral complementary spatial modulation of magnetization tagging using a spectral-spatial excitation for fat suppression in each cine frame. Midventricular short-axis and long-axis views of a line-tagged and a grid-tagged myocardium in a healthy subject. The tagline distance is 4 mm, and the temporal resolution is 35 ms. The time after the R-wave is indicated on the images. On the grid-tagged, short-axis view, 50 tagline intersections can be observed.

CSPAMM imaging. Simultaneously, the same authors proposed an extension to a previously reported analysis procedure[28] that enables relatively time-efficient analysis and quantification of both systolic and diastolic motion of the heart.[29] However, the acquisition times were lengthy and only practical in coached breathing patterns in well-trained subjects.

Complementary Spatial Modulation of Magnetization Sequence Development Approaches
Magnitude Reconstruction

The magnitude image CSPAMM reconstruction (MICSR) technique has been developed for improving CSPAMM tagging contrast and

persistence.[30] By reconstructing only magnitude images, MICSR yields tags with zero mean sinusoidal profiles, which obviates the need for acquiring phase calibration data or applying phase correction algorithms. Based on the MICSR technique, the same authors developed a method for trinary display of the resulting images, which emphasized the tagging persistence and presented a novel way for visualizing myocardial deformation.[30,31] MICSR was shown to have the following advantages: (1) a true sinusoidal tagging profile is created as opposed to rectified sinusoids; (2) a peak MICSR contrast is obtained between 200 and 500 ms after the R-wave, corresponding to the period in the cardiac cycle with the largest myocardial deformation (late systole to early diastole); (3) the tagging contrast is higher and persists for a longer period of time than

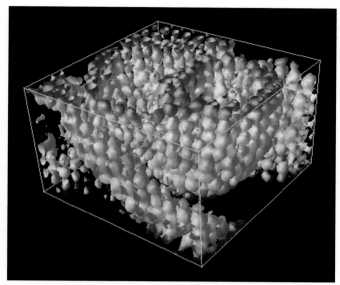

FIG. 22.5 Isosurface rendering of three-dimensional complementary spatial modulation of magnetization. A volume of 128 × 128 mm^2 is displayed. Tag spacing is 10 mm. (From Ryf S, Spiegel MA, Gerber M, Boesiger P. Myocardial tagging with 3D-CSPAMM. *J Magn Reson Imaging.* 2002;16:320–325, with permission.)

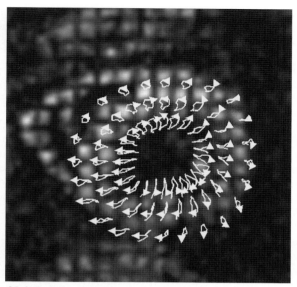

FIG. 22.6 End-diastolic apical complementary spatial modulation of magnetization acquired in a healthy adult subject. The grid-tagged image is overlain with the corresponding local trajectories. The arrows start at the beginning of systole and at end diastole.

in conventional CSPAMM; and (4) the images are optimized for processing with harmonic phase magnetic resonance (HARP) analysis.[28]

Real-Part Reconstruction

Kuijer et al.[32] presented a technique for improving the tagging contrast without increasing the scan time through real-part data reconstruction using an internal phase reference from the tagged images. The tagging efficiency of the proposed technique was similar to that of real-part reconstruction with a separate reference scan. However, compared with magnitude image subtraction, the tagging contrast-to-noise ratio was improved by 70% without increasing the scan time.

Fat Suppression in Complementary Spatial Modulation of Magnetization

An efficient fat suppression method (inherent fat cancelation) has been developed for CSPAMM imaging.[33] The inherent fat cancelation method makes use of the two acquisitions required for CSPAMM imaging by allowing for complementary and in-phase modulations of the water and fat spins, respectively; therefore, in the final CSPAMM image, the tagging contrast of water is doubled, while the tagging signal from fat is canceled. Compared with the spectral-spatial selective fat suppression,[34] the inherent fat cancelation method provides fat-suppressed CSPAMM images with high temporal resolution and short echo time without increasing the scan time.

Off-Resonance Insensitive–Complementary Spatial Modulation of Magnetization

Recently, CSPAMM has been combined with Fourier analysis of stimulated echoes (FAST) for quantification of LV systolic and diastolic function.[35] The developed technique provides a semiautomatic means for quick and quantitative assessment of LV systolic and diastolic twist and torsion. The developed technique requires a short scan time and provides quantitative assessment of systolic and diastolic LV twist, torsion, twisting rates, time-to-peak twist, duration of untwisting, and ratio of rapid untwist to peak twist.

Orthogonal Complementary Spatial Modulation of Magnetization

Orthogonal CSPAMM has been recently introduced to reduce the scan time in half while maintaining the CSPAMM advantage of removing the central nontagged (DC) signal peak in k-space.[36] Because CSPAMM is based on acquiring two separate SPAMM images (which are 180 degrees out of phase with each other) for producing a line-tagged image, then four separate SPAMM acquisitions would be required for producing a 2D grid-tagged CSPAMM image. The orthogonal CSPAMM sequence is based on rotating the tag orientation in the second SPAMM acquisition by 90 degrees relative to the first one, such that when the two images are subtracted to produce the final CSPAMM image, the DC signal peak is canceled (as in conventional CSPAMM), while a 2D grid-tagging is obtained, thus producing a CSPAMM grid-tagged image from only two SPAMM acquisitions.

Tagging Analysis

For the extraction of motion data from the tagged time series of images, sophisticated image analysis tools are needed. Although the identification of tags was very labor intensive and took hours in the early years, sophisticated algorithms that reduce quantification of tagged time series of cardiac images to seconds are now readily available,[28] and variants have been successfully implemented.[29] Analysis of tagged images involves the identification of the tags in each heart phase image. Using automated or semiautomated algorithms, the tags may be identified with an accuracy that exceeds the image resolution.[37] If the grid intersection points are identified for all heart phase images, local trajectories on the myocardium (Fig. 22.6) are defined, and motion-specific parameters (e.g., strain, rotation, rotation velocity, radial or circumferential shortening, or shear between epicardial and endocardial muscle layers of the myocardium) can be derived. Using this approach, studies of healthy subjects and patients with MI,[38] HCM,[39] and AS with pathologically hypertrophied hearts, as well as athletes with physiologic hypertrophy, were evaluated for apical untwisting during diastole.[40] Untwisting velocity, time-to-peak untwisting velocity, and early diastolic strain can be determined as indices of diastolic function. Time-to-peak untwisting velocity (untwisting time; Table 22.1) is defined as the time delay between the point in time of minimum inner cavity area and the maximum untwisting velocity (Fig. 22.7).

CLINICAL APPLICATIONS

Beyond the technical developments addressed earlier in this chapter, CSPAMM has been implemented in a large number of clinical applications. CSPAMM reproducibility has been studied in healthy subjects, where the results showed good intraobserver, interobserver, and interstudy reproducibility for measuring LV circumferential strain and twist, and less reproducibility for measuring radial strain.[41] Studies for measuring regional LV function are promising, as are those for examining the pattern of RV contractility. Heart rotation and torsion are equally interesting areas of study, as well as the effect of aging on

heart function. Other CSPAMM applications include CAD, ischemic heart disease, MI, HCM, interventricular synchrony, valvular diseases, postsurgical cardiac function evaluation, and congenital heart disease. In this section, we focus on applications related to studying diastolic cardiac function.

Ventricular Rotation

As mentioned previously, at the apex of the healthy heart, a counterclockwise rotation during systole can be seen (see Fig. 22.3, phases 1 to 9; see Fig. 22.7, phase 1). This systolic rotation is followed by a rapid untwisting during isovolumic relaxation (see Fig. 22.3, phases 10 to 15 and early diastole; see Fig. 22.7, phase 2). This untwisting phase is typically followed by the filling phase of the ventricles, during which little rotational component is seen (see Fig. 22.7, phase 3).[3,42] An identical separation of early diastolic apical untwisting and the filling phase of the ventricles is seen in highly competitive athletes with physiologically hypertrophied hearts. Neither the apical peak rotation angle nor diastolic untwisting time is changed in the hypertrophied hearts of athletes compared with healthy control subjects (see Table 22.1). However, among patients with LV hypertrophy, as a result of pressure overload/AS, a completely different apical rotation pattern is seen (see Fig. 22.7). The end-systolic peak rotation is significantly increased ($P < .01$) in comparison with the athletes or healthy subjects, and no separation of untwisting and filling can be seen during diastole. Untwisting and filling occur simultaneously, and the point in time of maximum untwisting velocity is significantly delayed in these patients ($P < .01$; see Fig. 22.7).

Pressure overload LV hypertrophy results in the addition of new sarcomeres in parallel.[43] Furthermore, an increase in the amount of collagen, with a consequently increased elastic stiffness, has been reported.[44] This rearranged fiber architecture, together with the increased stiffness of the muscle tissue, may explain the alterations of the diastolic rotation pattern with a prolonged and delayed apical untwisting in these patients. The prolongation of untwisting results in an overlap with early diastolic filling and presumably impedes normal filling. Thus, a prolongation of early diastolic untwisting may be responsible for the occurrence of diastolic dysfunction in these patients. In patients with

TABLE 22.1 **Peak Rotation at the Apex, Maximum Rotation Velocity During Diastolic Untwisting and Untwisting Time for 12 Aortic Stenosis Patients, 12 Athletes, and 11 Healthy Volunteers**[a]

Patients	Peak Rotation (Degrees)	Untwisting Velocity (Degrees/s)	Untwisting Time (% ES)
Aortic stenosis	12 ± 5	80 ± 29	32 ± 6
Athletes	6 ± 2	56 ± 8	17 ± 8
Volunteers	7 ± 2	55 ± 17	16 ± 8

[a]The untwisting time is related to the duration of systole. Data are expressed as mean ± 1 standard deviation.
ES, End systole.
Modified from Stuber M, Scheidegger MB, Fischer SE, et al. Alterations in the local myocardial motion pattern in patients suffering from pressure overload due to aortic stenosis. *Circulation.* 1999;100:361–368.

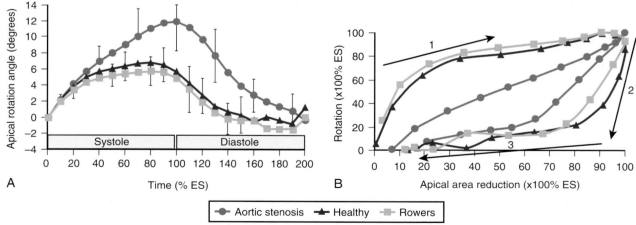

FIG. 22.7 (A) Cross-sectional apical rotation velocity of athletes, healthy adults, and patients with aortic stenosis (AS). The values are mean ± 1 standard deviation. The time axis is normalized to the end-systolic point of the cardiac cycle. The time point of maximum diastolic untwisting velocity *(arrows)* is delayed in the patients with AS compared with the athletes or the healthy control subjects. Apical rotation velocity is identical in athletes and control subjects. (B) Left ventricular (LV) rotation-area loop (apical plane) in healthy control subjects, rowers, and patients with AS. The loop is separated in isovolumic contraction (1), ejection (2), isovolumic relaxation (3), and LV filling. Both rotation and area change of the inner lumen at the apex are related to their maximum values (100%). *ES,* End systole.

MI, a prolonged untwisting phase with an overlap of diastolic untwisting and filling has also been observed[45] and end-systolic apical peak rotation is usually severely reduced.

In 2011, Russel et al.[46] used CSPAMM to study ventricular torsion in patients with recessive mutation causing familial HCM. The results showed that the mutation carriers have normal wall thickness, but increased LV torsion with respect to controls, which suggests that healthy carriers may be targets for clinical intervention at a preclinical stage to prevent the onset of future dysfunction.

Ventricular Hypertrophy

CMR assessment of diastolic function is beginning to be studied in broader populations. HCM has been studied using CSPAMM tagging.[39] CSPAMM was combined with the cardiac phase to order reconstruction (CAPTOR) technique[47] for quantifying regional indices of myocardial function throughout the cardiac cycle. The results showed distinct differences in strain in HCM compared with controls (Fig. 22.8). Specifically, although early systolic shortening was similar, the total systolic shortening was significantly reduced in the septal and inferior regions. Furthermore, early diastolic strain rate was reduced in all regions and no period of diastasis was observed in HCM. Therefore, the ventricular response to atrial systole could be seen as strain exceeding the end-diastolic reference.

A population-based study, the multiethnic subclinical atherosclerosis (MESA) study, showed evidence of diastolic dysfunction in asymptomatic individuals with LV hypertrophy.[48] Despite similar regional systolic strain and strain rate among those with and without LV hypertrophy, the regional diastolic strain rate was significantly reduced among those with LV hypertrophy. A provocative study in a small group suggested that diastolic untwisting dysfunction could be identified by SPAMM after a sedentary rest in previously active adult subjects.[49]

Aortic Stenosis

Among some of the early CSPAMM studies is one that studied the effect of AS on alterations in local myocardial motion patterns.[40] This study found that diastolic apical untwisting in patients with pressure overload as a result of AS is delayed compared with healthy controls or athletes who have a similar degree of hypertrophy as the patients. In another study by Nagel et al.,[50] the authors used CSPAMM to study cardiac torsion as well as systolic and diastolic wall motion in 12 healthy controls and 13 patients with severe AS. The results showed that during systole, the normal LV undergoes a clockwise rotation (when viewed from the apex) of -4.4 ± 1.6 degrees at the base and a counterclockwise rotation of $+6.8 \pm 2.5$ degrees at the apex. In patients with AS, however, this rotation was found to be reduced at the base and increased at the apex. Furthermore, the overall rotation velocity is decreased and maximal torsion is increased in AS. Recently, CSPAMM has been implemented for studying changes in myocardial strain following transcatheter aortic valve implantation (TAVI).[51] TAVI resulted in improved mid-LV circumferential strain and decreased myocardial twist. However, although systolic strain rate increased following TAVI, there was no significant change in diastolic strain rate.

Diastolic Heart Failure

CMR tagging has been used to illustrate changes in regional myocardial function in HF patients with preserved ejection fraction (HFpEF). In one study, LV function was examined in eight patients with HFpEF and eight normal subjects.[52] The HFpEF patients showed decreased LV filling rate, reversed early-to-atrial filling ratio (E/A), decreased peak strain, and early diastolic strain rate, compared with the normal subjects. In another study, 218 patients with LV hypertrophy and normal systolic function were studied using CMR tagging.[48] The study showed that HF progression begins as a regional myocardial dysfunction, which is affected by patterns of hypertrophy. The results revealed a direct relationship between regional diastolic dysfunction and increased LV mass. Although patients with LV hypertrophy were found to have less global systolic function than that in normal subjects, systolic strain was not affected. However, diastolic strain rate was significantly reduced with hypertrophy (1.5 ± 1.1 per second) compared with a group without hypertrophy (2.2 ± 1.1 per second, $P < .001$), regardless of age or gender.

Limitations

The additional value of CMR tagging applied for the quantification of diastolic function remains to be more fully investigated compared with

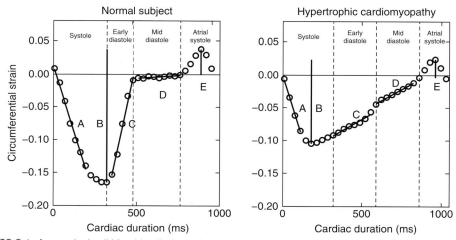

FIG. 22.8 Left ventricular (LV) midwall circumferential strain curve in the inferior wall in a normal subject *(left)* and a hypertrophic cardiomyopathy patient *(right)*. Indices of cardiac function are shown on the curves: *A,* systolic strain rate; *B,* total systolic strain; *C,* early-diastolic strain rate; *D,* mid-diastolic strain rate; and *E,* lengthening subsequent to atrial systole. Measures *B* and *E* were used to calculate the percent lengthening subsequent to atrial systole, defined as *E/B*. (From Ennis DB, Epstein FH, Kellman P, et al. Assessment of regional systolic and diastolic dysfunction in familial hypertrophic cardiomyopathy using MR tagging. *Magn Reson Med.* 2003;50:638–642, with permission.)

gold standard techniques. Currently, the CMR technique is not widely accessible to clinical cardiologists and the CSPAMM sequence is not currently available on all vendors' systems. Furthermore, because CSPAMM is based on a subtraction technique, scanning time is doubled and susceptibility to diaphragmatic drift or misregistration in serial breath-holds must be considered. However, with the availability of parallel imaging, EPI, or spiral imaging, the number of RF excitations for imaging can be minimized. As an alternative to CSPAMM, more conventional tagging[12,53] in combination with bSSFP may support an improved tagging contrast-to-noise ratio, as does 3 T imaging because of an increase in T1 (from ~850 ms at 1.5 T to ~1200 ms at 3 T for myocardium and from ~1200 ms at 1.5 T to ~1650 ms for blood at 3 T). For these reasons, access to early diastolic myocardial motion may be feasible, even without the availability of CSPAMM. Nevertheless, the investigation of heart wall motion is still the subject of basic research, and appropriate parameters for the quantification of diastolic dysfunction and threshold values for normal subjects remain to be fully defined.

CONCLUSION

The CSPAMM myocardial tagging technique is a noninvasive method for the quantification of local heart wall motion. Because of the suppressed fading of the tags and the accessibility to the diastolic phase of the cardiac cycle, CSPAMM is well suited for the characterization of the diastolic portion of the cardiac cycle. Moreover, by the application of the slice-following procedure, the effects of through-plane motion can be suppressed and the same tissue elements can be tracked. Because of the relatively high temporal resolution of the data, rapid cardiac motion components, such as apical diastolic untwisting, can be recorded.

The current data derived from CSPAMM myocardial tagging suggest that alterations in the diastolic phase of the cardiac cycle can be recorded readily. With the advent of parallel imaging, higher magnetic field strength, and more advanced imaging sequences, persistence of tags can be prolonged, enabling access to diastolic motion of the left ventricle. Although CMR myocardial tagging requires off-line computer analysis, image postprocessing time is now a matter of seconds and the technique may offer a new tool for the evaluation of diastolic wall relaxation in healthy and diseased states. Therefore CSPAMM, with its inherent ability to visualize both systolic and diastolic myocardial motion with or without true myocardial motion tracking, will continue to play a very important role in advancing regional heart function evaluation with CMR.

REFERENCES

A full reference list is available online at ExpertConsult.com

23

Magnetic Resonance Imaging of Coronary Arteries: Technique

Mehmet Akçakaya, Claudia Prieto, René M. Botnar, and Reza Nezafat

Despite significant efforts in prevention and treatment, coronary artery disease (CAD) remains the leading cause of death in the United States, accounting for one in every seven deaths.[1] Each year nearly 700,000 Americans are estimated to have a new myocardial infarction (MI), and nearly 325,000 to have a recurrent infarction. Furthermore, an additional estimated 165,000 will have their first silent MI.[1] The current clinical "gold standard" for the diagnosis of significant (≥50% diameter stenosis) CAD is catheter-based invasive x-ray angiography. More than a million catheter-based x-ray coronary angiograms are performed annually in the United States,[1] with a higher volume in Europe. However, these invasive tests have a relatively low yield, with less than 40% of patients referred for x-ray coronary angiography having obstructive CAD,[2] unnecessarily exposing these patients to the potential risks and complications of an invasive test that includes ionizing radiation and iodinated contrast.[3,4] To relieve symptoms or decrease pharmaceutical use, percutaneous coronary intervention in single vessel disease is commonly performed, but the greatest impact on mortality occurs with mechanical intervention among patients with left main (LM) and multivessel CAD. Thus alternative noninvasive imaging modalities, which allow direct visualization of the proximal and mid native coronary vessels for the accurate identification/exclusion of LM/multivessel CAD, are desirable.

Cardiovascular magnetic resonance (CMR) imaging is a very promising noninvasive tool for comprehensive early risk assessment, guidance of therapy, and treatment monitoring of CAD. CMR is considered the gold standard for the assessment of cardiac anatomy, biventricular systolic function, myocardial viability (late gadolinium enhancement [LGE]) and rest/stress myocardial perfusion.[5-8] Clinical research studies also have demonstrated its usefulness for quantitative myocardial tissue characterization (T_1 and T_2 relaxation time mapping), and its ability to differentiate between healthy and diseased tissue.[9,10] Coronary magnetic resonance imaging (MRI) is a noninvasive diagnosis alternative to catheter-based x-ray angiography among patients with suspected anomalous coronary artery disease[11] and coronary artery aneurysms.[12] Although coronary multi-detector computed tomography (MDCT) offers superior isotropic spatial resolution and more rapid imaging, coronary MRI has advantages over MDCT in several respects, including the absence of ionizing radiation or iodinated contrast, which facilitates follow-up scanning, as well as smaller artifacts related to epicardial calcium. Because of the advantages of coronary MRI and its diagnostic accuracy, coronary MRI is recommended and deemed appropriate in patients suspected of anomalous coronary artery disease by both the American College of Cardiology and American Heart Association.[13,14] However, CMR assessment of coronary lumen integrity and plaque burden/activity remains challenging. Nevertheless, CMR has shown great potential for coronary lumen,[15,16] plaque (with and without contrast agents)[17-19] and thrombus/hemorrhage[20,21] visualization. The combination of these techniques could add invaluable prognostic information for patients at risk or with known CAD. Thus technical developments are being investigated to allow coronary MRI to achieve similar diagnostic lumen accuracy as the current clinical gold standard, as well as plaque characterization. Main technical challenges include suboptimal spatial resolution (as a result of long acquisition times required), and coronary motion suppression with unpredictable scan times (depending largely on the breathing pattern of the subject). In this chapter, we will review the technical imaging strategies for MRI of coronary arteries, coronary vessel walls, and coronary veins. The clinical results of coronary MRI are addressed in Chapter 24.

CORONARY MAGNETIC RESONANCE IMAGING

The early approaches to coronary artery MRI were based on two-dimensional (2D) breath-hold electrocardiogram (ECG)-triggered segmented sequences.[22,23] Subsequently, three-dimensional (3D) free-breathing approaches have replaced 2D breath-hold approaches, enabling greater anatomical coverage and higher signal-to-noise ratio (SNR). Three-dimensional coronary MRI can be acquired using a targeted or whole-heart coverage of the coronary anatomies. In the targeted technique,[24] a double-oblique 3D volume aligned along the major axis of the left or right coronary artery (RCA) is acquired.[25-27] For the visualization of the RCA, the imaging plane passing through the proximal, mid, and distal coordinates of the RCA is identified and the targeted 3D coronary sequence is acquired in this orientation, typically with a 30-mm slab with 20 slices, using a segmented acquisition.[26,27] For the imaging of the left main (LM), left anterior descending (LAD), and left circumflex (LCX) coronary arteries, a 3D volume is interactively prescribed in the axial plane centered about the LM coronary artery (Fig. 23.1).[27,28] In the whole-heart coronary MRI technique,[29-43] an axial (or coronal) 3D volume encompassing the entire heart is sampled in a single acquisition, in a manner analogous to coronary MDCT. This facilitates the imaging setup via simpler slab prescription, and provides a more complete anatomical coverage, positioned ~1 cm above the LM and extending to the inferior cardiac border. However, based on single-center trials to date, it has not been shown to be superior to the targeted approach for CAD assessment (Table 23.1).

Targeted thin-slab 3D acquisitions have been acquired using both gradient recalled echo (GRE) and balanced steady-state free precession (bSSFP) sequences.[44] A thin-slab 3D targeted acquisition with a GRE sequence results in more homogenous blood pool signal, but is heavily dependent on the inflow of unsaturated protons.[45] Saturation effects will cause a local signal loss if coronary artery flow is slow or stagnant. This signal loss is often relatively exaggerated, as compared with the lumen

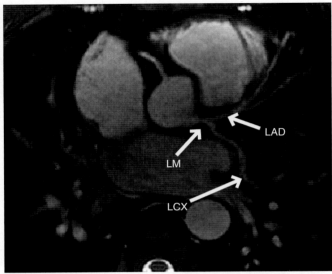

FIG. 23.1 Reformatted coronary artery magnetic resonance image of the left coronary system acquired using a targeted free-breathing acquisition with real-time navigator gating and tracking in a healthy adult subject. The transverse acquisition displays the left main *(LM)*, left anterior descending *(LAD)*, and the left circumflex *(LCX)* coronary arteries. The in-plane spatial resolution is 0.7×1.0 mm^2.

TABLE 23.1   Single-Center Echocardiogram-Triggered, Free-Breathing, Targeted Three-Dimensional and Whole-Heart Coronary Magnetic Resonance Imaging With and Without Contrast Agents

Study	Single-Center/ Multicenter	No. of Patients	Sensitivity	Specificity
Noncontrast 3D Targeted Coronary MRI				
Kim[24]	Multicenter	109	88%–98%	32%–52%
Bunce[126]	Single-center	46	50%–89%	72%–100%
Sommer[127]	Single-center	107	74%–88%	63%–91%
Bogaert[128]	Single-center	21	85%–92%	50%–83%
Noncontrast 3D Whole-Heart Coronary MRI				
Jahnke[129]	Single-center	21	79%	91%
Sakuma[41]	Single-center	39	82%	91%
Sakuma[40]	Single-center	131	82%	90%
Pouleur[130]	Single-center	77	100%	72%
Kato[15]	Multicenter	138	88%	72%
Contrast Enhanced 3D Whole-Heart Coronary MRI				
Yang[124]	Single-center	62	94%	82%
Yang[131]	Multicenter	272	91%	80%

3D, Three-dimensional; *MRI,* magnetic resonance imaging.

stenosis. Compared with GRE sequences, bSSFP provides intrinsically higher SNR because of its balanced gradients and improved blood-myocardium contrast attributed to its T_1/T_2 weighting,[46] with reduced sensitivity to inflow effects. Both GRE and bSSFP have been used for targeted 3D coronary MRI, where both have shown similar diagnostic accuracy for CAD.[46,47] For whole-heart noncontrast coronary MRI at

1.5 T, SSFP appears to be the sequence of choice as a result of its higher blood–myocardium contrast and superior inflow properties.[45]

Even with these technical advances, clinical acceptance of coronary MRI remains challenging because of coronary artery motion, long scan times, limited spatial resolution, suboptimal SNR and blood–myocardium contrast-to-noise-ratio (CNR). The technical challenges in coronary artery MRI are different from other CMR acquisitions as a result of unique issues including the coronary artery: (1) small caliber (3–6 mm diameter), (2) high level of tortuosity, (3) near-constant motion during both the respiratory and the cardiac cycles, and (4) surrounding signal from adjacent epicardial fat and myocardium.

Cardiac-Induced Motion

Bulk epicardial coronary artery motion is a major impediment to coronary CMR, and it can be separated into motion related to direct cardiac contraction/relaxation during the cardiac cycle and motion attributed to superimposed diaphragmatic and chest wall movement during respiration. The magnitude of motion from each component may greatly exceed the coronary artery diameter, leading to blurring artifacts in the absence of motion–suppressive methods.

To compensate for bulk cardiac motion, accurate external ECG synchronization with QRS detection is required, and vector ECG approaches are preferred.[48] Coronary artery motion during the cardiac cycle has been characterized using both catheter based x-ray angiography[49,50] and CMR.[51-53] Both the proximal/mid RCA and the LAD display a triphasic pattern, with the magnitude of in-plane motion nearly twice as great for the RCA. Coronary artery motion is minimal during isovolumic relaxation, approximately 350 to 400 ms after the R wave, and again at mid diastole (immediately before atrial systole). The duration of LAD diastasis is longer than that of the RCA, and it begins earlier in the cardiac cycle.[54] The duration of the mid diastolic diastasis period is inversely related to the heart rate and dictates the preferred coronary artery data acquisition interval.

As compared with MDCT in which the acquisition is constrained by gantry rotation, for coronary artery MRI the acquisition interval is adapted to the heart rate/diastasis interval using a patient-specific diastasis period. This can be readily identified by the acquisition of high temporal resolution cine dataset orthogonal to the long axis of the proximal/mid RCA and of the LAD. Semiautomated tools to identify the optimal data acquisition window have also been proposed.[55,56] For patients with a heart rate of 60 to 70 beats per minute, a coronary artery MRI acquisition duration of ~80 ms during each cardiac cycle results in improved image quality.[28] The duration must be further abbreviated (e.g., <50 ms) at higher heart rates, whereas with bradycardia, the acquisition interval can be expanded to 120 ms or longer. The use of patient-specific acquisition windows serves to reduce overall scan time.[57,58] Image degradation can be caused by sinus arrhythmia, leading to heart rate variability, which is common especially in younger adults.[59] An adaptive real-time arrhythmia rejection algorithm can correct for heart rate variability and improves coronary artery MRI quality.[56]

Respiratory-Induced Motion

The second major challenge for coronary artery MRI is compensation for bulk respiratory motion. With inspiration, the diaphragm may descend up to 30 mm and the chest wall expands, resulting in an inferior displacement and anterior rotation of the heart.[60] Several approaches have been proposed to minimize respiratory motion artifacts, including sustained end-expiratory breath-holding, chest wall bellows, respiratory navigators, fat navigators, and self-gating methods.

Prolonged (15–20 seconds) end-expiratory breath-holds were used to suppress respiratory motion in initial 2D coronary artery MRI methods.[61] Breath-holding offers the advantage of relative ease of implementation in compliant subjects, but it limits the temporal acquisition window, image spatial resolution, and anatomic coverage. Additionally, many patients are unable to adequately sustain a breath-hold. Furthermore, slice registration errors (attributed to variability in end-expiratory diaphragmatic position) are very common as is diaphragmatic drift during the breath-hold[61-64] and may occur in up to half of patients.[54] Supplemental oxygen and hyperventilation (separately or in combination) can be used to prolong the breath-hold duration,[63,64] but these methods may not be appropriate for all patients, and both diaphragmatic drift and slice registration errors persist.[64]

Diaphragmatic respiratory navigators, first proposed by Ehman[65] for abdominal MRI, enable free-breathing acquisitions without the stringent time constraints and patient cooperation requirements imposed by multiple breath-holds, and thus offer superior spatial resolution opportunities. Although the specifics of navigator implementation vary among CMR vendors, in the ideal implementation, the navigator can be positioned at any interface that accurately reflects respiratory motion, including the dome of the right hemidiaphragm (Fig. 23.2),[66,67] the left hemidiaphragm, the anterior chest wall, the anterior free wall of the left ventricle,[67,68] or even through the coronary artery of interest. The navigator should not cause an image artifact and should be temporally located immediately preceding the imaging portion of the sequence with data accepted (used for image reconstruction) only when the navigator indicates that the "interface" (e.g., diaphragm position) falls within a user-defined window. The dome of the right hemidiaphragm has become the preferred location[26,68] because of the simplicity and ease in set-up, where the motion of the right hemidiaphragm in the superior-inferior direction can be tracked. From CMR studies of cardiac border position during the respiratory cycle, it was observed that the ratio between cardiac and diaphragmatic displacement is ~0.6 for the RCA and ~0.7 for the left coronary artery at end-expiration,[60] although there is variability among subjects[62,69,70] and position (e.g., supine vs. prone imaging).[71] This rule-of-thumb offers the opportunity for prospective navigator gating with real-time tracking,[67,69] in which the position of the interface (diaphragm) is determined, and the slice position coordinates can then be shifted in real time (before the data collection)

to appropriately adjust spatial coordinates.[72] This technique allows for the use of wider gating windows and increased navigator efficiency, leading to shorter scan times. Real-time tracking implementations with a 5-mm diaphragmatic gating window are often used with a navigator efficiency approaching 50%.[69] Coronary artery MRI with real-time navigator tracking has been shown to minimize registration errors (as compared with breath-holding) while maintaining or improving the image quality.[69,73] It should also be noted that the quality of coronary artery MRI is improved by using consistent ECG timing, as well as respiratory suppression methodology for both the coronary localizing/motion scout images and for the coronary artery MRI acquisitions.[74]

A number of refinements to the navigator method have been proposed. Although a "fixed" superior–inferior correction factor of 0.6 (with no left–right or anterior–posterior correction)[72,75] is commonly used, significant individual variability has been observed.[62] A subject-specific tracking factor has been advocated and shown to improve the quality of coronary images when the subject-specific tracking factor differs from 0.6.[76] The use of multiple navigator locations, use of leading and trailing navigators, and use of navigators that provide guidance for affine transformations (i.e., 3D translations and rotations) of the slice prescription for each heart beat have been proposed.[37,77-79] The affine transformation permits use of larger navigator windows, and hence higher navigator efficiency. It has also been proposed that the heart itself be tracked,[34,80-82] such as with methods that track the epicardial fat to detect the heart position.[83-86] Navigator gating with fixed scan efficiency has also been studied, which results in imaging at a fixed scan time based only on heart rate and acquisition duration.[87] Novel k-space trajectories and various image reconstruction based methods, such as cross correlation of low resolution images, have also been proposed for respiratory motion compensation.[42,88-90]

Self-navigation methods have also been proposed to derive the respiratory-induced motion of the heart from the acquired data itself without the need of either a one-dimensional (1D) navigator echo or a heart-diaphragm tracking factor. Respiratory-induced displacements of the heart can be directly estimated from the repetitive acquisition of the central k-space point[91] or the central k-space line,[92-95] corresponding

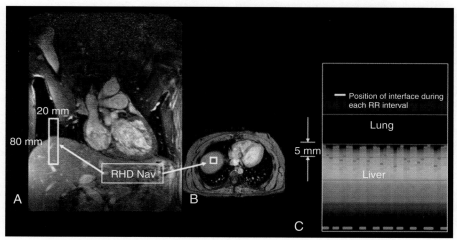

FIG. 23.2 Positioning and utility of the respiratory navigator. Coronal (A) and axial (B) thoracic images for positioning the navigator at the dome of the right hemidiaphragm *(RHD Nav)*. (C) Respiratory motion of the lung-diaphragm interface is recorded using a two-dimensional selective navigator with the lung (superior) and liver (inferior) interface. In this example, the maximum excursion between end-inspiration and end-expiration is ~11 mm. The position of the lung-liver interface at each RR interval is indicated by the broken line in the middle of (C). Data are only accepted if the lung-liver interface is within the acceptance window of 5 mm. Data acquired with the navigator outside of the window are rejected. Accepted data are indicated by the broken green line at the bottom of (C).

to zero-dimensional or 1D projections of the field of view. Similar to the 1D navigator echo approaches, self-navigation methods typically perform motion correction only in the foot-head translational motion. Another drawback of the self-navigation approach is that the inclusion of static structures, such as the chest wall, can degrade motion estimation and correction.

To overcome these problems and account for more complex motion, several 2D and 3D image-based navigator (so-called iNAV) approaches have been proposed for coronary artery MRI[96-103] (Fig. 23.3). In these approaches a low-resolution 2D or 3D image is acquired in every heartbeat before (or after) the coronary MRI data acquisition. The main advantage of this approach is that the moving heart can be spatially isolated from surrounding static tissues and the respiratory-induced cardiac motion can be directly estimated via (rigid or affine) image-registration of iNAVs at different respiratory positions. Self-navigation and image-based navigator methods can be used to gate the acquisition and correct for motion within a small gating window, as described for 1D navigator echoes. Furthermore, because these methods directly track heart motion/position, a much larger gating window can be used, or it can be removed entirely, thereby increasing the scan efficiency to, or close to, 100%. These promising approaches may lead to shorter and predictable scan times.

Image Quality Assessment

Epicardial fat and the myocardium surround the coronary arteries. Thus CNR can be improved by suppressing the fat and myocardium signals surrounding the coronary arteries. Frequency (spectrally) selective prepulses are applied to saturate signal from fat tissue, thereby allowing visualization of the underlying coronary arteries.[61,104] To differentiate myocardium and the coronary lumen, endogenous contrast preparation techniques are commonly used.[28,104-107] Two methods that can enhance the contrast between the coronary lumen and underlying myocardium are T2 preparation prepulses[28,105,106,108] and magnetization transfer contrast (MTC).[104,107] The former is often used for coronary artery MRI because it also suppresses deoxygenated venous blood, whereas the latter is used for coronary vein CMR.[109]

The limited SNR in coronary artery MRI, along with constraints on acquisition duration, restricts the spatial resolution in the acquisition. Spatial resolution requirements for clinical coronary artery MRI depend on whether the goal is to identify the origin and proximal course of the coronary artery (e.g., issues of anomalous coronary disease) or to identify focal stenoses in the proximal and middle segments.

The SNR of coronary MRI can be enhanced by higher B_0 field strength,[110] larger 3D spatial coverage,[43] vasodilator administration, and

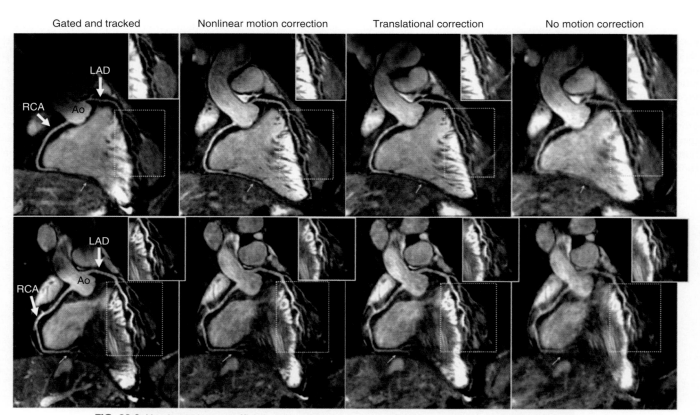

FIG. 23.3 Nearly 100% scan efficiency nonrigid motion correction coronary artery magnetic resonance image. This approach is based on beat-to-beat translation correction followed by respiratory bin-to-bin nonlinear motion correction. Reformatted images are shown for conventional navigator gated and tracked acquisition, nonrigid motion correction, translation correction only, and no motion correction for two different subjects. Blurring present in the no motion correction images is reduced with translation correction and sharpness further increased with the nonlinear motion correction approach *(boxes)*. The distal portions of both the right coronary artery *(RCA)* and the left anterior descending *(LAD)* coronary artery are particularly affected by motion *(arrows)*. The nonlinear motion correction approach has similar image quality to the conventional navigator gated and tracked acquisition; however, the latter requires significantly longer scan times (~2 to 3 times longer). *Ao,* Aorta.

contrast agents based on gadolinium chelates. The intrinsically higher SNR associated with higher magnetic field strengths may be advantageous for noncontrast coronary MRI. However, additional considerations, such as higher B_1 and B_0 inhomogeneity and higher specific absorption rate, affect certain aspects of coronary MRI, such as the diminished utility of bSSFP sequences at 3 T. Hence, GRE sequences, which are less sensitive to field inhomogeneity, as well as localized shimming[111] and contrast preparation techniques that deal with B_1 inhomogeneities[108,112] have been advocated.

The increased coverage of whole-heart coronary MRI can potentially improve the SNR, but this also increases the scan time. Thus the SNR gain is often counteracted by the need for accelerated imaging to reduce scan time, which carries an SNR penalty. Furthermore, whole-heart imaging suffers from saturation effects of the inflowing blood magnetization.[45] Despite these issues, excellent image quality of whole-heart coronary MRI has been shown in several studies,[40,43] and an example from a single-center study[40] is depicted in Fig. 23.4. Another technique to improve SNR

in coronary artery MRI is the administration of vasodilators because the increased coronary blood flow secondary to vasodilatation reduces the inflow saturation effects.[113,114] Fig. 23.5 demonstrates the impact of sublingual isosorbide dinitrate administration on 3D targeted coronary artery MRI up to 30 minutes after drug administration, in terms of subjective image quality and objective SNR and vessel sharpness.

The administration of exogenous gadolinium contrast agents (both extracellular[30,115,116] and intravascular[117-122]) that shorten the T1 relaxation time provides an alternative flow-independent approach to improve SNR and CNR. Because conventional extracellular contrast agents (e.g., gadopentetate dimeglumine [Gd-DTPA]) diffuse rapidly into the interstitial space, early contrast-enhanced coronary artery MRI studies focused on breath-hold coronary artery MRI to take advantage of the first passage of these agents.[116] However, both the breath-hold and first-pass aspects of such approaches limit the spatial resolution and are unsuitable for whole-heart coronary acquisitions.[123] Following the availability of a high relaxivity extracellular contrast agent, gadobenate dimeglumine

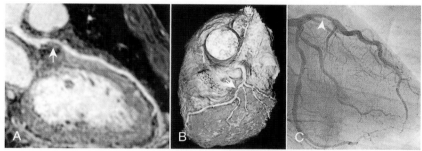

FIG. 23.4. Whole-heart coronary artery magnetic resonance image. (A) A stenosis in the left anterior descending (LAD) coronary artery is visualized using a curved multiplanar reconstruction *(arrow)*. (B) A three-dimensional view of LAD with stenosis is depicted in the volume-rendered image. (C) X-ray coronary angiography confirms proximal LAD stenosis *(arrowhead)*. (Modified from Sakuma H, Ichikawa Y, Chino S, et al. Detection of coronary artery stenosis with whole-heart coronary magnetic resonance angiography. *J Am Coll Cardiol.* 2006;48:1946–1950.)

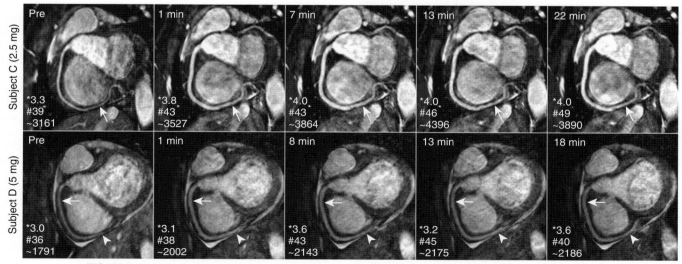

FIG. 23.5 Reformatted images from a targeted three-dimensional (3D) coronary magnetic resonance image of the right coronary artery (RCA). Images were acquired before and after sublingual isosorbide dinitrate administration on two healthy subjects using a 3D free-breathing balanced steady-state free precession following 2.5 mg *(top row)* or 5 mg doses *(bottom row)* as a function of time. Improved RCA vasodilation and signal enhancement can be observed in all images after isosorbide dinitrate *(arrows in top and bottom row)*. The enhanced signal-to-noise ratio following isosorbide dinitrate also allows for improved visualization of the distal segments.

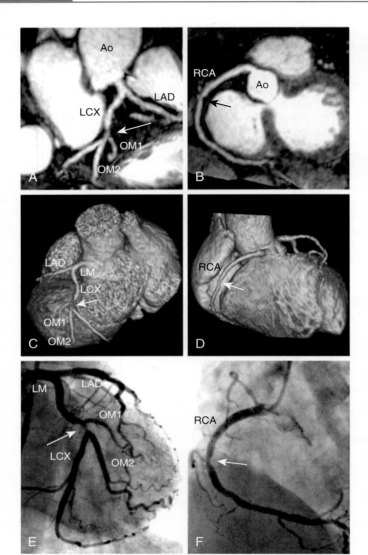

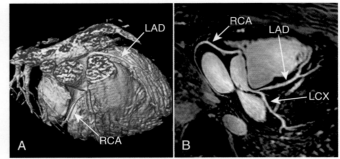

FIG. 23.7 Whole-heart balanced steady-state free precession coronary magnetic resonance image acquired with a bolus injection of gadobenate dimeglumine. (A) Three-dimensional volume rendering of the acquisition volume. (B) Corresponding reformatted whole-heart image. All three major coronary arteries and distal branches are clearly depicted. *LAD,* Left anterior descending coronary artery; *LCX,* left circumflex coronary artery; *RCA,* right coronary artery.

FIG. 23.6 Contrast-enhanced whole-heart three-dimensional coronary magnetic resonance image with a slow infusion of gadobenate dimeglumine contrast agent in a patient with atypical chest pain. (A, B) Contrast-enhanced whole-heart maximum intensity projection images show a significant stenosis in the proximal left circumflex *(LCX)* coronary artery and a nonsignificant stenosis in the middle right coronary artery *(RCA;* *arrows)*, respectively. (C, D) The volume-rendered images have the same findings in LCX and RCA *(arrows)*. These were consistent with the findings *(arrows)* of conventional coronary angiography (E, F). *Ao,* Aorta; *LM,* left main; *OM,* obtuse marginal artery. (Modified from Yang Q, Li K, Liu X, et al. Contrast-enhanced whole-heart coronary magnetic resonance angiography at 3.0-T: a comparative study with X-ray angiography in a single center. *J Am Coll Cardiol.* 2009;54:69–76.)

Furthermore, the bolus contrast injection method is advantageous in multiple ways because it simplifies the initiation time of coronary MRI acquisition compared with slow infusion, and it is compatible with late gadolinium enhancement imaging, which enables the assessment of coronary artery stenosis and myocardium viability using a single bolus contrast injection. Many patients with CAD also have renal dysfunction. The use of gadolinium contrast coronary MRI must consider the patient's renal function for issues related to nephrogenic systemic fibrosis and long-term retained gadolinium.

CORONARY MAGNETIC RESONANCE IMAGING— ADVANCED METHODS

The sensitivity and specificity of coronary MRI for detection of CAD remain moderate, based on single-center[40,41,124,126-130] (Table 23.1) and multicenter[15,24,131] studies (see Chapter 24), despite the tremendous technical improvements in the last two decades. Coronary motion, SNR and CNR remain as major impediments to coronary MRI, and these issues need to be addressed before clinical prime time for coronary MRI. To overcome some of these hurdles, several CMR centers continue with the development and implementation of novel approaches, including non-Cartesian acquisitions, accelerated imaging techniques, coronary vein MRI, and higher field imaging.

Non-Cartesian acquisitions provide efficient k-space traversals that lead to incoherent or less visually significant artifacts. Thus alternative non-Cartesian k-space acquisitions, including spiral and radial coronary MRI, have received attention. The use of spiral coronary artery MRI was first reported more than 2 decades ago.[132] Spiral acquisitions are advantageous to Cartesian acquisitions in several respects, including a more efficient filling of k-space, enhanced SNR,[46,133] and favorable flow properties. However, drawbacks of spiral trajectories include increased sensitivity to magnetic field inhomogeneity and longer image reconstruction. Interleaved spiral imaging is typically used because of reduced artifacts,[132-135] although a single-shot k-space trajectory can also be employed. Both breath-hold and free-breathing/navigator-gated 2D acquisitions can be performed with spiral coronary artery.[46,117,133,135] Compared with conventional Cartesian approaches, single spiral acquisitions (per RR interval) afford a near 3-fold improvement in SNR.[46,133] Hence, acquiring two spirals during each RR interval will halve the acquisition time, while maintaining superior SNR (vs. Cartesian acquisition) and CNR. Variable density spirals have also shown benefit.[90] Radial trajectories also enable more rapid acquisitions, while decreasing sensitivity

(Gd-BOPTA; MultiHance; Bracco Imaging SpA, Milan, Italy), improved whole-heart coronary artery MRI at 3 T was shown to be feasible using a T1-weighted inversion recovery (IR) GRE sequence with a slow infusion of Gd-BOPTA.[30] An example of a contrast-enhanced whole-heart coronary artery MR image from a CAD patient and the corresponding x-ray angiogram is shown in Fig. 23.6, demonstrating agreement between two modalities in detecting significant stenosis.[124] A bolus infusion of Gd-BOPTA for coronary MRI has also been reported,[125] and an example depicted in Fig. 23.7 shows a clear visualization of the three major coronary vessels in the reformatted and 3D-volume rendered images.

to motion. Data in healthy subjects appear promising[46,136-138] and may be particularly beneficial for coronary wall imaging.[82,139,140]

Parallel imaging techniques such as generalized autocalibrating partially parallel acquisition (GRAPPA)[141] or sensitivity encoding (SENSE)[142] are the most commonly used clinical acceleration technique for coronary artery MRI.[30,122,124,125] Resultant acceleration rates of up to 2-fold while using 5 to 16 element cardiac-coil arrays, and up to 4-fold acceleration rate using 32-channel coils have been achieved.[143,144] Currently, parallel imaging is considered the state-of-the-art accelerated imaging technique for whole-heart coronary artery MRI, and is commonly used for clinical imaging.

In addition to the non-Cartesian trajectories[145] described previously, compressed sensing (CS) has emerged as a robust alternative acceleration technique that exploits the sparsity of the image in a transform domain.[146,147] CS also requires an incoherent undersampling pattern, which can be achieved by random undersampling of k-space data in the k_y-k_z plane for 3D Cartesian acquisitions. In high-resolution coronary MRI, an advanced CS-based reconstruction strategy was shown to provide reconstructions with reduced blurring compared with conventional CS techniques[148] and was successfully used in contrast-enhanced whole-heart coronary MRI.[149] More recently, for highly-accelerated sub-millimeter resolution whole-heart coronary MRI, CS was shown to outperform parallel imaging at 6-fold accelerated imaging in a head-to-head comparison[150] (Fig. 23.8). CS can also be used in conjunction with non-Cartesian imaging, such as with spiral acquisitions, to enable whole-heart acquisitions in a single prolonged breath-hold[89] or with 3D radial trajectories.[151]

Coronary MRI at high fields has been an active area of research as a result of potential benefits in SNR and CNR. SNR is directly related to field strength (B_0), and thus 3 T imaging would offer the opportunity to double SNR compared with 1.5 T systems.[152] Although the vast majority of coronary artery MRI investigations have been performed on 1.5 T, clinical 3 T systems are commonly available and becoming the platform of choice for CMR. Technical challenges to 3 T include increased susceptibility artifacts, field inhomogeneities,[108] reduced T2*,[153,154] increased specific absorption rate (SAR), T1 prolongation, and the amplified magnetohydrodynamic effect.[48] At 3 T, free-breathing navigator and breath-hold 3D coronary artery MRI studies in healthy volunteers have demonstrated >50% improvement in SNR with impressive image quality using segmented k-space gradient echo or SSFP,[155] as well as spiral and contrast enhanced methods.[156-158] Coronary MRI at 3 T using SSFP sequences is challenging because of increased field inhomogeneity and high SAR; thus GRE sequences have become widely used for coronary CMR at 3 T. To reduce the impact of B_1 inhomogeneity at the high field strengths, improved preparation sequences such as adiabatic T2 magnetization preparation[108,112] and adiabatic fat saturation have also been used. Fig. 23.9 shows example coronary MRI acquired at 3 T using improved T2 magnetization preparation, which suppresses the

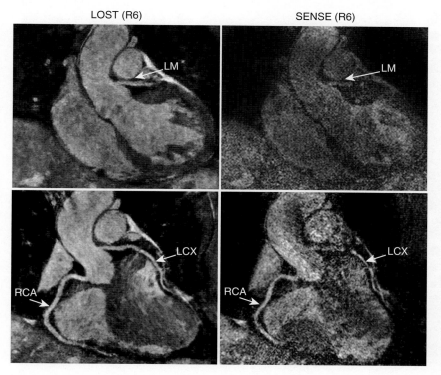

FIG. 23.8 Example images from two separate highly-accelerated sub-millimeter resolution whole-heart coronary artery magnetic resonance images. An example coronal slice *(top)* containing a cross section of the left main *(LM)* shows that sensitivity encoding *(SENSE)* images, acquired with 6-fold uniform undersampling *(right)*, suffers from noise amplification. In contrast, the LM is clearly visualized using an advanced compressed sensing–based technique (low-dimensional-structure self-learning and thresholding *[LOST]*, acquired using 6-fold random undersampling *(left)*. In the reformatted coronal images *(bottom)*, the proximal left circumflex *(LCX)* coronary artery cannot be tracked because of the high noise level in the SENSE reconstruction, but right coronary artery *(RCA)* and LCX branches are visualized with the LOST technique.

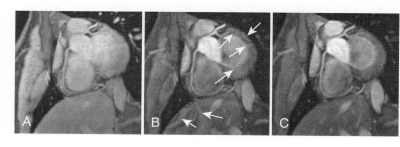

FIG. 23.9 Example reformatted three-dimensional coronary magnetic resonance image of the right coronary artery at 3 T (A) acquired with no T2-preparation; (B) with T2-preparation; and (C) with adiabatic T2-preparation. Arrows in B point to the artifacts resulting from T2-preparation sequence. The banding artifacts are suppressed in C, where the homogeneity of the signal is also improved.

banding artifact resulting from conventional T2 magnetization preparation. Coronary MRI at even higher field strengths, such as 7 T,[159] is even more challenging. Several technical issues, including coil design, motion compensation, and B_0 and B_1 field inhomogeneity, need to be addressed before clinical evaluation is possible. Finally, simultaneous black-blood LGE methods and bright-blood coronary MRI imaging are being explored as a means of improving scan efficiency for the comprehensive assessment of patients with known or suspected CAD.[159a]

Coronary Artery Wall Imaging

As with coronary artery lumen MRI, the first in vivo MRI demonstrating the coronary vessel wall were obtained using 2D fat-saturated fast-spin echo techniques.[139,160] A double inversion recovery (IR) preparation pulse was applied to obtain black-blood images and improved contrast between the blood and the vessel wall.[161] Further developments of the technique include the combination of the double IR preparation with fast-gradient echo readout techniques,[162] including spiral[163] and radial[140] acquisition trajectories. Examples of in-plane and cross-sectional coronary vessel wall images with double IR preparation and radial and spiral acquisitions are shown in Fig. 23.10 and Fig. 23.11, respectively. Clinical studies demonstrated outward positive remodelling with lumen preservation in patients with established CAD and increased vessel wall thickness in patients with type 1 diabetes and renal dysfunction.[18,164]

One limitation of black-blood approaches for coronary vessel wall is that these techniques rely on blood flow, which may be insufficient in patients with very low coronary flow or heavily calcified coronary plaque. Furthermore, these acquisitions are limited in coverage to 2D acquisitions or targeted 3D scans. Because the coronary arteries have

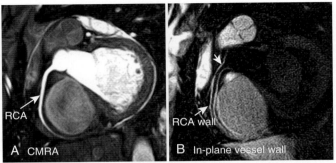

FIG. 23.10 (A) Coronary artery magnetic resonance image and (B) three-dimensional (3D) in-plane coronary vessel wall imaging using a local inversion preparation pulse and a 3D stack-of-stars (radial) scan with an in-plane spatial resolution of 0.9 mm × 0.9 mm and a slice thickness of 2.4 mm. *CMRA*, Coronary magnetic resonance angiography; *RCA*, right coronary artery.

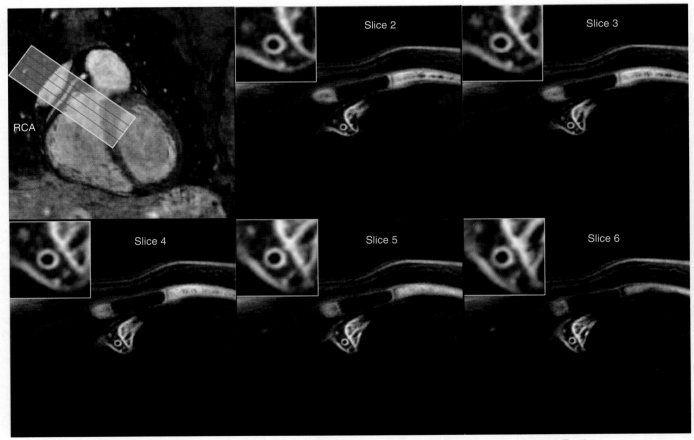

FIG. 23.11 Three-dimensional (3D) cross-sectional coronary vessel wall imaging performed at 3 T using a local inversion recovery preparation pulse and a 3D stack-of-spirals scan with in-plane spatial resolution of 0.6 mm × 0.6 mm and a slice thickness of 3 mm. To acquire cross-sectional slices of the vessel wall, the 3D imaging volume (6 slices) was positioned perpendicular to a relatively linear portion of the proximal/mid right coronary artery *(RCA)*. (Modified from Peel SA, Hussain T, Schaeffter T, et al. Cross-sectional and in-plane coronary vessel wall imaging using a local inversion prepulse and spiral read-out: a comparison between 1.5 and 3 Tesla. *J Magn Reson Imaging.* 2012;35:969–975.)

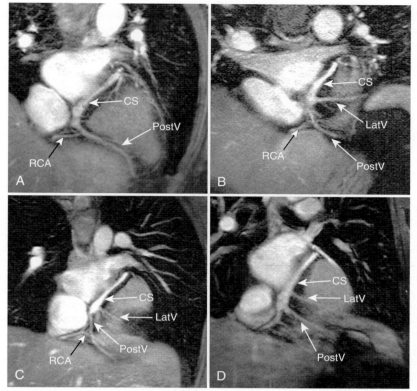

FIG. 23.12 (A–D) Example coronary vein cardiovascular magnetic resonance acquired using magnetization transfer contrast gradient recalled echo during the systolic rest period, depicting the variations in the coronary venous anatomy in four healthy adult subjects. Clear variations in the branching point, angle, and diameter of different tributaries of coronary sinus are observed, highlighting the potential for noninvasive assessment of the coronary venous anatomy in cardiac resynchronization therapy. For example, subject A has no visible lateral vein *(LatV)*. *CS*, Compressed sensing; *PostV*, posterior vein; *RCA*, right coronary artery.

a tortuous course, complicated scan planning is required. A 3D flow independent approach for vessel wall imaging was proposed based on an interleaved acquisition and subtraction of bSSFP data with and without a T2 preparation pulse.[165] This allows for nulling of arterial blood signal while maintaining myocardial and vessel wall signal. Although this approach provides simultaneously coronary lumen and vessel wall images, the required subtraction is particularly sensitive to respiratory motion corruption. Further recent improvements include the combination of this technique with an image-navigator based non-rigid motion correction approach.[166]

Coronary Vein Cardiovascular Magnetic Resonance

For several interventional cardiac procedures, including epicardial radio-frequency ablation,[167,168] retrograde perfusion therapy in high-risk or complicated coronary angioplasty,[169] arrhythmia assessment,[170,171] stem cell delivery,[172] coronary artery bypass surgery,[173] and cardiac resynchronization therapy (CRT),[174,175] there has been increased interest in imaging the coronary vein anatomy. In CRT, simultaneous pacing of the right ventricle and left ventricle (LV), or pacing the LV alone, results in hemodynamic improvement and restoration of a more physiological contraction pattern.[176] One of the technical difficulties of CRTs is achieving effective, safe, and permanent pacing of the LV. Transvenous coronary sinus pacing is the most common technique because it has the least procedural risk, but it is associated with long procedure times, extensive radiation exposure from fluoroscopy, implantation failure, and LV lead dislodgment. Two of the major difficulties of the transvenous approach are the small number of coronary vein

branches adjacent to an appropriate LV wall and the great variability in coronary vein anatomy.[175] Ideally coronary venous morphology should be assessed noninvasively before CRT procedure to determine whether epicardial or transvenous lead placement would be more appropriate.

The technical challenges of coronary vein CMR are similar to coronary artery MRI, and techniques developed for coronary artery MRI are widely applicable. Notable differences in coronary vein CMR include the MTC methods and optimal time window for imaging within the cardiac cycle, as well as more modest spatial resolution requirements because information regarding vein anatomy and vessel size are desired, but not focal stenoses. MTC has been used in coronary vein imaging, which is different than the T2 magnetization preparation commonly used in coronary artery MRI, for both targeted[109] and whole-heart[177] approaches. Fig. 23.12 shows an example of coronary vein CMR using a targeted approach with a MTC sequence. Contrast in coronary vein CMR can be improved by other means, including the use of intravascular contrast agents such as gadocoletic acid trisodium salt[178] or the use of high relaxivity extracellular contrast agents such as Gd-BOPTA.[125] For the optimal window of imaging, whereas coronary artery MRI is commonly performed during the mid diastolic quiescent period, coronary vein CMR is acquired in the end-systolic quiescent period as it coincides with the maximum size of the coronary veins.[109]

REFERENCES

A full reference list is available online at ExpertConsult.com

24

Coronary Artery Imaging: Clinical Results

Shiro Nakamori, Hajime Sakuma, and Warren J. Manning

Chapter 23 reviewed the technical issues and solutions for coronary artery cardiovascular magnetic resonance (CMR) imaging. This chapter reviews the clinical data comparing coronary artery CMR with invasive x-ray coronary angiography for identification of anomalous coronary artery disease (CAD), characterization of coronary artery aneurysms, detection of native vessel disease, and assessment of coronary artery bypass graft integrity. It also describes studies comparing CMR with coronary artery multidetector computed tomography (MDCT), the other principal noninvasive modality for imaging the coronary arteries. The majority of data represent single-center experience, with quantitative x-ray coronary angiography used as the reference standard for most of the larger single-center and few multicenter studies.

IDENTIFICATION OF ANOMALOUS CORONARY ARTERIES

As discussed in Chapter 23, using current whole-heart imaging with or without gadolinium contrast, the native proximal coronary arteries can be reliably visualized in nearly all subjects. Although unusual (<1% of the general population[1,2]) and most often benign, congenital coronary anomalies in which the anomalous segment courses anterior to the aorta and posterior to the pulmonary artery are well-recognized causes of myocardial ischemia and sudden cardiac death in children and young adults.[3,4] These adverse events commonly occur during or immediately after intense exercise and are believed to be related to compression of the anomalous segment, vessel kinking, or coexistent eccentric ostial stenoses.[3]

The ability of coronary artery CMR to reliably identify the major coronary arteries and their relationship to the ascending aorta and pulmonary artery immediately provides for its application for the identification and characterization of anomalous CAD. The spatial resolution requirements for identifying anomalous coronary vessels are less stringent than for defining native vessel stenoses, allowing for lower resolution and faster CMR imaging.

Projection x-ray angiography had traditionally been the imaging test of choice for the diagnosis and characterization of these anomalies. However, the presence of an anomalous vessel is sometimes suspected only after the procedure, particularly in a situation in which there was unsuccessful engagement of a coronary artery. In addition, the uncommon use of a pulmonary artery catheter has made characterization of the anterior or posterior trajectory of the anomalous vessels more difficult to appreciate on projection x-ray angiography.

Coronary artery CMR has several advantages compared with both coronary MDCT and x-ray angiography in the diagnosis of these coronary anomalies. In addition to being noninvasive and not requiring ionizing radiation or iodinated contrast agents, coronary artery CMR provides a definitive three-dimensional (3D) "road map" of the mediastinum (Fig. 24.1). Early studies applied two-dimensional (2D) breath-hold segmented *k*-space gradient echo coronary artery CMR,[5–7] although most centers now use targeted 3D[8–11] or whole heart[11–16] free-breathing navigator coronary artery CMR because of the superior reconstruction capabilities afforded by 3D datasets, with similar results. The ability to acquire these data using CMR without the use of ionizing radiation is likely to be of particular benefit in the generally younger population.[17]

In addition, noncontrast coronary artery CMR is likely preferred to avoid potential long-term issues related to retention of gadolinium.[18]

There have been at least eight published series[5–10,12,14,16] of patients who underwent a comparison of coronary artery CMR at 1.5 T or 3 T with x-ray angiography for suspected anomalous CAD. These studies have uniformly reported excellent accuracy, including several instances in which coronary artery CMR was determined to be superior to x-ray angiography (Table 24.1). Data also suggest coronary artery CMR evidence of a coronary anomaly carries important prognostic information[11] with the identification of the anomalous segment originating from the opposite sinus of Valsalva (see Fig. 24.1) as conveying an adverse prognosis. As a result, CMR is considered a class I indication for suspected anomalous CAD.[19] At experienced CMR centers, clinical coronary artery CMR is the preferred test for patients in whom anomalous disease is suspected, those with known anomalous disease that must be further clarified, and those with coronary anomalies associated with other cardiac anomalies (e.g., tetralogy of Fallot). Although MDCT has also been shown to be efficacious for this indication,[20–22] coronary artery CMR is often preferred because there is no need for ionizing radiation or intravenous contrast.

CORONARY ARTERY ANEURYSMS AND KAWASAKI DISEASE

Coronary artery aneurysms are relatively uncommon, but have received increasing attention because of their common occurrence in pediatric and young adult patients with a history of mucocutaneous lymph node syndrome (Kawasaki disease), a generalized vasculitis of unknown etiology usually occurring in children age >5 years. The prevalence of Kawasaki disease is highest among children of East Asian countries, with the greatest prevalence in Japan.[23] Infants and children with this syndrome may show evidence of myocarditis or pericarditis, with nearly 20% having coronary artery aneurysms. These aneurysms (Fig. 24.2) are the source of both short-term and long-term morbidity and mortality.[24] Fortunately, one-half of the children with coronary aneurysms during the acute phase of the disease have a normal-appearing coronary lumen on catheter-based x-ray angiography 2 years later.[24,25] Transthoracic echocardiography is often adequate for diagnosing and following these proximal and mid-vessel aneurysms in very young children, but this modality is deficient after adolescence and in obese children. These young adults are therefore often referred for serial catheter-based x-ray coronary angiography, with the accumulation of significant radiation

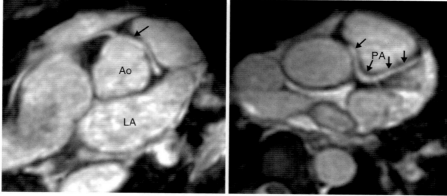

FIG. 24.1 Noncontrast whole heart 3 T coronary artery cardiovascular magnetic resonance imaging in a patient with an anomalous left coronary artery *(arrow)* from the right sinus of Valsalva. This is the malignant form of anomalous disease in which the anomalous segment courses between the anterior right ventricular outflow tract/pulmonary artery *(PA)* and posterior aorta *(Ao)*. *LA,* Left atrium.

TABLE 24.1 Coronary Artery Cardiovascular Magnetic Resonance for Anomalous Coronary Artery Disease

Investigator	Patients *(N)*	Correctly Classified Vessels
McConnell et al.[5]	15	14 (93%)
Post et al.[6]	19	19 (100%)[a]
Vliegen et al.[7]	12	11 (92%)[b]
Taylor et al.[8]	25	24 (96%)
Bunce et al.[9]	26	26 (100%)[c]
Razmi et al.[10]	12	12 (100%)
Tangcharoen et al.[15]	46 with congenital disease	46 (100%)
Piccini[16]	16	15 (94%)

[a]Including 3 patients originally misclassified by x-ray angiography.
[b]Including 5 patients unable to be classified by x-ray angiography.
[c]Including 11 patients unable to be classified by x-ray angiography.

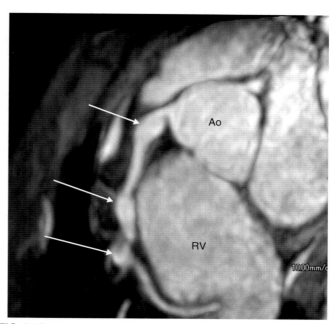

FIG. 24.2 Noncontrast whole heart coronary artery cardiovascular magnetic resonance in a child with Kawasaki disease and serial coronary artery aneurysms *(arrows)* involving the right coronary artery. *Ao,* Aorta; *RV,* right ventricle.

exposure over time. Coronary artery CMR data from two series of adolescents and young adults with coronary artery aneurysms have confirmed the high accuracy of coronary artery CMR for both the identification and the characterization (diameter and length [Fig. 24.3]) of these aneurysms[26–30] with addition of cine ventricular function and late gadolinium enhancement (LGE) for a comprehensive cardiac assessment.[28] Although not specifically examined in long-term follow-up studies, these data suggest that coronary aneurysms can now be effectively followed with serial CMR studies, including vessel wall inflammation.[29,30] Similar data have been reported for ectatic coronary vessels.[31]

NATIVE VESSEL CORONARY ARTERY STENOSES

Data support a broad clinical role for coronary artery CMR in the assessment of suspected anomalous CAD (and coronary artery bypass graft patency, which is addressed later), but data are not yet sufficient to support the use of clinical coronary artery CMR for routine identification of coronary artery stenoses among patients presenting with chest pain or for screening, even in high-risk patients. However, data suggest a role for coronary artery CMR among patients for the discrimination of ischemic versus nonischemic cardiomyopathy.

As discussed in earlier chapters, noncontrast gradient echo sequences show rapidly moving laminar blood flow as bright, whereas areas of stagnant flow or focal turbulence appear dark because of local saturation (stagnant flow) or dephasing (turbulence). Areas of focal stenoses appear as varying severity of "signal voids" in the coronary artery CMR, with the severity of signal loss related to the angiographic stenosis.[32] Because of time constraints of breath-hold, 2D breath-hold coronary artery CMR has relatively limited in-plane spatial resolution, but the technique has successfully shown proximal coronary stenoses in several clinical studies (Table 24.2).[32–35] When reported, the distance from the vessel origin to the focal stenosis on coronary artery CMR correlates closely with x-ray angiography findings.[32] However, there have been wide variations in the reported sensitivity and specificity of 2D coronary artery CMR, much of which may be attributable to technical and

TABLE 24.3 **Free-Breathing, Three-Dimensional, Gradient Echo Coronary Magnetic Resonance Imaging Using Prospective Navigators for Identification of Focal Coronary Stenoses 50% or More in Diameter**

Investigator	Subjects (N)	Technique	Sensitivity	Specificity
Prospective Navigators With Real-Time Correction Targeted Three-Dimensional Coronary Artery CMR				
Regenfus et al.[36]	50	TFE	94%	57%
Bunce et al.[37]	34	TFE	88%	72%
Moustapha et al.[38]	25	TFE	92%	55%
			90% (proximal)	92% (proximal)
Sommer et al.[39]	112	TFE	74%	63%
			88% (good quality)	91% (good quality)
Bogaert et al.[40]	19	TFE	85%–92%	50%–83%
Plein et al.[41]	10	TFE	75%	85%
Ozgun et al.[42]	14	TFE	91%	57%
		bSSFP	76%	85%
Dewey et al.[43]	15[a]	bSSFP	86%	98%
Maintz et al.[44]	12	TFE	92%	67%
		bSSFP	81%	82%
Ozgun et al.[45]	20	bSSFP	82%	82%
Jahnke et al.[46]	21	bSSFP	79%	91%
Paetsch et al.[59]	18	bSSFP	83%	77%
	18	Contrast	86%	95%
Sommer et al.[47]	18	TFE	82%	88%
Prospective Navigator With Real-Time Correction Whole Heart Steady-State Free Precession Coronary Artery CMR				
Sakuma et al.[50]	39	bSSFP	82%	91%
Jahnke et al.[51]	55	bSSFP	78%	91%
Sakuma et al.[52]	113	bSSFP	82%	90%
Nagata et al.[53]	62	32-channel SSFP	83%	93%
Klein et al.[54]	46	bSSFP	91%	54%
Pouleur et al.[55]	77	bSSFP	100%	72%
Greenwood et al.[56]	598	bSSFP	72% (M)/67% (F)	90% (M)/88% (F)
Nagata et al.[57]	67	bSSFP	87%	86%
Heer et al.[58]	59	bSSFP	86.7%	79.3%
1.5 T Self-Gated Postcontrast Whole Heart Coronary Artery CMR				
Piccini et al.[16]	40	Postcontrast bSSFP	71%	63%
3 T Whole Heart Coronary Artery CMR				
Sommer et al.[47]	18	TFE	82%	89%
Yang et al.[60]	69	Contrast IR-GRE	94%	82%

[a]Based on 60% of patients with good free breathing coronary magnetic resonance images.
bSSFP, Balanced steady-state free precession; *CMR*, cardiovascular magnetic resonance; *IR-GRE*, inversion recovery gradient echo; *TFE*, turbo field echo.

TABLE 24.4 **Multicenter Coronary Artery Cardiovascular Magnetic Resonance Trials**

Author	Field Strength	Patients (N)	Sensitivity	Specificity	PPV	NPV
Kim et al.[49]	1.5 T	109	93%	42%	70%	81%
Kato et al.[61]	1.5 T	138	88%	72%	71%	88%
Yang et al.[62a]	3 T	272	91%	80%		

NPV, Negative predictive value; *PPV*, positive predictive value.

study by Heer et al.[58] found that the combination of coronary artery CMR with adenosine stress perfusion improved overall accuracy from 78% to 92% for the detection of angiographically significant CAD. A 3T study by Zhang et al. involving 46 patients found the addition of contrast-enhanced coronary artery CMR resulted in higher sensitivity (100% vs. 76.5%) and accuracy (89% vs. 74%) with no change in specificity.[64]

Coronary Artery Cardiovascular Magnetic Resonance and Prognosis

Increasingly, validation of cardiac imaging is focused on the impact on outcomes. There are limited data on the prognostic valve of coronary artery CMR. Yoon and colleagues[65] studied 207 consecutive patients without prior known CAD using whole heart bSSFP free-breathing

TABLE 24.5 Comparison of Different Components of the Cardiovascular Magnetic Resonance Imaging Examination for Detection of Significant Coronary Artery Disease

CMR Component	Sex (N)	Sensitivity	Specificity
CE-MARC Trial; Modified From Greenwood et al.[56]			
LV function	393M	49.2%	92.9%
	235F	39.6%	95.1%
Perfusion	388M	75.4%	92.9%
	229F	81.1%	89.2%
LGE	392M	41.2%	94.4%
	235F	34.0%	97.8%
Coronary artery	349M	72.3%	90.3%
	208F	66.7%	87.7%
Heer et al.[58]			
Coronary artery	59	86.7%	79.3%
Coronary artery with perfusion	59	95.7%	88.9%
Gotschy et al.[91]			
Coronary artery	11	75%	79%
Coronary artery with perfusion and LGE	11	94%	82%

CE-MARC, Clinical Evaluation of Magnetic Resonance Imaging in Coronary Heart Disease; *CMR*, cardiovascular magnetic resonance; *LGE*, late gadolinium enhancement; *LV*, left ventricle.

coronary artery CMR at 1.5 T. Follow-up was available for a median of 25 months and 41% had CAD on coronary artery CMR (Fig. 24.5). The presence of a stenosis on coronary artery CMR had a univariate hazard ratio of 20.8 (multivariate 18)/12% risk of cardiac death (1.2%), unstable angina (4.8%), or late revascularization (8.3%) whereas the absence of a stenosis was associated with late revascularization in <1% of subjects.

COMPARISON OF CORONARY ARTERY CARDIOVASCULAR MAGNETIC RESONANCE WITH MULTIDETECTOR COMPUTED TOMOGRAPHY

Several studies have directly compared MDCT with coronary artery CMR for the detection of CAD (Table 24.6). Overall, these studies have suggested similar accuracy when interpretable segments were considered and superiority of 64-slice MDCT for patients with lower calcium scores with "intention to diagnose" analyses because of the superior ability of MDCT to acquire interpretable images. The first direct study by Gerber and colleagues[66] compared free-breathing, targeted noncontrast 3D coronary artery CMR with four-slice MDCT and showed slight superiority of coronary artery CMR for overall accuracy. A follow-up study of 52 patients performed by the same group with 16-slice MDCT showed equivalence with visual analysis.[67] Another 16-slice MDCT comparative study by Dewey and colleagues showed superiority of MDCT[68] for sensitivity, but the coronary artery CMR technique used free breathing or an inferior multiple-breath-hold approach. Interestingly, coronary artery CMR sensitivity (74%) was improved compared with an earlier report from this group,[43] suggesting a learning curve for coronary artery CMR. Patients expressed a preference for MDCT,[68] with the advantage of very rapid and simplified protocols at the expense of substantial

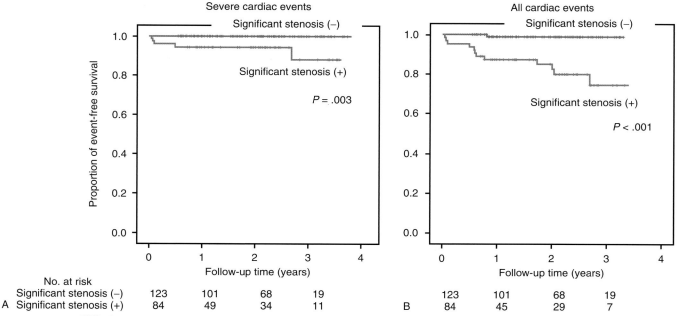

FIG. 24.5 Kaplan-Meier event free survival curves based on noncontrast three-dimensional whole-heart coronary artery cardiovascular magnetic resonance for (A) severe cardiac events and (B) all cardiac events. (Modified from Yoon YE, Kitagawa K, Kato S, et al. Prognostic value of coronary magnetic resonance angiography for prediction of cardiac events in patients with suspected coronary artery disease. *J Am Coll Cardiol.* 2012;60:2316–2322.)

TABLE 24.6 **Comparative Studies of Coronary Artery Cardiovascular Magnetic Resonance and Multidetector Computed Tomography[a]**

Investigator	CMR/CCT Method	Sensitivity	Specificity	PPV	NPV	Accuracy
Gerber et al.[66]	CMR:FB-SSFP	62%	84%[b]	49%	90%	80%[c]
	4-slice MDCT	79%[c]	71%	40%	93%	73%
Kefer et al.[67]	CMR:FB-SSFP	75%	77%	42%	93%	77%
	16-slice MDCT	82%	79%	46%	95%	80%
Dewey et al.[68]	CMR-BH/FB-SSFP	74%[b]	75%	95%	84%	—
	16-slice CT	92%	79%	95%	90%	—
Maintz et al.[69]	CMR-FB-SSFP	84%	95%	77%	95%	93%
	16-slice MDCT	82%	88%	68%	94%	87%
Pouleur et al.[55]	CMR-FB SSFP	100%	72%[c]	50%[c]	100%	78%[c]
	40/64-slice MDCT	94%	88%	70%	98%	90%
Liu et al.[74]	CMR-FB-SSFP	75%	81%	—	—	—
	64-slice MDCT	75%	48%[c]	—	—	—

[a]Reported values are from patient-based analyses for the detection of coronary artery disease.
[b]$P < .001$.
[c]$P < .05$.

BH, Breath-hold; *CMR*, cardiovascular magnetic resonance; *FB*, free breathing; *MDCT*, multidetector computed tomography; *NPV*, negative predictive value; *PPV*, positive predictive value; *SSFP*, steady-state free precession.

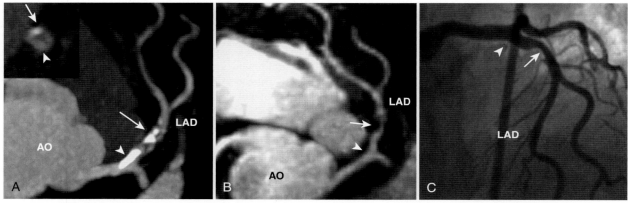

FIG. 24.6 (A) Extensive epicardial coronary calcium of the left anterior descending *(LAD)* coronary artery as visualized by multidetector computed tomography (MDCT). (B) Coronary artery cardiovascular magnetic resonance image. (C) X-ray coronary angiography. The proximal calcium deposit *(arrowhead)* obscures the lumen on MDCT but is seen on cardiovascular magnetic resonance as patent. The more distal calcium deposit *(arrow)* is identified as a stenosis on cardiovascular magnetic resonance image and the corresponding x-ray angiogram. *AO*, Aorta. (Modified from Liu X, Zhao X, Huang J, et al. Comparison of 3D free-breathing coronary MR angiography and 64-MDCT angiography for detection of coronary stenosis in patients with high calcium scores. *Am J Roentgenol.* 2007;189:1326–1332.)

radiation exposure and need for iodinated contrast. A third comparative study by Maintz and associates[69] of coronary artery CMR and a 16-slice MDCT showed superiority of coronary artery MDCT image quality and disease analysis on a coronary segment basis, but showed equivalence when only evaluable segments were included. Finally, a comparison of whole heart coronary artery CMR with 40-slice or 64-slice MDCT by Pouleur and coworkers[55] showed very high sensitivity of coronary artery CMR, but overall superiority of coronary artery MDCT. This is likely related to their "intention to diagnose" analysis and the classification of uninterpretable segments as "diseased" in a population with a low (22%) prevalence of CAD. Uninterpretable segments were more frequent for coronary artery CMR.

Epicardial calcium is associated with aging and with the development of coronary atherosclerosis. It is a marker for increased risk of adverse events associated with CAD.[70] The presence of epicardial calcium is a well-recognized limitation of coronary artery MDCT, with an exaggerated

appearance on imaging (frequently referred to as "blooming") that interferes with the accurate determination of coronary artery stenosis. Several trials using MDCT have excluded patients with substantial epicardial calcium[71] or have shown marked reduction in specificity for patients with Agatston calcium scores >400.[72,73] A comparative study of coronary artery CMR and 64-slice MDCT in patients with high calcium scores showed superiority of coronary artery CMR[74] (Fig. 24.6).

CORONARY ARTERY CARDIOVASCULAR MAGNETIC RESONANCE FOR CORONARY ARTERY BYPASS GRAFT ASSESSMENT

Assessment of coronary artery bypass graft patency is a common clinical issue.[75,76] Compared with the native coronary arteries, reverse saphenous vein and internal mammary artery grafts are relatively easy to image because of their relatively minimal motion during the cardiac

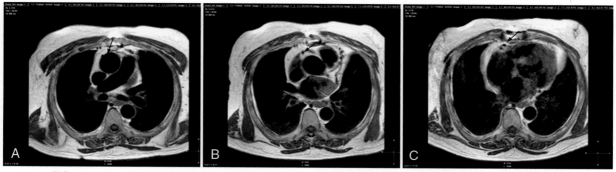

FIG. 24.7 Transverse fast spin echo images in a patient with previous coronary artery bypass grafting. (A) The proximal graft is identified *(arrow)*, with subsequent inferior sections (B) and (C) showing a patent graft *(arrows)*.

TABLE 24.7 Sensitivity, Specificity, and Accuracy of Coronary Artery Cardiovascular Magnetic Resonance for Assessment of Coronary Artery Bypass Graft Patency

Investigator	Technique	Grafts (N)	Patency	Sensitivity	Specificity	Accuracy
White et al.[77]	2D spin echo	72	69%	86%	59%	78%
Rubinstein et al.[82]	2D spin echo	47	62%	90%	72%	83%
Jenkins et al.[83]	2D spin echo	41	63%	89%	73%	83%
Galjee et al.[79]	2D spin echo	98	74%	98%	85%	89%
White et al.[78]	2D GRE	28	50%	93%	86%	89%
Aurigemma et al.[80]	2D GRE	45	73%	88%	100%	91%
Galjee et al.[79]	2D GRE	98	74%	98%	88%	96%
			66% (SVG)	92%	85%	89%
Molinari et al.[84]	3D GRE	51	76.5%	91%	97%	96%
Engelmann et al.[81]	CE-3D GRE	96 SVG	66%	92%	85%	89%
		37 IMA	100%	100%	100%	
Wintersperger et al.[85]	CE-3D GRE	39	87%	97%	100%	97%
Vrachliotis et al.[86]	CE-3D GRE	45	67%	93%	97%	95%

2D, Two-dimensional; *3D,* three-dimensional; *CE,* contrast-enhanced; *GRE,* gradient recalled echo; *IMA,* internal mammary artery graft; *SVG,* saphenous vein graft.

and respiratory cycle and the larger lumen of reverse saphenous vein grafts. Furthermore, their predictable and less convoluted course has allowed imaging of bypass grafts, even with less sophisticated CMR methods.

With schematic knowledge of the origin and touchdown site of each graft, conventional free-breathing electrocardiographic (ECG)-triggered 2D spin echo and noncontrast 2D gradient echo coronary artery CMR in the transverse plane have both been used to reliably assess bypass graft patency (Fig. 24.7 and Table 24.7).[77–86] Patency is determined by visualizing a patent graft lumen in at least two contiguous transverse images along its expected course (presenting as a signal void for spin echo techniques and bright signal for gradient echo approaches). If signal consistent with flow is identified in the area of the graft lumen, it is very likely to be patent. If a patent lumen is seen at only one level (e.g., for spin echo techniques, a signal void is seen at only one level), a graft is considered indeterminate. If a patent graft lumen is not seen at any level, the graft is very likely occluded. Combining spin echo and gradient echo imaging in the same patient does not appear to improve accuracy.[79] A 3D noncontrast[84] and contrast-enhanced coronary artery CMR has also been described for the assessment of graft patency,[85,86] with slightly improved results (see Table 24.7). The accuracy of ECG-triggered bSSFP sequences appears to be similar to that of spin echo and gradient echo approaches.[87]

TABLE 24.8 Diagnostic Accuracy of Submillimeter Coronary Artery Cardiovascular Magnetic Resonance for Saphenous Vein Graft Disease

	Sensitivity	Specificity
Graft occlusion	83% (36%–100%)	100% (92%–100%)
Graft stenosis ≥50%	82% (57%–96%)	88% (72%–97%)
Graft stenosis ≥70%	73% (39%–94%)	80% (64%–91%)

Modified from Langerak SE, Vliegan HW, de Roos A, et al. Defection of vein graft disease using high resolution magnetic resonance angiography. *Circulation.* 2002;105:328–333.

Limitations of coronary artery CMR bypass graft assessment include difficulties related to local signal loss and artifact as a result of implanted metallic objects (hemostatic clips, ostial stainless-steel graft markers, sternal wires, coexistent prosthetic valves and supporting struts or rings, and graft stents; Fig. 24.8). The inability to identify severely diseased yet patent grafts is also a hindrance to clinical utility and acceptance. Langerak and colleagues[88] found free-breathing navigator 3D gradient echo coronary artery CMR to be accurate for the assessment of

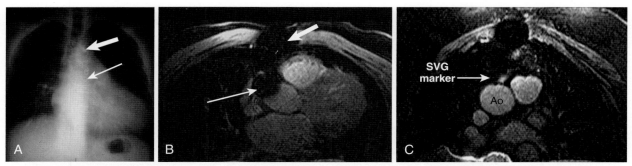

FIG. 24.8 (A) Posterior-anterior chest radiograph in a patient with coronary artery bypass grafts. Note the sternal wires *(thick arrow)* and the coronary artery bypass markers *(thin arrow)*. (B) Transverse coronary cardiovascular magnetic resonance image in the same patient. Note the large local artifacts (signal voids) related to sternal wires *(thick arrow)* and bypass graft markers *(thin arrow)*. (C) Barium and tantalum markers *(arrow)* result in the smallest artifacts. The size of the artifacts is reduced somewhat with spin echo and black-blood cardiovascular magnetic resonance. *Ao,* Aorta; *SVG,* saphenous vein graft.

saphenous vein graft stenoses, with very good agreement with quantitative x-ray angiography for the assessment of both graft occlusion and graft stenoses (Table 24.8). This group has also advocated assessment of rest and adenosine stress coronary artery flow assessment using the phase velocity CMR technique,[89,90] suggesting superior results for flow assessment.

CONCLUSION

Over the last two decades, coronary artery CMR has been transformed from a scientific curiosity to a clinically useful imaging tool in selected populations. Uses include the identification and characterization of anomalous coronary arteries, characterization of aneurysms, and assessment of coronary artery bypass graft patency. Coronary artery CMR also appears to be of clinical value for the assessment of native vessel-integrity in selected patients, especially those with suspected left main or multivessel disease. Normal findings on coronary artery CMR

strongly suggest the absence of left main or multivessel disease and also conveys an excellent prognosis. Overall, data suggest that successful coronary artery imaging is accomplished more often with MDCT, but when successfully obtained, accuracy is similar for CMR and MDCT. CMR is superior in patients with prominent epicardial calcium and has the advantage of avoiding ionizing radiation and iodinated contrast.

Technical and methodologic advances in motion suppression, along with improved surface coil design, faster acquisitions, and intravascular contrast agents continue to advance the field (see Chapter 23). Importantly, future studies comparing coronary artery CMR with fractional flow reserve and assessing outcomes will be needed for coronary magnetic resonance imaging to successfully transition to the clinical arena for the assessment of patients with suspected CAD.

REFERENCES

A full reference list is available online at ExpertConsult.com

25

Coronary Artery and Sinus Velocity and Flow

Jennifer Keegan and Dudley J. Pennell

A coronary stenosis may be observed during cardiovascular magnetic resonance (CMR) as an area of signal loss caused by turbulent flow, and although both the degree and the extent of signal loss are indicative of the severity of the stenosis, accurate quantification is not possible.[1] However, both phasic coronary artery blood flow and flow velocity may be affected by the presence of stenosis, and the ratio of coronary artery flow under maximal vasodilation to coronary artery flow at rest (coronary flow reserve) is a good indicator of the physiologic significance to the myocardium. This makes the measurement of coronary flow and velocity valuable. Measurements of instantaneous and mean coronary flow parameters are most commonly made using an intracoronary Doppler flow wire, positioned in the arterial lumen during x-ray contrast angiography. However, this is an invasive procedure, with a small but definite risk of complications, and the radiation dose to the patient is relatively high for a diagnostic test. The repeated use of such a technique to monitor disease progression or regression in response to drug therapy or lifestyle changes is therefore not acceptable. In addition, the presence of the Doppler wire may itself affect flow,[2] as may the stress to the patient resulting from the invasive nature of the procedure. Other techniques capable of assessing mean flow parameters include continuous thermodilution and positron emission tomography (PET), the former also requiring placement under x-ray contrast angiography, with the concomitant disadvantages, and the latter being relatively unavailable and expensive.

CMR has the ability to quantify blood flow noninvasively and has the potential to be a useful noninvasive alternative to the intracoronary technique. Since the 1980s, it has been used extensively for the assessment of phasic blood flow velocity and flow in a wide range of cardiovascular applications,[3,4] and it has the potential to be implemented in coronary flow studies. One of the main problems relating specifically to applying the technique to the coronary arteries is their small size (typically <5 mm in diameter), which, for current levels of in-plane resolution, results in only a few pixels across the vessel. This has implications for the accurate measurement of both vessel cross-sectional area and blood flow velocity. Vessel tortuosity is a further problem, giving rise to difficulties in accurately aligning the vessel so that flow is truly through-plane or in-plane, as required. This is exacerbated by the movement of the arteries with the cardiac and respiratory cycles. In addition, the temporal resolution of the velocity encoding sequence must be sufficiently good to minimize the blurring of the vessel as a result of motion within the period of acquisition and to resolve the phasic velocity profile. The low peak flow velocities in normal arteries at rest (typically <25 cm/s) present a further challenge and require highly sensitive velocity windows, whereas in the presence of stenoses, high velocities are present, together with complex flow, which may lead to signal loss. The combination of these problems is formidable, and it was only in the last 10 to 15 years that CMR techniques started to generate results. This chapter reviews the progress made to date and discusses potential future improvements.

INDIRECT ASSESSMENT OF TOTAL CORONARY FLOW AND FLOW RESERVE

Two indirect approaches for assessing total coronary flow and flow reserve by CMR have been reported, the first from velocity mapping of cardiac venous outflow and the second from velocity mapping in the aortic root.

Coronary Sinus Flow

Velocity mapping of coronary venous outflow is less problematic than velocity mapping in the coronary arteries because the coronary sinus has a much larger diameter (typically 7–10 mm), and also because effects of signal loss are unlikely because flow is less susceptible to turbulence. In the human heart, coronary sinus flow almost equals total coronary flow because approximately 96% of left ventricular (LV) venous blood flow drains into the right atrium via the coronary sinus.[5] van Rossum and colleagues were the first to show that blood flow in the coronary sinus could be measured using CMR.[6] This feasibility study assessed the ability of cine CMR velocity mapping to measure phasic and mean coronary venous outflow in the distal coronary sinus of 24 healthy subjects. The flow profiles were generally biphasic and primarily diastolic, with 37% of subjects showing some reverse flow immediately after the R-wave. The mean volumetric flow over the cardiac cycle was 144 ± 62 mL/min, similar to values reported in normal subjects using continuous thermodilution (122 mL/min).[7] Although phasic blood flow in the sinus may have been expected to be predominantly systolic, as in other venous structures, the authors suggested that the thin, compliant walls of the sinus, together with its drainage into the right atrium, where pressure varies considerably, may be responsible for the predominantly diastolic flow profile. These findings have been supported by other independent studies, both directly, using an ultrasonic transit time technique to measure phasic volumetric coronary sinus flow in conscious dogs,[8] and indirectly, by observing areas of signal void, caused by accelerating and turbulent flow near the entrance of the coronary sinus in the right atrium in early diastole, in conventional cine CMR in healthy subjects.[9]

Fig. 25.1 shows the typical image plane orientation for coronary sinus flow measurements together with a typical coronary sinus flow curve.

The imaging time for the feasibility study was typically 4 minutes, and this may be inappropriate when assessing sinus flow under pharmacologically induced maximal vasodilation. Kawada and associates[10] assessed the possibility of using a segmented k-space[11] gradient echo CMR approach to the acquisition so that all data could be acquired in <25 seconds. This had the further advantage that the full acquisition

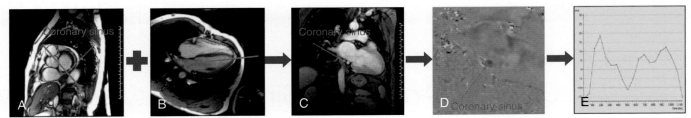

FIG. 25.1 Coronary sinus flow measurement. The coronary sinus is identified in the atrioventricular groove, on the basal slice of a short-axis stack (A). The plane for flow measurement is prescribed parallel to the long-axis of the heart on the 4-chamber view and perpendicular to the direction of flow in the coronary sinus, approximately 0.5 cm from the ostium (*green line*, A and B). The proximal coronary sinus is seen in cross-section on the phase contrast images (C and D). Flow versus time curves are generated by drawing a region of interest around the coronary sinus to calculate through-plane flow (E). (From Dandekar VK, Baumi MA, Ertel AW, et al. Assessment of global myocardial perfusion using cardiovascular magnetic resonance of coronary sinus flow at 3 Tesla. *J Cardiovasc Magn Reson.* 2014;16:24–33.)

could be performed in a single breath-hold, thereby eliminating the effects of respiratory motion. In a study of 9 healthy subjects and 29 patients with hypertrophic cardiomyopathy (HCM), data were acquired from an oblique coronal plane. Four reference and four velocity encoded views were acquired per data segment, giving a segment duration of 120 ms, but the temporal resolution was effectively improved by view sharing,[12] a technique whereby data are generated at intermediate time points from the preceding and following data segments. Hence, depending on the RR interval, velocity maps were obtained at up to 14 phases in the cardiac cycle. The authors observed the same biphasic velocity and flow profiles[6] in both healthy subjects and patients with HCM, with no significant difference noted between the baseline myocardial blood flow (coronary blood flow per unit mass of myocardium) in the two groups (0.74 mL/min per gram vs. 0.62 mL/min per gram). However, after intravenous administration of 0.56 mg/kg dipyridamole, the increase in myocardial blood flow in patients with HCM (0.62 mL/min per gram to 1.03 mL/min per gram) was less than that in the healthy subjects (0.74 to 2.14 mL/min per gram), resulting in significantly different coronary flow reserves for the two groups (1.72 ± 0.49 vs. 3.01 ± 0.75, respectively, $P < .01$). The authors concluded that, in healthy subjects, myocardial blood flow and coronary flow reserve, as measured by breath-hold phase velocity mapping, were similar to those found by other techniques; in addition, the CMR technique was able to distinguish between healthy subjects and patients with HCM. A more recent study in young HCM patients (22.3 ± 6.4 years) and age-matched subjects at risk of HCM has similarly shown that HCM patients (but not subjects at risk of HCM) have reduced myocardial blood flow response to adenosine-induced hyperemia, even in the absence of diastolic dysfunction or left ventricular outflow tract obstruction.[13] The breath-hold approach has also been used by Kennedy and colleagues[14] to show significant differences in the coronary flow reserve of healthy subjects (4.59 ± 0.58) and heart transplant patients with mild (2.15 ± 0.44, $P < .05$) and severe (2.21 ± 0.59, $P < .05$) coronary disease, as determined by posttransplant coronary angiography. It has also been used to show reduced coronary flow reserve in patients with high serum eicosapentaenoic acid (EPA) compared with those with low EPA,[15] and in those with heart failure with preserved ejection fraction compared with those with hypertensive left ventricular hypertrophy and controls.[16] At 3 T, the increased signal-to-noise ratio (SNR) available generally allows imaging of coronary sinus flow with higher spatial resolution or, particularly when used in combination with parallel imaging techniques, reduced breath-hold duration.[17] Imaging at 3 T has been used to determine the feasibility of flow reserve quantification using regadenoson, a relatively new selective adenosine A2A receptor agonist and to

investigate the role of aminophylline reversal.[18] It has also been used to show reduced coronary flow reserve in patients with surgically repaired tetralogy of Fallot, compared with healthy volunteers (1.19 ± 0.34 vs. 2.00 ± 0.43, $P = .002$)[19] and in two similar studies (one at 1.5 T[20] and one at 3 T)[21] to show that, whereas smokers and nonsmokers have similar baseline myocardial blood flows, smokers have a significantly reduced response to cold pressor testing (Fig. 25.2). A spiral k-space coverage phase velocity mapping sequence at 3 T has allowed the acquisition of data with a spatial resolution of 0.8 mm × 0.8 mm in an 11 to 15 s breath-hold with a temporal resolution of 60 to 69 ms and has been used to show myocardial blood flow increases in response to cold pressor testing in asymptomatic women.[22] A validation of the breath-hold approach was reported by Koskenvuo and associates, who compared myocardial blood flow measured by CMR with that measured by PET in both healthy subjects[23] and patients with coronary artery disease (CAD).[24] Good correlations were reported for myocardial blood flow in both subject groups (0.82 and 0.80, respectively), whereas for coronary flow reserve, the correlations were 0.76 and 0.5, respectively.

One issue with the breath-hold approach to measuring coronary sinus flow is that breath-holding changes intrathoracic pressure and affects cardiac output and venous blood flow.[25] Schwitter and coworkers[26] performed a validation of nonbreath-hold velocity mapping against PET. Although taking longer to acquire (typically 4 minutes), the nonbreath-hold technique has the advantages of higher spatial resolution (0.8 × 0.8 mm) and improved SNR through the acquisition of multiple averages. Furthermore, the high temporal resolution that is achievable is better suited for resolving the highly pulsatile flow profile and for minimizing the blurring effects of the extensive in-plane motion of the coronary sinus during the cardiac cycle. Unlike the initial study of van Rossum and coworkers,[6] this free breathing study used retrospective electrocardiogram (ECG) gating,[27] which enables data acquisition throughout the entire cardiac cycle, and respiratory ordered phase encoding,[28] which reduces the effects of respiratory motion. Scans were performed both before and after the administration of 0.56 mg/kg dipyridamole in 16 healthy subjects and 10 orthotopic heart transplant recipients and the results were compared with PET data. The mean difference between coronary flow reserve measured by PET and CMR was 2.2%, with limits of agreement of −27.2% and 31.6%. Correlation between CMR-measured myocardial blood flow (coronary sinus flow divided by myocardial mass) and PET was good ($r = 0.93$), although the slope was considerably less than unity (0.73). This underestimation of blood flow measured by CMR results from the fact that a variable part of the inferior and inferior-septal myocardium is drained by the middle cardiac vein, which either enters the coronary sinus just before

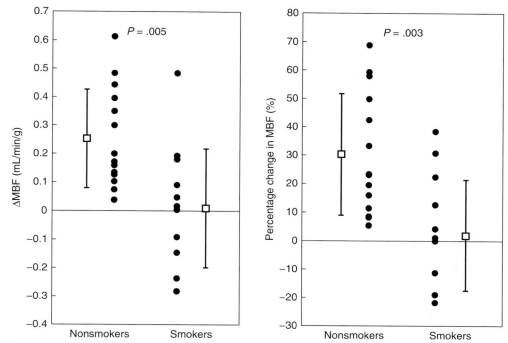

FIG. 25.2 Individual myocardial blood flow *(MBF)* Δ values and percent change of MBF in nonsmokers and smokers. The mean ΔMBF during the continuous performance test (CPT) in nonsmokers was 0.26 ± 0.18 mL/min per gram. The mean ΔMBF during the CPT in smokers was 0.02 ± 0.20 mL/min per gram and was significantly lower than in nonsmokers (*P* = .005). The mean percent change of MBF in smokers was significantly lower than in nonsmokers (3.6 ± 19.7 vs. 30.7 ± 21.3%, *P* = .003). (From Ichikawa Y, Kitgawa K, Kato S. Altered coronary endothelial function in young smokers detected by magnetic resonance assessment of myocardial blood flow during the cold pressor test. *Int J Cardiovasc Imaging.* 2014;30[suppl 1]:73–80.)

its orifice or empties directly into the right atrium.[29] If coronary sinus flow is divided instead by the mass of drained myocardium (as measured from a stack of short axis images), the correlation remains good (r = 0.95), whereas the slope approaches unity (1.05). Fig. 25.3 shows a regression plot of myocardial blood flow (sinus blood flow per unit mass of drained myocardium) measured by CMR and PET, with baseline flows normalized for rate-pressure product, together with a Bland-Altman plot. The mean differences between PET and CMR were 3.4% ± 12.8% at resting baseline and 3.9% ± 20.2% during hyperemia and were not significant. The authors have subsequently used this technique to show that administration of 17β-estradiol over 3 months without progestin coadministration does not improve coronary flow reserve in postmenopausal women.[30] A similar nonbreath-hold technique was used by Moro and colleagues at 3 T[31] to show that women have a higher increase in myocardial blood flow in response to cold pressor testing than men (0.73 ± 0.43 mL/g per minute vs. 0.22 ± 0.19 mL/g per minute, *P* = .0012).

A validation of nonbreath-hold CMR-measured coronary sinus flow has also been performed against flow probes in dogs by Lund and associates.[32] In this study, the correlation between coronary blood flow (measured as the sum of left anterior descending [LAD] and circumflex [LCX] coronary flow) with flow probes against coronary sinus flow measured with CMR was 0.98, with a nonsignificant mean difference of 3.1 ± 8.5 mL/min. Coronary sinus blood flow per unit mass of myocardium was 0.40 ± 0.09 mL/min per gram (CMR) compared with 0.44 ± 0.08 mL/min per gram (flow probes) and also was not significant. The authors went on to study patients with chronic heart failure and showed that coronary flow reserve was significantly reduced compared with that in healthy subjects (2.3 ± 0.9 vs. 4.2 ± 1.5, *P* = .01).[33] This has

been recently confirmed by Aras and colleagues[34] (coronary flow reserve 1.45 vs. 3 in patients with chronic heart failure and healthy subjects, respectively, *P* < .001). Similarly, Watzinger and coworkers[35] have shown significantly reduced flow reserve in patients with idiopathic cardiomyopathy compared with healthy subjects (2.19 ± 0.77 vs. 3.51 ± 1.29, *P* < .05). In all three studies, there were no significant differences in baseline flow between healthy subjects and those with disease (0.52 mL/min per gram vs. 0.46 mL/min per gram, *P* = not significant [NS]; 0.83 ± 0.26 mL/min per gram vs. 0.85 ± 0.30 mL/min per gram, *P* = NS; and 0.55 ± 0.19 mL/min per gram vs. 0.48 ± 0.07 mL/min per gram, *P* = NS).

These studies provide useful results, but have a number of important limitations. Cardiac and respiratory motion results in blurring of the sinus, and the small number of pixels covering the sinus (typically five across the diameter in diastole) results in considerable partial volume averaging in edge pixels, which is problematic for the accurate assessment of sinus cross-sectional area and for the determination of mean sinus flow velocity. As discussed, drainage of a variable part of the inferior and inferior-septal myocardium by the middle cardiac vein[28] results in underestimates of myocardial blood flow measured, and although this estimate is an indicator of total coronary blood flow, no regional assessment of either flow or flow reserve is possible with this technique.

Total Coronary Flow Reserve From Measurements in the Aortic Root

In 1993, it was proposed that coronary flow reserve might be derived from flow measurements made in the ascending aorta, which is less susceptible to cardiac and respiratory motion and partial volume effects

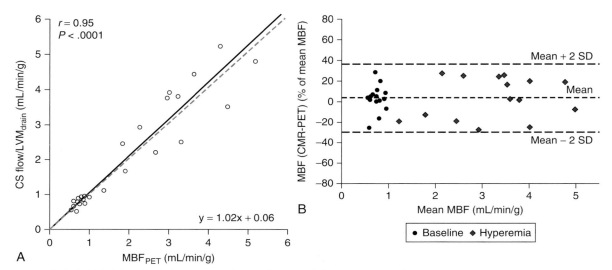

FIG. 25.3 (A) Correlation between estimate of myocardial blood flow *(MBF)* (mL/min per gram) derived from positron emission tomography *(PET) (x axis)* and magnetic resonance (MR) *(y axis)* measurements. For compressed sensing *(CS)* flow divided by drained myocardium, correlation with PET data is high and the slope of the regression line approximates unity *(dashed line)*. (B) Comparison of myocardial blood flow as measured by PET and MR (coronary sinus flow divided by drained myocardium mass) with baseline flow normalized for rate-pressure product (Bland-Altman analysis). Mean differences between PET and MR measurements during baseline (3.4% ± 12.8%) and hyperemia (3.9% ± 20.2%) were not significantly different. *CMR,* Cardiovascular magnetic resonance; *LVM,* left ventricular mass; *SD,* standard deviation. (From Schwitter J, DeMarco T, Kneifel S et al. Magnetic resonance-based assessment of global coronary flow and flow reserve and its relation to left ventricular functional parameters. *Circulation.* 2000;101:2696–2709.)

than the coronary arteries.[36] Coronary diastolic flow, which represents the bulk of coronary flow, can be estimated as the retrograde flow in the ascending aorta during systole and diastole minus the antegrade flow during diastole. A variable velocity encoding window was implemented to maintain the accuracy of velocity measurements during periods of both high flow in systole (window = 200 cm/s) and low flow in diastole (window = 30 cm/s).[37] Although it was suggested that the assessment of absolute diastolic coronary flow with this technique is inaccurate because of known errors associated with the velocity mapping technique, it was argued that these errors should be the same both pre-vasodilation and postvasodilation and therefore should be eliminated from the assessment of diastolic coronary flow reserve, defined in this instance as the difference (rather than the ratio) between the two measurements. In seven patients with abnormal findings on myocardial perfusion scintigraphy, the diastolic coronary flow reserve was −50 ± 76 mL/min compared with 260 ± 66 mL/min in eight healthy subjects. The principle of this technique was later refined by taking into account the motion of the coronary arteries during the cardiac cycle.[38] A model was developed describing the flow through five transverse parallel aortic slices extending from the base of the aortic valve to above the level of the coronary ostia. This was then solved mathematically, and in five healthy subjects, it was shown that the standard error in the measurement of total coronary artery flow was approximately 90 mL/min, or 30% of total coronary artery flow. The error in coronary flow reserve is higher because the errors in baseline and maximal vasodilation flow are additive. In addition, the assumption that flow is predominantly diastolic, although true in healthy subjects, may not hold in the presence of disease, introducing further unknown errors into the technique. A more recent attempt at measuring coronary artery blood flow in this way likewise found that the technique was compromised by poor reproducibility, although significant changes in coronary blood flow with hormone replacement therapy were observed.[39]

Direct Assessment of Coronary Artery Velocity

The problems associated with the assessment of flow velocity and coronary artery flow were discussed earlier and preclude the application of standard CMR techniques. As for coronary imaging, the major breakthrough for coronary flow techniques was the shortening of sequence duration to the extent that data could be acquired over a single breath-hold, effectively freezing respiratory motion and eliminating the resulting artifact. Further advances with navigator echo monitoring of the diaphragm position have allowed data to be acquired over multiple reproducible breath-holds or during free breathing, enabling increased spatial and temporal resolution and data averaging (resulting in higher SNRs). The following sections describe the approaches used to assess coronary flow velocity and flow.

Bolus Tagging

The first report detailing the imaging of coronary artery flow was made in 1991 in rat and mice hearts with bolus tracking.[40] With this technique, based on one previously implemented in vivo in the aorta and the carotid arteries,[41] a section of blood above the coronary ostia on the aortic root is tagged by the application of a slice-selective presaturation radiofrequency pulse, and imaging is performed after a delay. During this delay period, the tagged volume of blood washes into the coronary artery tree, where it is seen as a signal void. The mean velocity of the tagged blood can be calculated from the degree of tag movement and the wash-in delay time. The technique has also been developed for multibolus tracking using stimulated echoes,[42] and its application was demonstrated in a 3-mm diameter tube with laminar flow and in an isovolumetric perfused rat heart. Using this approach, an image of multiple boluses (typically three), each with a different wash-in time, can be obtained simultaneously to show the coronary artery tree. Again, the extent of the arterial pathway seen depends on the flow velocities in the tagged volumes and on the wash-in delay times, with short delays required for visualization of the proximal portions and longer delays for the mid- and distal portions. By tracking multiple boluses simultaneously in this way, this technique essentially results in images of blood flow.

Echo Planar Time-of-Flight Technique

Echo planar techniques are an attractive option for coronary artery investigations because of their fast imaging times, which reduce the effects of both cardiac and respiratory motion. In 1993, the first report detailing the use of an echo planar single-shot time-of-flight technique for assessing coronary artery flow velocity in 11 healthy subjects was reported.[43] In this study, short axis cardiac slices were acquired with an in-plane pixel size of 1.5 × 3 mm, each taking approximately 95 ms. Before the 90-degree slice selection radio frequency pulse, another 90-degree pulse was applied to saturate a thick band centered on the imaging slice. If increasing time delays are programmed between the saturation and slice select pulses, the signal intensity in the vessel changes as a result of blood wash-in through the slice. The rate at which it changes can be used to calculate the blood velocity at the time of imaging. The average velocity profile for the study group of 11 subjects is shown in Fig. 25.4 and illustrates the expected peak flow in early diastole. Using this technique, a separate breath-hold was required for velocity assessment at each time point in the cardiac cycle and it was not possible to image at time points of <200 ms from the R-wave because this time period is required for the application of saturation delays. This was not considered a problem for normal subjects because left coronary flow is predominantly diastolic. A further restriction of the technique is that the long echo time of the sequence (echo time [TE] 28 ms) may lead to signal loss at sites of turbulent flow. At such sites, there may also be a breakdown in the assumption of laminar flow required for the velocity calculations from the wash-in data. The authors reported that in nine subjects who were imaged during continuous hand and lower extremity exercise, eight showed an increase in diastolic velocity (increase over exercise period = 52 ± 24%). Isometric exercise does not produce a maximal physiologic stress response, and more recently, echo

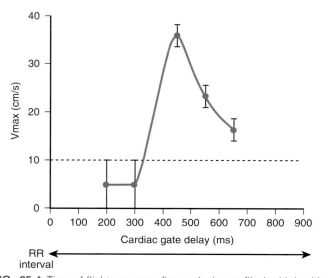

FIG. 25.4 Time-of-flight coronary flow velocity profile in 11 healthy subjects. For each subject and for each gating delay, a series of images with different saturation delays was acquired. (From Poncelet BP, Weisskoff RM, Weeden VJ, et al. Time of flight quantification of coronary flow with echo-planar MRI. *Magn Reson Med.* 1993;30:447–457.)

planar time-of-flight coronary flow velocity reserve has been measured using this technique in healthy subjects (N = 10) after the infusion of 0.56 mg/kg dipyridamole.[44] In these subjects, peak diastolic velocity was observed to increase from 22 ± 7 cm/s to 90 ± 40 cm/s, resulting in a coronary flow velocity reserve of 3.9 ± 1.5, with velocity returning to baseline (23 ± 5 cm/s) after the administration of aminophylline.

In this study, the authors acquired low-resolution, single-shot coronary images rather than using a segmented approach to build up higher-resolution images over a number of cardiac cycles. This was prompted by their observation of considerable variability in the beat-to-beat position of the LAD during both long and short breath-hold periods. This usually corresponded to a downward drift in vessel position as the breath-hold continued and could be as much as 6 mm (i.e., greater than the vessel diameter). It was unclear, however, how much of this movement was caused by poor breath-holding and how much was the result of beat-to-beat variations in cardiac contraction. Regardless of the cause, it would introduce blurring, which is largely avoided in a single-shot image. Beat-to-beat variations in flow, as opposed to spatial position, still have an effect on measured velocity because individual images must be acquired with different saturation delays in consecutive cardiac cycles to generate the wash-in curve. Therefore measured velocity is affected by changes over the breath-hold period. The importance of this study lies in its pioneering and largely successful approach to a previously unsolved problem. It has largely been superseded by phase velocity mapping approaches, as discussed later, which are more robust and have higher availability.

Gradient Echo Phase Velocity Mapping
Breath-Hold Techniques

Using a velocity encoded segmented k-space gradient echo technique, velocity maps may be acquired in a single breath-hold, thereby eliminating respiratory motion artifact. To accomplish this, the segment duration is typically on the order of 100 ms, and to minimize blurring as a result of cardiac motion, the acquisition is best performed in mid diastole, when the heart is relatively stationary. In addition to limiting the temporal resolution of the sequence, the need to perform data acquisition within a single breath-hold also limits the number of phase encoding steps that can be acquired, which in turn limits the spatial resolution and the SNR in the resulting images.

The first diastolic through-plane coronary artery phase velocity maps were reported by Edelman and coworkers in 1993.[45] These were acquired at 1.5 T using a fat-suppressed sequence consisting of a reference velocity compensated gradient waveform followed by a sensitized (velocity window = 150 cm/s) gradient waveform, each repeated four times in a cardiac cycle. TE was 8 ms and repetition time (TR) was 15 ms, resulting in a segment duration of 120 ms. The sequence was validated against a Doppler flow meter in vitro using both constant and mildly pulsatile flow in an 8-mm diameter tube and in vivo against a standard non-segmented velocity mapping sequence in the descending aorta of three healthy volunteers. Velocity maps were acquired over 24 cardiac cycles with in-plane pixel dimensions of 1.4 × 0.8 mm. In healthy subjects, mean flow velocities at rest in the mid portion of the right and left anterior descending coronary arteries were 9.9 cm/s and 20.5 cm/s, respectively. These values are lower than those found in Doppler flow studies, a finding that is to be expected because the small number of pixels across the vessel results in partial volume averaging of the velocity profile. In four subjects who received intravenous administration of adenosine, velocities increased by at least a factor of four, suggesting that CMR has the potential to assess the hemodynamic significance of a stenosis by measuring the flow response to vasodilation.

Another approach to quantifying the severity of stenosis is to perform in-plane coronary artery velocity mapping with a view to measuring increased velocity at the site of lumen narrowing. In-plane coronary artery velocity mapping was first performed in healthy volunteers by Keegan and associates,[46] using a sequence with TE of 10 ms, TR of 20 ms, and segment duration of 160 ms, which effectively limited acquisitions to the period of relative cardiac diastasis in early diastole. The in-plane resolution was 1.6×0.8 mm, and data were acquired over breath-holds of 24 to 32 cardiac cycles. The velocity sensitivity used was 50 cm/s and was achieved by phase map subtraction of two images, one sensitized so that flow velocities of 100 cm/s gave a phase shift of +2pi radians and the other sensitized so that flow velocities of 100 cm/s gave a phase shift of −2pi radians. This was shown to result in fewer blood flow artifacts than subtracting an image sensitized to flow velocities of 50 cm/s from a reference nonsensitized image. Through-plane and in-plane velocities measured with this technique were validated in vitro against a standard nonsegmented velocity mapping sequence in a 5.6 mm diameter tube with pulsatile flow having a maximum velocity of 30 cm/s and a maximum rate of change of velocity of 126 cm/s[2], comparable with the values expected in normal human coronary arteries at rest. Phantom work was also carried out to show the ability of the technique to measure a velocity increase at the sites of mild, moderate, and severe area-reducing stenoses and hence to quantify severity. However, although velocity increases at the sites of area-reducing stenoses have been observed with this approach,[3] the tortuous pathways and small caliber of the coronary vessels result in partial-volume-type effects being more problematic for in-plane than for through-plane velocity mapping. Furthermore, in-plane studies require a high degree of reproducibility in the breath-holding position, which is difficult to achieve without techniques such as navigator echo monitoring.

Navigator Techniques

The studies discussed earlier used breath-holding as a means of respiratory motion control, limiting the sequence parameters to allow the entire dataset to be acquired within the duration of a single breath-hold and requiring a high degree of patient cooperation, which is not always forthcoming. In addition, intervariations and intravariations in the breath-hold position may be problematic, and hemodynamic changes

occurring secondary to breath-holding, such as increases in intrathoracic pressure and heart rate, may themselves alter the blood flow being measured. A navigator echo approach under either prospective or retrospective control would enable data to be acquired during free breathing and would avoid these problems. Furthermore, temporal resolution of the sequence could be improved by reducing the segment duration, albeit at the expense of prolonged scan time.

The influence of temporal resolution was studied by Hofman and colleagues,[47] who compared the use of a segmented breath-hold technique (segment duration of 126 ms) with a retrospective respiratory gated technique[48] (reference and velocity sensitized view pair duration of 32 ms) for the assessment of flow velocity, vessel cross-sectional area, and volume flow in the right coronary arteries of six healthy subjects. Eight data averages were acquired, and the data were reconstructed with retrospective gating. The residual displacement of diaphragm positions in the reconstructed data was 3.9 mm. In-plane spatial resolution was 0.8×1.6 mm, and velocity sensitivity was ±25 cm/s. Vessel regions of interest were obtained semiautomatically from the magnitude images of the velocity compensated dataset by means of a seed growing algorithm and a 50% threshold. Velocity profiles generated from the retrospectively gated data for all six subjects (uncorrected for through-plane velocity of the vessel itself) are shown in Fig. 25.5A and show a sharp peak in systole, a minimum at end-systole, and a second peak in early diastole. The in-plane displacements of the vessels are shown in Fig. 25.5B and typically show peaks in systole and early diastole, with minimal displacement in mid to end-diastole. The authors have since reported a similar pattern of movement for the LAD.[49] During times of peak vessel displacement, motion blurring of the artery occurs and the breath-hold segmented images are consequently of poorer quality than those acquired with the retrospective respiratory gated short segment duration sequence (Fig. 25.6B). In diastole, however, when in-plane displacement of the vessel is low, the two techniques generate images of comparable quality (see Fig. 25.6A). This results in the breath-hold segmented k-space gradient echo sequence overestimating the instantaneous vessel cross-sectional area by as much as a factor of four, with an average increase in the time-averaged cross-sectional area of 90%. Based on this work,

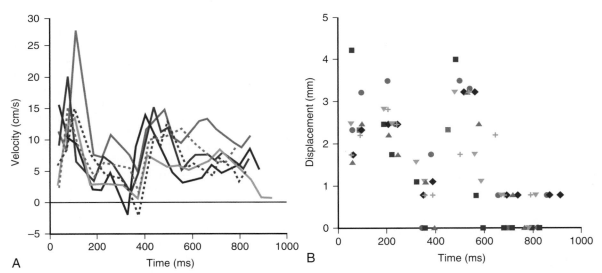

FIG. 25.5 Through-plane cross-sectional averaged velocity (A) and in-plane displacement (B) in the right coronary artery as a function of time in the cardiac cycle and as measured on respiratory gated acquisition (oversampling factor = 8) in six subjects. Different symbols represent different subjects. (From Hofman MBM, van Rossum AC, Sprenger M, et al. Assessment of flow in the right human coronary artery by magnetic resonance phase contrast velocity measurement: effects of cardiac and respiratory motion. *Magn Reson Med.* 1996;35:521–531.)

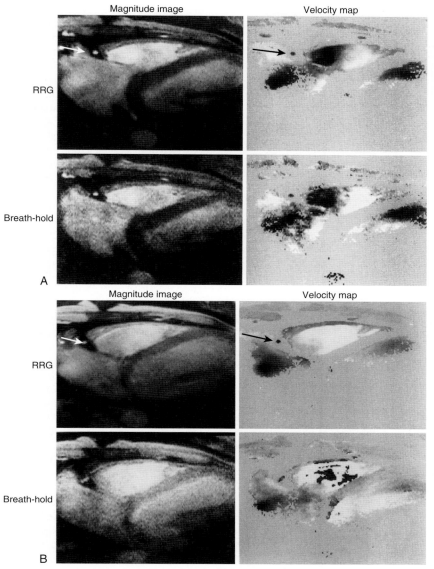

FIG. 25.6 Through-plane magnitude images and velocity maps for retrospective respiratory gated *(RRG)* acquisitions *(top)* and breath-hold acquisitions *(bottom)* acquired (A) in mid diastole (gating delay of 760 ms) and (B) in early systole (gating delay of 90 ms). In mid diastole, when in-plane displacement is low, good-quality images are obtained with both techniques. In early systole, however, when in-plane displacement is high, the long acquisition window of the breath-hold sequence results in considerable blurring of the artery *(arrows)*. (From Hofman MBM, van Rossum AC, Sprenger M, et al. Assessment of flow in the right human coronary artery by magnetic resonance phase contrast velocity measurement: effects of cardiac and respiratory motion. *Magn Reson Med.* 1996;35:521–531.)

the authors suggest that, for acceptable levels of blurring throughout the cardiac cycle, the acquisition window for studies of the left and right coronary arteries (RCAs) should be <90 ms and <25 ms, respectively. This is similar to the values derived by Marcus and coworkers,[50] who suggested an acquisition window of <58 ms and <23 ms for the left and right arteries, respectively.

A comparison between segmented *k*-space gradient echo phase velocity mapping and Doppler flow wire techniques has been performed in 26 angiographically normal coronary artery segments.[51] Both breath-holding and real-time slice-followed[52] navigator echo controlled free breathing CMR techniques (temporal resolution of 140 ms and 46 ms, respectively) were performed within 24 hours of the invasive procedure and the maximal coronary flow velocities in a 2 × 2 mm pixel region

of interest determined. Both CMR techniques were found to significantly underestimate flow velocity, although the correlations with invasive measurements were strong ($r = 0.70$ and $r = 0.86$, respectively). The navigator echo controlled technique was significantly more accurate than the breath-hold technique ($P < .02$), although this was at the expense of prolonged acquisition time. The underestimation of blood flow velocity by both techniques is largely caused by partial volume averaging of the spatial flow profile in the CMR studies, together with insufficient sampling of the temporal flow profile. The decreased accuracy of the breath-hold technique compared with the navigator echo-free breathing technique is likely to be caused by a combination of the longer acquisition window of the former, together with hemodynamic changes resulting from the breath-holding procedure itself. Fig. 25.7

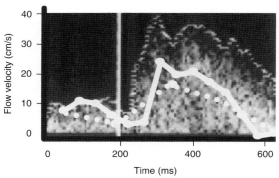

FIG. 25.7 Original tracing of an invasively determined flow curve of the left coronary artery compared with noninvasively determined flow curves in the same patient. The solid line shows the real-time adaptive navigator correction technique; the dotted line shows the breath-hold technique. (From Nagel E, Bornstedt A, Hug J, et al. Noninvasive determination of coronary blood flow velocity with magnetic resonance imaging: comparison of breath-hold and navigator techniques with intravascular ultrasound. *Magn Reson Med.* 1999;41:544–549.)

shows an example of the results obtained. Although still underestimating flow velocities, the significantly improved accuracy of the navigator echo-free breathing technique compared with the breath-hold technique provides a further step toward CMR assessment of coronary flow parameters, albeit at the expense of prolonged acquisition times. A navigator gated phase velocity mapping sequence has also been developed at 3 T and validated in a realistic flow phantom (4 mm diameter, mean flow velocity 15–20 cm/s) with simulated respiratory motion.[53] Using this technique, measured velocities were within 15% of actual velocities in vitro and subsequent in vivo studies in 9 healthy volunteers resulted in time-averaged flow velocities of 6.8 ± 4.3 cm/s in the left anterior descending artery, 8.0 ± 3.8 cm/s in the left circumflex artery and 6.0 ± 1.0 cm/s in the right coronary artery.

Interleaved Spiral Phase Velocity Mapping

Interleaved spiral imaging is an alternative technique for generating high-resolution images of the coronary arteries,[54] which, compared with those acquired using segmented gradient recalled echo (GRE), have higher SNRs and better temporal resolution.[55] This potentially enables velocity mapping in both the left, and the more mobile right, coronary arteries.[56] The results of breath-hold spiral, free breathing spiral, and breath-hold segmented GRE phase velocity mapping have been compared with those of free breathing GRE in healthy volunteers.[57] Eight left and eight right coronary arteries were studied and flow velocity profiles generated with each technique, with the free breathing GRE acquisitions being used as a gold standard. Flow profiles generated with the free breathing spiral sequence (100-cardiac-cycle acquisition, assuming 40% respiratory efficiency) agreed closely with those generated with the free breathing GRE sequence, taking 10 times longer to acquire for the same spatial resolution. By comparison, the breath-hold segmented GRE sequence did not resolve the sharp peaks in the temporal flow profiles of the RCA and, for the group as a whole, significantly underestimated peak systolic (88 mm/s vs. 252 mm/s, $P < .001$), peak diastolic (114 mm/s vs. 153 mm/s, $P < .01$) and mean (56 mm/s vs. 93 mm/s, $P < .001$) velocities. For the less mobile left artery, peak systolic, peak diastolic and mean velocities were also underestimated by the breath-hold segmented GRE sequence, but this only reached statistical significance for the peak systolic velocity (80 mm/s vs. 135 mm/s, $P < .01$). The breath-hold spiral sequence agreed reasonably well with the free breathing GRE sequence, although deviations were observed at times

of rapid cardiac movement. This was due to misregistration of the velocity encoded and reference datasets acquired consecutively in the same cardiac cycle in the breath-hold acquisition, whereas in the free breathing acquisition, they were acquired at the same time point on alternate cycles. In coronary blood flow studies, a region of adjacent myocardium is generally used as a marker of through-plane motion and is used to correct flow profiles. This is feasible for the left coronary artery, but for the RCA, the adjacent myocardium is too thin to provide a reliable correction. For this artery, epicardial fat surrounding the artery has been used for through-plane correction, with the fat signal provided from a fat-excitation image generated from a separate acquisition, or from one interleaved with the water-excitation image used for imaging flow.[58] Fig. 25.8 shows mean (± standard deviation [SD]) flow profiles before and after correction in the left ($N = 13$) and right ($N = 10$) coronary arteries of healthy subjects. The corrected flow profiles bear strong resemblances to those found in normal arteries using Doppler flow wire.[59]

Brandts and colleagues developed a spiral phase velocity mapping sequence at 3 T where the higher SNR allowed imaging with a spatial resolution of 0.8 mm × 8 mm, with a true temporal resolution of 33 ms in a 24 cardiac cycle breath-hold.[60] Using this technique, peak systolic and peak diastolic velocities in repeated breath-holds in the right coronary arteries of healthy volunteers showed a high reproducibility (mean difference (±SD of paired differences) being 0 ± 16.5 mm/s and 10.5 ± 14.3 mm/s, respectively). A similarly high reproducibility in peak systolic and diastolic velocities in patients undergoing clinical coronary angiography for shortness of breath or chest pain was also shown by Keegan and associates (1.7 ± 15.8 mm/s and 2.5 ± 11.6 mm/s).[61] In this study, the spatial resolution (1.4 mm × 1.4 mm) was sacrificed for a higher temporal resolution (19 ms) and shorter breath-hold duration (17 cardiac cycles) which enabled temporal details in the coronary artery velocity profiles to be resolved. Fig. 25.9 shows the high degree of inter–breath-hold reproducibility achieved with this technique in 5 right and 10 left coronary arteries. In a direct comparison with gold-standard Doppler guidewire studies in 23 vessels, CMR assessment of peak systolic velocity, peak diastolic velocity and mean velocity through the cardiac cycle underestimated Doppler values but the correlation between them was moderate to good ($R^2 = 0.57$, 0.64, and 0.79, respectively) (Fig. 25.10). In addition, CMR measures of the peak diastolic velocity to the peak systolic velocity showed a strong linear relationship with Doppler values ($R^2 = 0.71$ and 0.93 for left and right arteries, respectively) with a slope close to unity (0.89 and 0.90 for right and left arteries, respectively). In individual vessels, plots of CMR measured velocity at all cardiac phases against corresponding Doppler velocities showed a consistent linear relationship between the two, with high R^2 values (0.79 ± 0.13).

The advantages of high SNR, good temporal and spatial resolution, and ability to implement fat suppression give the spiral technique considerable promise, but more research is needed to investigate how the blurring of off-resonance material[62] and flow-direction-sensitive "implosion/explosion" artifacts in regions of poor homogeneity[63] affect the measurements.

Coronary Flow, Coronary Flow Reserve and Coronary Flow Velocity Reserve

The assessment of coronary flow, rather than flow velocity, is more difficult because of partial volume effects at the vessel boundary resulting in overestimations of the vessel cross-sectional area.

Validation and Feasibility Studies

The first directly validated measurements of coronary artery flow and coronary flow reserve using segmented GRE phase velocity mapping

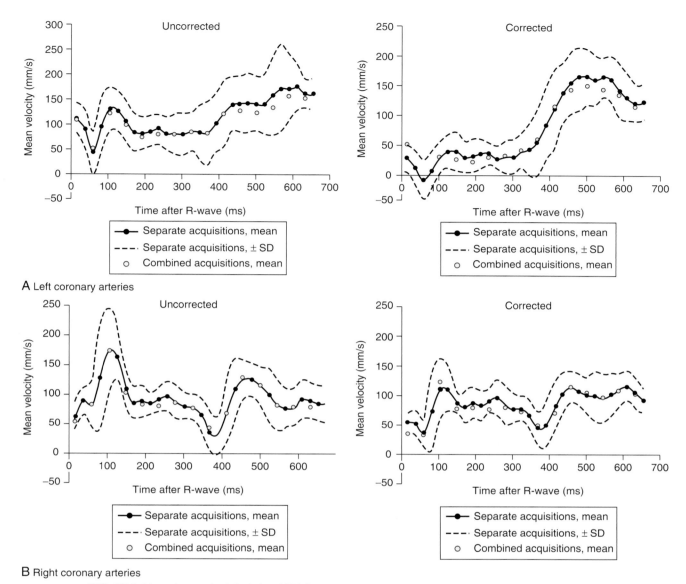

A Left coronary arteries

B Right coronary arteries

FIG. 25.8 Mean (± standard deviation *[SD]*) flow velocities as measured by the separate water-excitation and fat-excitation acquisitions in 10 left (A) and 13 right (B) coronary arteries both before *(left)* and after *(right)* correction for through-plane motion. Mean flow velocities determined from the combined water-excitation/fat-excitation acquisition are superimposed *(open circles)*. (From Keegan J, Gatehouse PD, Yang GZ, et al. Spiral phase velocity mapping of left and right coronary artery blood flow: correction for through-plane motion using selective fat-only excitation. *J Magn Reson Imaging.* 2004;20:953–960.)

were performed by Clarke and coworkers in dogs in 1995.[64] Nonmagnetic perivascular ultrasound probes were placed around the isolated LAD and LCX in eight ventilated dogs. A subcritical stenosis was generated in the LAD by placement of a polycarbonate resin constrictor. Breath-holding was effectively achieved by turning the ventilator off. Cine phase velocity mapping was performed using a sequence with TE of 11 ms and TR of 19.1 ms, with two to three reference and velocity sensitized view pairs per data segment. The segment duration was therefore 76 to 115 ms, allowing the acquisition of four to six image frames over the cardiac cycle. Images were acquired with an in-plane pixel size of 0.70 to 0.94 mm^2 over breath-holds of up to 40 seconds duration. The velocity sensitivity was ±138 cm/s. Data were acquired both before and after the administration of adenosine. A region of interest was drawn around the artery of interest in the magnitude image, and the mean velocity in that region on the corresponding velocity

map was calculated. In this study, the size of the region of interest was kept constant from frame to frame and only its position changed because the authors believed that the spatial resolution in the CMR image was insufficient to track phasic changes in the coronary arterial diameter. The results of a typical experiment are shown in Fig. 25.11A, and a plot of CMR flow reserve versus that measured by ultrasound is shown in Fig. 25.11B. For the LCX and LAD, mean CMR-measured flow reserves were 2.57 ± 0.92 and 1.38 ± 0.31, respectively (*P* = .011), compared with ultrasound-measured values of 2.55 ± 0.77 and 1.42 ± 0.31, respectively (*P* = .002). The mean difference between the two techniques was 0.01, with limits of agreement of +0.64 and −0.61. The authors concluded that, although the breath-hold period in this study is not feasible for the majority of patients and both temporal and spatial resolution are limited, the results of the phase velocity mapping technique agreed well with Doppler ultrasound, suggesting that it could be used for accurate,

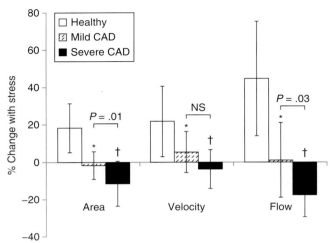

FIG. 25.18 Percent change (mean ± standard deviation) in coronary artery area, peak diastolic coronary flow velocity, and blood flow during isometric handgrip stress for healthy subjects (n = 20 *[open bars]*) and patients with single-vessel coronary artery disease *(CAD)* (n = 10). Brackets show comparisons between arteries with mild CAD *(hatched bars)* versus severe CAD *(solid bars)* within the same patients. *P* < .005, *P* < .001 versus healthy subjects. (From Hays AG, Hirsch GA, Kelle S, Gerstenblith G, Weiss RG, Stuber M. Noninvasive visualisation of coronary artery endothelial function in healthy subjects and in patients with coronary artery disease. *J Am Coll Cardiol.* 2010;56:1657–1665.)

noninvasive assessment of local coronary vasoreactivity.[88–91] To summarize the requirements, any technique must take into account the following factors:

1. *Spatial resolution:* For the assessment of volume flow, spatial resolution must be sufficiently good to measure the cross-sectional area throughout the cardiac cycle and to minimize partial volume averaging of flow velocities in edge pixels. These partial volume effects become larger as the vessel becomes smaller and the relative number of pixels in the boundary increases. The degree to which measured velocities are affected depends strongly on the relative magnitude of the stationary material included in the boundary pixels. Several studies have investigated these effects in small vessels. Hofman and associates[77] compared phase contrast measurements of time-averaged volume flow in the femoral arteries of dogs with measurements made by an ultrasonic transit time meter and found that the proportional difference between the techniques was 0.8% when the number of pixels across the vessel diameter was just three. Tang and colleagues[91] found that, for both in vitro and in vivo studies, volume flow accuracy increases with resolution, as expected, and errors are <10% when the ratio of pixel size to vessel radius is <0.5. This was also seen by Wolf and coworkers, who showed an error of 9% for five pixels across the vessel diameter.[92] Sondergaard and colleagues showed <18% error in measured flow rate for four pixels across the vessel diameter in vitro.[93] Arheden and associates[94] studied pulsatile flow in tubes with various spatial resolutions (but with a minimum of five pixels across the tube diameter) and found that overestimation of the size of the region of interest resulted in flow errors of <20%, provided that the imaging plane was within 10 degrees of

being perpendicular to the direction of flow. As has been noted, the effects of partial volume errors could potentially be reduced by using a complex difference, rather than phase difference, approach to the generation of velocity maps.[78]

2. *Temporal resolution:* The temporal resolution of the sequence used should be adequate to resolve the phasic velocity profile of coronary blood flow. This ability is determined by the number of views acquired per data segment in a segmented GRE acquisition. For accurate assessment of time-averaged parameters, measurements should be made throughout the entire cardiac cycle, with the accuracy increasing as the number of cine frames increases.[95] For segmented GRE acquisitions, these points favor the acquisition of small numbers of views per data segment, although this leads to long breath-hold periods or the need for navigator free breathing techniques. Alternatively, more rapid and efficient methods of *k*-space coverage may be used, such as interleaved rectilinear echo planar or spiral techniques. A further reason to reduce the duration of data acquisition is to minimize blurring of the vessel as a result of movement in the acquisition window, which leads to overestimation of the vessel cross-sectional area through partial volume averaging of edge pixels and underestimation of mean flow velocity.

3. *Velocity sensitivity:* The maximum velocity in normal coronary arteries at rest is typically <25 cm/s. Therefore the window used for resting studies should be narrow, approximately 50 cm/s, to allow measurement of these low velocities with maximum accuracy but without aliasing. For maximal vasodilation studies, the window should be increased accordingly.

4. *Through-plane movement of the vessel:* As has been noted, through-plane movement of the vessel through the cardiac cycle can affect instantaneous measurement of blood flow velocity and volume flow in that vessel considerably, although time-averaged measurements throughout the cardiac cycle are unaffected because the through-plane movement of the vessel averages to zero.

In addition, beat-to-beat variations in the position of the artery and of flow through the artery inevitably influence the results, and these variations may be exacerbated by breath-holding, particularly for long periods. Therefore a free breathing technique using navigator echoes may be the best approach and would also allow higher spatial and temporal resolution images, albeit with reduced scan efficiency and consequently longer scan duration. As discussed earlier, such a technique has been shown to significantly improve the accuracy of CMR velocity assessment compared with long segment duration breath-holding studies.[52] The long scan times could potentially be reduced by using a real-time phase encode reordering technique whereby the most significant central lines of *k*-space are acquired with the diaphragm position, as measured by a navigator echo, within a narrow range and the outermost lines acquired with the diaphragm position within a larger range. These techniques have already been successfully applied to coronary artery CMR.[96,97] Furthermore, real-time slice-following may also be implemented and could potentially result in improved scan efficiency by allowing the use of larger navigator windows without a reduction in image quality.

REFERENCES

A full reference list is available online at ExpertConsult.com

26

Coronary Artery Bypass Graft Imaging and Assessment of Flow

Constantin B. Marcu and Albert C. van Rossum

Since the report published in 1968 by Favaloro about the use of saphenous veins to restore coronary artery blood flow in 171 patients,[1] a large number of coronary artery bypass grafting (CABG) procedures have been performed worldwide. In the United States alone, 219,000 patients underwent a total of 397,000 CABG procedures in 2010.[2]

The left internal mammary artery (IMA) is frequently used as an arterial conduit to the left anterior descending (LAD) and its diagonal branches. Other arterial conduits include the right IMA placed to the right coronary artery (RCA) or LAD, the right gastroepiploic artery to the RCA, or the use of free radial artery grafts. Reversed saphenous veins are generally used for grafting to distal branches of the RCA and circumflex coronary artery (LCX) or to diagonal branches of the LAD.

The long-term results of aortocoronary bypass surgery depend largely on the maintenance of graft patency.[3] About 25% of venous grafts occlude within 1 year of surgery, whereas during the following 5 years there is a 2% annual occlusion rate, which increases to 5% yearly thereafter. Thus 50% to 60% of venous grafts are occluded after 10 years and only half of the remaining patent ones have no evidence of atherosclerosis.[4,5] The mechanisms responsible for venous graft occlusion are believed to be thrombosis in the early weeks after surgery, followed by intimal hyperplasia during the first year and accelerated atherosclerosis in the later stages.[6] Atherosclerotic changes develop comparatively in a smaller percentage of patients with IMA grafts. As a result, in situ arterial grafts occlude less frequently, up to 5% in the first year and 20% to 30% after 10 years, leading to an improved long-term survival.[5,7]

These graft attrition statistics result in the need for accurate evaluation of bypass graft patency and function, which often is required several times during the lifetime of any given patient.

IMAGING MODALITIES CAPABLE OF EVALUATING GRAFTS

Selective x-ray coronary angiography is the gold standard for assessment of graft anatomy and has the added advantage of simultaneous visualization of the native coronary arteries. Use of a Doppler-tipped guidewire during angiography provides hemodynamic information about graft function by assessing flow pattern at rest and after pharmacologically induced hyperemia.[8]

Selective coronary angiography is, however, invasive, uses ionizing radiation, iodine contrast, and has a small risk of complications such as coronary artery dissection, arrhythmia or stroke.

Two-dimensional (2D) Doppler echocardiography is restricted to evaluation of grafts placed on the LAD artery.[9,10]

Near infrared fluorescence complex angiography and perfusion analysis is a novel real-time imaging technology used to assess the physiologic response to grafting during the intraoperative phase of CABG and which may be useful in predicting subsequent graft failure.[11]

Cardiovascular magnetic resonance (CMR) and coronary computed tomography (CCT) are techniques which allow the direct evaluation of bypass grafts patency.[12-17] A unique feature of CMR is that in addition to standard anatomic imaging, blood flow velocity and volume can be quantified within the grafts. Thus the true physiologic status of the functional unit represented by a graft and its recipient vessel can be determined noninvasively.[18]

CARDIOVASCULAR MAGNETIC RESONANCE OF BYPASS GRAFTS

Over the years, several CMR techniques have been introduced to evaluate aortocoronary bypass grafts (Table 26.1).[19] The assessment strategy may include either anatomic (angiographic) or hemodynamic (flow volume, velocities, flow reserve) evaluation or a combination of these modalities. This is usually combined in clinical practice with evaluation of the myocardial function (cine CMR), tissue characterization (late gadolinium enhancement imaging for presence of myocardial fibrosis/infarction), and ischemia detection (pharmacologic first pass gadolinium contrast myocardial perfusion).

Whereas pulse sequences developed for imaging native coronary arteries are also applied for imaging bypass grafts, CABG imaging is associated with specific problems (different vessel anatomy and flow patterns and the presence of metallic vascular clips, ostial markers and sternal wires).

A majority of published clinical CMR studies addressed imaging the proximal portion of vein grafts. Proximal segments are less affected by bulk cardiac motion compared with distal graft segments or native coronary arteries, resulting in fewer motion artifacts, whereas the lack of direct contact with epicardial fat or myocardium results in higher contrast to surrounding tissues. Unfortunately, graft stenosis often occurs at the site of anastomosis with the native vessel where CMR encounters artifacts and resolution problems similar to those in imaging the native coronary arteries. Arterial grafts imaging poses additional problems because of vessel tortuosity and smaller caliber as well as presence of metallic artifacts from hemostatic clips and sternal wires.

BYPASS GRAFT ANATOMIC IMAGING TECHNIQUES

Conventional Spin Echo and Gradient Echo Imaging

The assessment of saphenous vein aortocoronary bypass graft patency has been one of the early indications for CMR. More than two decades ago several groups reported the feasibility of assessing graft patency using

TABLE 26.1 Detection of Bypass Graft Patency According to Different Cardiovascular Magnetic Resonance Techniques

Reference	Technique	No. of Grafts	Sensitivity (%)	Specificity (%)	Accuracy (%)
White et al.[20]	SE CMR	65	91	72	86
Rubinstein et al.[21]	SE CMR	44	92	85	89
Jenkins et al.[22]	SE CMR	60	90	90	90
Frija et al.[23]	SE CMR	52	98	78	94
White et al.[24]	Cine CMR	28	93	86	89
Aurigemma et al.[25]	Cine CMR	45	88	100	91
Galjee et al.[26]	SE CMR	98	98	85	96
	Cine CMR		98	88	96
	Combined		98	76	94
Kessler et al.[33]	3D navigator	19	87	100	89
Vrachliotis et al.[38]	3D CE MRA, ECG-triggered	44	93	97	95
Wintersperger et al.[37]	3D CE MRA Non–ECG triggered	76	95	81	92
Kalden et al.[30]	HASTE	59	95	93	95
	3D CE MRA ECG-triggered		93	93	93
Bunce et al.[40]	SSFP	79	84	45	78
	3D CE MRA ECG-triggered		85	73	84
Langerak et al.[35]	3D navigator Two observers	56	65–83	80–100	~80

CE MRA, Contrast-enhanced magnetic resonance angiography; *ECG*, electrocardiogram; *HASTE*, half-Fourier acquisition single-shot turbo spin echo; *SE CMR*, spin echo cardiovascular magnetic resonance; *SSFP*, steady state free precession.

conventional electrocardiogram (ECG)-triggered multislice spin-echo techniques.[20–23] On spin-echo images, patent grafts with good blood flow appear in consecutive imaging planes as conduits with a signal void. In contrast, stenotic grafts with slow flow or occluded grafts display intermediate signal intensity (Fig. 26.1). With selective x-ray angiography as the method of reference, the sensitivity of spin-echo CMR in predicting graft patency ranged from 90% to 98% with a specificity of 72% to 90%.

Using conventional gradient echo nonbreath-hold CMR, with a relatively long echo time (TE) and repetition time (TR), the sensitivity was in the same order of magnitude (88%–98%), with a somewhat higher specificity (86%–100%).[24–26] On gradient echo images blood flow within patent grafts appears bright (Fig. 26.2). On spin-echo images, signal voids from metal clips, stents or calcifications, can falsely mimic graft patency. These artifacts are accentuated, thus easier to detect, on gradient echo compared with spin-echo images, which decreases the number of false positive patent grafts (increases specificity). On the other hand, the number of false-positive occlusions might be expected to increase (decreased sensitivity).

Two-Dimensional Breath-Hold Cardiovascular Magnetic Resonance Angiography

This technique, first described for imaging coronary arteries, can also be applied for visualization of bypass grafts.[27] During a breath-hold lasting for 15 to 25 seconds, a segmented gradient echo image is acquired with 4 to 5 mm slice thickness and in-plane resolution of approximately 1 × 1.4 mm. The entire course of a bypass graft is covered by repeating the sequence multiple times. The procedure may become rather time consuming when multiple grafts have to be evaluated. Also, a high susceptibility to metallic materials used during surgery has been reported, with significant effects on diagnostic accuracy.[28] This technique has been used for evaluation of sequential grafts (Fig. 26.3).[29] High sensitivity and specificity were found for predicting patency of grafts to branches of the RCA, but the accuracy decreased in distal graft segments to branches of the LAD and was poor in distal segments to the LCX.[29]

Another 2D breath-hold approach uses a multislice half-Fourier acquisition single shot turbo spin echo (HASTE) sequence. Seven T2-weighted images are generated within a breath-hold of approximately 15 seconds, with a 1.3 × 1.4 mm in-plane resolution and 5 mm slice thickness. Using this technique, Kalden and colleagues reported a sensitivity and specificity of 95% and 93%, respectively, in predicting graft patency and good visualization of 83% of distal graft segments.[30] Because the HASTE sequence is less susceptible to metallic artifacts compared with gradient echo sequences, a remarkably high accuracy was found in detecting arterial graft patency (sensitivity of 90% and specificity of 100%). However, these figures must be interpreted with caution because the pretest probability of occluded arterial grafts is generally low. In that study, it is unclear how many of the 14 reported IMA grafts were occluded. In our personal experience, the HASTE sequence provides excellent visualization of coronary arteries and bypass grafts but rather poor detection of disease (Fig. 26.4). Accordingly, Kalden and colleagues noted that only two out of eight hemodynamically significant graft stenoses were detected using HASTE sequence.

Three-Dimensional Respiratory-Gated Cardiovascular Magnetic Resonance Angiography

A three-dimensional (3D) dataset of truly contiguous slices may be obtained with respiratory-gated gradient echo techniques. Gating to the respiratory cycle is achieved by using navigators that monitor the diaphragm position.[31] Magnetic resonance (MR) data acquired within a preset acceptance window of the respiration-induced diaphragm excursion are used for image reconstruction. The patient is allowed to breathe freely, at the expense of an increase in total imaging time. Several refinements of this gating procedure have been developed for imaging of the coronary arteries.[32]

Kessler and colleagues used respiratory-gated 3D MR angiography (MRA) with navigator guiding and retrospective data processing for imaging of bypass grafts.[33] In a relatively small number of 19 grafts, 13 out of 15 patent grafts and 4 out of 4 occluded grafts were correctly classified. Another study by Molinari and colleagues including 18 patients (51 grafts) which compared navigator guided 3D MRA with coronary

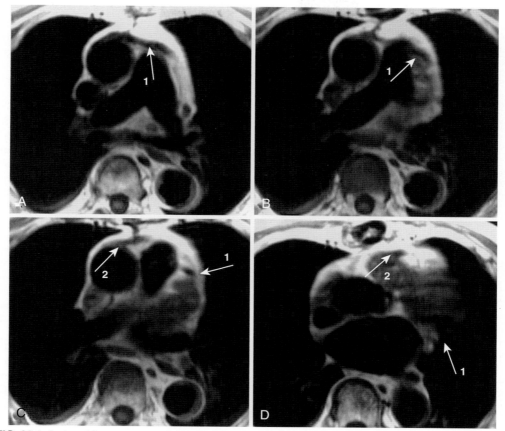

FIG. 26.1 Series of four transverse spin echo images of a sequential vein graft to the obtuse marginal branch of the circumflex (CX) artery *(1)* and a second vein graft to the left anterior descending artery (LAD) *(2)*. Patent grafts show low signal intensity. (A) Most superior image demonstrating the CX graft originating from the ascending aorta and overriding the main pulmonary artery. (B) More descending course of the CX graft left of the pulmonary artery. (C) LAD graft originating from the more proximal part of the ascending aorta. (D) Course of both grafts at the level of the left atrium.

angiography showed a sensitivity of 91%, the specificity of 97% for CMR in detecting occlusion versus patency of grafts.[34]

A study by Langerak and colleagues including 38 post-CABG patients (56 venous grafts) who underwent conventional angiography for recurrent angina, assessed the accuracy of contemporary high-resolution respiratory-gated 3D MRA in detecting vein graft disease.[35] The sequence used in the study included a T2-preparation prepulse (for muscle suppression), a fat suppression prepulse and had an acquisition window of 71 ms placed in mid diastole and at end expiration. A total of 50 out of 56 grafts were adequately visualized with a spatial resolution of 0.7 × 1 × 1.5 mm. The study reported sensitivities of 73% and 83%, with specificities of 80% to 87% and 98% to 100% in detecting grafts with ≥70% diameter stenosis and complete occlusion, respectively.

Three-Dimensional Contrast-Enhanced Breath-Hold Cardiovascular Magnetic Resonance Angiography

Breath-hold contrast-enhanced MRA is another technique which was first applied for aorta imaging.[36] The T1-shortening effect of the gadolinium-contrast agent on blood signal allows the obtaining of high vascular contrast when using short TR/TE gradient echo sequences. After intravenous injection of an interstitial gadolinium-contrast agent, a 3D spoiled gradient echo sequence with short TR/TE (4.4/1.4 ms or even shorter) is applied. Within a breath-hold of approximately 30 seconds, a 3D volume slab composed of 24 to 32 contiguous slices with

a total thickness of approximately 9 cm is imaged. Before acquiring the 3D volume slab, a single-slice 2D turbo gradient echo sequence is used to time the arrival of a contrast agent test bolus in the aorta. To maximize the contrast-enhancing effect, acquisition of the central *k*-space lines of the 3D imaging data is set to coincide with peak contrast arrival. This is achieved by introducing a time delay between contrast injection and start of the imaging sequence (delay = arrival time − ½ or ⅓ of acquisition time). Depending on the field of view, matrix size, number of partitions and slab thickness a spatial in-plane resolution of 1 × 1.5 mm with 2- to 3-mm section thickness is achieved. Each partition of the 3D acquisition yields a "source" image. Studies are evaluated by reviewing the source images and after postprocessing techniques such as maximum intensity projection and planar or curved reformatting (Figs. 26.5 and 26.6).[19]

Evaluation of aortocoronary bypass grafts using 3D contrast-enhanced MRA has been reported without and with ECG triggering.[30,37,38] Sensitivity, specificity, and accuracy for predicting graft patency varied between 93% and 95%, 81% and 97%, and 92% and 95%, respectively (Table 26.1). A lower specificity was found in the non–ECG triggered study.[37] Theoretically, one would expect ECG-triggered acquisitions to be superior for visualizing the sites of graft insertion on native coronary arteries. Although Kalden and colleagues specifically addressed this issue, they succeeded in pursuing distal anastomoses in only 64% of cases.[30] This might have been caused partly by the relatively long data collection

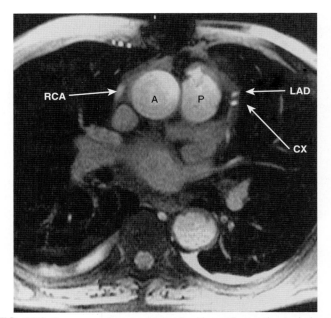

FIG. 26.2 Transverse image obtained with gradient echo technique. Cross sections of patent grafts to the right coronary artery *(RCA),* left anterior descending coronary artery *(LAD),* and circumflex coronary artery *(CX)* are indicated and demonstrate a high signal intensity. *A,* Aorta; *P,* pulmonary artery. (From van Rossum AC, Galjee MA, Post JC, Visser CA. A practical approach to CMR of coronary artery bypass graft patency and flow. *Int J Cardiac Imaging.* 1997;13:199–204, with permission from Kluwer Academic Publishers.)

window of 560 ms within each cardiac cycle, leading to residual blurring attributed to cardiac motion. The use of a shorter acquisition window of 120 ms, used for imaging coronary arteries of healthy volunteers,[39] has not been implemented yet in imaging bypass grafts.

Bunce and colleagues compared 3D contrast-enhanced MRA with the recently developed multislice balanced steady-state free precession (bSSFP) sequence for the assessment of 56 venous and 23 arterial bypass grafts patency in 25 patients.[40] Steady-state free precession (SSFP) had a temporal resolution of 336 ms, with a spatial resolution of $2.7 \times 1.4 \times 4.0$ mm, and 3D contrast-enhanced MRA had a temporal resolution of 440 ms with spatial resolution of $1.6 \times 1.6 \times 2.0$ mm. The two methods had similar accuracy (78% vs. 84%, $P =$ nonsignificant) for detection of coronary artery bypass graft patency, but there was a trend toward more false-positive findings for occlusion and reduced visualization of arterial grafts with SSFP angiography.[40]

IMAGING STRATEGY

The imaging strategy and image interpretation are facilitated when the surgical report is known before the CMR scan with respect to the number of grafts and insertion sites. Grafts descending to the perfusion area of the LCX, including obtuse marginal branches, generally originate most superiorly from the ascending aorta (Fig. 26.7).[27] The graft to the LAD system, including diagonal branches, originates inferiorly compared with most LCX grafts. Both types of grafts cross the pulmonary artery trunk in a left lateral and inferior course. Then the LCX graft proceeds posteriorly and inferiorly, whereas the LAD graft goes left and anteriorly. Grafts to the posterior descending artery of the RCA generally have the lowest origin from the ascending aorta and run inferiorly on the lateral

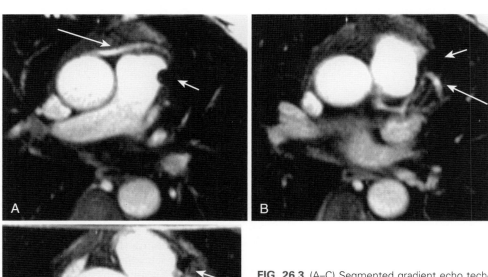

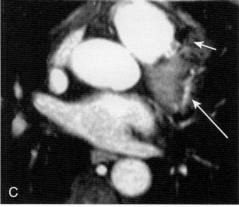

FIG. 26.3 (A–C) Segmented gradient echo technique, 1 image per breath-hold of 16 heartbeats. Patient with sequential graft from the aorta to the diagonal branch of the left anterior descending coronary artery (LAD) and obtuse-marginal branch of the left anterior descending coronary artery and left internal thoracic artery graft to the LAD. The tall arrow indicates bright segments of the sequential graft. The short arrow points at the dark signal loss of the ITA clip artifact. (From van Rossum AC, Bedaux WLF, Hofman MBM. Morphologic evaluation of coronary artery bypass conduits. *J Magn Reson Imaging.* 1999;10:734–740.)

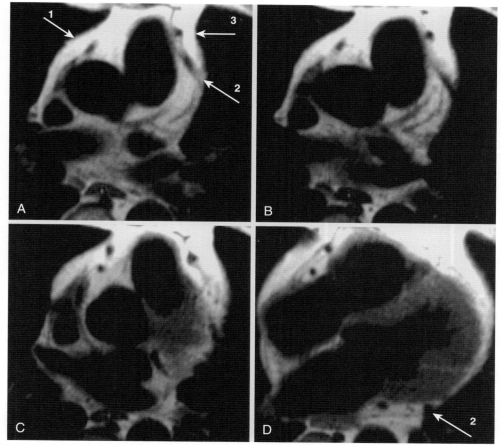

FIG. 26.4 Half-Fourier acquisition single shot turbo spin echo sequence, four out of five images obtained in a single breath-hold (A, B, C, D). Patient with single vein graft to the right coronary artery *(1)*, sequential vein graft to the first diagonal branch of the left anterior descending coronary artery (LAD) and obtuse marginal branch of the circumflex coronary artery *(2)*, and the left internal thoracic artery to the LAD *(3)*. In panels A and B, the native left main coronary artery, the LAD, and the great cardiac vein are visualized. In panels C and D, the right coronary artery is seen inferior to the graft in the right atrioventricular groove.

side of the right atrium. For assessment of patency and measurement of flow within a graft, CMR can best be performed at the proximal part of the graft. At this level, most grafts have a straight course, less motion, and are easily distinguished from native coronary vessels. The surface coil must be centered at the mid sternum level, which is somewhat more cranial compared with a standard cardiac study.

Since the widespread use of *k*-space segmented sequences and phased-array coils, most images can be obtained within a breath-hold. This decreases respiratory motion artifacts and increases image quality.

Because the course of a graft is more or less predictable, the choice of imaging planes can be fairly well standardized. An effective approach is first to acquire a set of multislice transverse images covering the ascending aorta and superior part of the heart. In our experience, one or two breath-hold multislice series using the HASTE sequence will be most informative (see Fig. 26.4). The images just superior of the pulmonary artery trunk will demonstrate in-plane views of proximal parts of LCX and LAD grafts, whereas the images at a lower level show cross sections of grafts to the left and right coronary arteries. Once the proximal course of the grafts has been localized, one may proceed with high-resolution single or multislice 2D imaging, in orientations following the more distal course of the grafts. The advantages of this approach are the short image reconstruction time and the immediate availability of the images. The disadvantage is that it requires patient cooperation

and may be subject to misregistration due to inconsistent breath-holding. Alternatively, 3D MRA techniques may be used to acquire larger imaging slabs covering the course of the grafts. The resolution is higher, and the acquisition time is shorter. However, the reconstruction time is longer than in 2D techniques, and interpretation requires some form of postprocessing. Notwithstanding these limitations, the 3D approaches are likely to become the first choice with improving technology.

CARDIOVASCULAR MAGNETIC RESONANCE QUANTIFICATION OF GRAFT FLOW AND FLOW RESERVE

Flow velocity and volume flow in bypass grafts can be measured by applying velocity-encoded phase-contrast cine CMR sequences, thus allowing the assessment of graft function in addition to a morphologic evaluation (Fig. 26.8).[41] Galjee and colleagues demonstrated that adequate velocity profiles throughout the cardiac cycle could be obtained in 85% of angiographically patent vein grafts, using nonbreath-hold CMR velocity mapping.[26] Graft flow velocity was characterized by a biphasic pattern, with systolic and diastolic peaks (Fig. 26.9).[26] Similar findings have been obtained by using invasive Doppler guidewire approaches and transthoracic Doppler echocardiography.[8,9] However, there are differences in resting phasic flow patterns between in situ IMA conduits

into stents (transforming them into intravascular antennas coupled to a surface coil) allows the visualization of stent lumen.[58] CMR-lucent stents are also under development.

However, even a clear demonstration of graft-segment patency or narrowing will often not suffice for clinical decision making. In most patients, there is a need to also know the status of the native coronary arteries. Narrowing of the recipient coronary artery may have developed beyond the anastomosis of a patent graft segment, and progression of disease in other native coronary arteries must be excluded. Thus CMR does not eliminate the need for conventional x-ray coronary angiography when a revascularization procedure is considered.

INDICATIONS

A clinical indication for CMR of bypass grafts may therefore exist only in patients in whom there is no immediate need to know the status of the native coronary arteries. Such a category consists, for example, of patients with chest pain shortly after CABG surgery. Also, late after CABG surgery, information about graft patency and function might be helpful in deciding whether to postpone coronary angiography in patients with ambiguous anginal complaints. Noninvasive monitoring of flow parameters may then be useful to detect a gradual increase of graft stenosis and decide to proceed with conventional angiography and percutaneous intervention, before the onset of a total occlusion. Similarly, flow measurements could be used after bypass graft percutaneous angioplasty for the early detection of restenosis.

Furthermore, CMR can be used as a screening procedure before angiography, providing a road map for the grafts to be visualized. This might considerably shorten the angiographic procedure with less exposure to ionizing radiation and lower total iodine contrast dose. A useful indication also appears to be the assessment of the patency of grafts that are not visualized during conventional angiography. Although this often indicates a proximal occlusion of the graft, failure of the catheter to find an aortic graft anastomosis may result in a false diagnosis of graft occlusion. In cases of doubt, MRA will rapidly confirm or discard this diagnosis. Also, when angiography has demonstrated a graft stenosis, it can be helpful for further management to assess the flow reserve of a graft. There are also occasions when CMR is useful in visualizing and assisting with further surgical planning for complications of vein grafting, such as aneurysm of the graft.[59]

Finally, vein graft imaging may have a role in research of bypass techniques and has been used to demonstrate the efficacy of aprotinin[60] during surgery and in comparison of techniques for vein graft stripping,[61] by demonstrating patency rates without the need for invasive angiography.

Notwithstanding these indications, the majority of patients after CABG require evaluation with respect to percutaneous or surgical revascularization. Unless CMR will be able to provide more detailed information regarding the status of native coronary arteries, a wide application of the technique is unlikely to occur. Continuing improvement in CMR of coronary arteries and bypass grafts may be expected with new developments in scanner hardware and software and the use of contrast agents. Most recent clinical guidelines and consensus documents give MRA a high grading for evaluation of coronary anomalies; however, in the case of aortocoronary bypass grafts, MRA alone receives class II indication or uncertain appropriateness.[62-64] However, when combined with stress first pass gadolinium-contrast myocardial perfusion CMR, most experts consider it an appropriate indication for patients who have undergone CABG and have recurrent symptoms suggesting myocardial ischemia.

CONCLUSION

There is clear evidence that conventional spin echo and gradient echo CMR are capable of assessing patency of venous aortocoronary grafts. With recent advances in breath-hold 2D and contrast-enhanced 3D techniques, the accuracy in detecting graft occlusion has further improved. Limitations are still present in evaluating distal graft segments and sequential grafts caused by insufficient spatial resolution, low SNRs and motion. Imaging of arterial grafts is complicated by the sternal wire and metallic clip artifacts. Recently, significant progress has been made in the assessment of graft flow patterns and flow reserve using phase contrast velocity-encoded CMR both at 1.5 T and 3 T. Clinically, these functional measurements may become useful for noninvasive monitoring of bypass graft narrowing progression before and even after percutaneous interventions.[48] However, the majority of patients undergo graft evaluation in preparation for revascularization procedures. In these cases knowing which venous grafts are completely occluded, although helpful, is still not sufficient because information on the status of the native coronary arteries is still required. A broader role for CMR in the evaluation of patients with aortocoronary bypass grafts may therefore be expected only after further improvement in CMR coronary angiography.

REFERENCES

A full reference list is available online at ExpertConsult.com

27

Atherosclerotic Plaque Imaging: Aorta and Carotid

Marc R. Dweck, Philip M. Robson, James H.F. Rudd, and Zahi A. Fayad

Although death rates in industrialized countries have been consistently falling since the 1980s, atherosclerosis is now raging throughout the developing world. As a consequence the complications of atherosclerosis have become the leading cause of mortality and morbidity worldwide. Fundamentally, atherosclerosis is an inflammatory disease, which affects medium and large arteries from the first decade of life until death. It has a predilection for certain arterial beds, with the carotid artery and aorta being the most common sites of plaque formation. In the carotid circulation, the end result can be an ischemic cerebral insult causing either temporary (transient ischemic attack [TIA]) or permanent (cerebrovascular attack [CVA]) symptoms. If unchecked, aortic atherosclerosis can predispose to dissection, intramural hemorrhage, aneurysm formation and downstream embolus. Importantly, because atherosclerosis is a systemic disease, assessments of the carotid arteries and aorta also provide surrogate information about disease burden and activity in the coronary circulation, providing prognostic information about the risk of myocardial infarction.[1]

PATHOBIOLOGY OF ATHEROSCLEROSIS

Atherosclerosis is characterized by the gradual accumulation of lipid, inflammatory cells, and connective tissue within the arterial wall. It is a chronic, progressive disease with a very long asymptomatic/subclinical phase. The first abnormality to develop is the fatty streak, caused by the collection of lipid and macrophages in the subendothelial space. Fatty streaks develop primarily in regions of low wall shear stress, which results in endothelial dysfunction and the production of less nitric oxide.[2] The major atherogenic risk factors including smoking, hypertension, and diabetes mellitus also all affect endothelial function,[3] impairing both its barrier function and secretory capacity. Ultimately the blood vessel wall becomes more permeable to blood-derived lipids and inflammatory cells in these regions, encouraging the early stages of atherosclerosis.

Once within the subendothelial space, low-density lipoprotein (LDL) becomes oxidized and attracts monocytes by triggering the release of monocyte chemoattractant protein-1 (MCP-1) from the overlying endothelial cells.[4] Endothelial adhesion molecules, including vascular cell adhesion molecule-1 (VCAM), intercellular adhesion molecule-1, E-selectin, and P-selectin, facilitate the internalization of further monocytes. Once they have escaped the blood pool, monocytes transform into macrophages and bind and internalize oxidative LDL via their scavenger receptors.[5] Eventually, the subendothelial accumulation of modified LDL and macrophage-derived foam cells leads to the formation of the atheromatous lipid core. The thrombogenic components of the lipid core become separated from blood in the lumen by the endothelialized fibrous cap, which consists predominantly of vascular smooth muscle cells (VSMCs) and connective tissue. VSMCs migrate from the arterial media and synthesize the extracellular matrix components of the cap, such as elastin and collagen. The cap also contains variable numbers of inflammatory cells, most importantly macrophages. As the plaque enlarges, the affected artery grows outward (by expansion of the external elastic lamina) so that lumen diameter and therefore blood flow is initially preserved; this is a process known as positive remodeling.[6] As the artery's wall stress increases with outward remodeling, further expansion eventually becomes impossible and the plaque then encroaches into the lumen. Ultimately this may cause angina by compromising blood flow to the myocardium.

Mature plaques may also become calcified, a process that preferentially affects the intima of the artery and is thought to occur as a healing response to inflammation and cell death within the plaque. Although the early stages of microcalcification are associated with high-risk inflamed atheroma, the latter stages of macrocalcification are by contrast associated with burnt-out stable disease. Very advanced plaques with a large necrotic core and associated hypoxia will also often be perforated by new blood vessels under the influence of angiogenic factors, a process called *neovascularization*, with similarities to that which occurs within growing tumors. However, these small arteries are structurally fragile and have a tendency to spontaneously hemorrhage, which can destabilize the plaque leading to increased plaque inflammation, rupture, and the precipitation of acute myocardial infarction.[7]

Atherosclerotic plaques may remain quiescent for decades. However, when they initiate clot formation in the vessel lumen, they can very quickly become life threatening. This occurs predominantly as a result of fibrous cap rupture, with consequent exposure of the thrombogenic and tissue factor-rich lipid core to circulating blood. Less commonly, there can be erosion of the endothelial cell layer overlying the fibrous cap, which in the context of an advanced thrombogenic response can also lead to intravascular thrombosis. It is estimated that endothelial erosion accounts for ~30% of myocardial infarctions.[8] Regardless of the mechanism, plaque disruption will lead to varying degrees of local platelet activation and thrombus formation, depending on the characteristics of the plaque and the thrombogenicity of the blood. Importantly, however, the majority of these plaque ruptures do not appear to result in overt clinical events but instead remain subclinical and responsible for abrupt plaque growth.[9]

It has become clear that the cellular and extracellular composition of the plaque is the primary determinant of plaque stability.[10] Lesions with a large lipid core, thin fibrous cap, positive remodeling, angiogenesis, microcalcification, and a preponderance of inflammatory cells compared with VSMCs are at the highest risk of rupture. Inflammatory cells, particularly macrophages, produce metalloproteinase enzymes, which break down matrix proteins, weakening the fibrous cap. In addition, they secrete inflammatory cytokines, in particular interferon γ, which inhibit VSMC proliferation and matrix production. Furthermore, VSMCs in the fibrous cap have a reduced proliferative capacity and a propensity to apoptosis.[11] Consequently, inflammation within the plaques promotes destruction of the fibrous cap, a propensity to plaque rupture, and subsequent thrombosis. However, this is balanced by the action of VSMCs, which nourish and repair the cap, promoting plaque stabilization. This dynamic balance between proinflammatory and healing responses across the vasculature ultimately governs a patient's risk of myocardial infarction or stroke. These processes are independent of the degree of luminal stenosis. Consequently, positively remodeled and angiographically invisible plaques can rupture to precipitate a fatal clinical event, while many large plaques that obstruct flow and cause angina may be stable and not life threatening. There is therefore an urgent need for imaging techniques that can discriminate "stable" from potentially "unstable" lesions in clinical practice. This chapter will investigate the role that cardiovascular magnetic resonance (CMR) imaging might play in this respect, with a focus on its ability to measure the total plaque burden, to investigate high-risk plaque characteristics, and to determine disease activity with advanced molecular techniques.

IMAGING ATHEROSCLEROSIS

CMR can make use of differences in tissue relaxation times (T1 and T2) and proton density, intrinsic material properties that affect the magnitude of the magnetic resonance (MR) signal, to generate soft-tissue contrast, providing detailed information about atherosclerotic plaque composition. This is readily feasible in the large and relatively immobile carotid arteries and thoracic aorta, with intensive research aimed at transferring these techniques into the more challenging coronary vasculature.

The aim of atherosclerotic plaque imaging is ultimately to identify vulnerable patients at high risk of myocardial infarction or stroke before symptoms and complications develop.[12] Similarly, early identification of disease might allow the implementation of pharmacologic treatment to halt or even reverse the process of plaque progression and possibly prevent rupture (e.g., with statin therapy).[13] Recently, rapid advances in CMR hardware, software, and molecular imaging tracers have seen CMR develop into a modality of considerable utility and versatility for imaging large vessel atheroma. In particular, assessments of atherosclerotic plaque burden offer powerful prediction of adverse cardiovascular events, whereas more advanced techniques aimed at evaluating high-risk plaque characteristics and disease activity hold promise in refining this risk prediction even further. Each of these features will be discussed in detail below.

ASSESSMENTS OF PLAQUE BURDEN

Simple measures of the atherosclerotic plaque burden in different vascular beds provide powerful prognostic information, presumably because the more plaques a patient has the more likely one will rupture or erode and cause an event. CMR can effectively image atherosclerotic plaque using high-resolution, black-blood, fast-spin echo sequences.[14] Preparatory pulses null signal in the blood pool and perivascular fat, improving contrast between the plaques and vessel lumen, and surrounding tissue, respectively. The atherosclerotic plaque burden can then be quantified using measurements of plaque thickness in two dimensions and plaque volume in three dimensions. In the aorta these measurements demonstrate a close correlation with transesophageal echocardiography[15] and with increasing numbers of cardiovascular risk factors.[16,17] Similar approaches have been used to measure plaque thickness and the plaque volume in the carotid arteries,[18] providing measures of atherosclerotic

burden that compare favorably with histology[19] and predict major adverse cardiovascular outcomes.[20]

Black-blood CMR also allows the early detection of subclinical atherosclerotic disease. Indeed CMR is particularly attractive for this purpose, given the absence of ionizing radiation, and has already proved useful in several large cohort studies. In asymptomatic subjects enrolled in the Framingham Heart Study (FHS), FHS coronary risk score was strongly associated with asymptomatic aortic atherosclerosis detected by CMR.[16] The prevalence and extent of aortic atherosclerosis increased with age. In a substudy of the Multiethnic Study of Atherosclerosis (MESA), CMR aortic wall thickness increased as a function of age, but males and black participants had the greatest wall thickness.[21] In another study of 102 patients undergoing x-ray coronary angiography, aortic atherosclerotic plaques were detected with a higher frequency in active smokers and in those with high levels of LDL-cholesterol, but the volume and area of aortic plaques correlated most strongly with age and the presence of hypertension. Interestingly, only atherosclerotic plaques located in the thoracic aorta were found to be associated with coronary artery disease (CAD).[17] Taken together, these studies confirm the strong correlation between the presence of cardiovascular risk factors and the incidence of aortic atherosclerosis. It should be noted, however, that there are racial and population differences in the response to individual risk factors, which presumably have a genetic basis.[21]

Another benefit readily appreciated by pharmaceutical companies and others wishing to study the effects of drugs on plaque progression (and regression) is the low coefficient of variability of CMR plaque volume measurements.[22,23] This translates directly into the requirement for lower patient numbers for studies investigating the impact of pharmaceutical agents on plaque volume, because any true drug effect will not be swamped by noise within the measuring technique. This was illustrated in two separate studies where high-dose statin regimens were shown to be superior to low-dose regimens in terms of atheroma burden reduction, an effect that could be demonstrated with only 20 patients per group.[24,25]

Subsequently, in the first double-blind, multicentric, dal-PLAQUE (safety and efficacy of dalcetrapib on atherosclerotic disease using novel noninvasive multimodality imaging) study, 130 patients were randomly assigned to placebo ($N = 66$) or 24 months treatment with the cholesterylester transfer protein (CETP) inhibitor dalcetrapib ($N = 64$). In patients receiving dalcetrapib, the absolute change from baseline relative to placebo in total vessel area was 4.01 mm^2 (90% CI, 7.23 to 0.80; nominal $P = .04$) over 24 months.[26]

PLAQUE CHARACTERISTICS

Plaques at risk of rupture have certain pathological characteristics, including inflammation, positive remodeling, a large necrotic core, angiogenesis, microcalcification, and a thin, fibrous cap. Each represents a potential imaging target, and although not all of these plaques will progress to rupture and even less will cause events,[27] emerging evidence suggests that identification of such plaques may identify patients at increased cardiovascular risk.[28] Again, CMR techniques aimed at resolving these characteristics are best suited to the carotid arteries.

Positive Remodeling

Similar black-blood imaging techniques as described earlier can be used to identify positive remodeling. Indeed, identification of positive remodeling in the aorta and carotids has been shown to identify patients with an increased risk of future adverse cardiovascular outcomes.[20] Moreover, positive remodeling is also detectable with CMR in individual coronary arteries,[29] although the relationship between this CMR finding and prognosis is yet to be established.[30]

Multicontrast Magnetic Resonance

Multicontrast CMR of the plaque is based on successive high-resolution black-blood fast-spin echo CMR sequences that null signal in the flowing blood and perivascular fat with preparatory pulses. Several sequences with different weightings are generally acquired (e.g., T1 weighted, T2 weighted, and proton density weighted [PDW]). Analysis of the various signal intensities in each of these sequences allows reasonable differentiation of plaque components. In particular, the lipid core, fibrous tissue, plaque hemorrhage, the fibrous cap, and the degree of calcification can all be identified and quantified according to their different relaxation properties on CMR.[31,32] In Fig. 27.1 an axial section through the thorax reveals a complex aortic plaque. Fig. 27.2 demonstrates a carotid plaque imaged at 3 T, with corresponding T1, T2, and PDW images displayed. A final example of multicontrast CMR showing different plaque components and automatic segmentation of these plaques using a *k*-means cluster algorithm is shown in Fig. 27.3.[33]

The lipid rich necrotic core can be identified in the carotid arteries and aorta using multicontrast weightings plus postcontrast T1-weighted imaging, with advances in CMR acquisition protocols allowing acquisition times to be reduced many-fold.[14] The necrotic core usually appears isointense to hyperintense on time-of-flight angiographic and precontrast T1-weighted images and has minimal contrast enhancement compared with the surrounding tissue on postcontrast T1-weighted images.[34] The combination of these images can therefore be used to identify and quantify the lipid necrotic core burden. Yuan et al. demonstrated that multicontrast CMR of human carotid arteries had sensitivity and specificity values of 85% and 92%, respectively, for the identification of a lipid core.[35,36]

Alterations in the lipid necrotic core burden with therapy have also been demonstrated and may be more sensitive to treatment effects than simple plaque burden measurements. The ORION trial assessed the impact of rosuvastatin on carotid plaque volume and composition in 43 patients treated for 2 years. Although no change in the plaque volume was observed, a reduction in the percentage of lipid necrotic core was demonstrated.[37] A subsequent study by Zhao and colleagues confirmed

the effect of lipid-lowering therapy on the lipid content of atherosclerotic plaque after just 1 year of treatment. Importantly, the observed reduction continued in to the second year of therapy and preceded any effects on vessel wall area.[34]

Imaging Acute Thrombus and Plaque Hemorrhage

Histopathological studies[38] suggest that intraplaque hemorrhage may play a role in triggering both plaque rupture and growth. A first study proved that multicontrast CMR could accurately image intraplaque hemorrhage in carotid atheroma using T2*-weighted sequences.[39] However CMR can also distinguish between recent and remote hemorrhage on the basis of its methemoglobin content using noncontrast T1-weighted gradient recalled echo sequences, incorporating fat and blood suppression. Methemoglobin is an intermediate breakdown product of hemoglobin formed 12 to 72 hours following hemorrhage. It therefore represents a key component of acute thrombus and is associated with a short T1 and high signal on T1-weighted imaging. This property allows CMR to detect fresh thrombus using T1-weighted images in a range of conditions including deep venous thrombosis and pulmonary embolism. This approach has been used in atherosclerosis to visualize regions of both intraplaque hemorrhage and endothelial thrombus related to plaque rupture/erosion. Indeed, the culprit carotid plaques of patients who have suffered a recent stroke consistently demonstrate this high T1-weighted signal.[40,41]

Early Imaging of Aortic Stenosis and Calcification

Histologic validation of this approach has also been provided using the carotid model in 63 patients undergoing endarterectomy. This demonstrated that high-intensity plaques had negative and positive predictive values of 70% and 93%, respectively, for the detection of complex carotid lesions with evidence of surface rupture and intraluminal or intraplaque hemorrhage.[42] Moreover, imaging of hemorrhage and thrombus in the coronary arteries, where the small size of the vessel wall makes multicontrast imaging challenging, are the targets of intense research[43-46] (see Chapter 3).

Importantly, unenhanced T1-weighted CMR imaging also appears to provide important prognostic information. In one study, the presence of high-intensity plaques in the carotid arteries predicted cardiac events, outperforming carotid intimal medial thickness and traditional cardiovascular risk factors.[47] This finding was corroborated in a subsequent meta-analysis of 8 studies incorporating data from 689 patients, which demonstrated a 6-fold increase in cerebrovascular events in patients with high-intensity carotid plaques.[48] The approach is also applicable to the coronary arteries, with high-intensity plaque again appearing to identify patients at increased risk of future coronary events.[49] Noncontrast T1-weighted imaging therefore holds major promise as a prognostic marker, and in studying the natural history of plaque hemorrhage and the prevalence and importance of subclinical atherosclerotic plaque rupture.

Angiogenesis

Pathological studies first revealed the central role of plaque neovascularization in contributing to atherosclerotic plaque vulnerability.[50] The presence of neovessels is strongly associated with plaque inflammation, macrophage content, and the likelihood of rupture,[51] presumably because they provide an alternative route for monocyte entry into the plaque and because of the propensity of these vessels to leak and rupture.

Gadolinium (Gd) chelates represent the most commonly used CMR contrast agents for imaging new plaque vessels. These paramagnetic agents increase the blood signal on CMR images after intravenous injection and are therefore good candidates for measuring plaque neovasculature. Such techniques have been used in oncology imaging to quantify new vessels associated with tumors.[52] Kerwin and colleagues demonstrated

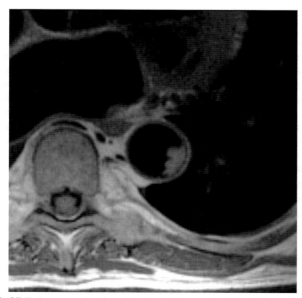

FIG. 27.1 An example of multicontrast plaque imaging with cardiovascular magnetic resonance. This axial section through the thoracic aorta demonstrates an eccentrically shaped plaque involving the lateral wall of the aorta.

USPIO imaging has also been used clinically to assess the antiinflammatory effects of novel therapies. The ATHEROMA (Atorvastatin Therapy: Effects on Reduction of Macrophage Activity) study randomized 47 patients with carotid stenosis >40% and increased USPIO uptake on baseline scanning to either 10 mg or 80 mg atorvastatin therapy for 12 weeks. A significant decrease in USPIO carotid plaque uptake was observed in the high-dose cohort but not the low-dose group.[74]

Macrophages within atherosclerotic plaques have also been targeted for imaging with Gd-loaded immunomicelles. These agents, with diameters between 20 and 120 nm, are composed of phospholipids, a surfactant, and an aliphatic chain with Gd-diethylenetriaminepentaacetic acid (Gd-DTPA) attached at the polar head group. The polar head group of the aliphatic chain can be attached to antibodies directly or via a biotin-avidin bridge. Using this model, we have made micelles that have over 10,000 Gd ions on each micelle surface and the ability to specifically target the macrophage scavenger receptor. Initial work demonstrated that these immunomicelles resulted in enhanced signal in murine atherosclerotic plaque.[75]

Endothelial Adhesion Molecules

Expression of endothelial adhesion molecules such as VCAM and selectins occurs early in the development of atherosclerosis, driving progressive macrophage recruitment in to the plaques. These are potential imaging targets in cardiovascular disease[76] and other conditions.[77] The ability to image VCAM was elegantly demonstrated by Kelly et al. They used a superparamagnetic fluorescent nanoparticle coupled to a payload peptide that was internalized by endothelial cells expressing VCAM. This was tested in ApoE-/- mice fed a high cholesterol diet and was highly specific for VCAM-expressing cells, compared with immunohistochemistry.[78]

CMR imaging of the selectin family of molecules has also been attempted, at least in vitro. Kang et al. showed that a monoclonal antibody fragment tagged with iron oxide nanoparticles was specific for human endothelial cells expressing E-selectin in culture, with an increased binding of 200 times compared with controls.[79] Intracellular adhesion molecule 1 (ICAM-1) receptors expressed on the cerebral arterial vascular endothelium have been imaged with CMR using antibody-conjugated paramagnetic liposomes.[80] CMR provided sufficient signal enhancement to determine the areas of increased expression, and binding was verified by fluorescent histopathology.

Angiogenesis

A novel agent targeting the integrin $\alpha_v\beta_3$ (specifically expressed on the endothelial surface of neovasculature) has been developed to identify regions in the vessel wall undergoing angiogenesis. Winter et al. demonstrated in a rabbit model of atherosclerosis that regions of neovascularization in plaques had a 47% increase in signal intensity on CMR after the injection of $\alpha_v\beta_3$-targeted nanoparticles.[81] Another epitope that has been successfully exploited for imaging plaque angiogenesis is fibronectin. The binding of an antifibronectin antibody was confirmed in ApoE-/- mice, both autoradiographically and by the use of a fluorescent probe, demonstrating specificity for the vasovasorum of the atheroscleorisc plaque.[82]

Thrombus

Intraluminal thrombosis represents the final step in the evolution of vulnerable atherosclerotic plaque and is therefore a candidate target for novel-specific CMR contrast agents. Histologic studies have demonstrated that superficial thrombus superimposed on a ruptured atherosclerotic plaque characterizes those plaques at high risk of ischemic events.[83] Moreover, a clinical study analyzed the histology of intracoronary thrombus aspirated from 211 patients with acute myocardial

infarction, demonstrating that >50% of the culprit thrombi were at least days or weeks old.[84] Presumably, microplaque rupture events with thrombus formation often predate the catastrophic rupture event that causes the clinical syndrome. The ability to detect these early warnings might therefore allow intense therapy or device placement to avert symptoms.

Aside from the T1-weighted CMR imaging approach described earlier, several molecular techniques have been taken to image thrombus with CMR. Yu et al. used a Gd-loaded nanoparticle coupled to a fibrin antibody and tested this against in vitro thrombus.[85] They demonstrated significant signal enhancement and confirmed tight binding of the antibody to the thrombus with scanning electron microscopy. A similar method, but using a different nanoparticle construct, was employed successfully by Winter.[81]

A fibrin-specific CMR contrast agent has also been designed. With this agent, thrombus resulting from plaque rupture has been identified using CMR in a rabbit model. In the 25 arterial thrombi induced by carotid crush injury, Botnar et al. demonstrated a sensitivity and specificity of 100% for in vivo thrombus detection.[86] Sirol et al. used the same fibrin-specific CMR contrast agent (EP-1242) in 12 guinea pigs to demonstrate that the signal intensity of the thrombus was increased by over 4-fold compared with noncontrast images. The detection of thrombi improved from 42% pickup precontrast injection compared with 100% detection after injection.[87] Finally, another experimental fibrin-targeted peptide (EP-2104R) for thrombus detection allowed discrimination between occlusive and nonocclusive thrombi, and tracking of intravascular thrombus as it aged and became more organized by fibrous tissue infiltration[88] (Fig. 27.4).

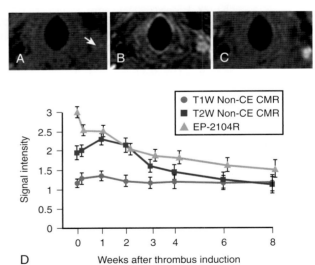

FIG. 27.4 Axial cardiovascular magnetic resonance *(CMR)* images of a rabbit carotid artery one week after thrombus induction, imaged using a double inversion recovery turbo-spin echo sequence. (A) T1-weighted *(T1W)* and (B) T2-weighted *(T2W)* images were obtained without any injection of contrast agent. White arrow indicates location of the thrombus. (C) T1W images obtained 30 minutes after EP-2104R injection. (D) Relative signal intensity changes (mean ± standard deviation) over time for T1W *(red circles)*, T2W *(blue squares)* and after EP-2104R injection *(yellow triangles)*. This gadolinium-based, fibrin-targeted CMR contrast agent demonstrates significant enhancement of the thrombus compared with T1W images (*P* < .001). (Modified from Sirol M, Fuster V, Badimon JJ, et al. Chronic thrombus detection with in vivo magnetic resonance imaging and a fibrin-targeted contrast agent. *Circulation.* 2005;112:1594–1600.)

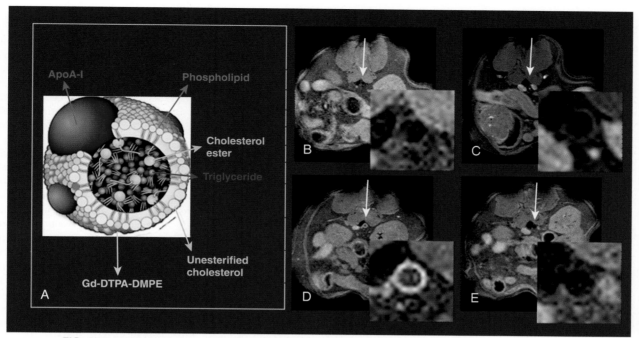

FIG. 27.5 (A) This represents the reconstituted high density lipoprotein (HDL)-like cardiovascular magnetic resonance contrast agent composed of an HDL-like particle and a phospholipid-based contrast agent *(Gd-DTPA-DMPE)*. Axial in vivo magnetic resonance images of the abdominal aorta in an 8-week-old mouse at 9.4 T before (B), 1 hour (C), 24 hours (D), and 48 hours (E) after the injection of recombinant HDL-like nanoparticles. The insets denote the magnification of the aortic region. *ApoA-I,* Apolipoprotein A1. (Modified from Frias JC, Williams KJ, Fisher EA, Fayad ZA. Recombinant HDL-like nanoparticles: a specific contrast agent for MRI of atherosclerotic plaques. *J Am Chem Soc.* 2004;126:16316–16317.)

Extracellular Matrix

Other novel CMR contrast agents have been found to accumulate within atherosclerotic plaques. For example, gadofluorine M is a lipophilic, macrocyclic, water-soluble, Gd chelate complex with a perfluorinated side chain. Both Sirol and Barkhausen separately demonstrated that gadofluorine M significantly increased signal intensity in rabbit aortic plaques compared with controls. A strong correlation was found between the intensity of CMR signal enhancement after the injection of gadofluorine and the presence of lipid-rich plaques on corresponding histologic sections.[89,90] This suggests a high affinity of gadofluorine M for atherosclerotic plaque. There is now emerging data that gadofluorine M is restricted to the extracellular space of plaques and may interact with resident proteins in the extracellular matrix milieu.

High-Density Lipoprotein Imaging

Our group developed another type of imaging agent based on a recombinant high-density lipoprotein (HDL) molecule that incorporates Gd-DTPA phospholipids.[91] The natural role of HDL in the body is to remove lipid from atherosclerotic plaque and return it to the liver (reverse cholesterol transport). Elevated levels of HDL are associated with a reduction in plaque rupture events, presumably because of this protective effect.[92] The recombinant HDL imaging agent has a small diameter (7–12 nm) allowing it to diffuse into atherosclerotic plaques; however, because it uses endogenous transport molecules, it does not trigger any immune reaction. Atherosclerotic plaques demonstrated a 35% increase of CMR signal intensity 24 hours after the injection of these recombinant HDL particles in an ApoE knockout mouse model. Furthermore, fluorescent recombinant HDL colocalized with macrophages present in atherosclerotic plaques with confocal microscopy. Fig.

27.5 demonstrates the enhancement of atherosclerotic plaques after the injection of recombinant HDL.

HYBRID POSITRON EMISSION TOMOGRAPHY/ CARDIAC MAGNETIC RESONANCE IMAGING

PET is a molecular imaging technique that is highly sensitive to the activity of specific disease processes that can be targeted with specially designed radiotracers. This sensitivity gives it major advantages over CMR-based molecular imaging techniques; however, PET remains limited by its low spatial resolution. With the availability of PET/CMR systems the capability now exists to combine functional information from PET with the anatomic detail and soft-tissue characterization of CMR, combining the major advantages of these two imaging approaches (Fig. 27.6). Once again the absence of radiation associated with MR means these hybrid systems offer considerable potential advantages to the more established and widely available PET/CT scanners.

Arterial inflammation is a key driver of atherosclerosis and, in particular, the precipitation of acute plaque rupture and adverse cardiovascular events. 18F-fluorodeoxyglucose (18F-FDG) is a glucose analog that identifies macrophages, which use substantially more glucose than neighboring cell types in the vasculature,[93] particularly in hypoxic conditions.[94] 18F-FDG uptake has been demonstrated to be increased in the culprit carotid plaques poststroke/TIA compared with asymptomatic contralateral lesions[95] and associated with cardiovascular risk factors.[96] Moreover early studies suggests that the detection of increased vascular 18F-FDG activity might identify patients with an adverse prognosis.[97,98]

Importantly the arterial 18F-FDG signal is modifiable with drug therapy, so that this technique is being increasingly employed as an end-point in trials assessing the antiinflammatory effects of novel

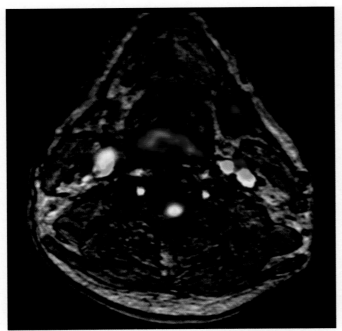

FIG. 27.6 Hybrid positron emission tomography/cardiovascular magnetic resonance image in the axial plane demonstrating increased 18F-fluorodeoxyglucose signal localizing to a region of carotid atheroma.

antiatherosclerosis drugs in the carotid arteries and thoracic aorta.[26,99,100] The effect of therapy can be detected as early as 3 to 6 months, which is well before changes can be observed using CMR alone. Widely available 18F-FDG is limited by its lack of specificity, leading to interest in more specific PET markers of inflammation[101,102] and tracers targeting other disease processes of interest such as angiogenesis, microcalcification, and plaque hypoxia.[103-107] With the advent of such novel tracers, PET/CMR holds major potential as an imaging tool for the study of carotid atheroma[108] and cardiovascular disease in general.[109]

CONCLUSION AND FUTURE DIRECTIONS

Thanks to the absence of ionizing radiation, CMR represents the imaging technology of choice for the noninvasive high-spatial resolution detection and serial monitoring of atherosclerotic plaques in the carotid arteries and aorta. High image quality and sensitivity to small changes in plaque size mean that there is little variance between measurements, permitting small sample sizes to be used in comparative studies. Thus multicontrast CMR is ideally suited for use in evaluation of novel antiatheroma drugs.

The development of functional molecular imaging of atherosclerosis may also help to reveal the key pathological steps that lead from a stable atherosclerotic plaque to an acute ischemic event. However, clinical studies have underscored the multiple locations of vulnerable and ruptured atherosclerotic plaques and the diffuse inflammation of the arterial tree in patients with acute ischemic events compared with stable patients. Therefore the concept of detecting infrequent vulnerable atherosclerotic plaques with imaging and treating them individually has started to shift to a more global process of identifying vulnerable patients at high risk of acute clinical events, irrespective of the arterial location.[110]

In the future, CMR atherosclerosis imaging may help to focus individual evaluation of cardiovascular risk and to optimize antiatherosclerotic therapies with hybrid PET/CMR allowing advanced multiparametric imaging.

ACKNOWLEDGMENTS AND FUNDING

M.R.D. is supported by the British Heart Foundation (FS/14/78/31020) and is the recipient of the Sir Jules Thorn Biomedical Research Award 2015. J.H.F.R. is part-supported by the NIHR Cambridge Biomedical Research Centre, the British Heart Foundation, the EPSRC, and the Wellcome Trust. ZAF is part supported by NIH/NHLBI R01 HL071021.

REFERENCES

A full reference list is available online at ExpertConsult.com

28

Atherosclerotic Plaque Imaging: Coronaries

Imran Rashid, W. Yong Kim, Claudia Prieto, Marcus R. Makowski, Warren J. Manning, and René M. Botnar

Coronary artery disease (CAD) is a leading cause of global mortality.[1] It results from atherosclerosis, which is a systemic and progressive disease involving the intimal layer of large- and medium-sized arteries. Atherothrombosis, defined as atherosclerotic plaque disruption (predominantly plaque rupture) with superimposed thrombosis, can lead to arterial occlusion and subsequent life-threatening conditions such as acute myocardial infarction (MI) or ischemic stroke. The concept of a "vulnerable plaque" was first introduced to distinguish unstable, rupture-prone plaques from plaques with a stable phenotype. Analyses of human coronary plaque have demonstrated that plaque rupture occurs at a higher frequency than clinical events, suggesting that prothrombotic conditions are also necessary for plaque rupture to trigger acute coronary syndromes.[2,3] As such, effective risk stratification algorithms need to include both local and systemic factors that confer increased risk of cardiovascular events. At present, clinical risk scoring systems are largely based on the assessment of traditional risk factors with the addition of noninvasive imaging or functional ("stress") testing for investigation of symptoms that are potentially ischemic in origin.[4] A limitation of this approach includes failure to detect specific features of coronary plaque that confer increased risk of rupture. The identification of high-risk patients might be further improved through the direct assessment of coronary plaque burden, high-risk characteristics, or disease activity, allowing for targeted administration of therapies that are likely to result in prognostic benefits.

Subclinical atherosclerosis can precede the development of clinical disease by many years or even decades, providing an opportunity to identify high-risk patients for targeted primary prevention therapies and ongoing clinical surveillance.[5] At present, multidetector computed tomography (MDCT) coronary angiography is often used for the assessment of low–intermediate risk patients with chest pain where its high negative predictive value allows for the exclusion of coronary artery disease in many individuals. MDCT also allows for the quantification of the overall atherosclerotic plaque burden and the identification of some vulnerable plaque characteristics, through patterns of positive remodeling, low x-ray attenuation, and spotty calcification. Cardiovascular magnetic resonance (CMR) imaging is a noninvasive modality with excellent contrast of soft tissues and the blood/vessel wall interface that has significant potential to assess coronary lumen integrity, plaque burden, and composition without the requirement for ionizing radiation. Advances in CMR data acquisition and gating techniques have improved image quality, which to date has been constrained by limited spatial and temporal resolution. As such, CMR is emerging as a promising modality for coronary artery imaging where its selective use in conjunction with myocardial perfusion imaging, viability, and ventricular function assessments, where CMR is the clinical reference standard, may allow for the complete assessment of suspected CAD with a single imaging modality. Furthermore, evolving molecular imaging techniques may allow for the assessment of disease activity, delineation of vulnerable plaque phenotypes and identification of novel therapeutic targets.

DIAGNOSTIC PERFORMANCE OF CORONARY MAGNETIC RESONANCE IMAGING

Studies have shown that coronary magnetic resonance angiography (CMRA) can identify significant coronary artery plaque (>50% stenosis) with a diagnostic accuracy comparable with MDCT.[6–8] Multiple single center studies have compared the accuracy of CMRA against invasive angiography culminating in a meta-analysis that showed a sensitivity of 87% and specificity of 70% for detection of >50% stenoses.[9–12] However, technical improvements in coil design, image acquisition/reconstruction, and motion compensation have allowed for a reduction in total imaging time for whole heart CMR coronary angiography to approximately 5 minutes with improved diagnostic accuracy (see Chapter 24).[8] Another study has demonstrated that noncontrast, free breathing, three-dimensional (3D) balanced steady-state free precession (bSSFP) whole heart imaging has a sensitivity of 91% and a specificity of 86%, with an area under the receiver operator curve (ROC) of 0.92 when compared with quantitative invasive angiography for the detection of hemodynamically significant plaque.[13] Furthermore, 3D cross-sectional imaging of the coronary vessel wall at 3 T has been able to achieve an in-plane resolution of 0.5 × 0.5 mm, which is comparable with MDCT (Fig. 28.1).

Technical Challenges

Imaging of the coronary vessel wall and lumen is more challenging and technically demanding than imaging of other vascular beds because of the following[14–16]:
1. Motion: myocardial contraction/relaxation and respiration
2. Small and tortuous vessels
3. Close proximity to epicardial fat, coronary blood, and myocardium
4. Requirement for high spatial resolution

CORONARY MAGNETIC RESONANCE IMAGING TECHNIQUES

In both noncontrast and contrast-enhanced CMR, the main limiting factor is imaging time. For coronary artery imaging, a compromise has to be made between imaging time, the spatial resolution achieved, and arterial coverage.

Because a high spatial resolution is paramount for diagnostic coronary artery imaging, longer scan times are necessary, which in turn

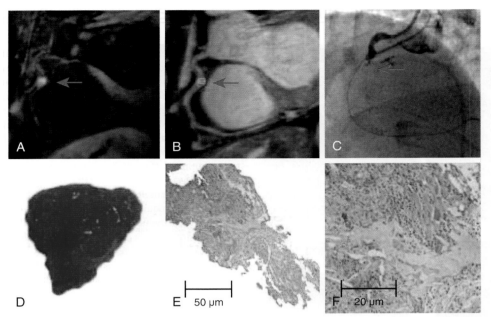

FIG. 28.6 Noncontrast cardiovascular magnetic resonance images of a patient with acute inferior myocardial infarction. T1-weighted images show increased in signal intensity (A) that colocalizes with the proximal right coronary artery when T1-weighted images are fused with bright-blood imaging (B). Invasive x-ray coronary angiography shows total occlusion of the proximal RCA (C) because of thrombus that was successfully aspirated (D). Subsequent histology confirmed the presence of acute thrombus with abundant platelets and erythrocytes that are the likely source of signal on T1–weighted images (E and F).

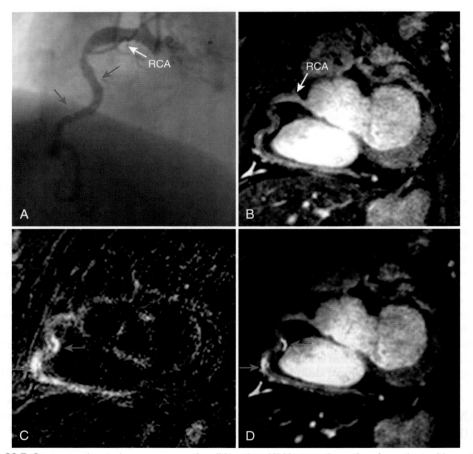

FIG. 28.7 Contrast-enhanced coronary vessel wall imaging. (A) X-ray angiography of a patient with unstable angina showing luminal irregularities *(red arrows)* of the mid right coronary artery *(RCA)*. (B) Multiplanar reformatted bright-blood imaging of the RCA and corresponding late gadolinium vessel wall enhancement demonstrating increased contrast uptake (C; *arrows*), indicative of an increased atherosclerotic plaque burden and possible inflammation. (D) Fusion of B and C. Areas of increased vessel wall uptake appear light orange *(arrows)*.

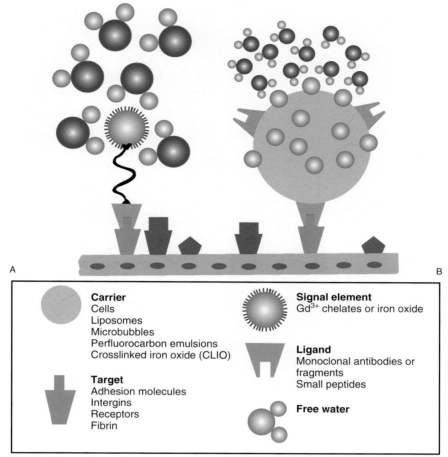

FIG. 28.8 Molecular cardiovascular magnetic resonance (CMR) imaging tracer characteristics. (A) CMR signal elements (Gd^{3+} or iron oxide) are conjugated to ligands such as monoclonal antibodies, antibody fragments, or small peptides that specifically bind to target sites. Gd^{3+}-based contrast agents achieve tissue contrast through shortening of T1-relaxation times of nearby protons; iron oxide promotes proton dephasing and can be detected as negative signal on T2* imaging. (B) Carrier molecules bound to multiple target-specific ligands and signal elements and are often used to maximize tracer concentration at target sites for enhanced tracer localization.

Progressive atherosclerosis results in increased deposition of extracellular matrix proteins in the neo-intima by smooth muscle cells and macrophages.[5] These include different types of collagen and elastin, which represent the most abundant extracellular matrix proteins.[78] An elastin-specific low-molecular weight CMR contrast agent (ESMA) has been shown to improve detection of atherosclerotic plaque and plaque burden.[79,80] This probe was shown to have favorable pharmacokinetic properties such as rapid biodistribution and fast clearance. In vivo measurements of plaque burden using ESMA in the ApoE-/- mouse model of atherosclerosis correlated with ex vivo histological assessment. Subsequent studies have similarly demonstrated good agreement between imaging and histology in a swine model of coronary remodeling following angioplasty and stent deployment[79,81] (Fig. 28.9).

Iron oxide particles differ from Gd-based contrast agents and to date they have not been used for characterization of coronary plaque. However, iron oxide-based tracers have been used extensively for the characterization of carotid and aortic atherosclerosis. These particles shorten T1 relaxation times; however, phagocytosis and accumulation in macrophages leads to more pronounced shortening of T2 and T2*, where it yields negative contrast or signal void on T2 and T2*-weighted images.[82] These particles exhibit higher relaxivity than Gd-based tracers and therefore are detected with greater sensitivity.[83] In contrast to Gd^{3+} they are fairly large and typically have slower clearance (5–30 nm particles) and more complex biodistribution.

HYBRID POSITRON EMISSION TOMOGRAPHY/CARDIOVASCULAR MAGNETIC RESONANCE

Positron emission tomography (PET) is the most sensitive molecular imaging modality with a wide variety of radiotracers that can be detected in the nano to picomolar range. The limitations of PET include the absence of anatomical information, relatively slow acquisition times, and susceptibility to physiologic motion. As CMR has superior soft-tissue contrast compared with computed tomography (CT), hybrid PET-MR platforms allow for the accurate in vivo localization of radiotracers and acquisition of multiple CMR contrasts, with the capacity to assess coronary intraplaque hemorrhage, thrombus, and edema as well as myocardial perfusion and fibrosis. Furthermore, CMR can be performed simultaneously with PET allowing for CMR-based PET motion correction.[83a] As such, PET-MR harnesses the complementary strengths of these modalities for improved image fusion, workflow, and multiparametric data analysis.

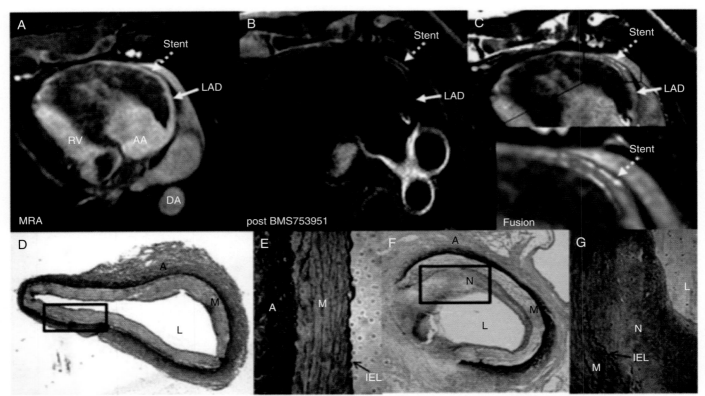

FIG. 28.9 Elastin imaging of coronary remodelling. (A) Comparison of coronary magnetic resonance angiography *(MRA)* with (B) delayed enhancement MRI. (C) Fusion of A and B of stented and control coronary vessel segments and corresponding histology (D–G). (B and C) Strong enhancement can be observed at the stent location *(dotted white arrow)*, whereas little to no enhancement is visible in the normal, noninjured proximal segment of the left anterior descending *(LAD)* artery *(solid white arrow)*. (D and E) Elastin von Gieson stain of noninjured coronary vessel segment shows intact internal elastic lamina *(IEL)* and circular arranged elastin fibers *(black)* in the media. (F and G) Elastin von Gieson stain of a stented vessel segment demonstrates disruption of IEL and neointima formation, with diffuse elastin deposition *(black dots)*. E and G are magnifications of insets in D and F. *A,* Adventitia; *AA,* ascending aorta; *BMS,* bare metal stent; *DA,* descending aorta; *L,* lumen; *M,* media; *N,* neointima. (From von Bary C, Makowski M, Preissel A, et al. MRI of coronary wall remodeling in a swine model of coronary injury using an elastin-binding contrast agent. *Circ Cardiovasc Imaging.* 2011;4:147–155.)

[18]F-flurodeoxyglucose (^{18}F-FDG) and ^{18}F-sodium fluoride (^{18}F-NaF) are PET radiotracers that have previously been used for plaque imaging. ^{18}F-FDG is a glucose analogue that accumulates in areas of increased metabolic activity. Increased ^{18}F-FDG signal has been demonstrated in carotid atherosclerotic plaque where the signal intensity correlates with areas of inflammatory cell infiltration.[84] However, ^{18}F-FDG imaging of coronary atherosclerosis is complicated by the relatively high metabolic activity of the surrounding myocardium that can obscure signal from the coronary vessel wall.[85] More recently, imaging of vascular microcalcification using ^{18}F-NaF has been shown to colocalize with culprit plaques in postacute MI patients.[86] Further studies will be required to assess the prognostic impact of ^{18}F-NaF PET in ischemic heart disease.

ASSESSMENT OF ENDOTHELIAL FUNCTION BY NONCONTRAST–CARDIOVASCULAR MAGNETIC RESONANCE

Endothelial dysfunction is an early feature of subclinical CAD and can be a predictor of adverse cardiovascular events.[87,88] Under physiological conditions, release of nitric oxide by endothelial cells induces local coronary vasodilation. Assessment of endothelial function requires assessment of the vasodilatory and flow responses to endothelial stressors.[87] Several studies have demonstrated that noncontrast CMR can noninvasively assess coronary vasodilation pre- and poststimulus.[89,90] An abnormal coronary vasodilatory response to isometric handgrip exercise has been shown to correlate with local plaque burden,[91] and the same technique can provide insight into systemic vascular endothelial function via assessment of the internal mammary artery.[92] Coronary artery distensibility,[93] coronary flow and flow reserves can also be assessed noninvasively with noncontrast CMR.[94,95] As such, in addition to the quantification and characterization of atherosclerotic plaque, CMR has the capacity to assess the impact of disease on coronary physiology, which is an important determinant of coronary ischemia.

CONCLUSION

Recent advances in CMRA have yielded improvements in spatial resolution and imaging times, highlighting the potential of CMR for comprehensive coronary assessment without the need for ionizing radiation.

In addition to plaque burden, noncontrast CMR can provide important information regarding plaque characteristics such as intraplaque hemorrhage and thrombus formation, through the T1-shortening effect of methemoglobin that has proven prognostic utility. Furthermore, CE-CMR and molecular imaging using hybrid PET-MR systems have the potential to identify active cellular and molecular processes that drive atherosclerotic disease progression. These may allow for the precise risk stratification of individuals with subclinical disease, in addition to the identification of novel therapeutic targets. Despite challenges, the quality and feasibility of coronary magnetic resonance imaging continues to improve, and its eventual use in combination with existing CMR reference standards such as myocardial perfusion, viability, and functional imaging raises the enticing prospect of comprehensive, single modality assessment of patients with ischemic heart disease.

REFERENCES

A full reference list is available online at ExpertConsult.com

29

Assessment of the Biophysical Mechanical Properties of the Arterial Wall

Raad H. Mohiaddin

Arteries are elastic tubes whose diameter varies with the pulsating pressure. In addition, they propagate the pulse created by ejection of blood by the heart, at a velocity that is determined largely by the elastic properties of the arterial wall. The vascular wall can be deformed by pressure and shear stress forces exerted by the blood as well as the tethering imposed by the surrounding tissues. Biophysical mechanical properties of the arterial wall play an important role in the pathogenesis of cardiovascular diseases. Sclerosis (or stiffness), for example, is an important aspect of atherosclerotic vascular disease that can be demonstrated in experimental disease both in animals[1] and in humans,[2] and regression of the disease leads to reduced stiffness.[3,4] Rupture of atherosclerotic plaque (a common mechanism of myocardial infarction) and aortic dissection can be viewed as mechanical failures in the diseased vessels. In addition, the effectiveness of interventional procedures such as angioplasty is often achieved by causing mechanical injury to the vessel wall, and the injury itself may lead to restenosis. A number of common conditions are associated with changes in arterial mechanical properties, although their importance is not always recognized.

Systemic hypertension is almost always associated with altered mechanical properties of the peripheral vasculature. Although it is not clear which of the two is the inceptive event, one begets the other, fostering a vicious cycle. Compliance (the reciprocal of the resistance offered to deformation) of the proximal aorta is reduced as a result. This causes waves reflected from the periphery to return prematurely and coincide with the incident or forward-traveling wave produced by the ventricle. This augments aortic systolic pressure, increases pulse pressure, and reduces diastolic pressure (because the reflected wave no longer contributes to diastolic pressure). Decreased subendocardial/subepicardial flow ratio has been demonstrated with reduced aortic compliance.[5] Thus decreased aortic distensibility may increase the risk of subendocardial ischemia in the presence of coronary artery stenosis, left ventricular hypertrophy, or both.

Aortic compliance represents an important determinant of left ventricular performance. Measurement of ventricular–vascular coupling takes into account the pulsatile load imposed on the left ventricle, as well as the systemic vascular resistance.[6] Metabolic disorders such as Ehlers–Danlos and Marfan syndromes,[7] diabetes mellitus,[8] familial hypercholesterolemia,[9] and growth hormone deficiency[10] are also known to alter arterial compliance.

Similarly, the distensibility of the pulmonary arteries is reduced in pulmonary hypertension. Postmortem studies of externalized pulmonary arterial strips have shown that the extensibility of the pulmonary trunk is decreased in pulmonary arterial hypertension.[11] The wall of an artery becomes less extensible, the more it is stretched from its natural length. An increased stretching of the circumference of the vessel will diminish the distensibility. When the pulmonary artery resistance increases in vivo, the vessels become more distended and less distensible. Indirect measurements of pulmonary artery compliance have suggested that pulmonary arterial distensibility decreases with rising pulmonary artery pressure.[12,13] The ability of cardiovascular magnetic resonance (CMR) to image flow within any medium-sized vessel in any plane provides a unique opportunity to study the pulmonary arteries. Distensibility and flow have already been assessed in patients with pulmonary arterial hypertension.[14,15]

In this chapter, the clinical importance of arterial biophysical function and its assessment by CMR will be examined in detail as a complement to Chapter 27.

ARTERIAL STRUCTURE

A normal artery consists of three morphologically distinct layers. The intima consists of a single continuous layer of endothelial cells bounded peripherally by a fenestrated sheet of elastic fibers. The media consists entirely of diagonally oriented smooth muscle cells, surrounded by variable amounts of collagen, elastin, and proteoglycans. The adventitia consists predominantly of fibroblasts intermixed with smooth muscle cells loosely arranged between bundles of collagen and proteoglycans. Each structural component has its own characteristic properties. Smooth muscle is the physiologically active element, and by contracting or developing force, it can alter the diameter of the vessel or the tension in the wall. The other components are essentially passive in their mechanical behavior. Elastin, which can be stretched to up to 300% of its length at rest without rupturing,[16] behaves mechanically more closely to a linear elastic material such as rubber than other connective tissue components do. When elastin fibers are stretched and released, they return promptly to their original state. Elastin fibers are important for maintaining normal pulsatile behavior, but they fracture at very low stresses and are probably much less important in determining the overall strength of the vessel wall. Collagen fibers, on the other hand, are much stiffer, but they are much stronger. The proportion of these components varies from artery to artery. In the thoracic aorta, the elastin forms 60% of total fibrous element, and collagen forms 40%. The collagen proportion increases with increasing distance from the heart, reaching 30% elastin and 70% collagen in the extrathoracic vessels.[17] The collagen-to-elastin ratio increases with age, which is one reason why vascular stiffness increases with age. The human thoracic aorta is supplied by vasa vasorum and grows by increasing the number of lamellar units. The abdominal aorta, in comparison, is avascular because it lacks vasa vasorum and grows by increasing the thickness of each lamellar unit. The avascular thickness and the elevated tension per lamellar unit of the abdominal aorta predispose it to atherosclerosis.

The distensibility of a blood vessel depends on the proportions and interconnections of these materials and on the contractile state of the vascular smooth muscle. Elasticity is a material's ability to return to its original shape and dimensions after deformation, the deformation being proportional to the force applied. This proportionality was first described by Hooke in 1676 and is known as Hooke's law. The point at which Hooke's law ceases to apply is known as the elastic limit, and when a solid has been deformed beyond this point, it cannot regain its original form and acquires a permanent distortion. With larger loads still, the yield point is reached when the deformation continues to increase without further load and usually rapidly leads to breakage. In purely elastic bodies, stress (the force per unit area that produces deformation) produces its characteristic strain (the deformation of a stressed object) instantaneously, and strain vanishes immediately on removal of the stress. Some materials, however, require a finite time to reach the state of deformation appropriate to the stress and a similar time to regain their unstressed shape. Blood vessels typically exhibit such behavior, which is called viscoelasticity.

DEFINITION OF VASCULAR WALL STIFFNESS

Vascular mechanics have been described by using different elastic moduli and assumptions and for different purposes. Several approaches have been described that use clinically available methods for in vivo characterization of the stiffness of the vessel wall. The ability to measure vascular stiffness has been greatly improved by the recent advances in imaging, such as high-frequency ultrasound and CMR.

The relationship between vascular wall deformation (strain) and the pressure exerted on the inner surface of the vascular wall (stress) is commonly used for the measurement of arterial wall biophysical properties (elastic modulus). A plethora of terminology for the description of different elastic moduli, which can be confusing, has been described.[18] The pressure–strain elastic modulus of the arterial wall (E_p) described by Peterson and colleagues[19] is commonly used. This elastic modulus that applies to an open-ended vessel in the absence of reflection is defined as $E_p = 2\Delta P/(\Delta V/V)$. This is the inverse of the fractional distensibility $\Delta V/V$ of the arterial lumen per unit pulse pressure ΔP.

Arterial compliance, C, which is defined as the change in volume ΔV per unit change in pressure ΔP, has been also used in the literature. It has been argued that this definition is appropriate to measurement of ventricular compliance and not to the compliance of an open-ended arterial segment. For the latter, the inverse of Peterson's modulus was suggested $1/E_p$.

The average arterial compliance of a particular vessel pathway can also be determined by measuring the speed of propagation of the pulse in the vessel pathway. The velocity of such waves depends principally on the distensibility of the vessel wall. In real terms, this pulse is measurable by the disturbances in pressure, flow, or vessel diameter that it causes. The propagation of flow waves has not been studied as extensively as that of pressure waves, partly because, unlike flow, accurate methods of pulsatile pressure measurements have been available for a long time and partly because the distinction between flow wave velocity and blood velocity has not always been clearly recognized. Blood velocity means the speed of an average drop of blood, whereas flow wave velocity means the speed with which motion is transmitted. The wave velocity is usually much faster than that of the blood itself. Although CMR is unable to assess pressure changes, alterations in the flow within (or diameter of) a vessel can be measured accurately.

MEASUREMENT OF ARTERIAL WALL STIFFNESS

Arterial stiffness, which describes the resistance of arterial wall to deformation, is difficult to measure because of the complex mechanical behavior of arterial wall. As a result, a bewildering number of choices

abound. Although smooth muscle tone is not considered, in vitro human arterial compliance has been measured from pressure–volume curves in postmortem arteries.[20–23] In vivo estimation of arterial wall compliance is more difficult, however, and has been performed by using indirect and invasive techniques, including pulse wave velocity measurements in animals and in humans,[24,25] the pressure–radius relationship using the Peterson transformer coil in animals,[26] x-ray contrast angiography in humans,[27,28] and ultrasonography.[29–31] The contributions of CMR to the assessment of arterial wall mechanics are discussed in the following paragraphs. Other noninvasive measures are forced to rely on the assessment of accessible and often superficial vessels. Under the assumption that central and peripheral arteries behave in a similar fashion, the properties of these arteries are then used as surrogates for those of central arteries. There is, however, considerable heterogeneity between peripheral and central sites. CMR circumvents this problem by allowing the study of central arteries. Its ability to identify anatomic landmarks suggests that reproducibility between studies should be improved, allowing more effective follow-up.

CARDIOVASCULAR MAGNETIC RESONANCE OF REGIONAL AORTIC COMPLIANCE

CMR provides a direct, noninvasive way of studying local aortic compliance.[32,33] High-resolution cine imaging or electrocardiogram-gated spin echo imaging in a plane perpendicular to the ascending and/or descending aorta allows measurement of aortic cross-sectional area during systole and diastole. Measurement of regional aortic compliance by CMR is calculated from the change in volume of an aortic segment and from aortic pulse pressure estimated by a sphygmomanometer at the level of the brachial artery. The lumen of the aorta is outlined manually on the computer screen to measure the change in aortic area (ΔA) between diastole and systole. Regional aortic compliance (C) (microL/mm Hg, m^3/Nm^{-2}) is calculated from the change in volume ($\Delta V = \Delta A \times$ slice thickness) of the aortic segment divided by the aortic pulse pressure (ΔP) measured by a sphygmomanometer (Fig. 29.1). Automatic measurement of aortic cross-sectional area is also possible.[34] Other indices of aortic stiffness that can be derived from these measurements include distensibility, Peterson's elastic modulus, and stiffness index β ([systolic blood pressure/diastolic blood pressure]/area strain).

The accuracy of the indirect measurement of the pressure change that is needed to compute compliance is limited because it ignores the changes in the pressure wave as it propagates through the arterial tree (a process known as amplification). Further, it is important to obtain this pressure data on patients who are ideally lying in the magnetic resonance imaging (MRI) scanner using CMR-compatible apparatus. Despite the limitations of the pressure measurement, there is a good correlation between measurement of local aortic compliance and measurement of global compliance from the speed of the propagation of the flow wave within the vessel.[35]

In addition, noninvasive pressure wave analysis using arterial applanation tonometry has been shown to provide an accurate and reproducible measurement of central vascular pressure measurements and can be used to overcome this limitation.[36]

CARDIOVASCULAR MAGNETIC RESONANCE OF FLOW WAVE VELOCITY

Flow wave velocity is defined as the speed with which a flow wave propagates along a vessel and is regarded as the purest measure of arterial stiffness. It is the quotient of distance traveled divided by the time taken for the flow wave to move between the two points and represents an average for that length of vessel (Figs. 29.2 and 29.3). The

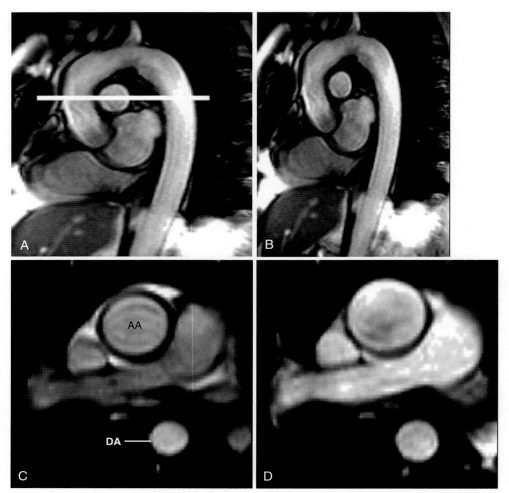

FIG. 29.1 (A) Oblique sagittal image of the ascending aorta, arch and descending thoracic aorta showing the sites where flow wave velocity and regional compliance are measured. The oblique transverse plane shown in the top image is represented in diastole (B) and systole (C). This shows the change in area of a 22-year-old healthy subject. *AA*, Ascending aorta; *DA*, descending aorta.

approach is dependent on assessment of path length traveled and accurate measurement of pulse arrival time. The latter requires recognition of equivalent features or points on leading edges of the proximal and distal flow waveforms (see Fig. 29.2), a process that is made complicated by alterations that occur in flow wave morphology and magnitude as it progresses down the vessel. Unlike noninvasive measurements that rely on linear, transcutaneous measurements, CMR makes no assumptions about the shape of the artery and can accurately measure the path length traveled.

Mohiaddin and colleagues showed the feasibility of using CMR phase-shift velocity mapping to measure aortic flow wave velocity in humans.[35] By taking advantage of the anatomy of the aorta, cine two-dimensional (2D) phase shift velocity maps were acquired with high temporal resolution in a single plane perpendicular to the ascending and descending aorta, and the time taken for the flow wave to travel between the two points was measured (Fig. 29.4). Instantaneous flow (in liters per second) in the mid-ascending aorta and mid-descending aorta was calculated by multiplying the aortic cross-sectional area and the mean velocity within that area. Pulse wave velocity (PWV) was calculated in meters per second from the transit time *(T)* of the foot of the flow wave (see Fig. 29.4) and from the distance *(D)* between

the two points obtained from an oblique sagittal image. The distance is determined manually on the computer screen by drawing a line in the center of the aorta joining the two points. In Fig. 29.4, the foot of the flow wave was defined by extrapolation of the rapid upstroke of the flow wave to the baseline as opposed to the midpoint of the upslope method used in Fig. 29.2.

Others have used different magnetic resonance flow imaging techniques to assess arterial compliance. Tarnawski and colleagues[37] used the comb-excited Fourier velocity-encoded method, previously reported by Dumoulin and colleagues,[38] to measure local arterial wave speed in the femoral artery in healthy men. In this method, simultaneous Fourier velocity-encoded data from multiple stations were acquired. The technique employs a comb excitation radiofrequency pulse that excites an arbitrary number of slices. This causes the signals from the spin in a particular slice to appear at a position in the phase-encoding direction, which is the sum of the spin velocity and an offset arising from the phase increment given to that excitation slice. Acquisition of spin velocity information occurs simultaneously for all slices, permitting the calculation of wave velocities arising from the pulsatile flow.

Hardy and colleagues[39] studied aortic flow wave velocity using a 2D CMR selective excitation pulse to repeatedly excite a cylinder of

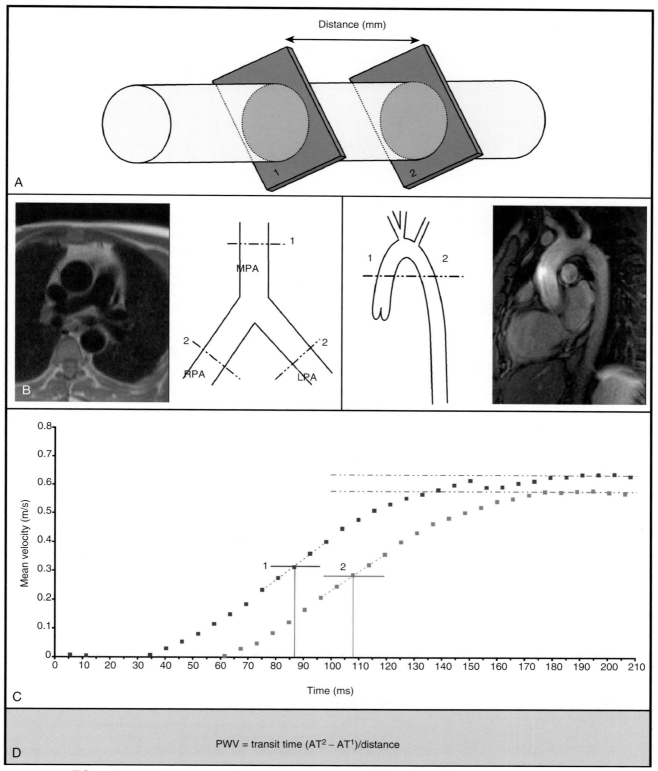

FIG. 29.2 Assessment of pulse wave velocity *(PWV)*. (A) Phase velocity acquisition across a vessel is undertaken at two points (1, 2), and the distance between the two is measured. (B) Examples of slice prescription are given for the proximal pulmonary arteries and aorta; note that coverage of the ascending aorta and descending aorta is enabled by a single slice. (C) Transit time is defined by the difference in arrival time *(AT)* for the flow wave at both points, and is divided by the distance to give pulse wave velocity (D). *LPA,* Left pulmonary artery; *MPA,* main pulmonary artery; *RPA,* right pulmonary artery.

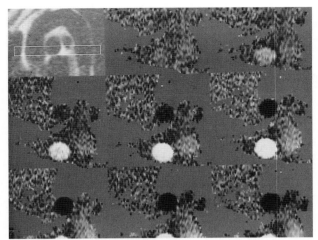

FIG. 29.3 Cine velocity mapping in a plane equivalent to that shown in Fig. 29.1. The first frame was acquired 50 ms after the R-wave of the electrocardiogram and represents the onset of left ventricular systole. The velocity maps indicate zero velocity as medium gray, caudal velocities in the descending aorta as light gray to white, and cranial velocities as darker shades of gray to black, gray level intensity being proportional to velocity.

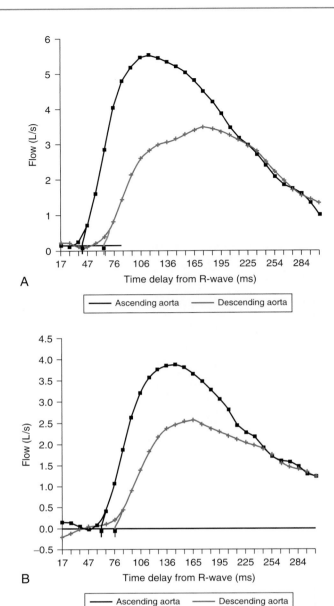

FIG. 29.4 The foot of the flow wave is defined by extrapolation of the rapid upstroke of the flow wave to the baseline, and this is performed for flow in both the ascending aorta and descending aorta. The transit time needed for the flow wave to propagate from a point in the mid-ascending aorta to a point in the mid-descending aorta can then be measured. The distance around the arch from the plane in the ascending aorta to the plane in the descending aorta can be measured from the oblique sagittal image shown in Fig. 29.1, and the flow wave velocity is calculated by division of this distance by the propagation time. (A) Transit time from a normal subject with good compliance. (B) Transit time from an elderly patient with poor compliance. Note that the transit time is significantly shorter in the patient with poor compliance. (From Mohiaddin RH, Firmin DN, Longmore DB. Age-related changes of human aortic flow wave velocity measured noninvasively by magnetic resonance imaging. *J Applied Physiol.* 1993;74:492–497.)

magnetization in the aorta, with magnetization readout along the cylinder axis each time. A toggled bipolar flow-encoding pulse was applied before readout to produce a one-dimensional (1D) phase-contrast flow image. Cardiac gating and data interleaving were employed to improve the effective time resolution to 2 ms. Wave velocities were determined from the slope of the leading edge of flow measured on the resulting M-mode velocity image. Aortic pulse wave velocity was also measured by the same group, using a combination of cylinder of magnetization with Fourier velocity encoding and readout gradients applied along the cylinder axis (aorta) (Fig. 29.5),[40] with the advantage of eliminating partial volume effects that hindered their previous approach, but the Fourier method has the drawback that it is no longer in real time and errors occur, owing to accumulation of flow data over several (typically 16 to 32) cardiac cycles. For both methods, the interleaved repeats needed to achieve high temporal resolution make them highly sensitive to physiologic variability.

In vitro experiments showed CMR measurements of pulse wave velocity in a tube phantom to be very reproducible and in good agreement with pulse wave velocity measurements made with a pressure catheter.[41] These methods have not been widely applied in clinical research, nor has their in vivo reproducibility been proven yet.

REFLECTED WAVES

When the incident pulse wave from the ventricle reaches the periphery, it may be reflected and return toward the heart as a backward-running wave. Reflected waves express properties of the peripheral circulation; if the peripheral resistance is elevated, reflected waves will be greater in magnitude and will return sooner. Because its shape and magnitude will be defined by the complex interaction between forward incident wave and backward reflected waves, the measured flow wave will also be altered in pathologic conditions. As a result, the timing and location of measurements become important considerations in the CMR assessment of arterial properties.

If work is concerned only with the structure of proximal arteries, measurement should be made as far from the periphery and as early in systole as possible to avoid the influence of reflections. These requirements become more demanding when the available length of vessel is limited (e.g., in the pulmonary arteries) or baseline data particularly noisy. Conversely, study of the influence of reflected waves on measured flow waves might provide interesting insights into the nature of the more distal vessels.

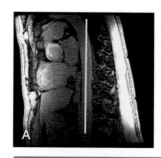

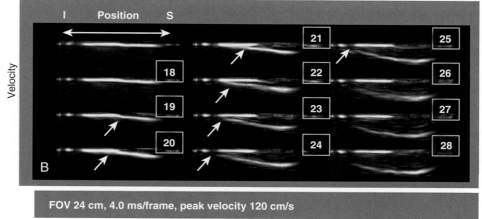

FOV 24 cm, 4.0 ms/frame, peak velocity 120 cm/s

FIG. 29.5 Fourier velocity measurements in a healthy subject. (A) In this method, the magnetic resonance signal is obtained from a column aligned with the descending aorta. (B) The position along the column is shown horizontally in each of the 12 cine frames. The velocity is shown by the vertical position of the signal. *FOV,* Field-of-view; *I,* inferior; *S,* superior.

CLINICAL USE OF CARDIOVASCULAR MAGNETIC RESONANCE FOR ASSESSING ARTERIAL WALL STIFFNESS

Mohiaddin and colleagues were the first to use CMR for measurement of aortic compliance.[42] They demonstrated that aortic compliance in asymptomatic subjects falls with age and that patients with coronary artery disease have abnormally low compliance (Fig. 29.6). The results suggested a possible role for compliance in the assessment of cardiovascular fitness and the detection of coronary artery disease. Because there is overlap between normal compliance and compliance in patients with coronary artery disease above the age of 50 years, the test cannot have perfect sensitivity and specificity. Below the age of 50 years, however, there is much less overlap and the test is more specific. Abnormally low aortic compliance has also been demonstrated in patients with aortic coarctation[43] and in patients with Marfan syndrome.[44] The same group also showed the feasibility of using CMR velocity mapping for measurement of aortic flow wave velocity. Aortic flow wave velocity increased linearly with age, and there was a significant difference between the youngest decade and the oldest decade studied. Flow wave velocity was negatively correlated with regional ascending aortic compliance measured in the same subjects (Fig. 29.7).

In a study employing a single-slice phase-contrast acquisition of the ascending, arch, proximal aorta, and distal thoracic aorta, Rogers and colleagues[45] demonstrated an age-related increase in PWV among their cohort. In addition, among the older patients, stiffness increased the more proximally the aorta was studied. The researchers ascribed these changes to the disproportionate effect of elastin degradation with age

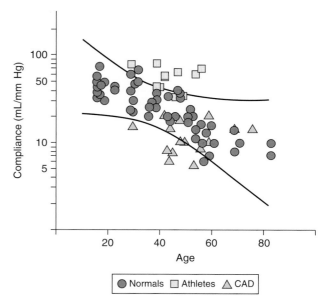

● Normals □ Athletes △ CAD

FIG. 29.6 Ascending aortic compliance displayed by using a logarithmic scale and plotted against age in three groups: normals, athletes, and patients with coronary artery disease *(CAD).* The 95% confidence limits are shown for the normals. The athletes' compliance is abnormally high, and that in coronary disease patients is abnormally low. (From Mohiaddin RH, Underwood SR, Bogren HG, et al. Regional aortic compliance studied by magnetic resonance imaging: the effects of age, training, and coronary artery disease. *Br Heart J.* 1989;62:90–96.)

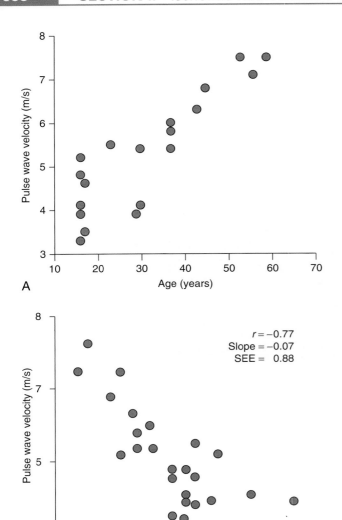

FIG. 29.7 Flow wave velocity is directly proportional to age (A) and inversely proportional to regional aortic compliance (B). *SEE,* Standard error of the estimate. (From Mohiaddin RH, Firmin DN, Longmore DB. Age-related changes of human aortic flow wave velocity measured noninvasively by magnetic resonance imaging. *J Applied Physiol.* 1993;74:492–497.)

on the more proximal parts of the aorta, where the elastic to collagen ratio is at its greatest.

More recently, Voges and colleagues provided normal CMR values for cross-sectional areas, distensibility and pulse wave velocity of the thoracic aorta in children and young adolescents, which may serve as a reference for the detection of pathological changes of the aorta.[46]

Regression of atheroma with reduction of cholesterol levels is recognized to occur, but less is known about reversal of sclerosis. Noninvasive indices of sclerosis have largely been based on carotid ultrasound measurements. Forbat and colleagues[47] measured aortic compliance, coronary calcification, and carotid intimal–medial thickness during reduction of cholesterol level in hypercholesterolemic patients with and without coronary artery disease. All received fluvastatin for 1 year. Aortic compliance was assessed by using CMR, and the coronary calcification score was determined by electron beam computed tomography. Carotid intimal–medial thickness was measured by carotid ultrasound. The authors showed an improvement in aortic compliance over 1 year,

which indicates that the lipid changes induced by fluvastatin (an increase in high-density lipoprotein [HDL] level, decrease in very-low-density lipoprotein level, and improvement in low-density:high-density lipoprotein ratio) beneficially influenced vascular pathophysiology. In the patients who were studied with carotid ultrasound means, carotid intimal–medial thickness decreased from 1.09 to 0.87 mm ($P = .004$), corroborating these results.

Kupari and colleagues[48] measured aortic elastic modulus by CMR in asymptomatic subjects and correlated these measurements with physical activity, ethanol consumption, systolic blood pressure, fasting blood lipids, and serum insulin. They showed that the average value of the ascending and descending aortic elastic modulus was associated positively and statistically significantly with blood pressure, physical inactivity, serum insulin, and HDL. The elastic modulus was associated negatively with the ratio of low-density lipoprotein (LDL) cholesterol to HDL cholesterol. No association between aortic elastic modulus and either smoking or ethanol consumption was demonstrated in this study. The same group demonstrated a higher aortic elastic modulus in patients with Marfan syndrome than in healthy subjects, indicating a relative decrease in the distensibility of the thoracic aorta.[49] Kupari and colleagues also demonstrated that aortic flow wave velocity was more reproducible (interobserver and intraobserver) than measurement of the pulsatile aortic area change or the elastic modulus. However, interstudy reproducibility has not been tested.[50]

Adams and colleagues demonstrated abnormal aortic distensibility and stiffness index in patients with Marfan syndrome using CMR.[50] These findings were confirmed by Groenink and associates using a CMR derived measure of distensibility and aortic PWV. Arrival time was determined by the point at which flow had reached half its maximum value.[51] Beta-adrenergic blocking agents may reduce the rate of aortic root dilation and the development of aortic complications in patients with Marfan syndrome. This may be as a result of beta-blocker induced changes in aortic stiffness. To investigate this, Groenink and colleagues used CMR to measure aortic distensibility and aortic pulse wave velocity to assess aortic stiffness in Marfan syndrome and healthy volunteers before and after beta-blocker therapy.[52] They showed that in both groups, mean blood pressure decreased significantly but only the Marfan syndrome patients had a significant increase in aortic distensibility at multiple levels and a significant decrease in pulse wave velocity after beta-blocker therapy. The same group[53] sought to explain why some of these patients responded to beta-blockers whereas others did not. Cross-sectional assessment of aortic area was made at the level of the pulmonary bifurcation by CMR and plotted against a surrogate for central aortic pressures (using a finger arterial blood pressure–derived brachial blood pressure). Using pressure-area lines, a subgroup with a transition point (a departure from a linear pressure-area relationship) was identified in 6 out of 32 patients. It was suggested that this point represented the recruitment of collagen to load-bearing elements. These patients demonstrated a trend toward reduced distensibility, although this relationship might have been stronger had the study group been larger. It was hypothesized that patients in whom the transition point is seen at higher blood pressures might experience greater improvements in distensibility with beta-blockade than those whose transition points occurred at lower blood pressures.

Savolainen and colleagues[54] used CMR and indirect brachial artery blood pressure measurements to assess aortic elastic modulus in patients with essential hypertension before therapy and after 3 weeks and 6 months of therapy with cilazapril (an angiotensin-converting enzyme inhibitor) or atenolol (a beta-1-adrenergic blocker). The authors concluded that 6 months of treatment with either cilazapril or atenolol reduces the stiffness of the ascending aorta in essential hypertension. No statistically significant differences between the effects of the two drugs were observed. Honda and associates used CMR to measure aortic distensibility in patients with systemic hypertension and demonstrated that the antihypertensive drugs nicardipine and alacepril have a beneficial effect on aortic distensibility.[55] Resnick and colleagues[56] assessed aortic distensibility, left ventricular mass index, abdominal fat (subcutaneous and visceral), and free magnesium levels in the brain and skeletal muscle by CMR. In patients with essential hypertension, the following were concluded: Systolic hypertension and increased left ventricular mass index may result from arterial stiffness; arterial stiffness may be one mechanism by which abdominal visceral fat contributes to cardiovascular risk; and decreased magnesium contributes to arterial stiffness in hypertension.

Chelsky and coworkers[57] used CMR to measure aortic compliance in nine premenopausal women before and after menotropin therapy. They demonstrated that a short-term rise in estrogen induced by menotropin treatment was associated with an increase in aortic compliance. Aortic size was not significantly increased within this time frame.

Rider et al. demonstrated that HIV infection is an independent predictor of aortic stiffness as measured by CMR. However, because of the observational nature of this study, it is not possible to confirm causality or mechanisms which might underlie the increase of aortic stiffness in patients with HIV.[58]

Bogren and colleagues[59] used CMR to study pulmonary artery distensibility in healthy subjects (Fig. 29.8) and in patients with pulmonary arterial hypertension (Fig. 29.9). The distensibility was found to be significantly lower in pulmonary arterial hypertension than in normal subjects, but there was no age-related difference. The results also demonstrated a small retrograde flow (2%) in the pulmonary trunk of normal subjects close to the pulmonic valve. Antegrade plug flow occurred in most normal subjects but varied among individuals. There were also other variations in the flow pattern among normal individuals. All patients with pulmonary arterial hypertension had a markedly irregular antegrade and retrograde flow and a large retrograde flow (average 26%).

Changes in the cross-sectional area of the pulmonary artery in a magnitude image from a phase velocity sequence have been measured to derive pulmonary artery PWV[60–62] values for normal subjects and for patients with pulmonary hypertension.[62] In the latter group, maximum and minimum values for mean pulmonary artery pressure (mPAP) were predicted that "framed" the actual mPAP reliability.[62]

Finally, Stefanides and colleagues have showed that aortic stiffness has prognostic power in determining the likelihood of future cardiac events (Fig. 29.10).[63] This interesting study merits further examination because it uses a simple marker of disseminated arterial disease that is

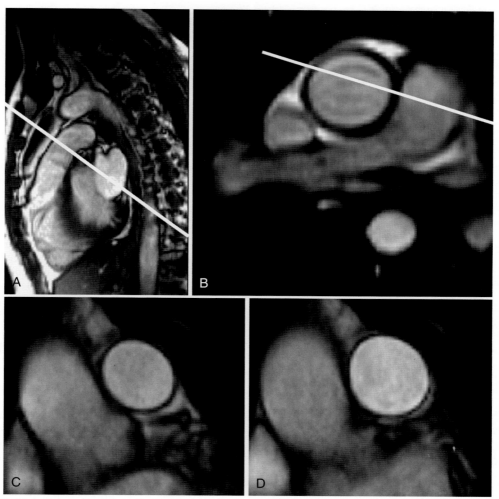

FIG. 29.8 Right ventricular outflow tract image (A) and oblique sagittal and transverse image (B) of the main pulmonary artery, showing the sites where main pulmonary artery distensibility was measured *(white lines)*. In the bottom row, the change in the main pulmonary artery cross-sectional area between diastole (C) and systole (D) demonstrated a large change in a 25-year-old healthy subject.

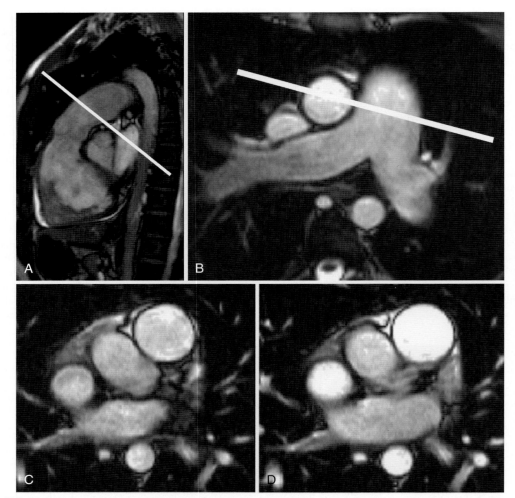

FIG. 29.9 Right ventricular outflow tract image (A) and oblique sagittal and transverse image (B) of the main pulmonary artery, showing the sites where main pulmonary artery distensibility was measured *(white lines)*. In the bottom row, the change in the main pulmonary artery cross-sectional area between diastole (C) and systole (D) demonstrated little change in a patient with pulmonary hypertension.

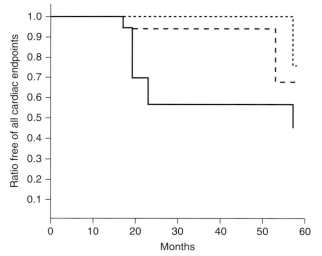

FIG. 29.10 Relationship of aortic stiffness to occurrence of any cardiac end point, with the study population divided into terciles ($P = .001$). (From Stefanides C, Dernellis J, Tsiamis E, et al. Aortic stiffness as a risk factor for recurrent acute coronary events in patients with ischaemic heart disease. *Eur Heart J.* 2000;21:390.)

easy to measure in large populations. More recently, Maroules and colleagues showed that in 2122 Dallas Heart Study participants without cardiovascular disease, CMR measures of total arterial compliance and aortic distensibility may be stronger predictors of nonfatal cardiac events, whereas pulse wave velocity may be a stronger predictor of nonfatal extracardiac vascular events (Fig. 29.11).[64]

ASSESSMENT OF ENDOTHELIAL FUNCTION

Brachial artery reactivity (BAR) testing has been proposed as a biomarker of endothelial function.[65] In the normal subject, release of a previously occluded brachial blood pressure cuff results in postischemic hyperemia (Fig. 29.12)[66] and subsequent increased shear stress of the local arterial wall. This, in turn, causes the release of endothelium-derived nitric oxide, a potent vasodilator. The extent to which nitric oxide is released (itself dependent on the amount produced and stored locally) can be indirectly assessed by measuring the degree of vessel dilation resulting from this provocation. Additionally, endothelium-independent function can be assessed by using dilation mediated by glyceryl trinitrate (GTN) (normally administered sublingually).

The noninvasive, uncomplicated, and well-tolerated nature of this examination makes it an attractive endpoint in epidemiologic studies. This

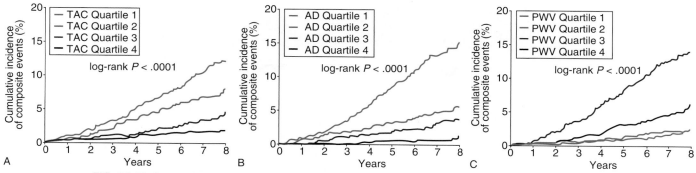

FIG. 29.11 Cumulative incidence curves for composite cardiovascular events based on quartile of (A) total arterial compliance *(TAC)*, (B) ascending aortic distensibility *(AD)*, and (C) arch pulse wave velocity *(PWV)*. (From Maroules CD, Khera A, Ayers C, et al. Cardiovascular outcome associations among cardiovascular magnetic resonance measures of arterial stiffness: the Dallas Heart Study. *J Cardiovasc Magn Reson.* 2014;16:33.)

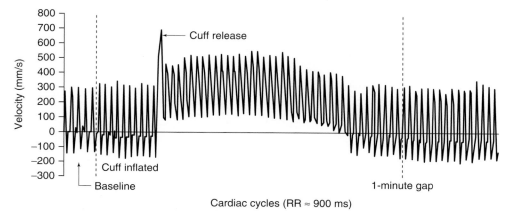

FIG. 29.12 Mean velocity in real time shown graphically for 72 cardiac cycles. The first 5 cardiac cycles are before cuff inflation. Imaging was suspended for the cuff inflation and a 5-minute delay. The next 10 cycles were acquired with the cuff inflated and show a shorter forward peak (i.e., reduced forward flow) in the waveform, although the peak velocity does not reduce. The occlusion cuff was placed more than 10 cm distal to the imaging plane. Note the increased reverse flow during the occlusion. After release of the cuff, the forward peak is longer, and the reverse flow changes to forward flow. Both effects recover to baseline after approximately 40 seconds. (From Mohiaddin RH, Gatehouse PD, Moon JCC, et al. Assessment of reactive hyperemia using real time zonal echo planar flow imaging. *J Cardiovasc Magn Reson.* 2002;4:283–287.)

has been further strengthened as alterations in flow-mediated response (by ultrasound) have been shown to precede clinical manifestations of disease. These findings suggest a useful role for this biomarker as a screening tool in the future, allowing risk stratification and intervention at an earlier stage than might previously have been thought possible.

Although the peripheral location of the brachial artery allows ultrasound ready access to such a measure, CMR can also be employed in a similar fashion. In this way, BAR can be used as an adjunct, combining with more routine measures of ventricular and vascular function to provide a powerful means by which to evaluate patients in research (Fig. 29.13). CMR offers other advantages over ultrasonography for this measure because it is more reproducible and less operator dependent.[67] This has logistical and economic consequences for researchers undertaking such work because it allows sample size to be reduced without compromising the ability to identify statistically significant changes. Also, CMR measures the true cross-sectional area, whereas ultrasound usually measures diameter only. In addition, assessment of reactive hyperemic response using real-time CMR flow imaging has been shown to be associated with cardiovascular increased risk.[68]

CMR has been used to demonstrate perturbations of endothelial function in a variety of different scenarios. Sorenson and coworkers[67]

were able to demonstrate impairment of flow-mediated dilation, whose degree was inversely related to circulating levels of estradiol, in patients who were given depot medroxyprogesterone acetate when compared with controls. Weismann and colleagues[69] showed that brachial artery flow-mediated dilation was significantly reduced in smokers in comparison with nonsmokers. As with Sorenson and colleagues' work, impairment of dilation was endothelium-dependent only because the degree of GTN-mediated dilation was similar in the two groups. Conversely, reduced endothelium-independent (but not endothelium-dependent) function has been demonstrated in young elite rowers.[70]

ARTERIAL WALL SHEAR STRESS

The use of detailed anatomic model and boundary conditions, such as the inlet and outlet flow, captured in CMR are important for the generation of a patient-specific computational fluid dynamic (CFD) simulation. The CFD method allows the calculation of features and properties such as wall shear stress (WSS) and mass transfer rate, which are difficult to measure directly with imaging but are important to the understanding of basic hemodynamics. CFD is the technique of using numerical methods to solve equations that govern the fluid flow. The basic

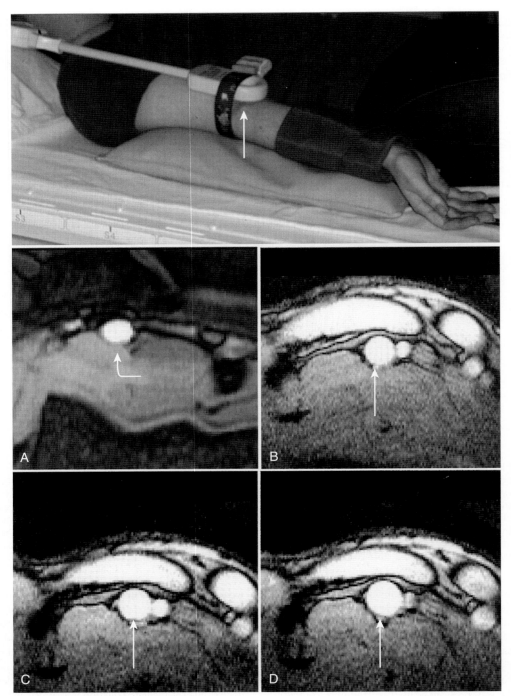

FIG. 29.13 Assessment of brachial artery reactivity. The top panel demonstrates the arrangement of the surface coil and cuff on a subject's right arm whose motion is restricted by sandbags. The transaxial plane in which the brachial artery is at its most superficial (A) is used to prescribe a plane perpendicular to the brachial artery (B). Arterial reactivity is then assessed through peripheral reactive hyperemia (C) and sublingual glyceryl trinitrate (D). Arrows indicate the brachial artery position in the top panel and the cross section of the brachial artery in A–D. (From Sorenson MB, Collins P, Ong PJL, et al. Long-term use of contraceptive depot medroxyprogesterone acetate in young women impairs arterial endothelial function assessed by cardiovascular magnetic resonance. *Circulation.* 2002;106:1646–1651.)

premise of CFD is to split the domain to be analyzed into small volumes or elements. For each of these, a set of partial differential equations is solved, which approximates a solution for the flow to achieve the basics of conservation of mass, momentum, and energy for each volume or element. The three basic equations are solved simultaneously, with any additional equations implemented in a particular model to obtain the

flow velocities and pressure and therefore any derived quantities, such as shear stress. CFD has been extensively used to model physiologic flow and arterial WSS, particularly in the carotid bifurcation, in attempts to better understand the mechanism of atherosclerosis in this region[71] and to give insight into the pathogenesis of arterial aneurysms.[72] WSS is defined as the mechanical frictional force exerted on the vessel wall by flowing blood and is the product of the blood viscosity with the velocity gradient at the vessel wall. Low or oscillating arterial WSS is correlated with atherosclerosis.[73]

In the aorta, once an aneurysm is formed, fluctuation in blood flow within it can induce vibrations of the aneurysm wall that can contribute to progression and eventual rupture. Volume flow measured by CMR alone is not yet capable of sufficient spatial and temporal resolution for accurate measurement of WSS. Simulation with CFD provides more information than current diagnostic tools. In particular, it allows the determination of the shear stress level, which in turn helps in identifying regions that are susceptible to aneurysm formation, growth, and rupture. The only criterion that has been used so far for the selection of surgical patients has been the maximum diameter and the rate of change of aortic diameter.[74] This is based on Laplace's law for hollow circular pipes, which states that the maximum stress within the arterial wall is proportional to the radius. Works in literature suggest that the peak wall stress is a more reliable parameter for the assessment of the rupture risk of aortic aneurysms. Fillinger and colleagues reported that the peak wall stress in aneurysms has a higher sensitivity and specificity for predicting the rupture than maximum diameter.[75] CMR and CFD are promising tools for stress and velocity patterns simulation using patient-specific flow condition. Figs. 29.14 and 29.15 show how the stress pattern and values are influenced by the shape of the aneurysm and the presence of intraluminal thrombus.

CMR four-dimensional (4D) velocity mapping has been used to study flow patterns in the heart and great vessels,[76] and to derive WSS

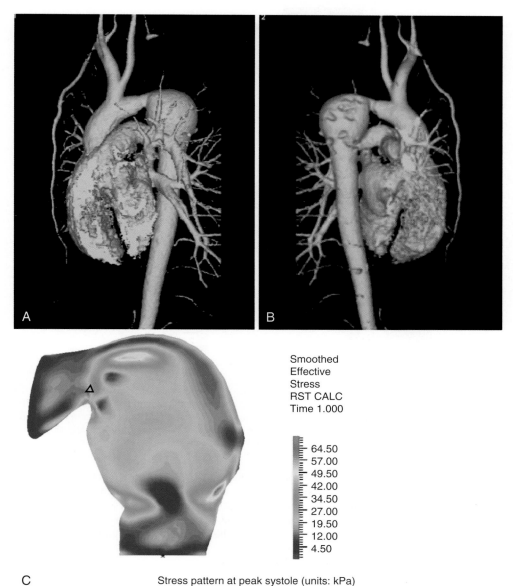

Smoothed
Effective
Stress
RST CALC
Time 1.000

64.50
57.00
49.50
42.00
34.50
27.00
19.50
12.00
4.50

Stress pattern at peak systole (units: kPa)

FIG. 29.14 (A) Surface-rendered contrast-enhanced magnetic resonance angiography in the left anterior oblique and right anterior oblique views in a patient with aortic arch aneurysm at the site of previous coarctation repair (left subclavian artery flap). (B) The aortic arch morphology was segmented from the cardiovascular magnetic resonance (CMR) images, and the inflow–outflow flow conditions were extracted from CMR flow mapping. (C) Stress pattern at peak systole (units: kilopascals [kPa]). Regions of high shear stress *(arrowhead)* are found in the aortic arch and at the entry of the aneurysmal bulge in the first model, with low values only in the distal region of the aneurysm.

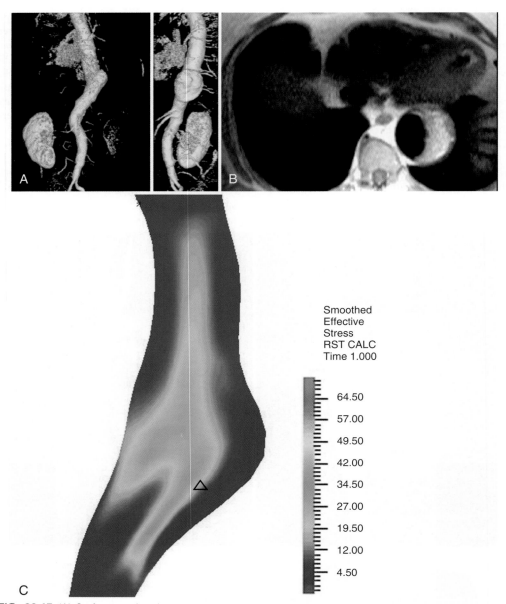

FIG. 29.15 (A) Surface rendered contrast-enhanced magnetic resonance angiography in the coronal and sagittal views in a patient with atherosclerotic aneurysm in the distal descending thoracic aorta. (B) The aneurysm contains a large crescent-shape mural thrombus. (C) Stress pattern at peak systole (units: kilopascals). Low values of shear stress throughout the aneurysm are noted where the thrombus appears to absorb part of the pressure load resulting in low stress in the wall *(arrowhead)*.

in the normal and dilated thoracic aorta.[77] Increase in ascending aorta diameter was found to significantly correlate with the presence and strength of supraphysiologic helix and vortex formation in the ascending aorta, as well as with decrease in systolic regional WSS and increase in oscillatory shear index.

CONCLUSION

Atherosclerosis consists of two components, the most often discussed being atherosis, relating to plaque genesis and composition. Sclerosis is often the forgotten partner in clinical practice, but measurement of vessel wall stiffening has now been shown to be useful both diagnostically and prognostically. Coupled with CMR's powerful role in excluding secondary causes of hypertension and accurately assessing ventricular

function, CMR is an ideal tool for its investigation, and further studies of the clinical role of parameters of sclerosis can be expected. The capability of CMR to assess brachial artery reactivity and to measure WSS, in conjunction with CFD, will enhance further its role in the studies of the biophysical properties of the arterial wall.

ACKNOWLEDGMENTS

The author acknowledges the helpful contributions of Peter Gatehouse, PhD, and William Bradlow, MD, in the preparation of this manuscript.

REFERENCES

A full reference list is available online at ExpertConsult.com

30

Valvular Heart Disease

Philip J. Kilner and Raad H. Mohiaddin

As an imaging modality, cardiovascular magnetic resonance (CMR) offers unrivaled versatility and freedom of anatomic access. In relation to heart valve disease, its relative strengths include the following:

- Depiction by cine imaging of valve movements and jet flow in planes, or stacks of planes, of any orientation.
- Measurement of right as well as left ventricular volumes and mass by multislice cine imaging.
- Measurement of volume flow and regurgitant fraction (pulmonary and aortic, at least) by phase contrast velocity mapping.
- Assessment of the context and consequences of heart valve disease using the wide fields of view, multiple image slices, and the versatility of tissue characterization available to magnetic resonance.

So although CMR is generally regarded as a second-line imaging modality after echocardiography for the assessment of heart valve disease,[1] it can have important contributions to make toward decision making in regard to the timing and nature of surgical intervention, particularly in cases in which there have been inconclusive or conflicting findings, perhaps owing to inadequate echocardiographic access, or in which heart valve dysfunction is one aspect of more complex congenital or acquired pathology.[2] And potentially, at least, CMR offers several possible methods for the measurement of valve regurgitation,[3–6] although work is still needed to optimize and standardize acquisition protocols and to fully validate the techniques used.

If CMR is to become established as a reliable second-line modality, several potential weaknesses or pitfalls need to be recognized and avoided or corrected:

- The slice thickness (typically 6 mm) and the dimensions of voxels (typically about $6 \times 1.5 \times 1.2$ mm^3) of cine and velocity map acquisitions need to be borne in mind.
- The images are not usually acquired in real time but are reconstructed from data gathered over several heart cycles during a breath-hold. For these reasons, valve leaflets are not always well seen, especially if there is arrhythmia; nor is CMR effective for visualizing the smaller, more mobile vegetations of endocarditis, although it can be useful for identifying an abscess or false aneurysm.
- It is important to attempt to depict valve and jet structure by cine imaging in several planes and orientations, not just one; appearances and, potentially, interpretation can differ considerably between images of a particular valve acquired in different planes (Fig. 30.1). Contiguous stacks of cine images are valuable for covering all parts of the mitral or tricuspid valves.

- The accuracy of phase velocity mapping cannot be taken for granted.[7] For jet velocity mapping, the dimensions of the voxels can be large in relation to the size and shape of a narrow or fragmented jet, leading to possible inaccuracies because of signal loss, partial volume averaging, and other artifacts. For the measurement of volume flow, particularly for the calculation of regurgitant fractions, surprisingly large inaccuracies have been found to occur as CMR systems have been "improved" to allow more rapid acquisition in the last 10 years, because of eddy currents and concomitant gradients.[7,8] The severity of the problem can vary considerably according to the hardware and software that are used and can change between the upgrades of a system. The uncertainties do not end there, however. The sequence parameters and imaging plane that are needed have to be chosen appropriately relative to the characteristics of flow under investigation if artifacts are to be minimized.
- Measurements of biventricular volume and function are not necessarily as reliable and straightforward as has often been implied, particularly if there is arrhythmia or the right ventricle is structurally abnormal owing to congenital heart disease or previous surgery, and volume analysis remains time consuming and to some extent subjective. The methods of acquisition and analysis need to be specified appropriately for comparisons over time or between patients.
- In general, the unrivaled versatility of CMR is a strength, but it is also a challenge. There is an ongoing dilemma between continuing development on the one hand and standardization on the other.

With these cautionary remarks in mind, the aim of this chapter is to describe some important underlying principles and to guide users to the CMR techniques that we and others have found the most informative.

Stenotic and regurgitant lesions of each heart valve are considered later, and an overview of measures of the severity of valve dysfunction is given in Table 30.1, which is adapted from the 2006 American College of Cardiology/American Heart Association Guidelines for the Management of Patients with Valvular Heart Disease.[1] It is important to realize that right-sided valve lesions, particularly pulmonary or tricuspid regurgitation, differ from their counterparts on the left. Although echocardiography has become well established in the assessment of valvular lesions of the left heart, CMR, with phase velocity mapping, has particular strengths in relation to the assessment of valvular and perivalvular lesions of the right heart.

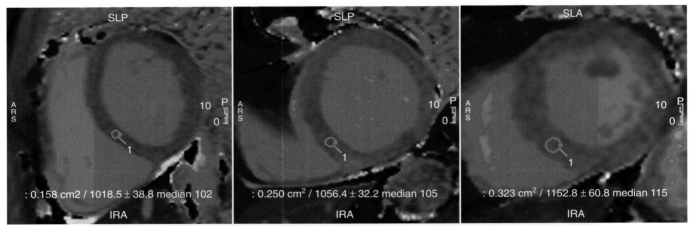

FIG. 30.17 Native T1 maps obtained in the mid short-axis view of the left ventricle using Siemens 448B modified Look-Locker inversion sequence on a 1.5 T Siemens Avanto scanner. Left image is from a healthy volunteer (septal T1 = 1018.5 ms); middle image is from a patient with moderate aortic stenosis (septal T1 = 1056.4 ms); right image is from a patient with severe aortic stenosis (septal T1 = 1152.8 ms). (Courtesy Dr. Vassiliou Vassilis, Royal Brompton Hospital, London.)

CONCLUSION

For investigation of valvular heart disease, the important strengths of CMR lie in visualization and quantification of regurgitation; the measurement of ventricular volumes, function, and mass; and the investigation of associated congenital or acquired pathology. Freedom of access and free orientation of planes, together with ability to measure post-stenotic jet velocities, also give CMR a role in cases such as calcified AS, in valvular dysfunction of the right heart including ventriculopulmonary conduits, and in patients with chest deformity or lung abnormality where ultrasonic access may be limited. In addition, CMR techniques for assessment of focal and diffuse myocardial fibrosis in valvular heart disease are unique biomarkers that have the potential to provide valuable prognostic information in patients with valvular heart disease as well as for optimal timing of aortic valve replacement in asymptomatic patients.

ACKNOWLEDGMENTS

We wish to thank our colleagues at the CMR Unit of the Royal Brompton Hospital for their help and support and the British Heart Foundation and CORDA, the Heart Charity, for support and grants.

REFERENCES

A full reference list is available online at ExpertConsult.com

31

Role of Cardiovascular Magnetic Resonance in Dilated Cardiomyopathy

Brian P. Halliday, Upasana Tayal, and Sanjay Prasad

Dilated cardiomyopathy (DCM) is defined as a disease of the myocardium characterized by left ventricular dilatation and systolic impairment that cannot be exclusively explained by abnormal loading conditions (such as hypertension or valvular heart disease) or coronary artery disease.[1,2] The true prevalence is debated because of a lack of large contemporary population studies.[3] The original Olmsted County study, performed between 1975 and 1984, estimated the prevalence to be in the region of 1 in 2700 individuals.[4] However, the calculated prevalence of hypertrophic cardiomyopathy in the same study has since been shown to be a gross underestimate, possibly explained by the fact that echocardiography was still a developing technique.[5] Recent reports have estimated the prevalence to be closer to 1 in 400 people in the United States.[3] Nevertheless, DCM is a commonly encountered condition, representing the most frequent indication for cardiac transplantation and a common cause of heart failure and sudden cardiac death (SCD). Despite therapeutic advances, 3-year treated mortality rates are estimated to be 12% to 20%.[6,7] Definitive early investigation giving a prompt and accurate diagnosis is therefore essential for the expedient introduction of targeted therapy. We will discuss the benefits of cardiovascular magnetic resonance (CMR) in the investigation of DCM after a brief overview of our current understanding of the disease.

BACKGROUND

DCM represents the final common phenotype of a diverse range of genetic and acquired insults (Table 31.1).[8,9] In 20% to 35% of cases, at least one first-degree relative is affected; in 20% to 40% of cases, a causative genetic mutation can be demonstrated with modern techniques.[2,3,10–12] Mutations in over 50 genes have now been linked with the disease, the majority of which occur in autosomal genes.[12–14] In a small proportion of cases the mutations are associated with broader syndromes, most commonly neuromuscular disorders such as Duchenne muscular dystrophy.[15] Inheritance is generally autosomal dominant, although often marked by reduced penetrance and variable expressivity.[3] In contrast to hypertrophic cardiomyopathy, mutations associated with DCM occur in a diverse range of genes responsible for many different cellular functions. The most common mutations occur in genes encoding sarcomeric proteins, with mutations found less commonly in genes responsible for the function of ion channels, the cytoskeleton, and the nuclear envelope (see Table 31.1).

Truncating variants of the large titin gene, *TTN*, are the most common mutations causing DCM.[16] Titin is the largest protein in the human body, spanning the length of the sarcomere, and it acts to generate and regulate contractile force.[17–19] Advances in genetic sequencing have enabled more detailed study of *TTN* mutations and their role in DCM and other cardiac pathology. Truncating variants of *TTN* have now been identified in 25% cases of familial DCM, 18% of sporadic cases

and <1% of unaffected controls.[16,20] Mutations in the *LMNA* gene, which encodes the lamin A/C protein, part of the nuclear envelope, are also associated with DCM.[21] These mutations are characterized by a highly penetrant and malignant form of the disease that requires aggressive treatment at an early stage given high rates of sudden death and advanced heart failure.[22,23] Aside from variants in *LMNA*, the identification of DCM disease-associated mutations holds most significance for relatives of the proband, enabling cascade screening and discharge from follow-up if found to be mutation carrier negative. Cascade screening and the identification of mild disease in asymptomatic individuals enables early diagnosis, disease monitoring, and appropriate intervention. There is also huge opportunity for targeted genetic-based interventions with the development of gene editing techniques.

The most common acquired causes of DCM include exposure to toxins such as excess alcohol and cardiotoxic chemotherapies.[1,8,9] The toxic effects of these agents appear to be dose-dependent and cardiac dysfunction often resolves after toxin removal.[24] A previous episode of viral myocarditis is another common cause and is thought to evolve into DCM in up to 30% of cases.[25] Less common, noninfective autoimmune inflammatory conditions can also present with a DCM phenotype. Given the heterogeneity of response to these environmental insults, it appears likely that individual susceptibility is linked to genetic factors.

Peripartum cardiomyopathy (PPCM) is a rarer form of the disease characterized by the development of a DCM in the last trimester of pregnancy or in the first 6 months postpartum. Many studies have linked the development of this condition to an abnormally cleaved segment of prolactin which is toxic to cardiomyocytes.[26–28] A strong genetic component to the condition has, however, also been demonstrated.[29–31] In one study, women with PPCM were found to have a similar burden of genetic variants, particularly in *TTN* (15% of the cohort), compared with a population with idiopathic DCM.[29] Similarly, undiagnosed DCM has been found to be more common in first-degree relatives of patients with PPCM.[31] This neatly demonstrates that PPCM and DCM have a common genetic etiology, which may be unmasked in the presence of specific environmental triggers.

In summary, DCM is the result of a complex interplay between genetic abnormalities, such as variants in *TTN*, and environmental factors including hemodynamic, inflammatory, and toxic insults. The interaction between these factors may help to explain the variable penetrance and reduced expressivity of mutations and the heterogeneous response of different individuals to environmental insults.

TREATMENT

The current treatment strategies for dilated cardiomyopathy focus on the use of neurohormonal medical therapies and cardiac resynchronization

TABLE 31.1

Genetic[a]	Acquired
Sarcomeric	**Toxins**
TTN (25%, titin)	Chemotherapy (anthracyclines,
MYH6 (4%), *MYH7* (4%) (myosin	monoclonal antibodies)
heavy chain)	Alcohol
TNNC1 (<1%), *TNNT2* (3%),	Recreational drugs (cocaine,
TNNI3 (<1%) (troponin)	amphetamines, anabolic steroids)
MYPN (3%–4%, myopalladin)	
	Infectious Insults
Nuclear Envelope	Viral myocarditis (parvovirus, human
LMNA (6%, lamin A/C)	herpes virus, Coxsackie)
	HIV
Cytoskeleton	Chagas disease (*Trypanosoma cruzi*)
DMD (N/A, dystrophin)	
DES (<1%, desmin)	**Peripartum**
	Autoimmune
Ion Channels	Giant cell myocarditis
SCN5A (2%–3%, sodium channel	Multisystem disease (systemic lupus,
protein type 5 subunit)	Churg-Strauss)
Mitochondrial	**Endocrine**
TAZ (NA, tafazzin)[b]	Pheochromocytoma
	Hypo- and hyperthyroidism
Sarcoplasmic Reticulum	
PLN (<1%, phospholamban)	**Iron Overload**

[a]Gene listed followed by prevalence and protein encoded in brackets.[2,3]
[b]X-linked genes, remainder of genes are autosomal.

therapy to treat and prevent heart failure, and implantable cardioverter defibrillators (ICDs) to prevent sudden cardiac death from malignant ventricular arrhythmia.[32–35] Evidence strongly supports the use of neurohormonal therapies such as beta-blockers and angiotensin-converting enzyme inhibitors in patients with reduced left ventricular ejection fraction (LVEF), and cardiac resynchronization therapy in patients with reduced LVEF and prolonged QRS duration.[32–35] Data on the use of primary prevention ICD therapy in DCM are, however, slightly less convincing.[36,37] Current guidelines recommend consideration of ICD therapy in patients with severely depressed ejection fraction, although this single-criterion approach lacks sensitivity and specificity.[32,34] In clinical trials investigating the benefit of ICD therapy in patients with severely reduced LVEF, only 5% of patients received appropriate therapies per year.[36–39] This demonstrates that the majority of patients currently receiving primary prevention devices on the basis of guidelines do not gain benefit. Conversely, large population studies have shown that 70% to 80% of SCD sufferers do not have a severely reduced LVEF.[40,41] Additional parameters, which identify patients at risk of SCD, will allow us to improve the selection of patients for ICD therapy.[42–44] We discuss the potential of CMR techniques in risk stratification.

CARDIOVASCULAR MAGNETIC RESONANCE ASSESSMENT OF DILATED CARDIOMYOPATHY

Morphology and Function

Diagnosis and subsequent management of patients with DCM relies on detailed assessment of left ventricular morphology and function. LVEF is currently the sole arbiter in the selection of patients for device therapy; therefore precise measurement is crucial.[32,34] CMR allows accurate and reproducible assessment of LV volumes, mass, and ejection fraction without the need for geometrical assumptions and is therefore considered the gold standard noninvasive technique (Fig. 31.1).[45,46] Analysis of regional function and myocardial strain can also be assessed using myocardial tissue tagging and feature tracking.[47,48] Analysis of longitudinal strain using myocardial feature tracking has been shown to predict adverse outcomes, independently of other predictors such as LVEF and late gadolinium enhancement (LGE), in patients with DCM.[47] Analysis of wall thickening and end-systolic wall stress and visualization of impaired fiber shortening can also be performed.[45,49,50]

Right ventricular (RV) size and function is abnormal in between 30% and 60% of cases of DCM.[51,52] This is thought to be secondary to intrinsic myocardial dysfunction and increased afterload related to a rise in pulmonary vascular resistance. CMR provides the gold standard noninvasive assessment of both RV size and function because of its three-dimensional capabilities.[53,54] Accurate assessment can be challenging using other forms of imaging, such as echocardiography, because of its complex and variable shape. Reduced RV ejection fraction on CMR is an independent predictor of all-cause mortality and adverse heart failure outcomes.[51] This supports a role for its use in prognostication of patients with DCM.

CMR also allows accurate quantification of left atrial (LA) volume using the biplane area-length method (Fig. 31.2).[55] This compares favorably against other noninvasive imaging methods because of its excellent endocardial border definition and multiplanar imaging ability, even in the presence of atrial fibrillation.[56–59] LA size is often increased in cases of DCM secondary to pressure overload from LV diastolic impairment, functional mitral regurgitation, and atrial fibrillation. It has been proposed that the degree of LA enlargement acts as a barometer of diastolic dysfunction and, consequently, there has been interest in the use of LA size to predict heart failure outcomes.[58] Indeed, it has been demonstrated that indexed LA volume calculated using CMR independently predicts cardiac transplant-free survival in DCM.[60] A cutoff value of >72 mL/ m^2 has been shown to predict a 3-fold increase in adverse outcomes in patients with DCM.[60]

Functional mitral regurgitation is also a common consequence of DCM secondary to mitral annular dilatation and leaflet tethering secondary to LV impairment. A long-axis cine stack and a short-axis cine image across the valve allows accurate assessment of all parts of the valve apparatus, including individual leaflet scallops, chordae, and papillary muscles.[61] Mitral regurgitant volume can be calculated by estimating the aortic forward flow volume, using phase contrast flow imaging, and subtracting this from the total LV stroke volume.[59,60] This method has been validated against volumes calculated from echocardiographic indices and catheterization data with good intertechnique agreement.[62,63] Once again, the accurate assessment of the degree of functional mitral regurgitation provides important prognostic information in DCM.[64]

Given the accuracy in functional assessment, CMR has been proposed as the method of choice for the follow-up of patients with DCM after pharmacologic and surgical intervention.[65,66] Given the favorable interobserver variability compared with other methods of assessment, the use of CMR in clinical trials can reduce the sample size required, reducing the overall cost and time needed to complete the research.[67] Moreover, it may be possible to avoid repeated studies using less precise methods, which are inconsistent. More precise adjustment of therapy and reduction of admission for repeat studies are likely to overcome the additional costs of a CMR study.

Tissue Characterization

Apart from accurate and reproducible assessment of cardiac morphology and function, the major advantage of CMR in the assessment of DCM is its ability to perform tissue characterization using LGE. This allows the detection and quantification of myocardial fibrosis. We also

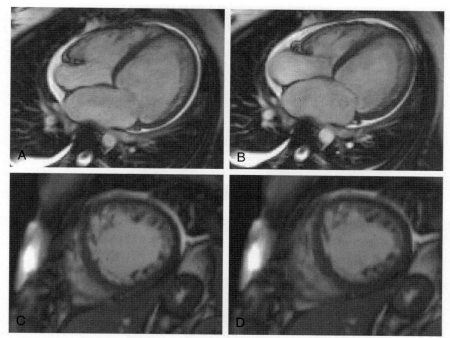

FIG. 31.1 Steady-state free precession images demonstrating biventricular dilatation with severe left ventricular systolic impairment, a small pericardial effusion, and right pleural effusion: (A) four chamber, end diastole; (B) four chamber, end systole; (C) mid-ventricular short axis, end diastole; (D) mid-ventricular short axis, endsystole.

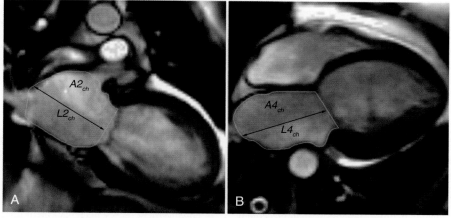

FIG. 31.2 Left atrial volume measurement using the biplane area-length method. The endocardial border is traced in two-chamber (2_{Ch}; A) and four-chamber views (4_{Ch}; B) in end systole, excluding pulmonary veins and left atrial appendage. The left atria length is measured from the midpoint of the mitral valve, perpendicularly, to the top of the atrium. (From Gulati A, Ismail TF, Jabbour A, et al. Clinical utility and prognostic value of left atrial volume assessment by cardiovascular magnetic resonance in non-ischaemic dilated cardiomyopathy. *Eur J Heart Fail.* 2013;15:660–670, with permission.)

discuss the potential role of the more recently developed T1 mapping technique, the use of which is currently confined to research.

Fibrosis

One of the histologic hallmarks of DCM, common to all causes of heart failure, is myocardial fibrosis.[68–70] There are two main forms of fibrosis detected histologically: interstitial fibrosis and replacement fibrosis (Fig. 31.3). Interstitial fibrosis describes an increase in the collagen volume fraction with expansion of the extracellular matrix, whereas replacement fibrosis describes discrete areas of myocardial scarring resulting from myocyte cell death.[68] Fibrosis is promoted through activation of the renin–angiotensin–aldosterone and the beta-adrenergic axes, both consequences of heart failure. Injurious stimuli and toxins also play an important role by activating inflammatory cascades, leading to the production of reactive oxygen species.[71] These pathways result in activation of myofibroblasts, with upregulation of transforming growth factor beta, altered activity in matrix metalloproteinases, and, ultimately, the production of collagen.[71,72]

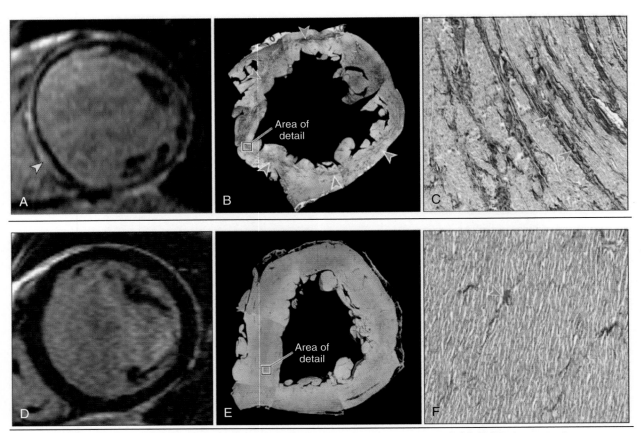

FIG. 31.3 (A) Late gadolinium enhancement cardiovascular magnetic resonance (LGE CMR), demonstrating extensive midwall enhancement *(arrowhead)*. (B) Picrosirius red staining in the corresponding postmortem macroscopic specimen, demonstrating bands of collagen *(arrowheads)* in the same distribution as the LGE. (C) Replacement fibrosis *(arrowheads)* on microscopic examination. (D) LGE CMR, demonstrating absence of LGE. (E) Picrosirius staining of the corresponding macroscopic postmortem specimen without staining for collagen. (F) Small amounts of perivascular interstitial fibrosis *(arrowhead)* without replacement fibrosis. (From Gulati A, Jabbour A, Ismail TF, et al. Association of fibrosis with mortality and sudden cardiac death in patients with nonischemic dilated cardiomyopathy. *JAMA.* 2013;309:896–908, with permission.)

Fibrosis is associated with adverse ventricular remodeling and increased all-cause mortality.[71] It has also been shown to provide an important substrate for the maintenance of re-entry ventricular arrhythmias.[73–77] An electroanatomical mapping study demonstrated that inducible ventricular arrhythmia and a history of sustained ventricular tachycardia (VT) only occurred in those patients with replacement fibrosis on LGE CMR.[78] Additionally, in each of the cases with inducible arrhythmia, its origin was mapped to the location of the LGE on CMR.[78] Fibrosis has also been associated with fractionated electrograms, slowed conduction, and conduction block during electrophysiology studies.[76,79] Each of these abnormalities has been associated with an increased risk of sustained VT and ventricular fibrillation.[76,79] The combination of fibrosis interspersed with areas of surviving myocardium has been correlated with the generation of re-entry wavefronts.[73,76,80] Moreover, the targeting of isthmuses of surviving myocardium has been shown to eliminate ventricular arrhythmia.[81,82] The combination of fibrosis and areas of viable myocardium has therefore been proposed to act as a substrate for re-entry arrhythmia.[73,76,80] All of these observations strongly support a role for fibrosis in the generation of ventricular arrhythmia.

Noninvasive detection of fibrosis using CMR therefore provides an opportunity to identify patients with DCM at high risk of sudden arrhythmic death. Treatments targeted at preventing or reversing fibrosis also provide important future therapeutic possibilities.

Late Gadolinium Enhancement Cardiovascular Magnetic Resonance and Midwall Replacement Fibrosis

LGE CMR identifies midwall enhancement in around 30% of patients with DCM, typically occurring in a linear distribution in the septum (see Fig. 31.3).[7,83,84] Histologic validation has confirmed that this pattern of enhancement represents replacement fibrosis.[7,84] The mass of fibrosis can be quantified using semiautomated software and validated methods. The most commonly used methods are the full width at half maximum (FWHM) and the >2 standard deviation (>2 SD) approach.[85] The FWHM method quantifies regions of myocardium with a signal intensity >50% of the maximally enhanced region, whereas the >2 SD approach includes regions with a signal intensity >2 SD above the signal intensity of a reference area of normal myocardium.

Given the suboptimal sensitivity and specificity of current LVEF-based criteria for sudden death risk stratification, there has been interest in the incremental value of adding the presence and extent of mid-wall fibrosis, as determined by LGE CMR, to the model. The largest study to date reported all-cause mortality and SCD/aborted SCD rates of 27% and 30%, respectively, in patients with midwall fibrosis, compared with 11% and 7% in patients without fibrosis.[7] Multivariable analysis confirmed that the presence of midwall fibrosis was an independent predictor of all-cause mortality and SCD/aborted SCD. The adjusted hazard ratio (HR) for the SCD composite endpoint was 4.6 in those patients with fibrosis ($P < .001$), whereas the adjusted HR for every 1% increment in the mass of fibrosis was 1.1 (95% confidence interval [CI] 1.05–1.16; $P < .001$). The same study demonstrated that the addition of mid-wall fibrosis to an LVEF-based strategy improved overall risk stratification. This finding has been replicated in similar studies and a large meta-analysis.[84–91] It has also been demonstrated that LGE quantification by both the FWHM and 2 SD methods provides robust prognostication for the prediction of adverse events.[85] It has been demonstrated that an LGE extent of >6.1% by 2 SD and >4.4% by FWHM predicts adverse events with the greatest sensitivity and specificity.

Altogether, current evidence strongly supports a role for LGE CMR in improving the selection of patients who may benefit from ICD therapy, by identifying those patients at highest risk of adverse arrhythmic outcomes. LGE CMR appears to add robust incremental value to the current LVEF-based approach. The added value of LGE mass quantification appears less convincing, possibly because of interobserver and intraobserver variability. Another explanation may be that, rather than the overall mass of fibrosis, it is the size of the border between areas of fibrosis and surviving myocardium that is most relevant to overall arrhythmic risk. As discussed, isthmuses of surviving myocardium within fibrotic areas appear to play an important role in the generation of re-entry wavefronts.[73,76,80–82] Therefore the size of the area where these two components interact may reflect arrhythmic risk more accurately.

Confirming the Diagnosis

The use of LGE CMR is also key to confirming the diagnosis of DCM in suspected cases. A study investigating the use of LGE CMR in patients with a suspected diagnosis of DCM, based on angiographic and echocardiographic findings, demonstrated that, in fact, 13% of patients had subendocardial enhancement indicating previous myocardial infarction.[92] This demonstrates that coronary angiography misdiagnoses a proportion of patients as having a nonischemic etiology when in fact they have suffered previous asymptomatic infarction. It is recognized that around 25% of patients with myocardial infarction do not present to hospital. A proportion of these patients have unobstructed coronary vasculature on angiography, presumably with infarction secondary to embolic phenomenon or plaque rupture with subsequent re-canalization (see Fig. 31.4E). This leads to the subsequent incorrect diagnosis of a nonischemic etiology. The correct diagnosis of this subgroup of patients, mislabeled by coronary angiography, is crucial given the different clinical courses and management strategies with regards to ischemic and dilated cardiomyopathies. Subsequent to this, LGE CMR has been shown to be at least as sensitive and specific as invasive angiography in diagnosing the cause of LV impairment in patients presenting with heart failure.[93] This demonstrated a 97% diagnostic accuracy for LGE CMR compared with a 95% diagnostic accuracy for coronary angiography. This supports the role of LGE CMR as the initial diagnostic test in patients presenting with heart failure and LV systolic impairment of uncertain etiology. Fig. 31.4 correlates the findings of LGE CMR and coronary angiography from the study, demonstrating the different possible combinations of findings from CMR and angiography and the subsequent diagnoses. LGE and T2* sequences also allow the diagnosis of other pathologies, such as sarcoidosis and myocardial iron overload, which can occasionally present with a DCM phenotype, requiring different management strategies, and which are not easily diagnosed using other imaging modalities.[94,95] Sarcoidosis is discussed in further detail later.

RESEARCH TECHNIQUES

T1 Mapping and Interstitial Fibrosis

Recent advances in T1 mapping techniques now allow the direct quantification of T1 relaxation times of each myocardial voxel, enabling the construction of T1 maps.[96,97] T1 mapping can be performed

preadministration and postadministration of gadolinium contrast. Using precontrast and postcontrast T1 values and hematocrit measurement, the extracellular volume (ECV) fraction can subsequently be calculated.[96] The extent of interstitial fibrosis has been shown to correlate well with ECV fraction and native T1 times.[98] This has led to the possibility of quantifying the degree of interstitial fibrosis in DCM using a noninvasive technique. It has potential advances over the qualitative LGE technique, which relies on subjective interpretation. Moreover, given the fact that the LGE technique relies on regional differences, there is the potential to miss diffuse myocardial fibrosis, which can appear as "nulled" normal myocardium. T1 mapping also offers opportunities for monitoring the response to therapies with potential antifibrotic properties. Studies have reported elevated native T1 values and ECV fractions in DCM, compared with controls.[98–100] Elevation of ECV in even mild phenotypes of DCM, compared with controls, has been demonstrated.[99,101] This raises the possibility of using T1 mapping for the diagnosis of borderline cases.

A large study on patients with DCM has demonstrated that native T1 values independently predicted all-cause mortality and a composite of adverse heart failure outcomes.[102] However, despite the association between outcome and native T1 values, it did not demonstrate an independent association between ECV and outcomes. This may be explained by heterogeneities in the methods of ECV calculation, including the timing at which postcontrast images were taken and also the timing of hematocrit measurement relative to the study.[103] This demonstrates the need for standardized precise protocols for T1 mapping for future research and clinical practice.

Perfusion Imaging

Studies have demonstrated a reduction in myocardial blood flow in patients with DCM.[104] Many theories have been proposed to explain this phenomenon despite visually normal epicardial coronary arteries. These mainly focus on dysfunction of the microvessels or increased oxygen diffusion distance because of interstitial fibrosis.[105,106] The degree of myocardial blood flow impairment has been strongly correlated with prognosis.[104,107] However, what has been less clear is whether abnormal perfusion is responsible for the adverse prognosis because of myocardial oxygen deprivation or is merely a marker of disease severity. A study using blood oxygen level-dependent CMR, however, has improved our current understanding of the pathophysiologic relevance.[108] This study assessed myocardial oxygenation and myocardial perfusion reserve during adenosine stress in patients with DCM compared with controls. Although myocardial perfusion reserve was reduced in patients with DCM, compared with controls, oxygenation during stress was not significantly different. Moreover, resting cardiac energetics in patients with DCM were not affected by oxygen administration. This suggests that the perfusion deficit is not sufficient to cause a reduction in oxygenation during stress and also that the resting impairment in energy metabolism is not secondary to a myocardial oxygen deficit. This also indicates that the reduction in perfusion observed in DCM is merely a marker of disease severity rather than a significant pathophysiologic driver.

Metabolic Imaging

Investigation of myocardial energetics in DCM is largely confined to research. Magnetic resonance (MR) spectroscopy allows the level of myocardial adenosine triphosphate (ATP) and phosphocreatine (PCr) to be determined.[109] Both compounds are involved in high-energy metabolism and a reduced ratio of PCr:ATP indicates a myocardial energy deficit. The use of MR spectroscopy therefore enables myocardial energetics to be assessed. In patients with DCM, the PCr:ATP ratio has been shown to strongly correlate with outcomes and therapies such as angiotensin-converting enzyme inhibitors have been linked with an improvement in the ratio.[109] Studies on exercise training have also

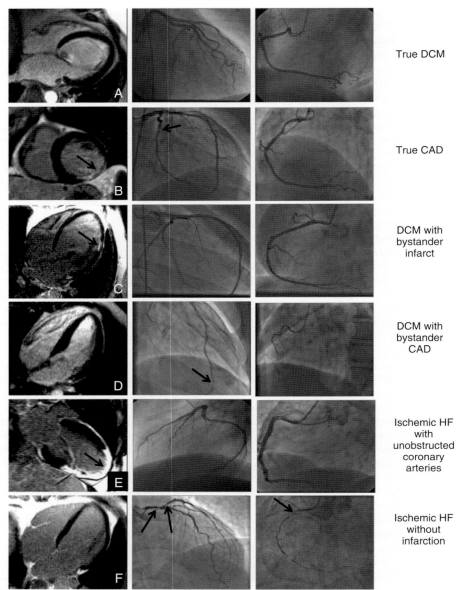

FIG. 31.4 Late gadolinium enhancement cardiovascular magnetic resonance (LGE CMR) and corresponding coronary angiography in patients presenting with heart failure *(HF)* and left ventricular dysfunction of unknown cause. (A) True dilated cardiomyopathy *(DCM)* with unobstructed epicardial arteries and no LGE on CMR. (B) True coronary artery disease *(CAD)* with a subendocardial inferolateral LGE, consistent with a circumflex territory infarct and a tight proximal circumflex stenosis *(arrows)*. (C) DCM with a subendocardial LGE *(arrow)* representing a bystander infarct and unobstructed epicardial arteries. (D) DCM without subendocardial LGE and bystander coincidental distal coronary disease *(arrow)*. (E) Ischemic cardiomyopathy with large apical infarct *(arrow)* on LGE and unobstructed coronary arteries. (F) Ischemic cardiomyopathy with severe proximal CAD *(arrows)* but no infarction on LGE CMR. (From Assomull RG, Shakespeare C, Kalra PR, Lloyd G, Gulati A, Strange J, et al. Role of cardiovascular magnetic resonance as a gatekeeper to invasive coronary angiography in patients presenting with heart failure of unknown etiology. *Circulation.* 2011;124:1351–1360, with permission.)

confirmed that although training improves LV function, there is no adverse effect on energetics with no change in PCr:ATP ratio.[110,111]

LEFT VENTRICULAR NONCOMPACTION CARDIOMYOPATHY

Left ventricular noncompaction cardiomyopathy (LVNC) is characterized by prominent trabeculations, deep intratrabecular recesses, and compact and noncompact layers of myocardium (Fig. 31.5).[112] It can occur as a primary myocardial abnormality and also in the context of congenital heart defects such as Ebstein anomaly and hypoplastic left heart syndrome. Genetic abnormalities are thought to account for 30% to 50% of cases, with sarcomeric mutations being the most common.[113] Clinical events include arrhythmia, ischemia, heart failure, and sudden death.

The true prevalence of the disease is controversial but has been estimated at between 0.05% and 0.26%.[114,115] Diagnostic criteria have

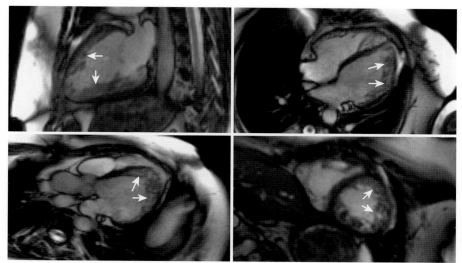

FIG. 31.5 Cardiovascular magnetic resonance (CMR) in a patient with ventricular noncompaction. Steady-state free precession (SSFP) images in a two-chamber view *(top left panel)*, three-chamber view *(bottom left panel)*, four-chamber view *(top right panel)*, and mid short axis *(bottom right panel)*. All mid and apical segments, except the septum, reveal a significant amount of noncompacted wall with a thin compact wall *(arrows)*. The left ventricular volume is increased, and its systolic function is substantially impaired.

been proposed on the basis of the ratio of noncompact myocardium to compact myocardium. The most commonly used CMR criteria uses a ratio of greater than 2.3:1 in end diastole.[116] Prominent trabecular patterns, meeting diagnostic criteria for LVNC, have, however, been demonstrated in healthy populations exposed to hemodynamic loads such as pregnant women and athletes.[117,118] This demonstrates the difficulties in differentiating LVNC from normal variants.

Morphology and Function

A spectrum of LVNC phenotypes exist with varying morphologies.[112] A dilated phenotype similar to DCM is the most common, characterized by cavity dilatation, eccentric hypertrophy, and systolic dysfunction. Benign phenotypes with normal cavity size, mass, and systolic function and, less commonly, hypertrophic phenotypes characterized by wall thickening, increased mass, and varying levels of systolic and diastolic dysfunction are also recognized.

Steady-state free precession (SSFP) cine imaging allows the easy recognition of the morphologic abnormalities together with accurate calculation of volumes, mass, function, and compact to noncompact myocardium ratios. A perpendicular orientation of the imaging plane to the wall should be carefully ensured because tangential orientation may lead to overestimation of the relative extent of the noncompacted wall. To visualize the trabecular meshwork without having partial volume effects induced by intratrabecular blood, a high temporal and spatial resolution should be used. Although some trabeculation may be a normal variant, the recognition of additional abnormalities such as an abnormally thin compact myocardial layer with abnormal systolic motion is important. The calculation of trabeculated LV mass may also prove a useful diagnostic technique.[119] One study has demonstrated that a trabeculated mass of >20% has a 94% sensitivity and specificity for the diagnosis of LVNC. Studies have demonstrated the superiority of CMR imaging over two-dimensional echocardiography in the assessment of LVNC.[120] CMR was shown to provide more complete evaluation of each myocardial segment and identified noncompacted layers more readily.

Tissue Characterization

Similar to DCM, LGE is a common finding in LVNC, being found in up to 55% of patients.[121] The most common pattern is septal midwall enhancement followed by insertion point (20%), subendocardial (13%), and transmural (10%).[121] In one study there was no relationship between the pattern of noncompaction and the distribution of LGE. Although LGE corresponds to reductions in LVEF, there are no data correlating LGE with adverse clinical outcomes yet.

CARDIAC SARCOIDOSIS

The incidence of myocardial involvement in systemic sarcoid varies with geography, with estimations of ~25% in the United States and >50% in Japan.[122–124] It accounts for between 13% and 25% of deaths because of the disease, primarily caused by sudden death and congestive heart failure.[122–126] The histologic hallmark of the disease is the presence of noncaseating granuloma which can be patchy and, consequently, missed with endomyocardial biopsy. Accurate diagnosis therefore requires a multimodality approach, including CMR.

Morphology and Function

Cardiac sarcoid can mimic a variety of phenotypes, most commonly DCM and less commonly hypertrophic and ischemic cardiomyopathies. It frequently produces LV dilatation with regional and global hypokinesia and wall thinning. Granulomatous inflammation may also lead to an increase in wall thickness, mimicking LV hypertrophy. SSFP sequences allow the accurate and reproducible assessment of ventricular morphology and function.

Tissue Characterization

Together with accurate assessment of morphology and function, CMR allows the detection of underlying acute and chronic disease. Acute inflammation and active disease can be identified using T2-weighted triple inversion recovery spin echo sequences and early gadolinium-enhanced images.[127] LGE allows the assessment of scar and fibrosis and

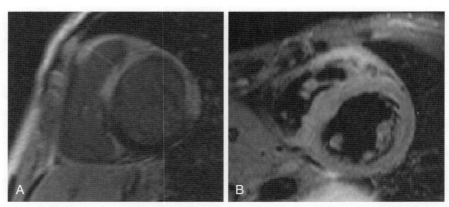

FIG. 31.6 A case of biopsy-proven cardiac sarcoid with dense, almost transmural subepicardial late gadolinium enhancement in a shepherd's crook distribution (A) without corresponding signal intensity change of short inversion time inversion recovery imaging (B) indicative of chronic disease.

in combination with T2-weighted imaging can differentiate active from chronic disease.[94] Comparison with positron emission tomography–computed tomography (PET–CT) demonstrates similar sensitivities for both modalities but a higher specificity with CMR.[94,128,129]

LGE occurs in a wide variety of patterns, including midwall, subepicardial, subendocardial, and transmural (Fig. 31.6).[94,125,130] A shepherd's crook pattern has been recognized with enhancement extending from the anterior RV-free wall round to the anterior RV insertion point and the LV septum (see Fig. 31.6). A coronary distribution of enhancement has been demonstrated in 48% of cases despite the absence of coronary disease on angiography and demonstrates the ability of sarcoid to masquerade as other disease processes.[94,125,130] The presence of LGE has been strongly correlated with adverse prognosis with a 30-fold increased risk of death and aborted SCD.[130,131] Studies have suggested that LGE imaging may also be used to assess the response to steroid therapy and also as a guide for endomyocardial biopsy.[132] T1-mapping offers potential advantages in the future for detecting diffuse processes missed by current techniques, which rely on the comparison of signal intensity with a reference area of normal myocardium.

In summary, CMR imaging allows rapid, high-resolution, noninvasive and reproducible assessment of the underlying pathologic changes and functional consequences associated with cardiac sarcoid and is therefore considered the gold standard technique.

CONCLUSION

In conclusion, the ability of CMR to provide accurate and robust assessment of morphology and function, together with tissue characterization, in a single noninvasive test offers many advantages in the assessment of DCM. It enables accurate diagnosis, with exclusion of other ischemic and nonischemic processes and provides the clinician with the ability to stratify risk and prognosis more accurately through the accurate assessment of chamber size and function, and the detection and quantification of myocardial fibrosis.

REFERENCES

A full reference list is available online at ExpertConsult.com

32

T1 and T2 Mapping and Extracellular Volume in Cardiomyopathy

Thomas A. Treibel and James C. Moon

Cardiovascular magnetic resonance (CMR) exploits the inherent difference between tissues in their configuration of atoms by generating differing signals—the fundamental tissue properties T1, T2, and T2*. Whereas differences in these parameters had to be previously visualized by weighted sequences, they can now be measured in a single breath-hold with T1, T2, or T2* displayed as pixel maps where each color-coded pixel carries the absolute value. Furthermore, if T1 is measured before and after contrast, the myocardial extracellular volume (ECV) is mapped, representing the percentage of tissue that is extracellular water, a surrogate for the process holding water, be it fibrosis, amyloid, or edema. In turn, T2 mapping is a highly attractive technique for characterization of myocardial tissue in the disease state accompanied by inflammation. T1, T2, and ECV change in disease, each being differentially sensitive to pathologic processes (Fig. 32.1). The technique potential is best considered in rare (infiltrations), common (edema), and ubiquitous (diffuse fibrosis) disease processes.

TISSUE CHARACTERIZATION: MOVING BEYOND LATE GADOLINIUM ENHANCEMENT

The key single technique that stimulated the greater adoption of CMR into routine clinical practice was scar imaging. The late gadolinium enhancement (LGE) technique was first used in infarction, but it has proved to be reproducible[1] and robust enough for use in a multicenter clinical trial,[2] and it has established itself as the gold standard method in both ischemic and nonischemic heart diseases, including cardiomyopathy,[3] myocarditis,[4] aortic stenosis-induced pressure-overload hypertrophy,[5] and infiltrative diseases.[6] However, LGE is a difference test between normal and abnormal myocardium, and therefore is not able to characterize and quantify diffuse myocardial disease or inform on how nonscarred areas are adapting to the increased workload or whether they are at risk of generating new scar. There are many pathways active in normal myocardium, and these change with different pathologic processes. Each parameter may be differently sensitive to these. Multiparametric tissue characterization is therefore an attractive strategy for noninvasive "biopsy" and "whole heart" sampling, avoiding potential morbidity and mortality of actual biopsy.[7]

HISTOLOGIC VALIDATION OF T1, T2, AND EXTRACELLULAR VOLUME

Extracellular tracers for measuring the interstitium were first described in the 1960s.[8] In the 1970s, Poole-Wilson et al.[9] used ^{51}Cr-EDTA in an ex vivo heart model with photographic paper to measure the myocardial extracellular volume. Early in vitro work by Kehr et al.[10] on human myocardium obtained postmortem compared T1 values, calculated from the inversion recovery signal curves, with collagen volume fraction, determined by the picrosirius red method, and showed a significant correlation between the two methods. In 2010, Flett et al.[11] developed an at equilibrium extracellular volume technique and validated it in patients with severe aortic stenosis and hypertrophic cardiomyopathy (HCM). The ECV showed a high correlation with the collagen volume fraction of biopsies obtained intraoperatively in this cohort. This work has been replicated in transplant hearts, shorter protocols, and with newer, faster T1 mapping sequences (Tables 32.1 and 32.2).[12,13]

NATIVE T1, POSTCONTRAST T1, AND EXTRACELLULAR VOLUME

Native T1

Native T1 measures the intrinsic signal from the combined cellular and interstitial compartments of the myocardium.[14] The advantages are that it does not require an exogenous gadolinium-based contrast agent. Native T1 relaxation time is prolonged with collagen (fibrosis),[11] edema,[15] and amyloid[16] and is shortened with reduced fibrosis,[17] iron,[18] fat,[19] and hemorrhage.[20] Given that native T1 measures both interstitium and myocyte T1, a signal from the interstitium alone is somewhat diluted by the myocyte signal, so subtle differences (diffuse fibrosis) are harder to detect. Moreover, capillary density, capillary vasodilatation, and "partial voluming" between blood pool and myocardium are also measured, potential biases if the signal sought is the matrix or myocyte compartments alone. Native T1 time is different with field strength and sequence design[21] and varies between scanners, making comparison of native and postcontrast values between centers challenging. Currently, several groups have developed T1 phantoms to facilitate multicenter trials (Hypertrophic CardioMyopathy Registry [HCMR][22]) or develop reference standards (T1 mapping and ECV standardization in CMR [T1MES] program[23]).

Postcontrast T1

After administration of gadolinium, T1 is dominated by, and inversely proportional to, the concentration of tissue gadolinium. Measuring T1 after contrast provides a value linked to the interstitium and has been applied to patients with heart failure.[24] Postcontrast T1 also varies with gadolinium dose, time post bolus, and importantly, patient-specific factors such as heart rate, clearance rate, body composition, and hematocrit.

Extracellular Volume Fraction

If the change in T1 precontrast and postcontrast is measured in both blood and myocardium after sufficient equilibration of the contrast distribution, the partition coefficient can be calculated. By adding in the blood compartment contrast volume of distribution (1 − hematocrit), the myocardial ECV is derived (Fig. 32.2). ECV is a more stable

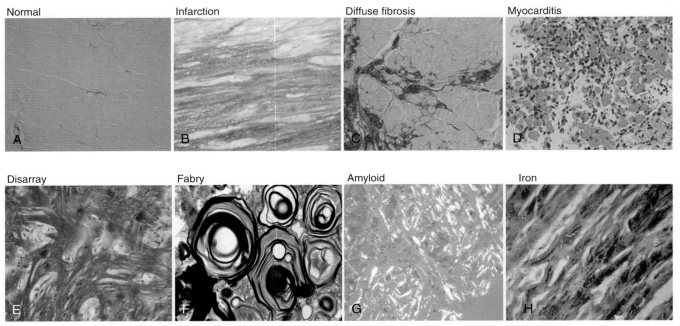

FIG. 32.1 Histopathological findings on myocardial biopsy. (A–H) Eight different pathologies that can potentially be characterized by cardiovascular magnetic resonance multiparametric mapping and may allow us to understand the underlying pathophysiologic processes of several diseases.

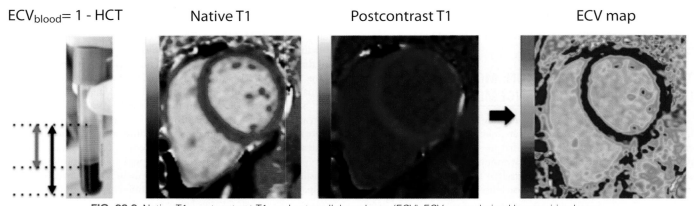

FIG. 32.2 Native T1, postcontrast T1, and extracellular volume *(ECV)*. ECV maps derived by acquiring hematocrit *(HCT)*, native T1, and postcontrast T1 modified Look-Locker inversion recovery of the short axis of a healthy volunteer.

TABLE 32.1 Histologic Validation Cohorts in T1 and T2 Mapping

Reference	Year	Population	N	Parameter	Sequence
Iles et al.[24]	2008	DCM	25	Postcontrast T1	1.5 T; IR VAST
Flett et al.[11]	2010	AS/HCM	26	ECV	1.5 T; EQ-CMR; multibreath-hold FLASH IR
Sibley et al.[100]	2012	DCM/IHD/HCM/amyloid	47	Postcontrast T1	1.5 T, IR Look-Locker
Mascherbauer et al.[88]	2013	HFpEF	9	Postcontrast T1	1.5 T, IR FLASH
White et al.[37]	2013	AS	18	ECV	1.5 T; EQ-CMR; ShMOLLI
Miller et al.[13]	2013	DCM/IHD (transplant)	6	ECV	1.5 T, MOLLI
Bull et al.[96]	2013	AS	19	Native T1	1.5 T; ShMOLLI
Lee et al.[106]	2015	AS	20	Native T1	3 T, MOLLI
De Meester et al.[107]	2015	AS/AR/MR	31	T1 and ECV	3 T, MOLLI
Kammerlander et al.[132]	2016	Mixed HF	36	ECV	1.5 T, MOLLI
Lurz et al.[53]	2016	Myocarditis	129	T1/T2/ECV	1.5 T and 3 T, MOLLI

AR, Aortic regurgitation; *AS,* aortic stenosis; *CMR,* cardiovascular magnetic resonance; *DCM,* dilated cardiomyopathy; *ECV,* extracellular volume fraction; *EQ,* equilibrium contrast; *HCT,* hematocrit; *HCM,* hypertrophic cardiomyopathy; *HF,* heart failure; *HFpEF,* heart failure with preserved ejection fraction; *IHD,* ischemic heart disease; *IR,* inversion recovery; *MOLLI,* modified Look-Locker inversion recovery; *MR,* mitral regurgitation; *ShMOLLI,* shortened modified Look-Locker inversion.

TABLE 32.2 Overview of T1, T2, and Extracellular Volume Fraction Mapping in Myocardial Disease[a]

Biological Process	Characteristic Disease	T1 Signal	T2 Signal	ECV Signal	Histological Validation	Main References[a]
Fibrosis						
Focal	Myocardial infarction, no hemorrhage	↑↑↑	↑↑↑	↑↑↑		Verhaert et al. 2011[108]; Ugander et al. 2012[109]
Diffuse	Aortic stenosis	—	↓	—	☑	Flett et al., 2010[11]; Bull et al., 2013[96]; Chin et al., 2014[110]; Singh et al., 2015[111]
	Systolic heart failure	↑	↑[b]	↑		Iles et al., 2008[24]; Su et al., 2014[113]; Bohnen et al., 2015[112]
	Diastolic heart failure	↑		↑		Su et al., 2014[113]
	Hypertrophic cardiomyopathy	↑	—	↑	☑	Ho et al., 2013[114]; Puntmann et al., 2013[101]
	Nonischemic dilated cardiomyopathy	↑	↑	↑		Puntmann et al., 2013[101]; Barison et al., 2015[115]
	Mitochondrial cardiomyopathy	↑	↑	↑		Lee et al., 2014[116]
	Diabetes	↑		↑		Wong et al., 2013[117]
	Hypertensive heart disease	↑		—		Kuruvilla et al., 2015[92]; Treibel et al., 2015[91]
	Obesity			↑		Shah et al., 2013[118]
	Congenital heart disease	↑		↑		Plymen et al., 2013[119]
Inflammatory	Rheumatoid arthritis	↑↑		↑↑		Ntusi et al., 2015[80]
	Systemic sclerosis	↑↑	↑[c]	↑↑		Ntusi et al., 2014[79]; Barison et al., 2015[120]
	Systemic lupus erythematosus	↑↑↑	↑	↑↑		Puntmann et al., 2013[78]; Zhang et al., 2015
Edema						
Regional	Acute myocarditis	↑↑↑	↑↑	↑↑		Ferreira et al., 2013[77]; Hinojar et al., 2015[121]
	Takotsubo cardiomyopathy	↑↑	↑↑	↑↑		Thavendiranathan et al., 2012[122]
Global	Acute myocarditis	↑↑	↑↑	↑↑	☑	Ferreira et al., 2013[77]; Hinojar et al., 2015[121]
	Antisynthetase syndrome	↑↑	↑↑	↑↑		Sado et al., 2016[82]
	Active systemic capillary leak syndrome	↑↑		↑↑		Ertel et al., 2015[123]
	Acute cardiac allograft rejection	—/↑	—/↑	—		Miller et al., 2014[124]
Infiltration						
Amyloid	AL amyloid	↑↑↑		↑↑↑		Banypersad et al., 2015[64]
Glycosphingolipid	TTR amyloidosis	↑↑	↑↑	↑↑↑		Fontana et al., 2014[125];
	Anderson-Fabry disease	↓↓		—		Messalli et al., ,2012; Thompson et al. 2013[126]; Sado et al., 2014[19]
Iron	Thalassemia major	↓↓↓				Hanneman et al., 2015[127]
	Sickle cell disease	↑/↓				Alam et al., 2015[128]
	Hereditary hemochromatosis	↓↓				Alam et al., 2015[128]
	Myocardial infarction, with hemorrhage	↓↓	↓↓	↑↑		Verhaert et al., 2011[108]; Pedersen et al., 2012[129]
Toxins	Uremia in chronic kidney disease	↑		↑		Edwards et al., 2014[130]
	Anthracycline toxicity	↑/—	—	↑/-		Tham et al., 2013[131]

[a]Reference list is nonexhaustive—several other references may exist that are not listed here.
[b]If myocardial hemorrhage accompanies acute infarction.
[c]In acute heart failure.

ECV, Extracellular volume; —, no significant change; ↑, significant increase; ↓, significant decrease; ▢, unreported to date.
Modified from Captur G, Manisty C, Moon JC. Cardiac MRI evaluation of myocardial disease. *Heart*. 2016;102(18):1429–1435.

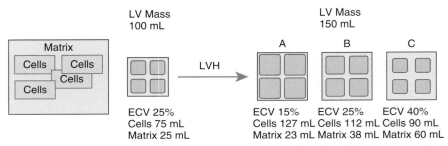

FIG. 32.3 Extracellular volume *(ECV)* divides the myocardium into cell and matrix components. In diseases with global homogeneous hypertrophy and extracellular matrix expansion, the ECV fraction may offer limited information, because it just depicts the ratio between cell and matrix volumes. By multiplying the left ventricular mass *(LVM)* with the global ECV, matrix volume (LVM * ECV) and cell volume (LVM * [1 – ECV]) can be derived, respectively. *LVH,* Left ventricular hypertrophy.

and biologically significant biomarker, as well as a more robust parameter than T1.[25,26]

Extracellular Volume Fraction Dichotomizing the Myocardium Into Cell and Matrix Components

ECV divides the myocardium into two compartments (extracellular and cellular) and, therefore allows noninvasive quantification of the myocardial matrix volume and its counter-part, cell volume (Fig. 32.3). The cell volume represents intact myocardial cellular components, proving a way to measure the myocyte volume (note that this also includes fibroblasts, blood cells, macrophages, etc.). How these change in disease (e.g., left ventricular hypertrophy [LVH]) is important. For example, in transthyretin-related (TTR) hereditary amyloidosis and light-chain amyloidosis, both have a massive matrix increase, but TTR has more matrix and 20% higher cell volume suggesting compensatory hypertrophy, which may permit more tolerance of the amyloid burden.[27] By modeling water exchange, there is also some evidence that the contrast kinetics could be used to obtain cell size-dependent parameters, particularly if very high doses of gadolinium contrast are used.[14]

T1 Mapping Evolution

The T1 mapping field is rapidly advancing to the point of widespread clinical utility. The first to T1 mapping was Messroghli in 2004 with a pulse-sampling scheme known as MOLLI (modified Look-Locker inversion recovery),[28] replacing previous multibreath-hold approaches. This was refined, including new MOLLI variants, shortened modified Look-Locker inversion recovery (ShMOLLI; a shortened variation with long T1 advantages[28–30]), saturation recovery variants such as saturation recovery single-shot acquisition (SASHA; offering complete heart rate insensitivity[30]) or hybrid approaches (accelerated and navigator-gated Look-Locker imaging for cardiac T1 estimation [ANGIE], quantification using an interleaved Look-Locker acquisition sequence with T2 preparation pulse [QALAS], SAturation Pulse Prepared Heart rate independent Inversion-REcovery sequence [SAPPHIRE][31–33]). Incremental developments such as respiratory motion correction[34] gradually increased accuracy and precision.[31,35] For ECV, contrast regimes were simplified from bolus followed by infusion or multi-timepoint sampling to a single precontrast and single postcontrast T1 map.[36,37] Split contrast dose protocols suitable for stress perfusion imaging have been validated.[38] ECV maps are now routine in some centers.[39] ECV quantification is less field and sequence sensitive than native T1 mapping but ECV standardization is ongoing. Most recently, it was a found that a synthetic ECV can be automatically generated during scanning, in which the hematocrit of blood is inferred from the T1 of the blood pool (as the relationship between hematocrit and R1 [1/Blood T1] is linear), removing the need for a blood test.[40] Finally, magnetic resonance fingerprinting

may offer more rapid multiparametric tissue characterization in the future by providing myocardial T1, T2, and proton spin density in a single breath-hold.[41]

For clinical use, these developments need to transition to standardized methodologies to diagnose disease; define mechanistic pathways of disease affecting the interstitium, the myocyte, or both; change therapy; and employ ECV as a surrogate endpoint in trials of drug development. This is the aim underpinning the first T1 mapping consensus statement.[42] Our conceptual models are simple, but there is more going on; effects such as magnetization transfer, diffusion distance and time, contrast mechanisms, transcytolemmal water exchange rate, flow, T2 or T2* relaxation will require further investigation.[43,44] Part of this development requires global approaches. Quality control systems, commercial sequences, megaregistries (e.g., Global CMR Registry, HCM Registry, UK Biobank) are in progress, and will provide high volumes of new insights in what is now the most active CMR research area.[22,45]

Continuous Improvement Versus Stability

For a "feel" for the potential of mapping in different pathologic processes compared with health, transform the absolute difference into the maximum possible signal-to-noise ratio (SNR) in standard deviation (SD) units in severe but not extreme disease (a measure of effect size). Provided minimal systematic bias by disease-tracking confounders, such as heart rate or anemia, an SD change of 2 suggests the technique can detect between-group differences for biologic insights, >4 and it could determine the choice of therapy in individuals, and >6 said therapy could be monitored during treatment. A measured value consists of combined biologic and measurement variability. Considerable ongoing work is reducing the measurement variability, so the above SD changes are increasing with technical development.

T2 MAPPING AND MYOCARDIAL EDEMA

Cardiovascular magnetic resonance can assess myocardial edema by early gadolinium enhancement (EGE), T2-weighted imaging, LGE, multiparametric mapping (T1 precontrast, T1 postcontrast, T2 mapping), and the hybrid novel positron emission tomography/magnetic resonance imaging (PET/MRI) technique for myocardial inflammation. T2-weighted CMR has become established for the detection of myocardial edema,[46] has been a particularly valuable tool for the discrimination of acute from chronic myocardial infarction,[47] and has been investigated in health and disease.[48–51] But as for T1, T2-weighted sequences are prone artifacts, have low sensitivity,[52] and require either reference signal intensities in skeletal muscle (assuming that is normal) or are sensitive only to regional changes. As a result of different hardware or sequence parameters, reference values differ considerably. Furthermore, local myocardial wall motion and heart rate influence local myocardial T2 values.[51] Although T2 acquisition at 3 T has the potential benefit of increased signal, it offered the same diagnostic accuracy as 1.5 T in the MyoRacer study.[53] Using a turbo gradient spin echo sequence at 1.5 T, Bönner et al.[54] showed that T2 mapping was highly reproducible, and that female sex and aging were accompanied by increased myocardial T2 values, but found no influence of heart rate or regional strain. T2 mapping is therefore good for the characterization of myocardial tissue in ischemia or inflammation, as described later.

T1 MAPPING IN HEALTH AND DISEASE

T1 mapping appears robust in detecting disease characterized by high T1 and ECV (Figs. 32.4, 32.5, and 32.6), such as amyloidosis,[16] or marked native T1 contrast diseases such as Fabry disease ([FD]; where fat storage makes native T1 fall)[19]; little biopsy histologic correlation is available in these diseases, however. For smaller expansions, reference ranges are needed. It is not exactly clear yet what these need to be. Gender appears to make a difference, but age has a much smaller or possibly no contribution[55] once partial volume issues are accounted for. Here, the ratio of pathophysiologic signal-to-measurement error is a key determinant of test performance. Liu et al.[56] reported on T1 and ECV data using older T1 techniques from 1231 participants aged 54 to 93 years of the Multi Ethnic Study of Atherosclerosis (MESA) study, where women had significantly higher native T1 and partition coefficient as well as lower postcontrast T1 times than men. When hematocrit was available,

ECV was higher in women than in men ($28.1 \pm 2.8\%$ vs. $25.8 \pm 2.9\%$; $P < .001$). ECV correlated with age, however, with an R^2 of 0.021 ($P = .012$); that is, 98% of the variability of T1 was attributable to factors other than age.

A recent study investigating physiologic hypertrophy in an athlete's heart using T1 mapping showed that hypertrophy was caused by an expansion of the cellular compartment while the extracellular volume becomes relatively smaller, hinting that ECV quantification may have a future role in differentiating physiologic from pathologic left ventricular hypertrophy (LVH), which is a major result if confirmed.[17]

INFILTRATIVE CARDIOPATHIES: AMYLOID, IRON OVERLOAD, FABRY DISEASE

Infiltrations (iron, FD, amyloid) are important because although rare, expensive therapies are available that need noninvasive targeting and/or development. Furthermore, they provide insights into more complex and more common polygenic diseases because these diseases have very high signal changes on multiparametric mapping. The only pathology that causes T2* to fall is iron (−7 SD), although cobalt and chromium have been described in the liver[57]; T1 only falls substantially in two currently known diseases (see Fig. 32.4B and C), FD (−6 SD) and iron (−15 SD), with one study suggesting a small fall in athletic adaption (−1 SD). Amyloid native T1 elevation is marked (+8 SD; see Fig. 32.4D and E), and ECV elevation in amyloidosis (amyloidosis—where the amyloid is the cause of disease rather than a bystander) is always above

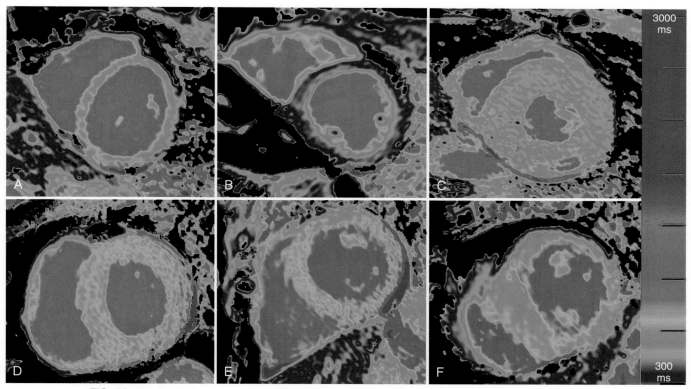

FIG. 32.4 Native T1 in health and disease. Native T1 maps (shortened modified Look-Locker inversion) in the basal short axis of: (A) a healthy volunteer—the myocardium appears homogenously green and the blood is red; (B) severe iron overload—the myocardium appears blue as the T1 is low from iron; (C) Fabry disease—the myocardium has a lower T1 *(blue)* because of intracellular lipid accumulation, except in the inferolateral wall, which is red because of fibrosis; (D) transthyretin amyloidosis (ATTR)—the myocardium has a higher T1 *(red)*; (E) light chain (AL) amyloidosis—the myocardium has a very high T1 with less hypertrophy than ATTR; and (F) hypertrophic cardiomyopathy—there is asymmetrical septal hypertrophy with right ventricular insertion point scar *(red)*.

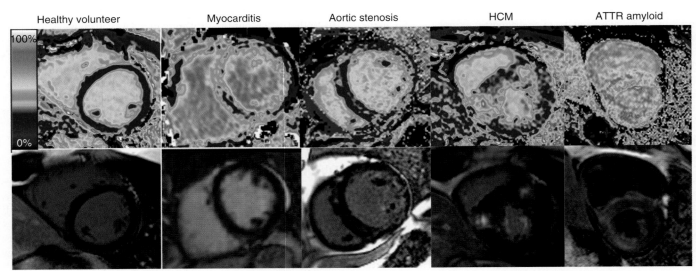

FIG. 32.5 Examples of extracellular volume (ECV) in health and disease. ECV maps *(top row)* and corresponding late gadolinium enhancement (LGE, *bottom row)* in the short axis of a healthy volunteer: the myocardium appears homogenously blue. Global myocarditis—note, because of the homogenous edema, there is no focal LGE, but the ECV map shows diffusely elevated ECV. Aortic stenosis—the ECV maps depicts ECV elevation corresponding to scar in the LGE image. Hypertrophic cardiomyopathy *(HCM)*—the ECV maps shows ECV elevation corresponding to scar in the right ventricular insertion points in the LGE image. Transthyretin amyloidosis *(ATTR)*—the blood:myocardial interface is lost in the ECV map because the ECV is as high as in the blood pool (i.e., ~60%)—the LGE images show classical global enhancement.

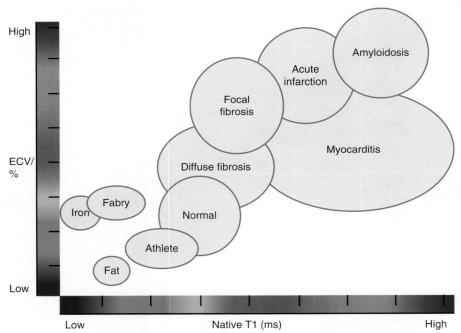

FIG. 32.6 Native T1 versus extracellular volume *(ECV)* in different pathologies. (Modified from Martin Ugander "Fibrosis and Edema" presentation, SCMR 2014.)

45%, a level seemingly impossible in other diffuse diseases (although more needs to be known about global myocarditis). Mapping in these diseases has important benefits: it may offer superior reproducibility (T1 in iron[18]), earlier disease detection (T1 is low in 50% of FD subjects without LVH[19]), or tracking change with therapy (amyloid[58]).

Amyloidosis

Cardiac amyloidosis is a rare condition characterized by a progressive infiltrative cardiomyopathy in which deposits of amyloid accumulate in the ventricular myocardium, almost always of either immunoglobulin light-chain (amyloid light-chain [AL]) or transthyretin (amyloid transthyretin-related [ATTR]) type, the latter being wild type or mutant. Advances in echocardiography, bone tracer scintigraphy, and CMR mean the noninvasive diagnosis of cardiac amyloidosis is maturing and biopsy is no longer needed in many circumstances.[59] Prognosis is often poor, and treatments are substantially influenced by cardiac involvement. CMR with phase-sensitive LGE has characteristic findings in cardiac amyloidosis and provides incremental information on the outcome even after adjustment for known prognostic factors; transmural involvement represents advanced cardiac amyloidosis with poor prognosis.[60] The marked interstitial expansion is also reflected on T1 and ECV mapping: Native T1 is significantly elevated in both AL and ATTR amyloidosis[16,55,61]—useful in a population with a high prevalence of renal failure. Karamitsos et al.[16] studied 53 patients with AL amyloidosis and compared native T1 and LGE to biomarker and echocardiographic criteria. They found that native T1 yielded a 92% accuracy for cardiac amyloidosis with possible or definite involvement and that it appeared more sensitive than LGE. Similarly, Fontana et al.[27] found that native T1 has a similar diagnostic accuracy in TTR amyloidosis but with a lower maximal T1, which has led to the (as yet unproven) hypothesis that the rapid deposition of amyloid fibrils in AL may be associated with myocardial edema. T2 mapping data is currently awaited in cardiac amyloid, although results from T2-weighted imaging have been conflicting, with one study showing no difference in T2[62] and another study showed a lower T2 ratio in cardiac amyloid, related to poorer survival (although no differentiation between AL and ATTR was made).[63]

ECV is a more direct marker of extracellular expansion, has high diagnostic accuracy for the diagnosis of cardiac amyloidosis, and predicts survival.[64] ECV has therefore been incorporated as a surrogate endpoint in clinical trials in amyloidosis (ClinicalTrials.org: NCT01777243/ NCT01981837).[58] When confronted with a patient with LVH, a very elevated T1 or ECV helps distinguish amyloidosis from hypertension or HCM.

Fabry Disease

FD is a rare but treatable X-linked disorder resulting in sphingolipid deposition in a number of different organs. Cardiac manifestations include LVH, arrhythmias, and valvular disease, and cardiovascular disease is now the primary cause of death in FD.[65] Early treatment with enzyme replacement therapy (ERT) may reverse or slow disease progression. Native T1 mapping can identify patients early, potentially helping target costly enzyme therapy. Two groups independently demonstrated lower myocardial T1 values in FD.[66,67] Furthermore, T1 mapping can discriminate against other diseases with hypertrophy, with no overlap in T1 values,[66] and has excellent reproducibility.[68] Pseudonormalization in T1 values (mixed extracellular fibrosis and lipid) and subsequent prolongation in T1 (burnt-out fibrosis) may provide an insight into disease progression. Furthermore, recent data by Nordin et al.[69] comparing T1 and T2 mapping, LGE as well as high-sensitivity troponin T (hs-TnT) and N-terminal pro b-type natriuretic peptide in FD with HCM, chronic myocardial infarction and healthy control, showed elevated T2 values in areas of LGE in FD. This highly correlated with hs-TnT, suggesting that FD with LGE is a chronic inflammatory cardiomyopathy.

Cardiac Siderosis

The impact of T2* measurement is discussed in Chapter 33. CMR linked to therapy has had a dramatic impact in reducing morbidity and mortality in cardiac iron loading, Cardiac iron loading has largely been the domain of T2* measurement sequences, which are histologically validated,[70] and can track iron levels with chelation. Cardiac siderosis, however, prolongs all three CMR parameters: T1, T2, and T2*.[71] Sado et al.[18] showed in 88 patients that T1 mapping correlates well with

T2* and was more reproducible than T2*. T2* mapping appears robust and simplifies analysis,[72] but performance in difficult cases remains undefined. Abdel-Gadir et al.[73] performed 126 scans in two 12-hour days in Thailand, with an average scan time of 8.3 minutes for combined T1 and T2* mapping that could be analyzed within 1 minute. Although the combined T1 and T2* acquisition is similar in duration to a T2* scan alone, further work is needed to establish the clinical value of such an approach.[74] An ultrafast mapping approach is being pursued in 18 countries and 28 sites globally.[75]

MYOCARDIAL EDEMA

Edema occurs in acute infarction and myocarditis (Fig. 32.7) but may be more ubiquitous—if we could detect it. It is also a therapeutic target. It can be intracellular or extracellular, and although it increases native T1 and ECV, T2 appears specifically sensitive with high elevations. Global inflammation by T2 can be found in acute heart failure, tracking histologic inflammation, and in connective tissue diseases. Whilst there is increasing recognition of global myocarditis, LGE is likely only seeing the tip of the iceberg.

Myocarditis

The diagnosis of myocarditis still represents a diagnostic challenge due to the variable clinical presentation, the invasive nature, and the limited availability of the gold standard of endomyocardial biopsy (EMB). CMR offers the ability to make a morphologic, functional, and tissue assessment in myocarditis, and this distinguishes it from other diagnostic modalities. However, it has lower sensitivity for pan-myocarditis or borderline cases.[52] Traditionally, T2-weighted imaging has been used to detect free water, and T1-weighted images precontrast and postcontrast for hyperemia based on historic studies at 0.35 T.[76] The Lake Louise criteria (LLC),[52] consisting of late enhancement sequences, T2-weighted edema images, and T1-weighted sequences before and after contrast injection (early enhancement), have been developed to standardize the diagnostic pathway, but they are now old, and new approaches are not included. The LLC can be challenging in a heart failure population with chronic significant overlap in symptoms and CMR findings. Multiparametric mapping techniques and quantification of the ECV have been suggested to overcome some limitations of the LLC, creating high expectations about their diagnostic utility. A recent study comparing T2-weighted imaging, late gadolinium, and T1 mapping at 1.5 T in 50 patients with myocarditis showed that native T1 mapping detected myocardial edema with higher sensitivity when compared with T2-weighted (note: nonquantitative) imaging[77] and with a 91% diagnostic accuracy when compared with LLC. In the recently published MyoRacer Trial, Lurz et al.[53] assessed the diagnostic performance of a comprehensive CMR protocol against EMB, including the LLC, native T1 mapping, quantification of ECV, and T2 mapping. In acute cases, native T1 yielded the best diagnostic performance, as defined by the area under the curve (AUC) of receiver-operating curves (AUC 0.82) followed by T2 (AUC 0.81), ECV (AUC 0.75), and LLC (AUC 0.56). In chronic cases, only T2 mapping has acceptable diagnostic performance in patients with chronic symptoms.

Connective Tissue Disease

In addition to viral myocarditis, other systemic inflammatory disorders can affect the myocardium. T1 mapping and ECV detect myocardial inflammation and fibrosis that in systemic lupus erythematosus, systemic sclerosis, and rheumatoid arthritis[78–80] and may be able to guide treatment. T1 and ECV have been used to identify cardiac involvement in other diseases such as systemic capillary leak[81] and antisynthetase syndrome—both are rare but potentially fatal.[82]

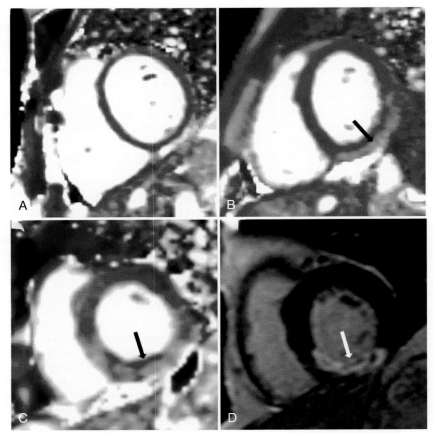

FIG. 32.7 T2 mapping in health and disease. T2 mapping in a normal volunteer (A). High T2 value in patient with myocarditis—here epicardial edema (B). Edema in acute myocardial infarction (C)—here patchy because of microvascular obstruction—see late gadolinium enhancement (D). (From Maestrini A. New generation cardiac parametric mapping: the clinical role of T1 and T2 mapping. *Magnetom Flash*. 5:2013 [Siemens]; https://www.healthcare.siemens.co.uk/magnetic-resonance-imaging/options-and-upgrades/clinical-applications/myomaps/use.)

Sarcoid Myocarditis

Sarcoidosis is a systemic granulomatous inflammatory disease with unknown etiology that can affect the heart either in isolation or as part of a multisystem disease. Typical cardiac manifestations include arrhythmias, heart failure, and/or sudden cardiac death. Sarcoidosis causes LV impairment from scar. Acutely, this is inflammatory. CMR using the LGE technique alone is unable to inform on whether there is disease activity that may potentially be treatable with immunosuppression. ^{18}F-Fluorodeoxyglucose positron emission tomography (FDG-PET) may be useful, but it is unlikely to be able to monitor the response to therapy because of the radiation dose. Mapping may help. To date, exploration has been limited, and further work is needed.

DIFFUSE FIBROSIS IN HEART FAILURE

Heart failure is a significant cost to health care services worldwide and yet its pathophysiology remains unclear, in part because of inadequate animal models but also because of the complexity of biochemical processes that are involved. Nevertheless, extracellular matrix (ECM) expansion is an important element of adverse remodeling either reflecting end-stage disease or signaling further deterioration. Importantly, diffuse fibrosis can be reversed by current therapies,[83,84] and new therapies show promise.[85] T1 and ECV rise in fibrosis, with ECV appearing the better test (~ +3 SD vs. 4 SD change). The ECV is shown to track fibrosis and is a major therapeutic target. It is prognostic, and in unselected patients it predicts outcomes as strongly as left ventricular ejection fraction[11,86] in some cohorts—results that, if generalizable, place the measured ECV as a fundamental myocardial property.

From a trial perspective, therefore, T1 mapping is a useful surrogate for an established pharmacologic target. From a clinical standpoint, ECV appears to be an important short-term prognostic marker, predicting mortality at 2 years and acute heart failure admissions in diabetics.[86,87] Mascherbauer et al.[88] showed in a cohort of heart failure with preserved ejection fraction that postcontrast T1 is associated with prognosis. In an unselected cohort, ECV was associated with hospitalization for heart failure, death, or both; was more strongly associated with outcomes than nonischemic LGE; improved the classification of persons at risk; and improved model discrimination for outcomes.[89]

DIFFUSE FIBROSIS IN PRESSURE OVERLOAD HYPERTROPHY

Arterial hypertension and aortic stenosis (AS) are attractive diseases for T1 mapping because they are common, lead to diffuse myocardial fibrosis, and are amenable to treatment (e.g., antifibrotic antihypertensives such as an angiotensin-converting enzyme [ACE] inhibitor or aortic valve replacement [AVR], respectively).

Arterial Hypertension

Recent data exploring the utility of T1 mapping in arterial hypertension and hypertensive heart disease have emerged,[90-92] but differences in native T1 and ECV have been found to be small (with significant overlap between hypertensive and control) and occurred only in those patients with LVH. Our own group concluded erroneously that the changes were at the detectable limit, but we underappreciated that the ECV may be unchanged if fibrosis is accompanied by a proportional increase in cell hypertrophy (i.e., proportional increase in cell and matrix volume).[91]

Aortic Stenosis

The timing for surgery in asymptomatic severe AS remains unclear despite a number of studies in the last decade.[93] AS is not just a disease of the valve. Graham Steell[94] noted in 1906 that it is the "reaction of the heart muscle" that is the "unmixed evil." Reflecting this, severe fibrosis by biopsy at the time of surgery was associated with worse outcome and more limited postoperative improvement in systolic and diastolic function.[95] Because fibrosis development seems to correlate with symptoms and systolic function, ECV as an imaging surrogate has the potential to provide a new marker to time surgery.[11,96] Multiple studies are currently underway due to report in the next few years and should provide prospective information on the utility of T1 mapping in AS (ClinicalTrials.org NCT01658345, NCT02174471, and NCT01755936). In severe AS patients, ECV has been found to be elevated, but, interestingly, LVH regression 6 months after AVR was cellular rather than fibrosis regression.[97] Recent data by our group (RELIEF-AS Study) found that at 1-year post-AVR, LV mass regressed by 20%, which was the result of a 17% reduction in fibrosis volume and a (higher) 23% reduction in cell volume. The greater cellular regression led to an increase in ECV; native myocardial T1 was unchanged. These data support the position that human diffuse fibrosis is dynamic and that this is measurable by CMR, a key biological result and proof-of-concept for drug development targeting myocardial fibrosis.[98]

GENETIC CARDIOMYOPATHIES

Cardiomyopathy encompasses a broad range of diseases from hypertrophic, dilated to noncompaction. The phenotypic variety makes each difficult to characterize; myocardial fibrosis is often the common denominator, regardless of pathophysiology. This can be either reactive and interstitial, such as present in idiopathic dilated cardiomyopathy (DCM), or replacement fibrosis after myocyte necrosis, as in HCM.[99] Previously, myocardial biopsy was the only means to establish fibrosis, but this carries its own risk, is prone to sampling error, and does not reflect the extent within the whole heart.

Dilated Cardiomyopathy

In DCM, prolonged native T1 has been histologically validated in small numbers of patients[100] and both native T1 and ECV are more extensively validated against normal populations.[55,101,102] Partially voluming of blood is a particular challenge in this population where only 3 to 4 pixels may cover the thin ventricular wall and bundle branch block may add to this complication (a typical voxel size is ~ $2 \times 2 \times 8$ mm^3).

Hypertrophic Cardiomyopathy

T1 mapping with ECV measurement as a novel imaging biomarker of diffuse myocardial fibrosis has been explored in HCM. HCM has also been similarly validated for both ECV and native T1 against normal populations.[37,90,101] Puntmann et al.[101] found that native T1 had a higher discriminatory performance than ECV.[103] This may hint that a high field strength or magnetization transfer weighting may improve native T1 mapping for the detection of fibrosis, here in HCM. Others have shown that T1 mapping abnormalities are larger than the LGE extent.[102] More work will be needed to understand these results. Wong et al.[104] have observed a preliminary association between ECV and B-type natriuretic peptide (BNP), and Ho et al.[105] reported that an ECV elevation is an early phenomenon, occurring in preclinical HCM (sarcomeric HCM mutation carriers without left ventricular hypertrophy). Finally, we await the results of the large 40-center observational study of HCM, HCMR, which is currently well on the way to completing recruitment, organized by Kramer and Neubauer to characterize prognostic markers in HCM, including T1 mapping markers of diffuse fibrosis (ClinicalTrials.gov identifier NCT01915615).[22]

CONCLUSION

Multiparametric myocardial characterization with T1, T2, and ECV has the potential to play a big role in a variety of clinical settings. The ability to distinguish multiple new pathologic processes such as fat storage, inflammation, diffuse fibrosis, and amyloid is a major advance (see Fig. 32.6). This information is beginning to be understood and incorporated into clinical practice. But it will take time to fully use these techniques to develop new drugs and change patient care and outcomes. Current challenges include restricted (although increasing) accessibility, nonstandardized reference values for normal and abnormal myocardium (addressed by current phantom studies), and nonuniformity of technique amongst vendors. We anticipate it will be the gold standard for diagnosis and treatment monitoring in rare diseases, where there are high disease-related changes and clinical need, and a drug development imperative will catalyze its standardization. Subsequently, this should provide the development platform for more robust methods for diffuse fibrosis. Combined, the potential is of better mechanistic insights into disease processes. It should eventually lead to improved diagnostic pathways, prognostication, and monitoring of therapy.

REFERENCES

A full reference list is available online at ExpertConsult.com

33

Cardiac Iron Loading and Myocardial T2*

Mark A. Westwood and Dudley J. Pennell

CONDITIONS ASSOCIATED WITH CARDIAC IRON LOADING

There are several conditions that can potentially lead to cardiac iron loading with cardiac complications. Cardiac iron loading can occur via two distinct mechanisms: first, primary disruption of iron regulation (genetic hemochromatosis syndromes) where excess gastrointestinal absorption is slow and symptoms often present in middle age; and, second, via transfusional iron overload where the iron accumulation rate is much faster and children can develop cardiac iron accumulation within a few years of initiating regular transfusion therapy. Excess iron cannot be naturally excreted in humans because of the lack of such a regulatory excretory pathway.

The most common pathology leading to severe iron accumulation is thalassemia major (TM). This is a genetic condition with severe reduction or absent production of the beta-globin chain constituent of hemoglobin A (HbA). Excess alpha-chains result from ineffective erythropoiesis, and there is a life-threatening anemia by 2 years of age. Not only does this require treatment with regular, lifelong, repeated blood transfusions, but it is compounded by a mild increase in gastrointestinal iron uptake related to hepcidin suppression.[1] TM occurs predominantly where malaria is endemic because heterozygote genetic hemoglobin mutations confer resistance. In other parts of the world it occurs primarily through immigration.

The detail of the hemoglobinopathy plays a role in the pattern and pathology of transfusion-dependent iron loading. For example, in the less severe condition of thalassemia intermedia, pulmonary hypertension and thrombosis play a greater clinical role and iron loading occurs at a later age.[2,3] In sickle cell disease (SCD), the defining clinical features include sickle cell crises (intermittent attacks of severe pain), pulmonary hypertension, thrombosis, and stroke.[4] Even where SCD patients are transfused to prevent cardiovascular complications, extrahepatic iron deposition is lower compared with other transfusional anemias. Conversely, in Diamond-Blackfan anemia, where the intrinsic bone marrow activity is low, patients are very prone to nonhepatic tissue iron accumulation.

PREVALENCE OF CARDIAC IRON OVERLOAD AND CARDIOMYOPATHY

The introduction of chelation therapy in the 1960s with deferoxamine changed the natural progression of TM patients receiving regular transfusions, where the most common cause of death was heart failure at a very young age.[5] Despite initially promising data and an increased life expectancy with the introduction of deferoxamine, cardiac iron overload continued to dominate, accounting for 70% of deaths.[6,7] However, as shown in a UK cohort, by the year 2000 the median age at death was 35 years because by this time patients had been exposed to regular chelation therapy from a young age.[6,8,9] Improving survival with deferoxamine by later birth cohort has been confirmed in other countries.[9,10] In the current millennium, data using T2* from TM patients across the world show that cardiac iron overload continues to be common, using definitions from T2* cardiovascular magnetic resonance (CMR) of severe cardiac iron loading of <10 ms, and mild-to-moderate cardiac iron loading of 10 to 20 ms (Table 33.1). The prevalence of cardiomyopathy is more difficult to measure. It can be estimated from either the prevalence of clinical heart failure or the presence of detectable left ventricular (LV) dysfunction, with the latter being higher in any given population. Prevalence generally increases with age and decreases with a more recent year of birth. For example, in a cohort of patients born before 1976, 37% had heart disease as defined by need for inotropic or antiarrhythmic medications,[6] but in a survey in 2004 the number of TM patients of all ages receiving cardiac medication was only 10%.

MECHANISMS OF CARDIAC IRON ENTRY AND TOXICITY

The mechanism of human cardiac iron loading is incompletely understood. In vitro and animal studies suggest cardiac entry of iron is mediated by calcium channels,[11–14] and indeed nifedipine hinders iron uptake into cardiac cells.[15] Accumulation of myocardial iron eventually leads to increased levels of intracellular free iron. The toxicity of free iron is mediated via several mechanisms (Fig. 33.1)[16,17]: (1) membrane damage caused by lipid peroxidation; (2) mitochondrial damage and perturbation of the respiratory enzyme chain[18,19]; (3) altered electrical function, including ryanodine release channel interference[20,21]; (4) cardiac fibrosis, which was reported as prominent in early autopsy studies[22,23]; and (5) changes in gene expression.[24] Iron that is safely stored in ferritin or hemosiderin is nontoxic, yielding hearts with low T2* and normal function. However, high iron stores predispose patients to development of cardiac dysfunction in the future. The result is that the natural history and clinical course in untreated patients is one of a long asymptomatic phase of progressive myocardial iron accumulation with sudden onset of either malignant arrhythmias or acutely impaired myocardial function in early adulthood. There was a significant mortality once symptomatic,[5,25] and 5-year survival for patients presenting in heart failure was only 48%.[26] One factor behind this is that although evidence suggested that intensive iron chelation therapy could completely restore cardiac function in most patients with asymptomatic cardiac dysfunction and even some clinical heart failure,[27–29] there was a risk of relapse caused by a lag between the clearance of cardiac iron and improvements in systolic function.[27–29] Even in asymptomatic patients, treatment of severe cardiac siderosis by aggressive chelation therapy is associated with improvements in ventricular function.[30] Improved life expectancy for TM patients in the United Kingdom has resulted from

TABLE 33.1	Incidence of Cardiac Iron Overload From Published Data Around the World			
Country	Sample Size	Severe T2* <10 ms	Mild-to-Moderate T2* 10–20 ms	Normal T2* >20 ms
United Kingdom[47]	109	20%	43%	37%
Hong Kong[145]	180	26%	24%	50%
Turkey[146]	28	46%	39%	14%
Australia[147]	30	37%	27%	37%
Oman[148]	81	24%	22%	54%
United States of America[149]	141	13%	21%	66%
Italy[150]	167	13% (<8 ms)	52% (8–20 ms)	35%
Italy[151]	220		30% <20 ms	66%
Greece[152]	159		68% <20 ms	32%
Worldwide survey[153]	3445	20%	22%	58%
Egypt[154]	89		25% <20 ms	75%
Pakistan[155]	83	47%	16%	37%
Indonesia[156]	162	5%	10%	85%

Modified from Pennell DJ, Udelson JE, Arai AE, et al; American Heart Association Committee on Heart Failure and Transplantation of the Council on Clinical Cardiology and Council on Cardiovascular Radiology and Imaging. Cardiovascular function and treatment in β-thalassemia major: a consensus statement from the American Heart Association. *Circulation.* 2013;128:281–308.

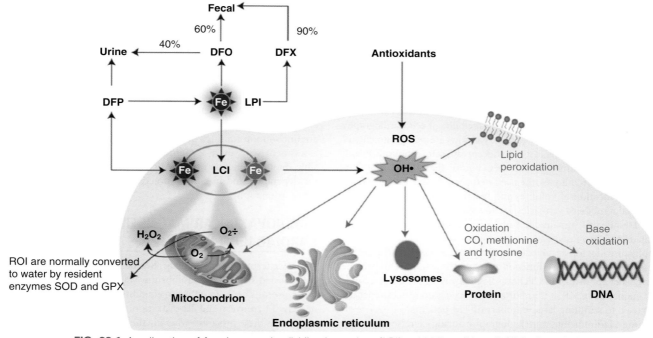

FIG. 33.1 Amelioration of free iron species (labile plasma iron *[LPI]* and labile cell iron *[LCI]*) by iron chelators and antioxidants. LPI is penetrating through the cell membrane with a consequent accumulation of LCI. Both LPI and LCI react with reactive oxygen intermediate *(ROI)* producing noxious reactive oxygen species *(ROS)*, for example, *OH'* radicals, which are highly reactive and oxidize DNA, proteins, and lipid components of the cell. Deferiprone *(DFP)* chelates LCI alone or in combination with LPI by deferoxamine *(DFO)*. Deferasirox *(DFX)* mainly removes LPI. (From Rachmilewitz EA, Giardina PJ. How I treat thalassemia. *Blood.* 2011;118:3479–3488.)

the increasing availability of T2* CMR and earlier escalation of therapy.[31] Even with modern-day chelation regimens, it is important to avoid stage IV heart failure in thalassemia as in-hospital mortality remains in excess of 50%.

Of significant clinical interest is that cardiac iron loading is commonly associated with endocrinologic complications including hypothyroidism, diabetes, hypoadrenalism, growth hormone deficiency, and hypoparathyroidism. This suggests a common or similar iron uptake mechanism. In untreated cardiac iron accumulation, historical series also showed more cardiac complications, such as pericarditis and myocarditis, that occurred in addition to heart failure and arrhythmias.[5,32] Chelation seems to have has altered this, with myocarditis and pericarditis now being unusual. Chelation has also led to a significant reduction in the historical occurrence of dense replacement fibrosis of myocytes, even in those who die from heart failure, although occasional small patches of fibrosis may be present.[5,23,32–34] In the modern era of chelation therapy, dilated cardiomyopathy (with restrictive features) and arrhythmia (predominantly atrial fibrillation) persist. Ventricular arrhythmias are more common in severe cardiac iron loading. Iron deposition throughout the myocardium in TM patients is nonuniform, being preferentially deposited in the subepicardium, but no systematic variation occurs between myocardial regions such that iron deposition in the interventricular septum is highly representative of total cardiac iron. There are other cardiac changes such as decreased left atrial (LA) function,[35] impaired right ventricular (RV) function,[36] impaired diastolic function,[37–39] and impaired endothelial function.[40–42]

ASSESSMENT OF THE HEART IN THALASSEMIA MAJOR

New-onset electrocardiogram (ECG) abnormalities are usually evident in TM patients with heart failure[43] and may include supraventricular arrhythmias, ECG findings suggesting right heart involvement, new-onset T-wave inversion, and small QRS complexes. In patients without heart failure, an abnormal ECG was found in 46%.[44] It is not known if progressive alterations in ECG tracings occur before heart failure develops, casting doubt over the use of serial ECG monitoring to assess disease progress. A chest x-ray may show cardiomegaly, signs of congestive heart failure, and, on occasion, extramedullary hematopoiesis. B-type natriuretic peptide is significantly increased in documented LV diastolic dysfunction, which may be helpful.[30,45,46] Exercise stress testing may be able to unmask subclinical LV dysfunction in TM, but results are influenced by many other factors, and it seems to have questionable value.

Before the development of CMR-derived T2*,[47] cardiac function was the key marker of disease progression despite a number of factors limiting its use. The limitations and reproducibility of echocardiography around operator experience and acoustic windows are well documented[48] but should be tempered against the widespread, safe, economical, and routinely available nature of this test. Before the advent of three-dimensional (3D) techniques, the need to make geometric assumptions for the quantification of volumes and mass, which often break down in abnormal remodeled ventricles, led to significant interobserver variability.[49] Despite this, impaired resting LV function by echocardiography correlated with increased cardiac mortality over 12 years.[50] Echocardiography provides less accurate quantification than CMR, and accuracy decreases with worsening LV function as geometric assumptions become an ever-greater approximation. Echocardiography is the preferred second-line technique after CMR. It is important that echo is done in experienced centers used to scanning large numbers of TM patients.[51]

Although radionuclide ventriculography during exercise can detect preclinical myocardial dysfunction in patients with iron overload,[52] concerns over radiation dose in young people, considerable intercenter variation, and the availability of other techniques have limited the use of this technique. Similarly, cardiac computed tomography (CT) can assess cardiac function,[53] and to some extent liver iron concentration,[54] but use of this technique is also limited because of concerns over repeated ionizing radiation exposure.

CMR is noninvasive, reliable, and free of ionizing radiation. Although increasingly seen as a mainstream cardiology investigation, the widespread use of CMR is limited by the cost and claustrophobia, although the latter is less of an issue with new-generation wide-bore scanners. The limitation with implanted cardiac devices is progressively being overcome. For the assessment of LV and RV function, the lack of geometric assumptions optimizes accuracy and reproducibility. Indeed, CMR is widely accepted as the gold standard for all biventricular measurements and indices. Routine use of steady-state free precession (SSFP)-based acquisitions

for cine imaging with end-expiratory breath-hold are acquired in the four-chamber and two-chamber long-axis views along with contiguous short-axis cines from the atrioventricular ring to the apex. The optimal end-diastolic volume (EDV) and end-systolic volume (ESV) are derived from LV volume/time curves generated from all frames of all cines and should include systolic valve tracking to adjust for systolic valve descent. LV mass should be calculated using the epicardial and endocardial borders of the LV in the end-diastolic frame. Papillary muscles should be included in the LV mass and excluded from the LV volumes. This method of volumetric assessment then has the benefit of having recognized normalized values for gender, body surface area, and age for both the LV,[55] and the RV.[56] These covariates have substantial impact on the normal ranges. Even where this stringent analysis method is not possible, CMR is more reproducible than other techniques, particularly where patients can be followed over time to allow longitudinal analysis of data.[57,58]

Consequent to the low hemoglobin from anemia, an adaptive response leads to increased cardiac output, usually through an increase in EDV, stroke volume, and heart rate. TM therefore represents a chronic, high-output state produced by volume-loaded ventricles (high preload) with the ejection fraction increased caused by a decreased afterload and an increased preload. Because of this state, the appropriate normal ranges to use are those derived from nonanemic TM patients because for both the LV[59] and the RV[60] there are differences compared with standard normal cohorts. Pediatric normal ranges are also available.[61,62] The hyperdynamic circulation also leads to an increased LV mass. The same pattern is true for the RV indices, but the differences are not as marked.[60] Using these adjusted "normal for TM" ranges may enhance diagnostic accuracy for detection of cardiomyopathy.

Whereas CMR offers several other techniques such as late gadolinium enhancement for the detection of myocardial fibrosis and myocarditis, and myocardial perfusion imaging for coronary artery disease, these are uncommon findings in this group of patients and routine cardiac assessment with these techniques is not advocated.[63] Although possible, diastolic function using CMR is time consuming and more operator dependent and in clinical practice is more readily assessed using echocardiography.[64,65]

CARDIOVASCULAR MAGNETIC RESONANCE OF CARDIAC IRON USING T2*

In simple terms, radiofrequency (RF) pulses cause spinning protons to be deflected from their equilibrium state. Immediately after this RF pulse, protons begin to return to equilibrium by two separate processes: namely, T1 recovery and T2 relaxation. Magnetic field inhomogeneity accelerates these processes whereby the protons return to equilibrium. As myocardial stores increase in the heart, ferritin breakdown increases into particulate hemosiderin, which is a form of ferrihydrite (hydrated iron oxide). The hemosiderin to ferritin ratio is significantly higher in cardiac siderosis than in normal hearts.[66] It is this particulate intracellular iron that markedly increases magnetic field inhomogeneity and thereby accelerates both T1 and T2 relaxation. Because the influence on these parameters as a result of particulate iron is much greater than normal field inhomogeneity, changes in these parameters become a biomarker for myocardial iron deposition. Magnetic resonance (MR) relaxometry is the use of specific MR sequences that repeatedly sample image data every few milliseconds from which relaxation or recovery curves can be derived. These techniques do not require contrast media.

Given that it is increased field inhomogeneity which is affected by increased iron deposition, it follows that the sequence most sensitive to this parameter should be chosen. Gradient echo sequences are much more susceptible to field inhomogeneity than spin echo sequences and

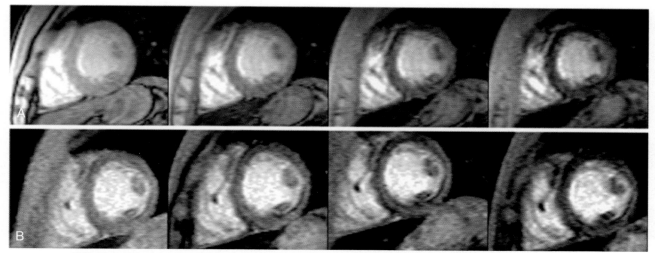

FIG. 33.2 T2* multiecho images. (A) A single breath-hold was used and (B) multiple breath-holds were used to acquire images of the myocardium with increasing echo time (TE). Note the better registration of the position of the diaphragm with the breath-hold technique. The signal intensity of the myocardium falls as the TE increases according to the myocardial T2*. (From Westwood M, Anderson LJ, Firmin DN, et al. A single breath-hold multiecho T2* cardiovascular magnetic resonance technique for diagnosis of myocardial iron overload. *J Magn Reson Imaging.* 2003;18:33–39.)

are particularly affected by particles of hemosiderin iron. Gradient echo sequences measure T2*, whereas spin echo sequences measure T1 and T2. In addition, a T2* multiecho gradient echo can repeatedly sample image data at different echo times (TE) in a single 10-second to 15-second breath-hold from which T2* can be derived, and such sequences are T1 independent (Fig. 33.2). A gating delay of 0 ms after the R-wave ensures all images are obtained at the same point in the cardiac cycle and removes any variability caused by changing heart rates. Such sequences are well validated, initially with "bright-blood" images and then subsequently with "black-blood" images, further refining reproducibility and reducing artifacts.[67–69] T2* and T2 are related by the formula $1/T2* = 1/T2 + 1/T2'$, where $T2'$ represents magnetic inhomogeneity. There is no particular advantage to a multislice method, which has been reported,[70,71] because iron concentration in the septum is representative of mean total iron concentration.[72–74]

The method of calculation of T2* values from raw datasets may be prone to error if care is not taken. Susceptibility artifacts at tissue borders, such as the lung myocardial interface and near the great cardiac veins in the anterior and posterior interventricular grooves, need to be minimized. For this reason, for routine analysis of T2*, a full-thickness region of interest (ROI) in the interventricular septum should be chosen to measure mean signal intensity for each echo time, thereby avoiding the above areas. Care is needed to ensure that the blood-pool signal and other artifacts are excluded from the ROI, which can be easier with a black-blood image. Signal intensity is plotted against TE, and a monoexponential decay curve is fitted to derive T2*, which represents the time taken for the signal intensity to decay to 37% of its initial value (Fig. 33.3). The signal intensity (SI) at each echo time is given by the following equation (where SI_0 represents the signal intensity at time zero and TE represents the echo time):

$$\text{Signal intensity (SI)} = SI_0 \cdot e^{-TE/T2*} \qquad \textbf{Eq. 33.1}$$

In severe myocardial iron loading, the myocardial signal obtained from the images with longer echo times becomes predominantly background noise, motion, and blood-pool artifacts. Because the true decay at these low signal values is masked by these effects, this will affect T2* calculations and may lead to spuriously high values. The simplest way to deal with these points at long TE, which are in effect just noise, is to delete them from the analysis and curve fitting, which is known as truncation (Fig. 33.4).[75] To ensure the most robust analysis, dedicated and validated analysis software is preferable.

T2* is highly robust and has a high interobserver and intraobserver reproducibility as well as high reproducibility between different studies performed a few hours or days apart and across different sites and scanner platforms.[76–78] Critically this means that T2* measurements at 1.5 T are independent of the scanner, site, or country where they were obtained. Although it is also possible to derive T2* using a 3 T scanner, clinical experience is much more limited in TM, and there are potentially more artifacts.[79,80] Current recommendations are that that clinical T2* MR is performed at 1.5 T. Finally, in very simple terms, increasing cardiac iron will lead to a decrease in the measured cardiac T2* value.

Although T2* has become the established technique for the assessment of myocardial iron loading, previous work used the ratio of signal intensity between the myocardium and skeletal muscle on a T2-weighted spin echo image. Because T2-weighted images are less susceptible to field inhomogeneity (indeed part of the refocusing of the RF pulse in a spin echo image is designed to mitigate effects attributed to field inhomogeneity), small changes in imaging parameters had a significant effect on results, and reproducibility was poor. It is, however, possible to construct multiecho spin echo sequences from which T2 can be derived in a similar way to T2*. Although T2 does shorten with increasing myocardial iron load, T2 assessment has not been validated to the same extent as T2*, and is not routinely used.

Similarly, T1 can be used to assess myocardial iron. T1 is measured using an inversion-recovery sequence with T1 representing the time taken for the magnetization to recover to 63% of its equilibrium value following an 180-degree RF pulse and a series of inversion-recovery images can be acquired with a range of inversion times. As with T2* multiecho, a modified Look-Locker inversion (MOLLI) sequence can produce a map of T1 values for the heart in a single breath-hold. T1 mapping techniques are increasingly being used for clinical assessment

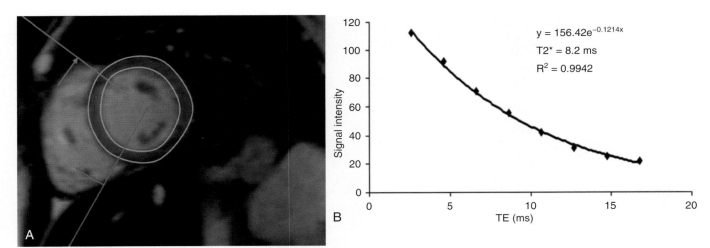

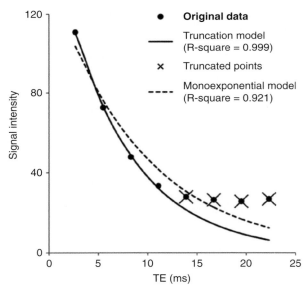

FIG. 33.3 (A) Image analysis software is used to measure the signal intensity of the interventricular septum. The endocardial and epicardial contours are drawn, and the full thickness septal region of interest is shown as the arc between the red and green radial lines, which is a region of interest that is not perturbed by susceptibility effects from deoxygenated hemoglobin in the anterior and inferior cardiac veins, nor the lung interface. (B) Decay curve and T2* calculation. The plot of septal signal intensity against echo time *(TE)* can be fitted with an exponential curve yielding the decay constant T2*. (A, From He T, Zhang J, Carpenter JP, et al. Automated truncation method for myocardial T2* measurement in thalassemia. *J Magn Reson Imaging*. 2013;37:479–483. B, From He T, Gatehouse PD, Kirk P, et al. Black-blood T2* technique for myocardial iron measurement in thalassemia. *J Magn Reson Imaging*. 2007;25:1205–1209.)

FIG. 33.4 Truncation curve analysis. When myocardial T2* is very short, the myocardial signal may decay to near the level of noise by the third or fourth echo time *(TE)*. The later points in the graph simply measure noise, but this has the unwanted effect of not allowing the exponential line-fit to drop to zero, which artificially increases the calculated T2* value, making it incorrect. This can easily be determined because the curve does not fit the first time points properly. Software tools are therefore used to truncate the signal values at long TE, so that the exponential curve fits the first points correctly. This gives a significantly lower T2* value, which is more accurate and in this example increases the *R-square* of fit from 0.921 to 0.999. (From He T, Zhang J, Carpenter JP, et al. Automated truncation method for myocardial T2* measurement in thalassemia. *J Magn Reson Imaging*. 2013;37:479–483.)

in a range of pathologies such as cardiac amyloidosis. For cardiac iron assessment, T1 does not yet provide any additional clinical value to T2*.[81] T1 yields improved reproducibility at normal levels of myocardial iron loading,[82] but this has no current clinical value in TM. Low native (noncontrast) T1 values are seen in two conditions affecting the heart: namely, myocardial siderosis and Anderson-Fabry disease. The normal range for T1 in noniron loaded hearts is approximately 800 to 1000 ms, but is variable and can require different centers to perform T1 mapping on normal subjects to establish local "normal" values, which is a significant limitation when compared with T2* techniques.[81]

T2*, PREDICTION OF HEART FAILURE, AND PROGNOSIS

Serum ferritin measurements are simple to undertake and are widely available. Although trends in ferritin are useful in monitoring the direction of body iron loading, they do not fully predict cardiac iron loading and, critically, a low ferritin measurement does not predict the future absence of heart failure.[6,50,83] In particular, a single ferritin measurement can be misleading and does not reflect cardiac iron burden. There is a similar problem with liver iron, where single liver iron measurements in patients on long-term iron chelation may be misleading because they do not correlate with cardiac iron levels.[27] Over time, poor liver iron control probably increases the risk of cardiac iron loading.[83,84] Similarly, noncompliance with chelation therapy leading to elevated serum ferritin levels (and thereby elevated liver iron) is a major predictive factor for cardiac iron loading in patients.[85] Therefore high liver iron levels per se may not be the best way to view the cardiac risk associated with liver iron loading, and although control of liver iron over time is likely to be important in prevention of cardiac iron accumulation, a low liver iron does not guarantee absence of cardiac iron loading.[86] Early on in the development of myocardial T2* the differential

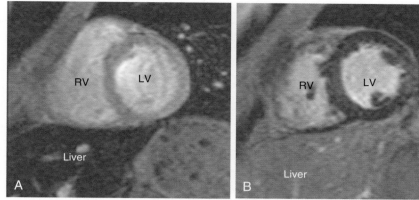

FIG. 33.5 Disparate heart and liver loading. (A) A dark liver signal but normal myocardium, indicating iron loading in the liver but not the heart. (B) The reverse is shown, with normal liver signal but dark myocardium indicating cardiac iron loading in the absence of liver iron loading. The latter patient is at risk from heart failure, but in previous decades before T2* cardiovascular magnetic resonance (CMR), it is the former patient who would have received intensified iron chelation treatment. This disparate iron loading between organs helps explain the high mortality burden from heart disease that occurred before T2* CMR was available to directly identify patients at risk of heart failure. *LV,* Left ventricle; *RV,* right ventricle. (From Anderson LJ, Holden S, Davis B, et al. Cardiovascular T2-star [T2*] magnetic resonance for the early diagnosis of myocardial iron overload. *Eur Heart J.* 2001;22:2171–2179.)

organ iron loading became apparent and disparate loading between the liver and heart was revealed as the reason for the limitations of these biomarkers (Fig. 33.5).

An increased risk of clinical heart failure has been demonstrated for patients with a falling left ventricular ejection fraction (LVEF) or absolute values below the lower limit of the normal range.[50,87] Limitations of the use of LVEF are that it requires meticulous attention to detail, but more importantly, changes in LVEF are a late event compared with falling T2* levels <20 ms and with low-to-moderate levels of cardiac iron, the change in LVEF is modest if at all present. Although absolute LVEF measurements vary between centers, volumetric analysis by CMR is superior to echocardiography.[57,58] There is a tipping point at which a marked deterioration in LVEF will occur with only a slight additional increase in cardiac iron loading. Because it is free iron that is toxic (but T2* measures storage iron in the form of hemosiderin) with intensive chelation treatment the LVEF will improve rapidly. However, the storage iron loading of the heart will only have decreased marginally in this time period. Prolonged periods of chelation are therefore required to remove all the stored iron in the heart. Although most focus has been on deteriorating LV function, myocardial iron deposition is also strongly associated with RV dysfunction.[88]

Cardiac T2* has been directly calibrated to human cardiac iron concentration (Fig. 33.6).[73,74] The practical and commonly used lower limit of normal is 20 ms, although it is not appropriate to consider cardiac iron as a dichotomous variable. Historical data suggest the upper limit of normal for cardiac iron is approximately 0.5 mg/g dry weight.[89] The probability of a reduced EF increases as cardiac iron increases,[47] and a cardiac T2* <10 ms predicts heart failure.[90] In one study, 98% of patients who developed heart failure had a myocardial T2* <10 ms and patients with a cardiac T2* <6 ms had a 50% likelihood of development of heart failure within 12 months (Fig. 33.7).[90] A normal cardiac T2* has a very high negative predictive value for exclusion of heart failure for at least 12 months. T2* is the most significant predictor of the development of heart failure compared with liver iron or serum ferritin.[90]

The high basal cardiac output in TM masks subtle but significant alterations in systolic function and a significant deterioration in LVEF

occurs at a late stage of the iron overload; hence, myocardial T2* is the most appropriate biomarker to use to assess risk. In a cohort of 652 TM patients followed up for 1 year where 80 episodes of heart failure occurred, the mean LVEF assessed by CMR within a median time of 158 days from heart failure event was 43.1%.[90] In nearly all patients, the myocardial T2* was <10 ms and the mean T2* was 6.7 ms. Furthermore, the risk of developing heart failure within 1 year without intensifying chelation therapy rises rapidly as the myocardial T2* progressively falls below 10 ms. For severe myocardial iron loading, a myocardial T2* value <6 ms conferred a relative risk of 270 compared with T2* values >10 ms for heart failure within 1 year. No additional prognostic information was provided from other biomarkers of cardiac iron (serum ferritin or liver iron). Receiver operating characteristic curve analysis shows that T2* is significantly superior in predicting heart failure compared with serum ferritin and liver iron, and should therefore always be used.[90] From this, the currently accepted T2* "risk ranges" for cardiac complications are T2* of <10 ms, representing high risk, 10 to 20 ms intermediate, and >20 ms low risk.

Although myocardial T2* assesses the risk of heart failure, the key next step is to change therapy to reduce that risk. Once a low T2* has been identified, it is necessary to intervene with intensive chelation treatment to lower cardiac iron quickly. This greatly reduces the risk of developing heart failure, which is important because once heart failure is established, it can precipitate an irreversible spiral of progressive deterioration in cardiac function, leading to death. Randomized controlled trials indicate that combining deferiprone with deferoxamine has the highest cardiac iron clearance rate and improves ventricular function. Intervention with intensified chelation appears to be very effective, as evidenced by a 71% reduction in cardiac deaths in the 5 years after the introduction of myocardial T2* in the United Kingdom in 1999 (Fig. 33.8).[91]

HEART FAILURE CAUSED BY CARDIAC IRON LOADING

Because the historical death rate from heart failure was 50% within 1 year, the current emphasis is to intervene early to prevent heart failure.[5,25]

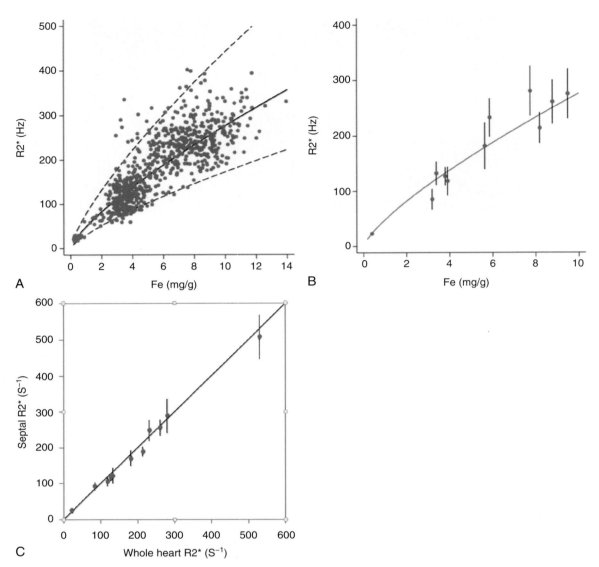

FIG. 33.6 Calibration of T2* to human iron. (A) The calibration of human R2* (equal to the reciprocal of T2*) for >500 myocardial samples against iron concentration measured by emission spectroscopy. The relation is [Fe] = 45 • T2*$^{-1.22}$. (B) A similar graph but using the mean whole-heart iron R2* (*N* = 11) vs. iron concentration. (C) The relation between whole-heart R2* and the septal R2* for each heart, confirming that using a septal region of interest alone was highly representative of average whole-heart iron concentration. (From Carpenter JP, He T, Kirk P, et al. On T2* magnetic resonance and cardiac iron. *Circulation*. 2011;123:1519–1528.)

In 52 patients with mean LVEF 36%, there was 48% survival after 5 years with no change in iron chelator and use of cardiac medications.[26] Data to guide optimal management of iron chelator treatment are sparse as there are few trials in acute heart failure. One follow-up study showed a mortality of only 1 in 7 patients in acute heart failure treated with continuous uninterrupted intravenous deferoxamine for 12 months.[27,92] The only randomized controlled trial in acute heart failure in TM was terminated early after only 23% recruitment.[93] It is therefore very underpowered and the results are difficult to interpret. It showed that the EF after 1 year on combination treatment of deferoxamine with deferiprone (EF + 8.4%) was higher (but not significantly higher) than the standard of care of monotherapy with deferoxamine (EF + 4.1%). It is critical to remember that even with a preserved LVEF, without escalation in therapy, the prospective risk for developing heart failure in 1 year is 47% if cardiac T2* is <6 ms, with a relative risk of 270 compared with

patients having a T2* >10 ms (only 1 out of 80 episodes of heart failure occurred in a trial over 7 years in patients with a myocardial T2* >10 ms).[90] Because the relative risk of overt heart failure is so great and coupled with a poor prognosis,[28] many centers treat patients with a myocardial T2* <6 ms and those with overt heart failure with the same intensified chelation regimens. Many symptoms that are common in anemia are also typically present in heart failure, which makes the diagnosis of heart failure difficult on clinical grounds, and this further cements the rationale for this approach.[94] Traditional signs of heart failure may appear late and may further delay treatment.[30,94] Sepsis may precipitate sudden, acute heart failure, possibly by disrupting iron stores and is the second leading cause of death in TM patients with severe cardiac iron loading.[95,96]

Patients with moderately severe cardiac iron loading (T2* between 6 and 10 ms) require intensified, but not necessarily maximal, chelation

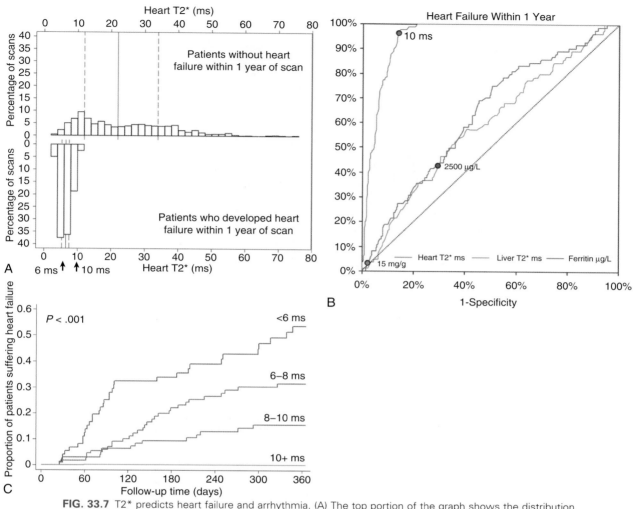

FIG. 33.7 T2* predicts heart failure and arrhythmia. (A) The top portion of the graph shows the distribution of myocardial T2* in patients who had a baseline cardiovascular magnetic resonance (CMR) scan and did not develop heart failure within 1 year. Note that the mean T2* was ~22 ms and there was a broad range of values. The lower portion of the graph shows the distribution of patients who did develop heart failure within 1 year of the baseline T2* CMR scan. Note the strong leftward shift of value, with a mean of ~7 ms. Nearly all patients had a T2* value <10 ms, and therefore this threshold is used clinically to indicate "high-risk" of cardiac events. (B) Receiver operating curve analysis of the relative power of cardiac T2*, serum ferritin, and liver iron to predict future heart failure. Cardiac T2* greatly outperformed the conventional measures. Note the relative strength of performance of conventional thresholds of serum ferritin of 2500 μg/L, liver iron of 15 mg/g dry weight, and cardiac T2* of 10 ms. (C) Kaplan-Meier curves of the incremental likelihood of developing heart failure according to the cardiac T2* value. Patients with a T2* <6 ms had an approximately 50% likelihood of developing heart failure over 1 year. (From Kirk P, Roughton M, Porter JB, et al. Cardiac T2* magnetic resonance for prediction of cardiac complications in thalassemia major. *Circulation.* 2009;120:1961–1968.)

therapy. Patients with mild-to-moderate cardiac iron loading (T2* between 10 and 20 ms) can be managed more conservatively by modification of chelator dose, improving patient compliance, or alternative chelating agents. Any reduction in cardiac function with the presence of any myocardial iron loading warrants escalation in chelation therapy, even in asymptomatic cases.[87] Patients with myocardial iron loading where ventricular function measurements show a trend of deterioration (even though the absolute values may remain in the normal range) require intensification of chelation. If this fails to stabilize the situation, then a change in iron chelator regime is required. In general, annual assessment of myocardial T2* is sufficient unless there is severe iron loading where more frequent assessment is required. More frequent assessment is also required if there is an impaired LVEF.

TREATMENT OF THALASSEMIA MAJOR AND IRON CHELATORS

Iron chelating agents have two functions: first, to tightly bind iron and prevent it acting as a catalyst for redox reactions; and second, to allow iron to be transported and then excreted from the body. Hence, iron chelators should reduce tissue iron levels, prevent excessive organ iron accumulation, and neutralize toxic labile iron pools. For a chelating

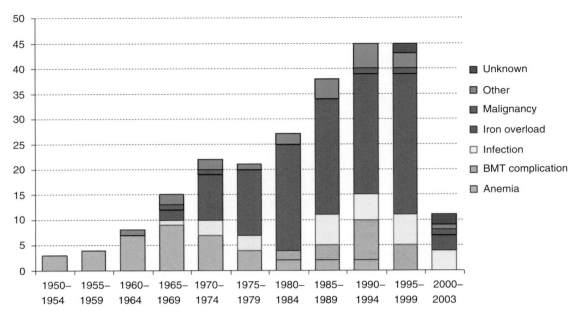

FIG. 33.8 UK mortality graph in thalassemia major (TM). The vertical axis shows the number of deaths in the United Kingdom in TM patients for each 5-year period from 1950 to after 2000. The portion of each column in red is the deaths from cardiac iron overload. After the introduction of cardiac T2* cardiovascular magnetic resonance in 1999, the mortality rate from cardiac iron overload fell by 71%. *BMT,* Bone marrow transplantation. (From Modell B, Khan M, Darlison M, et al. Improved survival of thalassaemia major in the UK and relation to T2* cardiovascular magnetic resonance. *J Cardiovasc Magn Reson.* 2008;10:42.)

TABLE 33.2 Main Features of Iron Chelators

Drug	FDA Approved	EU Approved	Route	Typical Chronic Dosing	Frequency	Excretion	Main Adverse Effects
Deferoxamine	Yes	Yes	SC (IV in heart failure)	20–50 mg/kg/d	8–14 h infusion for 5–7 days/week	60% urine 40% feces	Sensorineural deafness, visual disturbance, skeletal abnormality, growth retardation
Deferiprone	Yes	Yes	Oral	75–100 mg/kg/d	×3/d	75%–90% urine	Agranulocytosis, GI disturbance, arthropathy
Deferasirox	Yes	Yes	Oral	20–40 mg/kg/d	×1/d	~90% feces	Rash, GI disturbance, rise in creatinine

EU, European Union; *FDA,* US Food and Drug Administration; *GI,* gastrointestinal; *IV,* intravenous; *SC,* subcutaneous.

agent, diffusion through biologic membranes and hence the absorption from the gastrointestinal tract and the cellular penetration are governed not only by molecular size but also by lipophilicity and net molecular charge.[97] There are three commercially available iron chelators, each with very different properties.

The oldest iron chelator is deferoxamine, which was the first approved for use in the 1960s. It is not absorbed effectively by the gastrointestinal tract. This property, coupled with a short plasma half-life,[98] necessitates parenteral administration (usually subcutaneous) as a prolonged infusion or for severe iron loading a continuous infusion. Compliance is markedly adversely affected by the need for long parenteral administration. Other side effects include local infusion site reactions (induration, erythema, swelling, and itching), ophthalmologic and audiologic complications, renal toxicity and even, in high doses, adult respiratory distress syndrome.[99]

The next chelator to be marketed was deferiprone. This is rapidly absorbed from the upper gastrointestinal tract and is administered three

times daily orally because of its short half-life.[100] The iron–chelator complex is renally excreted.[100] Minor side effects include gastrointestinal symptoms (nausea, vomiting, and abdominal pain) and a transient increase of liver enzymes. Agranulocytosis and neutropenia are more serious side effects that can necessitate either temporary or permanent cessation of therapy.

Most recently, deferasirox has been developed. This is rapidly absorbed from the gastrointestinal tract and, because of a longer half-life, once daily administration is possible.[101] The main route of excretion is fecal.[102] Minor side effects include transient gastrointestinal disturbances (nausea, vomiting, diarrhea, and abdominal pain), diffuse maculopapular skin rash, and increased alanine aminotransferase (ALT) and serum creatinine.[101] More severe side effects include Fanconi syndrome and auditory and ocular toxicities. The main features of the common iron chelators are summarized in Table 33.2.

All three commonly used chelators remove cardiac iron if given in adequate doses and there is good patient compliance. However, each medication has advantages and disadvantages and optimal therapy must be tailored to each patient. There are many reviews on this subject.[103–105] The following recommendations are specific to patients with detectable, asymptomatic cardiac iron overload. There are several randomized trials of cardiac iron treatment using chelating agents. The introduction of deferoxamine in the 1970s had a profound effect on reducing mortality in TM,[106] which was then followed by deferiprone, which has been associated with reduced cardiac mortality in the United Kingdom, Italy, Cyprus, and Hong Kong.[91,107–111] The drastic improvement in cardiac mortality is probably multifactorial, including early identification of patients at cardiac risk from cardiac T2*, improved compliance with chelation therapy, and the use of specific agents alone or in combination.[91]

From a cardiac perspective, deferoxamine is only able to slowly remove cardiac iron with rates varying from 1.1% to 2.2% per month up to nearly 5% for constant 24/7 intravenous infusions.[27,112] Long-term infusions are inconvenient and uncomfortable, leading to reduced patient compliance. Although deferoxamine is the conventional chelating agent for TM, a change in therapy is probably warranted if compliance is poor. Deferiprone monotherapy offers superior cardiac protection,[113–115] and improves survival compared with deferoxamine monotherapy.[111] In the only prospective randomized study comparing deferoxamine and deferiprone monotherapy, deferiprone reduced cardiac iron at nearly double the rate of deferoxamine.[112] Deferiprone is therefore suitable for patients with cardiac siderosis, either as monotherapy or in combination with deferoxamine.[116] It is noteworthy that the use of either deferoxamine or deferasirox alone in mild-to-moderate cardiac iron loading does not improve LVEF,[112,117–119] which is in contrast to deferiprone, which does improve LVEF.[112,113,115,120] Deferasirox monotherapy can be used in patients with cardiac iron loading and preserved systolic function with clearance rates similar to deferoxamine.[121–123] Currently, there are few data on the use of deferasirox in patients with severe cardiac iron loading or a reduced LVEF.

There is evidence of a synergistic effect between deferiprone and deferoxamine,[19,124] and these agents have been successfully combined to improve cardiac and hepatic iron clearance.[125,126] Combination therapy can rapidly improve myocardial iron loading with an associated improvement in LVEF and has been shown to lead to a near doubling in the rate of increase of myocardial T2* when compared with deferoxamine monotherapy.[30,116,127–130] This accelerated cardiac iron clearance is associated with improved outcomes in severe cardiac iron loading.[110] Combination therapy is used for moderate-to-severe cardiac iron loading or where there is LV impairment. Although it is possible to combine deferiprone and deferasirox, currently there are relatively limited data on the utility of this combination.[131,132] Combination deferoxamine and deferasirox has also been tested.[133] American Heart Association guidelines on the heart in TM, the use of T2*, and the treatment of cardiac iron loading have been published,[134] and expert opinion[135] and numerous national guidelines are in accord with these.[136–141]

EMERGING CHALLENGES AND TREATMENTS

As we now enter an age of much improved survival, and patients with TM are entering their sixth decade of life and more, new challenges to cardiac health emerge. Diabetes caused by iron infiltration of the pancreas is a common finding in TM and is a risk factor for coronary artery disease. There is endothelial dysfunction even in the absence of iron loading. The prevalence of coronary artery disease in this population, which will occur as they age, is unknown. Additionally, the risk of arrhythmias such as atrial fibrillation (AF) attributed to altered hemodynamics in the left and right atrium is unknown but may also be higher than that in the general population. T1 mapping is able to assess myocardial iron and to characterize diffuse fibrosis, which does still occur with severe iron loading. However, these two processes have the opposite effect on T1 values, which may lead to challenges in interpretation of T1 values. The prognostic value of iron loading as assessed by T1 mapping is yet to be determined. Although recent trials on the use of amlodipine to block cardiac iron uptake in TM are of great interest,[142,143] much more work is needed to understand the prevention of heart failure. Finally, the ultimate goal would be to eradicate the defect in hemoglobin synthesis and, with advances in gene therapy such as *CRISPR-Cas9* gene editing, so far demonstrated in stem cells from patients with sickle cell anemia,[144] clinical trials are being planned.

REFERENCES

A full reference list is available online at ExpertConsult.com

34

Arrhythmogenic Right Ventricular Cardiomyopathy[a]

Anneline S.J.M. te Riele and David A. Bluemke

Arrhythmogenic right ventricular cardiomyopathy (ARVC) is a heritable heart muscle disease characterized by fibrofatty replacement of, predominantly, the right ventricular (RV) myocardium, which predisposes patients to potentially life-threatening arrhythmias and ventricular dysfunction.[1] Affected patients typically present between the second and fourth decade of life with arrhythmias coming from the RV.[2] ARVC is an unusual condition, with an estimated prevalence of 1 in 1000 to 1 in 5000 Caucasian individuals.[3,4] Approximately 60% of index cases harbor mutations in genes encoding the cardiac desmosome, a structure that provides mechanical connection between cardiomyocytes.[2,5] The defective mechanical connections in ARVC may structurally be represented by global or regional contraction abnormalities, ventricular enlargement, and/or fibrofatty replacement. As such, accurate evaluation of cardiac morphology and function is essential for ARVC diagnosis and management.

ARVC constitutes a diagnostic challenge for the cardiovascular magnetic resonance (CMR) physician. The variation in shape and contraction patterns of the normal RV complicates identification of early, subtle RV disease. In addition, many imaging centers have little experience with evaluating ARVC, and gaining experience is difficult because of the low prevalence of disease. Missing a diagnosis of ARVC may prove to be fatal, whereas overdiagnosis may lead to therapeutic repercussions in essentially healthy individuals. Despite these challenges, CMR is generally acknowledged to be the "best" noninvasive test for ARVC diagnosis and to distinguish ARVC from other cardiomyopathies. Thus the aim of this chapter is to review current knowledge of ARVC that is useful for CMR interpretation of individuals suspected of this disease. Our emphasis will be on ARVC diagnosis and management, including diagnostic criteria, CMR acquisition/analysis, and common regional morphologic and functional abnormalities in ARVC.

A HISTORICAL PERSPECTIVE ON ARRHYTHMOGENIC RIGHT VENTRICULAR CARDIOMYOPATHY

The first comprehensive clinical description of ARVC dates back to 1982, when Marcus and colleagues[1] described a cohort of 24 patients with arrhythmias originating from the RV and (right) heart failure. Using echocardiography, angiography, and histologic specimens obtained at surgery, they described ARVC as a regional RV disease with paper-thin RV myocardium, myocardial cell loss, and abundant subepicardial fat. The abnormal RV regions were traditionally thought to be located to the so-called triangle of dysplasia (i.e., RV inflow tract, RV apex, and RV outflow tract [RVOT]).[1] In subsequent years, several ARVC manuscripts have focused on gross or histologic evidence of myocardial cell loss with fibrofatty replacement.[6–8] It is important to note that these observations were made in tertiary centers, without the advantage of genetic testing and without sensitive diagnostic criteria. Over the last decade, several collaborative efforts in the United States and Europe have significantly enhanced our understanding of (the role of CMR in) ARVC diagnosis, clinical characteristics, and management. These advancements are reviewed here.

DIAGNOSIS OF ARRHYTHMOGENIC RIGHT VENTRICULAR CARDIOMYOPATHY

Diagnosis of ARVC is challenging because no single modality is sufficiently specific to establish an ARVC diagnosis. Therefore multiple sources of diagnostic information are combined in a complex set of diagnostic criteria. Definite ARVC diagnosis is based on the presence of major and minor criteria encompassing structural, histologic, electrocardiographic, arrhythmic, and family history criteria (Box 34.1).[9] These "Task Force" criteria (TFC) were first established in 1994 and updated in 2010 to improve (1) the specificity of the TFC by including quantitative metrics for diagnosis; and (2) sensitivity of the TFC in individuals who have a high likelihood of inherited/genetic disease. Structural criteria for ARVC diagnosis may be based on echocardiography, angiography, or CMR. However, echocardiographic evaluation of the RV is difficult because of its complex geometry,[10] and a recent study has shown that echocardiographic evaluation of subtle RV changes may be unreliable.[11] In addition, angiography is invasive and should not be employed as a first-line screening test for ARVC. In contrast, CMR allows for noninvasive multiplane morphologic and functional evaluation, as well as tissue characterization in a single investigation, and has emerged as the imaging modality of choice in ARVC.[12]

Cardiovascular Magnetic Resonance Task Force Criteria and Their Derivation

The diagnostic TFC for CMR require the presence of both qualitative findings (RV regional akinesia, dyskinesia, dyssynchronous contraction) and quantitative metrics (decreased ejection fraction *or* increased indexed RV end-diastolic volume) (see Box 34.1).[9] Quantitative values for RV volume and function for TFC were derived from a comparison of ARVC probands with normal healthy volunteers that were included in the Multi-Ethnic Study of Atherosclerosis (MESA).[13] To ascertain cutoff

---

[a]Modified from Te Riele AS, Tandri H, Bluemke DA. Arrhythmogenic right ventricular cardiomyopathy/dysplasia (ARVC/D): cardiac magnetic resonance update. *J Cardiovasc Magnet Reson.* 2014;16:50.

BOX 34.1 Revised 2010 Task Force Criteria for Arrhythmogenic Right Ventricular Cardiomyopathy

Global or Regional Dysfunction and Structural Alterations
Major
Two-Dimensional Echocardiography Criteria

Regional RV akinesia, dyskinesia, or aneurysm *and* one of the following measured at end diastole:
- PLAX RVOT ≥32 mm (PLAX/BSA ≥19 mm/m²), or
- PSAX RVOT ≥36 mm (PSAX/BSA ≥21 mm/m²), or
- Fractional area change ≤33%

Cardiovascular Magnetic Resonance Criteria

Regional RV akinesia or dyskinesia or dyssynchronous RV contraction *and* one of the following:
- RV EDV/BSA ≥110 mL/m² (male) or ≥100 mL/m² (female), or
- RV ejection fraction ≤40%

Right Ventricular Angiography Criteria

Regional RV akinesia, dyskinesia, or aneurysm

Minor
Two-Dimensional Echocardiography Criteria

Regional RV akinesia or dyskinesia or dyssynchronous RV contraction *and* one of the following measured at end diastole:
- PLAX RVOT ≥29 to <32 mm (PLAX/BSA ≥16 to <19 mm/m²), or
- PSAX RVOT ≥32 to <36 mm (PSAX/BSA ≥18 to <21 mm/m²), or
- Fractional area change >33% ≤40%

Cardiovascular Magnetic Resonance Criteria

Regional RV akinesia or dyskinesia or dyssynchronous RV contraction *and* one of the following:
- RV EDV/BSA ≥100 to 110 mL/m² (male) or ≥90 to 100 mL/m² (female)
- RV ejection fraction >40 to ≤45%

Tissue Characterization of Wall
Major
Residual myocytes <60% by morphometric analysis (or <50% if estimated), with fibrous replacement of the RV free wall myocardium in ≥1 sample, with or without fatty replacement of tissue on endomyocardial biopsy

Minor
Residual myocytes 60% to 75% by morphometric analysis (or 50% to 65% if estimated), with fibrous replacement of the RV free wall myocardium in ≥1 sample with or without fatty replacement of tissue on endomyocardial biopsy

Repolarization Abnormalities
Major
Inverted T waves in right precordial leads (V1, V2, and V3) or beyond in individuals >14 years of age (in the absence of complete RBBB)

Minor
Inverted T waves in V1 and V2 in individuals >14 years of age (in the absence of complete RBBB) or in V4, V5, and V6

Inverted T waves in leads V1, V2, V3, and V4 in individuals >14 years of age in the presence of complete RBBB

Depolarization/Conduction Abnormalities
Major
Epsilon wave (reproducible low-amplitude signals between end of QRS complex to onset of T wave) in the right precordial leads (V1, V2, or V3)

Minor
Late potentials by SAECG in ≥1 of 3 parameters in the absence of a QRS duration of ≥110 ms on standard ECG:
- Filtered QRS duration (fQRS) ≥114 ms
- Duration of terminal QRS <40 μV ≥38 ms
- Root-mean-square voltage of terminal 40 ms ≤20 μV

Terminal activation duration ≥55 ms measured from the nadir of the end of all depolarization deflections, including R', in V1, V2, or V3 in absence of complete RBBB

Arrhythmias
Major
Nonsustained or sustained VT of LBBB morphology with superior axis

Minor
Nonsustained or sustained VT of RVOT configuration, LBBB morphology with inferior axis or of unknown axis

>500 PVCs per 24 hours on Holter monitoring

Family History
Major
ARVC in first-degree relative who meets Task Force Criteria

ARVC confirmed pathologically at autopsy or surgery in first-degree relative

Identification of pathogenic mutation categorized as associated or probably associated with ARVC in the patient under evaluation

Minor
History of ARVC in first-degree relative in whom it is not possible to determine whether the family member meets Task Force Criteria

Premature sudden death (<35 years of age) due to suspected ARVC in first-degree relative

ARVC confirmed pathologically or by current Task Force Criteria in second-degree relative

ARVC, Arrhythmogenic right ventricular cardiomyopathy; *BSA*, body surface area; *ECG*, electrocardiogram; *EDV*, end-diastolic volume; *LBBB*, left bundle branch block; *PLAX*, parasternal long axis; *PSAX*, parasternal short axis; *PVCs*, premature ventricular complexes; *RBBB*, right bundle branch block; *RV*, right ventricular; *RVOT*, right ventricular outflow tract; *SAECG*, signal-averaged electrocardiogram; *VT*, ventricular tachycardia.
Modified from Marcus FI, McKenna WJ, Sherrill D, et al. Diagnosis of arrhythmogenic right ventricular cardiomyopathy/dysplasia: proposed modification of the task force criteria. *Circulation.* 2010;121:1533–1541.

values, RV dimension and function from 462 normal MESA participants were compared with 44 probands in the North American ARVC registry.[9] Major criteria (RV ejection fraction ≤40% *or* indexed RV end-diastolic volume ≥110 mL/m² for men and ≥100 mL/m² for women) were chosen to achieve approximately 95% specificity. Cutoffs with high specificity invariably result in lower sensitivity; this accounts for the major CMR criteria sensitivity of 68% to 76%.[14] Minor criteria (RV ejection fraction 40%–45% *or* indexed RV end-diastolic volume 100–110 mL/m² for men and 90–100 mL/m² for women) had a higher sensitivity (79%–89%), but a consequently lower specificity (85%–97%).[14]

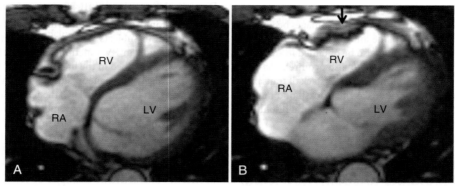

FIG. 34.2 Regional contraction abnormality in the subtricuspid region. End-diastolic (A) and end-systolic (B) images show the so-called accordion sign *(arrow)* in an arrhythmogenic right ventricular cardiomyopathy mutation carrier. Regional dyssynchronous contraction in the subtricuspid region is a readily recognized qualitative pattern of abnormal right ventricular contraction. *LV,* Left ventricle; *RA,* right atrium; *RV,* right ventricle.

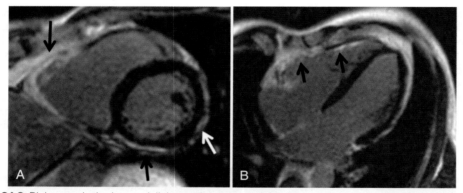

FIG. 34.3 Right ventricular late gadolinium enhancement (LGE) in arrhythmogenic right ventricular cardiomyopathy. The short-axis image (A) shows LGE in the right ventricle as well as the left ventricle *(black arrows).* The lateral wall of the left ventricle shows thinning because of fatty replacement *(white arrow)* that was confirmed on T1-weighted images. The long axis view (B) shows diffuse LGE involving the free wall of the right ventricle *(black arrows).*

Late Gadolinium Enhancement

Myocardial late gadolinium enhancement (LGE) is a well-validated technique for assessment of myocardial fibrosis, and has frequently been associated with ARVC: RV LGE has been observed in up to 88% of ARVC patients,[28,32] whereas LV LGE was reported in up to 61% of cases.[28,33,34] A characteristic example is shown in Fig. 34.3. Given that one of the pathologic hallmarks of ARVC is fibrofatty replacement of the myocardium, it is important to note that LGE is not incorporated in the current diagnostic TFC. Although the Task Force did recognize the presence of LGE in many patients with ARVC, several limitations withheld its inclusion in the TFC. First, detection of LGE in the RV is greatly hampered by the thin RV wall. In ARVC, RV wall thinning is pronounced, which makes the LGE technique less reliable than for the LV. Second, distinguishing fat from fibrosis by LGE sequences is challenging, which makes its interpretation highly subject to the CMR physician's experience. Last, LV LGE is nonspecific and has a wide differential diagnosis. LGE may be observed in many mimics of ARVC, such as sarcoidosis, myocarditis, amyloidosis, and dilated cardiomyopathy (DCM).

However, keeping these limitations in mind, LGE may be very useful in ARVC evaluation. Tandri et al.[32] showed excellent correlation of RV LGE with histopathology and inducible ventricular arrhythmias on electrophysiologic study. Identification of LGE by CMR may therefore provide guidance for electrophysiologic studies and endomyocardial biopsy. LGE CMR is also extremely useful when ARVC is excluded as a result of other cardiomyopathy such as sarcoidosis. In our opinion, the presence of LGE represents a late stage of ARVC; when LGE is present, multiple other findings of advanced disease are typically present, such as RV dilatation and dysfunction.[28] Importantly, before LGE can be included in a future iteration of the TFC, more data regarding the specific patterns of LGE that distinguish ARVC from other cardiomyopathies are necessary. Also, improved methods to determine fibrosis in the thin RV wall are needed. Until such a method emerges, the presence of LGE should be considered as diagnostic confirmation, not sole evidence of ARVC disease expression.

Left Ventricular Involvement

The advent of genetic testing and use of sensitive TFC have significantly increased our awareness of the phenotypic spectrum of ARVC, which also includes nonclassical (e.g., left-dominant and biventricular) phenotypes. As a result, we now know that some ARVC subjects have early and predominant LV involvement.[34,35] LV involvement has even been reported in 76% of ARVC subjects, of whom the majority had advanced disease.[36] The disease is therefore increasingly being referred to as "arrhythmogenic cardiomyopathy."[34,37]

In 2010, Jain led a study investigating LV regional dysfunction using CMR tagging, and found that LV peak systolic strain was lower in ARVC

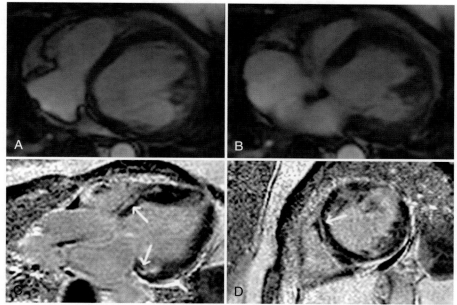

FIG. 34.4 Horizontal long-axis (A–B) bright-blood and late gadolinium enhancement images (C–D) in an arrhythmogenic right ventricular subject with predominant left ventricular abnormalities. Note a dilated left ventricle in the bright-blood images. Late enhancement is observed in a midmyocardial pattern in the basal septum and basal lateral wall (*arrows* in C–D).

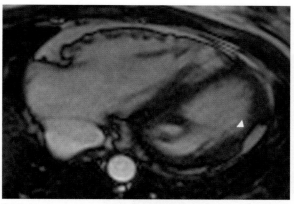

FIG. 34.5 Horizontal long-axis bright-blood image in an arrhythmogenic right ventricular cardiomyopathy patient revealing left ventricular lateral wall fatty infiltration with myocardial wall thinning (*arrowhead*).

subjects compared with controls.[38] Sen-Chowdhry et al.[34] recently published data supporting a genetic association between left-dominant ARVC and classical right-sided ARVC. In their study, the authors showed that one-third of genotyped ARVC patients with a left-dominant phenotype have a pathogenic mutation in the ARVC-related desmosomal genes. Phenotypic variations of predominant RV and LV involvement even coexisted in the same family.

LV involvement in ARVC typically manifests as LGE, often involving the inferior and lateral walls without concomitant wall motion abnormalities.[29,39] Fig. 34.4 shows an example. Septal LGE is present in more than 50% of cases with left-dominant ARVC, in contrast with the right-dominant pattern in which septal involvement is unusual. In addition, LV fatty infiltration was shown to be a prevalent finding in ARVC, often involving the subepicardial lateral LV and resulting in myocardial wall thinning (Fig. 34.5).[29,40] Future studies are necessary to confirm these data, and further our understanding of LV abnormalities in ARVC.

Misdiagnosis of Arrhythmogenic Right Ventricular Cardiomyopathy Using Cardiovascular Magnetic Resonance

Misdiagnosis of ARVC is a well-recognized problem. A prior study has shown that more than 70% of patients who were referred to Johns Hopkins Hospital from outside institutions with a diagnosis of ARVC did not actually meet diagnostic TFC.[41] In many cases, CMR misinterpretation is the cause of overdiagnosis in ARVC.[41,42] It is important to realize that, although CMR may be regarded as the standard of reference for evaluation of RV morphology and function, the use of CMR alone is not the "gold standard" for ARVC diagnosis. Rather, the TFC prescribe the use of multiple diagnostic tests.[9] Great caution must be employed when the only abnormality in a presumed ARVC patient is found on CMR because it is uncommon for ARVC patients to have a normal electrocardiogram (ECG) and Holter monitor but an abnormal CMR.[43,44]

ARVC misdiagnosis may occur because of an over-reliance on a single morphologic imaging finding, such as fatty replacement.[41,42] The focus on fatty replacement in ARVC evaluation is understandable because fibrofatty replacement of the myocardium is a unique pathologic hallmark of ARVC. However, intramyocardial fat also occurs physiologically in older, obese patients (Fig. 34.6). In addition, multiple reports have shown that CMR detection of intramyocardial fat was not reproducible even among experienced readers, constituting an important cause of misdiagnosis.[45–47] An apparently benign condition, lipomatous infiltration of the RV anterior wall shows abundant RV fat but does not demonstrate regional wall motion abnormality, which is otherwise required for ARVC diagnosis.[46] In summary, replacement of the myocardium by fat is not specific for ARVC in the absence of functional abnormalities.[48]

Furthermore, normal variants may mimic ARVC. A comprehensive description of ARVC mimics is available elsewhere.[49] In short, important normal variants previously mistaken for ARVC are pectus excavatum,[50] apical-lateral bulging of the RV free wall at the insertion

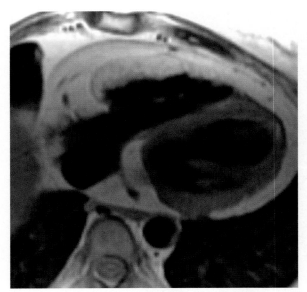

FIG. 34.6 A 45-year-old female with abundant lipomatous replacement of the anterior right ventricular wall by fat. This condition appears to be associated with obesity and abundant pericardial and mediastinal fat. Right ventricular wall motion was normal.

of the moderator band,[51] and the "butterfly apex," a normal anatomic variant of separate RV and LV apices causing the RV apex to look dyskinetic.[49] We have found the butterfly appearance of the apex to be more common on horizontal long-axis views at inferior levels (Fig. 34.7). In addition, a prominent band of pericardial connective tissue joining the RV free wall to the posterior sternum may lead to misinterpretation of RV wall motion; this "tethered" portion of the RV free wall remains static in location and may be misinterpreted as RV dyskinesia (Fig. 34.8).

In our experience, sarcoidosis is the most common mimic of ARVC, but other disorders, such as DCM and myocarditis, may also have diagnostic overlap with ARVC.[52,53] Table 34.2 shows a list of clinical features and CMR findings of conditions potentially confused with ARVC.[54] Compared with DCM, patients with (left-dominant) ARVC often have significant ventricular arrhythmias, disproportionate to the morphologic abnormalities and impaired LV systolic function. In addition, inflammatory processes, such as (viral) myocarditis, may mimic ARVC.[53] In myocarditis, T2-weighted imaging may detect tissue edema, which is usually absent in ARVC. In addition, fast spin echo T1-weighted images during the first minutes after contrast injection may be useful to detect myocardial hyperemia and muscular inflammation suggestive of myocarditis.[53] In equivocal cases, invasive studies, such as electroanatomic mapping and endomyocardial biopsy, may provide a more definite diagnosis.

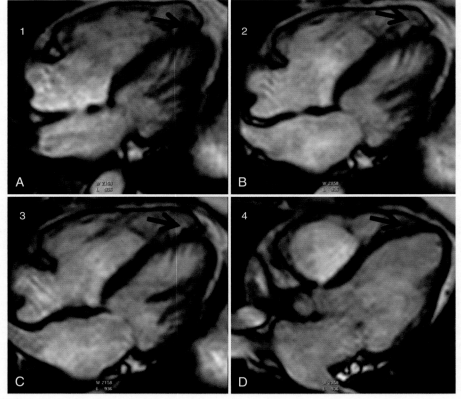

FIG. 34.7 Butterfly apex as a normal variation. Stack of horizontal long-axis views from inferior (A) to superior (D) in a control subject. Note the appearance of a butterfly apex on inferior views (*arrows* in A–C). This appearance is not seen on the more superior view (D). This is a normal variant.

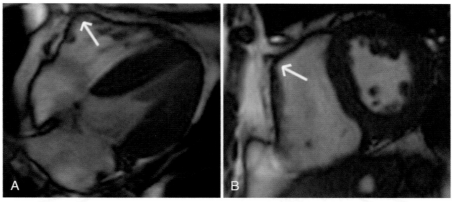

FIG. 34.8 Misdiagnosis of arrhythmogenic right ventricular cardiomyopathy: axial (A) and short-axis (B) bright-blood images in a control subject. Note the "tethering" of the mid right ventricular free wall to the anterior chest wall *(arrows)*, giving the right ventricle a dyskinetic appearance.

TABLE 34.2 Clinical Findings of Conditions Considered in the Differential Diagnosis of Arrhythmogenic Right Ventricular Cardiomyopathy

Condition	Finding
Sarcoidosis	Clinical findings: more common in women, African-Americans, and Northern European (Scandinavian) whites. Usually nonfamilial disease pattern. May present with extracardiac manifestations (often pulmonary/mediastinal lymphadenopathy, but any organ system may be involved). ECG may show PR interval prolongation and/or high-grade atrioventricular block. CMR findings: pulmonary granulomas, mediastinal lymphadenopathy, decreased LV function/heart failure, LGE (nonischemic pattern) in the interventricular septum.
Myocarditis	Clinical findings: may present with a viral prodrome with fever, myalgia, respiratory and gastrointestinal symptoms, new-onset atrial or ventricular arrhythmias, complete heart block, or acute myocardial infarction-like syndrome with chest pain, ST-T changes, and elevated cardiac enzymes. CMR findings: increased T2 signal due to tissue edema (acute phase), concomitant pericardial involvement, subepicardial patchy myocardial LGE (nonischemic pattern).
DCM	Clinical findings: variable. May be familial. Ventricular arrhythmias usually occur in the context of impaired LV systolic function and morphologic abnormalities. CMR findings: dilated LV with reduced function, midwall LGE enhancement in the septum.
Athlete's heart	Clinical findings: clinical history is indicative; subjects are typically engaged in intense and repetitive endurance type sports. Physical examination may show low heart rate, especially in young athletes. CMR findings: balanced dilatation of cardiac chambers, increased ventricular wall thickness (<15 mm), absence of regional ventricular dysfunction or regional wall motion abnormalities; lack of LGE on CMR.
Idiopathic RVOT VT	Clinical findings: benign, nonfamilial condition, only one VT morphology (LBBB with inferior axis), sinus rhythm ECG normal. CMR findings: normal.
Brugada syndrome	Clinical findings: ECG reveals RBBB and persistent ST segment elevation in the right precordial leads (spontaneous or after provocative drug challenge). Arrhythmias often occur in a sedentary setting (after a meal or at rest due to high vagal tone). Imaging findings: traditionally considered to be normal, although structural disease is increasingly reported.

CMR, Cardiovascular magnetic resonance imaging; *DCM,* dilated cardiomyopathy; *ECG,* electrocardiogram; *LBBB,* left bundle branch block; *LGE,* late gadolinium enhancement; *LV,* left ventricular; *PET,* positron emission tomography; *RBBB,* right bundle branch block; *RVOT,* right ventricular outflow tract; *VT,* ventricular tachycardia.
From Te Riele ASJM, Tandri H, Sanborn DM, Bluemke DA. Noninvasive multimodality imaging in arrhythmogenic right ventricular dysplasia/cardiomyopathy. *JACC Cardiovasc Imaging.* 2015;8(5):597–611.

GENETIC BACKGROUND OF ARRHYTHMOGENIC RIGHT VENTRICULAR CARDIOMYOPATHY

Beginning with the seminal discovery of plakoglobin in 2000, the past decade has witnessed the identification of mutations in five genes encoding the cardiac desmosome.[5] In recent reports, desmosomal mutations are found in up to 60% of ARVC cases.[2] A cartoon representation of the desmosome is shown in Fig. 34.9. Among US ARVC patients, the most common gene involved is plakophilin-2, followed by desmoglein-2, desmocollin-2, and desmoplakin.[2,55] Prevalence of mutations is similar in Europe, although desmoplakin mutations are more prevalent in the United Kingdom and Italy.[56,57] Desmosomes are complex multiprotein structures providing mechanical and electrical continuity to adjacent cells. Mechanical uncoupling in ARVC is accompanied by cell death and regional fibrosis, which causes the monomorphic arrhythmias typically associated with ARVC.[58] In addition, electrical uncoupling through

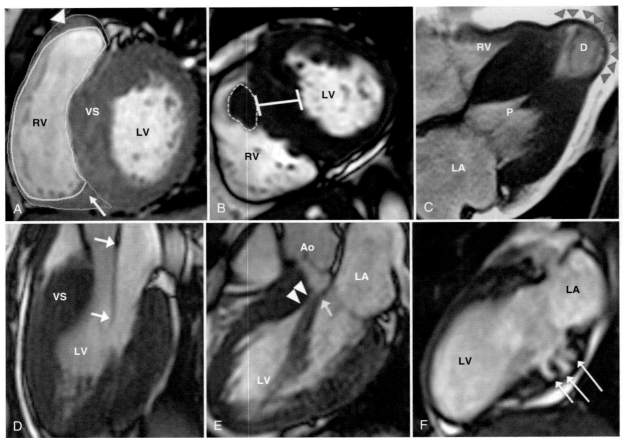

FIG. 36.4 Cardiovascular magnetic resonance (CMR) end-diastolic images demonstrating diversity of the phenotypic expression within hypertrophic cardiomyopathy (HCM). (A) Increased wall thickness in the superior segment *(arrowhead)* and inferior segment *(arrow)* of the right ventricular (RV) free wall. (B) Prominent and hypertrophied crista supraventricularis *(outlined structure)* and RV muscle structure. It is important not to include this muscle structure in the measurement of ventricular septum because this can lead to overestimation of maximal left ventricular (LV) wall thickness. (C) Medium-sized LV apical aneurysm *(arrowheads)* and maximum wall thickness at midventricular level with muscular apposition of the ventricular septum and LV free wall producing distinct proximal *(P)* and distal *(D)* chamber. (D) Elongation of the anterior mitral valve leaflet *(arrows)*, contributing to LV outflow obstruction in this patient. (E) Muscular midcavitary obstruction attributable to the insertion of anomalous anterolateral papillary muscle directly into anterior leaflet *(arrow)*, contacting the midventricular septum in systole *(arrowheads)*. (F) Asymptomatic genotype-positive, phenotype-negative patient with three deep myocardial crypts in the basal inferior LV wall. *Ao,* Aorta; *LA,* left atrium; *LV,* left ventricle; *RV,* right ventricle; *VS,* ventricular septum. (A, Modified from Maron MS, Hauser TH, Dubrow E, et al. Right ventricular involvement in hypertrophic cardiomyopathy. *Am J Cardiol.* 2007;100:1293–1298. D, Modified from Maron MS, Olivotto I, Harrigan C, et al. Mitral valve abnormalities identified by cardiovascular magnetic resonance represent a primary phenotypic expression of hypertrophic cardiomyopathy. *Circulation.* 2011;124:40–47. F, From Maron MS, Rowin EJ, Lin D, et al. Prevalence and clinical profile of myocardial crypts in hypertrophic cardiomyopathy. *Circ Cardiovasc Imaging.* 2012;5:441–447.)

HF symptoms.[4] Obstructive patients with advanced symptoms refractory to medical management become candidates for septal reduction interventions with surgical myectomy (or, alternatively, alcohol septal ablation) for relief of LVOT gradients.[1,2]

Given the importance of LVOT obstruction in dictating management strategies in HCM patients, accurate and reliable measurements of the pressure gradients remain critical. CMR allows for visualization of SAM and septal contact, but it is limited in reliably measuring dynamic LVOT pressure gradients in HCM.[1,9] Therefore TTE, via continuous wave Doppler, remains the preferred technique for assessing outflow gradients.[1]

Selection and Planning for Septal Reduction

CMR has emerged to have an important role in the morphologic evaluation of the LVOT and anomalies contributing to the mechanism of subaortic obstruction, including elongated mitral valve leaflet lengths[19] (Fig. 36.4D), anomalous insertion of the anterior papillary muscle directed into the mitral leaflet[28] (Fig. 36.4E), and muscle bundles that extend from the apex and attach into the basal anterior septum.[29] The identification of these features may be missed by TTE, yet are important because they potentially alter the septal reduction strategy in favor of surgical myectomy, as a percutaneous approach using alcohol septal

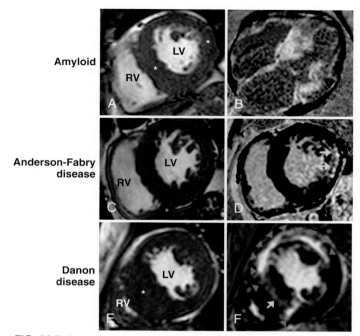

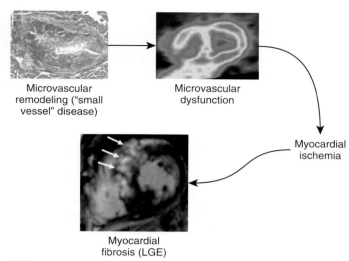

FIG. 36.6 Proposed mechanism for late gadolinium enhancement *(LGE)* in hypertrophic cardiomyopathy (HCM). Structurally abnormal intramural coronary arteries are responsible for microvascular ischemia. Over time, myocyte cell death and a process of repair with replacement fibrosis can be imaged as LGE in HCM.

FIG. 36.5 Cardiovascular magnetic resonance (CMR) for differentiation of etiology of left ventricular (LV) hypertrophy. (A) 64-year-old male with concentric LV hypertrophy (maximum LV wall thickness of 18 mm in septum and 14 mm in lateral wall). (B) Late gadolinium enhancement (LGE) image in the same patient demonstrates early contrast washout with transmural LGE in septum and lateral wall *(arrows)* features consistent with cardiac amyloid. The patient underwent cardiac biopsy confirming the diagnosis of amyloid. (C) A 44-year-old female with concentric LV hypertrophy (maximum wall thickness of 16 mm in septum and 13 mm in the lateral wall). (D) LGE image in the same patient demonstrates LGE confined to the basal inferolateral wall *(arrows)*, a location of LGE typical for Anderson-Fabry disease. The patient underwent genetic testing, which demonstrated pathogenic mutation in the GLA gene, confirming the diagnosis of Anderson-Fabry disease. (E) A 21-year-old male demonstrated massive LV hypertrophy (wall thickness of 32 mm) confined to the ventricular septum *(asterisk)*. (F) LGE images in the same patient demonstrated transmural LGE throughout the anterior and lateral walls *(arrowheads)* with mid-myocardial LGE throughout the septum *(arrow)* in a pattern atypical for HCM. Genetic testing was sent and revealed a pathogenic mutation in the LAMP2 gene, consistent with Danon cardiomyopathy. *LV,* Left ventricle; *RV,* right ventricle.

ablation is unable to intervene on these specific structural abnormalities[9,30] (see Fig. 36.2).

The identification of these morphologic abnormalities also may alter preoperative surgical planning because they dictate a specific surgical strategy[9,30] (see Fig. 36.2). Specifically, mitral valve leaflets are substantially increased in length in one-third of HCM patients and contribute to LV outflow obstruction, particularly when the leaflet length exceeds 2-fold the transverse dimension of the outflow tract at end systole.[17,30] In obstructive HCM patients with this abnormality, surgical strategy may be altered to perform extended myectomy trough and mitral valve repair (with plication) to eliminate SAM and the outflow gradient with less extensive septal hypertrophy (wall thickness ≤17 mm). CMR also allows for the reliable identification of anomalous and direct papillary muscle insertion into the anterior mitral leaflet, an uncommon but important mechanism of muscular obstruction,[28] which dictates a specific surgical approach with deep, extended muscular resection well beyond the contact point of the mitral valve and ventricular septum as well as reduction in papillary muscle thickness.[31] Similarly, apically

displaced accessory anterolateral or double bifid papillary muscles can tether the plan of the mitral valve toward the septum, contributing to the mechanism of obstruction.[30,32] The surgeon can address these abnormalities by resecting these muscles to ensure a complete abolishment of obstruction.

PATHOPHYSIOLOGY AND CLINICAL PROFILE OF LATE GADOLINIUM ENHANCEMENT IN HYPERTROPHIC CARDIOMYOPATHY

Histopathology

Areas of LGE in HCM are considered to represent the end result of a pathophysiologic cascade in which blunted myocardial blood flow due to abnormal intramural coronary arteries results in myocyte cell death and reparative processes of fibrosis (imaged as LGE)[33] (Fig. 36.6). This principle is supported by imaging studies in which myocardial blood flow is decreased during stress in areas occupied by, and directly adjacent to, regions of myocardial fibrosis as assessed by LGE.[34]

A number of histopathologic studies have identified LGE to represent fibrosis.[35,36] In ventricular septal tissue removed from HCM patients at the time of surgical myectomy, there is a stronger association between the extent of interstitial and replacement fibrosis assessed by histologic examination and LGE seen on preoperative CMR studies.[36] In addition, case reports of explanted HCM hearts have demonstrated strong correlation between areas of LGE on pretransplant CMR and replacement fibrosis by histologic evaluation.[35]

Clinical Profile

Up to 60% of all HCM patients demonstrate some LGE, which, when present, occupies an average of 9% of total LV myocardial volume.[37] Virtually any pattern, distribution, and location of LGE can be observed in HCM, although in general the location of LGE does not correspond to a coronary vascular distribution[37–41] (Fig. 36.7). Most commonly, LGE is located in both the ventricular septum and the free wall (in over 30% of patients), but less commonly can be confined to the apex and the areas of RV insertion into the interventricular septum.[42,43] LGE can also occur in other myocardial structures outside of the LV wall, including the RV wall, and papillary muscles.[32] Transmural extent of

LGE is not uncommon, occurring in one-half of patients.[42] A significant but modest relationship exists between hypertrophy and LGE: patients with LGE have greater maximal LV wall thickness and LV mass index than patients without LGE. On an individual patient basis, there is a relationship between the segmental LV wall thickness and LGE.[42,43] In contrast, prevalence and extent of LGE are no different across different genders or across different age ranges, including in elderly (≥65 years old) and younger (≤35 years old) HCM patients.[37]

LATE GADOLINIUM ENHANCEMENT AND PROGNOSIS

Sudden Cardiac Death

HCM remains the most common cause of sudden death in young patients.[1,2,7] Currently, American Heart Association/American College of Cardiology (AHA/ACC) guidelines recommend the identification of high-risk patients based on the presence of five noninvasive conventional risk factors,[1] whereas more recently the European Society of Cardiology (ESC) has promoted a risk score based on a mathematical formula taking into account numerous clinical variables.[2] However, current risk stratification strategies do not recognize all HCM patients at risk for sudden death, underscoring the need to identify additional markers of risk to more reliably identify high-risk patients, for whom LGE has been promoted.[37–41]

Early cross-sectional studies demonstrated a strong association between the presence of LGE and ventricular tachyarrhythmias on ambulatory 24-hour Holter ECG in HCM, with LGE conferring up to a 7-fold increased risk for ambulatory nonsustained ventricular tachyarrhythmias compared with HCM patients without LGE[44] (see Fig. 36.7). These results suggested that ventricular tachyarrhythmias emanate from regions of structurally abnormal myocardium, providing the rationale for a number of longitudinal LGE outcome studies. When combining the data together in a pooled manner, the presence of LGE is associated with an increased risk for sudden death.[45] However, LGE is common in HCM, with a prevalence of over 50% (and up to 70% in some select populations). Thus assessing LGE only in a binary fashion (presence vs. absence) is not a practical strategy as a risk marker because it would lead to over implantation of primary prevention ICD devices.[9]

Three large studies have been completed evaluating the extent of LGE and sudden death risk. When analyzed in a pooled manner, a strong relationship is evident between the amount of LGE and the risk of a sudden death event[45] (Table 36.1). The largest of these studies by Chan et al.,[37] a multicenter study employing a core laboratory analysis of almost 1300 HCM patients followed for an average of 3 years after CMR, demonstrated a statistically significant relationship between the amount of LGE and sudden death events as well as total mortality (see Fig. 36.7), with extensive LGE (≥15% of LV mass) associated with a 2-fold greater risk of sudden death events compared with patients with no LGE (Fig. 36.8), including in patients without any of the conventional sudden death risk markers. In addition, in patients with ≥1 conventional risk factor, the extent of LGE strengthened the current sudden death risk model by providing information that improved the ability to identify both high-risk and low-risk patients. On the other hand, patients without LGE had a relatively benign course and were at low risk for adverse events[37] (see Fig. 36.8). When data from this study were combined with Ismail et al.,[41] the other large study that adjusted for other variables known to impact sudden death risk, the extent of

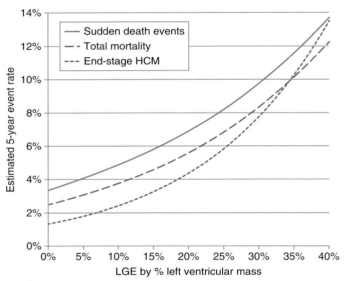

FIG. 36.7 Predicted 5-year event rates relative to the percentage of late gadolinium enhancement *(LGE)* for the risk of end-stage hypertrophic cardiomyopathy *(HCM)* with systolic dysfunction, sudden death events, and total mortality. (From Chan RH, Maron BJ, Olivotto I, et al. Prognostic value of quantitative contrast-enhanced cardiovascular magnetic resonance for the evaluation of sudden death risk in patients with hypertrophic cardiomyopathy. *Circulation.* 2014;130:484–513.)

TABLE 36.1   Metaanalysis for Late Gadolinium Enhancement and Sudden Death

Study	Unadjusted HR, per 10% LV Mass	95% CI	P	Adjusted HR, per 10% LV Mass	95% CI	P
SCD						
Bruder et al.[39]	1.7	1.2–2.5	< .01	NA	NA	NA
Ismail et al.[41]	1.5	1.1–2.1	.007	1.2	0.8–1.7	.2
Chan et al.[37]	1.5	1.2–1.8	< .0001	1.4	1.1–1.9	.002
Pooled	1.5	1.3–1.8	< .0001	1.3	1.1–1.6	.005
HF Death						
Ismail et al.[41]	1.5	1.0–2.1	.028	NA	NA	NA
Chan et al.[37]	1.7	1.1–2.7	.01	NA	NA	NA

CI, Confidence interval; *HF*, heart failure; *HR*, hazard ratio; *LGE*, late gadolinium enhancement; *LV*, left ventricular; *NA*, not available; *SCD*, sudden cardiac death.
Modified from Weng Z, Yao J, Chan RH, et al. Prognostic value of LGE-CMR in HCM: a meta-analysis. *JACC Cardiovasc Imaging.* 2016;9:1392–1402.

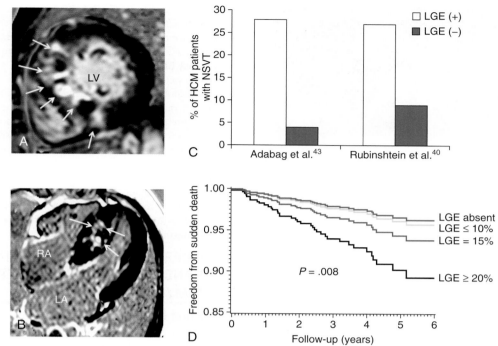

FIG. 36.8 Relationship between late gadolinium enhancement *(LGE)* and sudden death risk in hypertrophic cardiomyopathy *(HCM)*. (A and B) LGE CMR images in two different HCM patients, each with extensive LGE *(arrows)* throughout the ventricular septum. (C) Nonsustained ventricular tachycardia *(NSVT)* on 24-hour Holter electrocardiogram (ECG) is 7-fold more common in HCM patients with LGE compared with those without LGE. (D) Relation between extent of LGE and sudden death events in 1293 patients with HCM. *LV,* Left ventricle; *RV,* right ventricle. (Modified from Chan RH, Maron BJ, Olivotto I, et al. Prognostic value of quantitative contrast-enhanced cardiovascular magnetic resonance for the evaluation of sudden death risk in patients with hypertrophic cardiomyopathy. *Circulation* 2014;130:484–513.)

TABLE 36.2 Adjusted Hazard Ratios for Sudden Cardiac Death Using Data From Chan et al.[37] and Ismail et al.[41]

LGE %	Pooled HR$_{adjusted}$ Point Estimate	95% CI
0	1.0	—
1	1.03	1.01–1.05
10	1.36	1.10–1.69
15	1.59	1.15–2.20
20	1.86	1.21–2.86
30	2.5	1.33–4.83
40	3.4	1.46–8.16

CI, Confidence interval; *HR,* hazard ratio; *LGE,* late gadolinium enhancement.
Modified from Weng Z, Yao J, Chan RH, et al. Prognostic value of LGE-CMR in HCM: a meta-analysis. *JACC Cardiovasc Imaging.* 2016;9:1392–1402.

LGE remained a strong independent predictor of sudden death events (Table 36.2).

It is not possible to make reliable associations between the pattern of LGE and the outcome in HCM, a result of the enormous diversity observed in the distribution of LGE in this disease. Indeed, the only reliable LGE pattern seen in HCM is the relatively specific pattern of LGE confined to the RV insertion area (either anterior, inferior, or both)[42–44] (Fig. 36.9). However, neither the presence nor the extent of LGE in the RV insertion area of the LV appears to be a reliable predictor of adverse HCM-related events, including sudden cardiac death (SCD)[46] (see Fig. 36.9). This is probably related to the morphologic observation that the LGE in the RV insertion point is composed primarily of expanded extracellular space with interstitial fibrosis embedded within disorderly arranged myocytes without replacement fibrosis.

Based on these observations, it is now reasonable to consider incorporating the results of LGE CMR in the assessment of sudden death risk in patients with HCM[1,2,9,38–45] (Fig. 36.10). First, extensive (≥15% LV volume) LGE identifies HCM patients at increased risk for sudden death (even without a conventional risk factor) and could be deserving of consideration for primary prevention ICD.[1,9,37,45] In addition, extensive LGE can act as an arbitrator to help resolve decision making regarding ICD when sudden death risk remains ambiguous after standard risk stratification because it can serve as an arbitrator toward ICD placement. In contrast, the absence of (or minimal) LGE is associated with lower risk for sudden death and should provide a measure of reassurance and can arbitrate away from device therapy in ambiguous risk situations, potentially avoiding unnecessary ICD.[37] Further insights into the role of LGE in the management of at-risk HCM patients will emerge from the completion of the international multicenter Hypertrophic Cardiomyopathy Registry (HCMR) study.[47]

Heart Failure

A small subset of nonobstructed HCM patients are at risk for developing progressive HF symptoms refractory to pharmacologic treatment. These patients constitute two distinct subgroups: patients with impaired LV systolic function and adverse LV remodeling associated with extensive

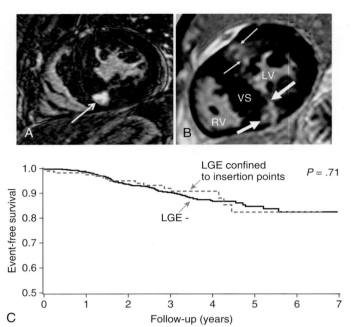

FIG. 36.9 Significance of right ventricular (RV) insertion point late gadolinium enhancement *(LGE)* in hypertrophic cardiomyopathy (HCM). (A and B) The confluence of the RV wall and ventricular septum (RV insertion point) is a common area for LGE in HCM and can occur in either the anterior, inferior (A) *(arrow)* or both (B) *(thin arrow,* anterior; *thick arrow,* inferior) insertion points. (C) Kaplan-Meier event-free survival curves comparing 134 patients with HCM and LGE confined to the RV insertion areas compared with 745 patients with HCM without LGE, demonstrating no significant difference in HCM-related event-free survival. *LV,* Left ventricle; *RV,* right ventricle; *VS,* ventricular septum. (Modified from Chan RH, Maron BJ, Olivotto I, et al. Significance of late gadolinium enhancement at right ventricular attachment to ventricular septum in patients with hypertrophic cardiomyopathy. *Am J Cardiol.* 2015;116:436–441.)

LV fibrosis (ejection fraction [EF] <50%; end stage),[48] and patients with preserved LV systolic function with little or no remodeling.[1,2] Extensive LGE has been observed as an emerging marker to prospectively identify HCM patients with preserved systolic function who are at increased risk for future development of end stage (see Fig. 36.7).[37,41,45] Patients who develop end stage are at increased risk for advanced HF symptoms at some point in their clinical course, often necessitating consideration for heart transplant.[47] In support of this principle, pooled data for the two largest LGE follow-up studies in HCM demonstrated a significant increase in risk for HF death with increasing amounts of LGE[45] (see Table 36.1).

QUANTIFICATION OF LATE GADOLINIUM ENHANCEMENT

Numerous techniques have been proposed to quantify the extent of LGE in HCM. At the time of this writing, there are no expert consensus recommendations regarding the preferred strategy. The most widely used approaches include semiautomated algorithms that identify high signal intensity LGE pixels in the LV wall after applying a grayscale threshold a number of standard deviations (SDs) above the mean signal intensity within a remote region containing normal "nulled" myocardium (i.e., 2, 4, 5, or 6 SDs) and the full width at half maximum (FWHM) method (pixels with a signal intensity >50% of the maximum intensity

of the brightest region of hyperenhancement).[49,50] In an individual patient with HCM there may be significant differences in amount of LGE identified depending on which SD threshold is chosen, with 2 SDs resulting in a 2-fold greater amount of LGE compared with 6 SDs.[49]

However, higher grayscale thresholds (6 SDs) and FWHM have appeared to yield the closest approximation to the extent of LGE identified visually and the most reproducible.[36,48] In addition, higher grayscale thresholding methods (such as 5 or 6 SDs) have been shown to provide the best representation of total fibrosis burden as demonstrated by histopathologic analysis of ventricular septal tissue removed in HCM patients undergoing surgical myectomy.[36] Of note, grayscale threshold can also be performed manually and adjusted to define areas of visually identified LGE. This method was used to assess the extent of LGE in the Chan et al.[37] multicenter LGE study in predicting sudden death events because it correlates well to the amount LGE quantified using high grayscale threshold cutoffs, has excellent reproducibility, and is less time consuming to perform.

OTHER CARDIOVASCULAR MAGNETIC RESONANCE TECHNIQUES IN HYPERTROPHIC CARDIOMYOPATHY

Myocardial Perfusion

In HCM, the intramural coronary arterioles are structurally abnormal, with small lumen resulting in blunted myocardial blood flow (MBF) during stress (i.e., microvascular dysfunction). CMR perfusion sequences can assess MBF at rest and during pharmacologic stress (typically adenosine, regadenoson, or dipyridamole) with superior spatial resolution. Regional differences in MBF have been observed within LV segments, with MBF reduced in the subendocardial layer compared with subepicardium, and the degree of abnormal perfusion related to the magnitude of wall thickness.[51] In addition, MBF also appears reduced in LV segments with LGE, suggesting that microvascular dysfunction may be responsible for myocardial ischemia-mediated myocyte death, and ultimately repair in the form of replacement fibrosis.[51] However, sufficient longitudinal follow-up studies with stress CMR in HCM have not been completed. Therefore the clinical significance and management implications of CMR MBF abnormalities remain uncertain.

Myocardial Tagging

Diastolic function is abnormal in nearly all HCM patients and is the major etiology of HF symptoms in nonobstructive patients with preserved LV systolic function. Proposed mechanisms for this dysfunction in HCM include myocardial disarray, microvascular ischemia, interstitial and replacement fibrosis, as well as LV hypertrophy. Myocardial tagging SPAMM offers the opportunity to quantify diastolic function in CMR by examining myocardial mechanical parameters, such as strain and torsion, and has been demonstrated to be abnormal within HCM.[52] These abnormalities are correlated both to magnitude of LV hypertrophy as well as areas of LGE in HCM. Of important note, these features can be abnormal even in areas free of hypertrophy and without LGE, demonstrating the multifactorial etiologies of abnormal diastolic function within HCM. Although of potential research interest, to date, tagging has not been shown to be associated with clinical outcomes within this disease and thereby has an uncertain role in clinical evaluation and management of HCM patients. As mentioned earlier, SPAMM may also be useful in discriminating physiologic hypertrophy from aortic stenosis due to HCM.[23]

Native T1 Mapping

Native T1 mapping and extracellular volume fraction (ECV) are novel, emerging CMR techniques that provide a noninvasive assessment of

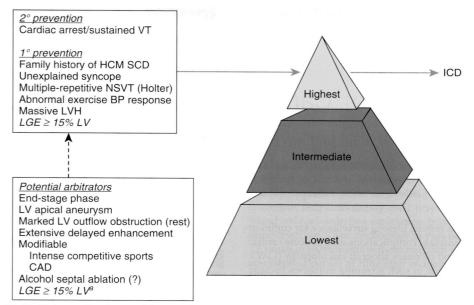

2° prevention
Cardiac arrest/sustained VT

1° prevention
Family history of HCM SCD
Unexplained syncope
Multiple-repetitive NSVT (Holter)
Abnormal exercise BP response
Massive LVH
LGE ≥ 15% LV

Potential arbitrators
End-stage phase
LV apical aneurysm
Marked LV outflow obstruction (rest)
Extensive delayed enhancement
Modifiable
    Intense competitive sports
    CAD
Alcohol septal ablation (?)
LGE ≥ 15% LV[a]

Highest → ICD
Intermediate
Lowest

FIG. 36.10 Risk stratification model currently used to identify hypertrophic cardiomyopathy *(HCM)* patients at the highest sudden cardiac death *(SCD)* risk who may be candidates for implantable cardioverter defibrillators *(ICDs)* and SCD prevention. Primary risk markers and potential arbitrators appear in boxes at the left. [a]Extensive late gadolinium enhancement *(LGE)*, while a primary risk marker, can also be used as an arbitrator when conventional risk assessment is ambiguous. *BP,* Blood pressure; *CAD,* coronary artery disease; *LV,* left ventricular; *LVH,* left ventricular hypertrophy; *NSVT,* nonsustained ventricular tachycardia; *VT,* ventricular tachycardia.

expanded extracellular space within the myocardium, based on the measurement of regional absolute T1 time of myocardial tissue, and which are rapidly evolving with the current emergence of multiple sequences and imaging strategies.[53] In this regard, the measurement of the T1 time before administration of any gadolinium contrast agent allows for measurement of a native T1 value. In contrast, ECV is a technique that measures the proportion of the myocardium that is occupied by the extracellular space and is a proposed marker of interstitial fibrosis, performed by measuring the change in relaxivity of myocardium and plasma before and at multiple time points after administration of gadolinium. Within each of these strategies are multiple methods for measuring absolute T1 values,[54] making it difficult to correlate findings between published studies. Despite these limitations, there remains much interest applying T1 mapping within HCM because diffuse interstitial fibrosis is an important morphologic component of the disease process that may not be reliably detected using LGE, which more reliably detects focal replacement fibrosis. In this regard there have been small-scale studies which have found significant correlations between ECV values and collagen volume fraction quantified from histopathology obtained from LV tissue obtained from HCM patients.[55]

The early clinical experience with T1 mapping in HCM has largely been confined to differentiating HCM from other cardiovascular disease with LV hypertrophy and in the evaluation of HCM family members. In this regard, both ECV and native T1 values have been found to be significantly higher in HCM patients compared with patients with LV hypertrophy secondary to systemic hypertension or cardiac amyloidosis. However, overlap occurs between groups, potentially limiting utility of the technique for reliable diagnosis in these clinical scenarios.[53] In contrast, encouraging observations have been demonstrated in reliably differentiating HCM from Anderson-Fabry disease using native T1 values.[56] It remains uncertain if ECV (or native T1 values) can be used to identify HCM family members who are G+P- and therefore

at risk for developing clinical disease with LV hypertrophy, although initial experience is encouraging.[20,53] To date there has been no demonstrated link to T1 mapping and outcomes within HCM, but these data are being gathered by the HCMR.[47] Thus continued investigation applying T1 mapping to HCM is necessary to determine if this technique has a role within risk stratification of HCM patients for sudden death or development of HF, and perhaps, more importantly, if this technique provides incremental value beyond LGE or as an alternative to LGE for patients who are not candidates for gadolinium due to renal dysfunction.

CONCLUSION

Over the last decade, CMR has become an important imaging technique in the evaluation of HCM patients and is uniquely suited to characterize the incredibly diverse phenotypic expression associated with this complex genetic heart disease. CMR provides information that can impact a variety of clinical management issues ranging from diagnosis and family screening, to procedural planning for invasive septal reduction therapy. Extensive LGE has emerged as a potential novel marker dictating the HCM clinical course along two divergent adverse pathways—risk for sudden death with preserved EF and for advanced HF with systolic dysfunction—and therefore may identify patients who may be candidates for primary prevention ICD therapy as well as those at risk for future development of end-stage phase. Data regarding native T1 and ECV are expected in the coming years. These observations help justify an important complementary role for CMR in the routine clinical assessment of HCM patients.

REFERENCES

A full reference list is available online at ExpertConsult.com

38

Cardiac and Paracardiac Masses

Herbert Frank, Teresa Sykora, and Francisco Alpendurada

Cardiovascular magnetic resonance (CMR) provides a noninvasive and three-dimensional (3D) assessment of masses involving the cardiac chambers, the pericardium, and extracardiac structures. CMR has become an established method to yield complementary diagnostic information and to guide cardiac surgeons in the design of an appropriate therapeutic strategy. The goals of CMR for assessing cardiac and paracardiac masses are to confirm or to exclude a mass initially suspected by echocardiography,[1] to assess the location, mobility, and its relationship to surrounding tissues,[2] to image the degree of vascularity,[3] to distinguish solid from fluid lesions,[4] and to determine tissue characteristics and the specific nature of a mass.[5]

TECHNICAL CONSIDERATIONS

For adequate image quality with reduced motion artifacts, CMR is performed using electrocardiogram (ECG) gating.[1] Alternatively, the navigator techniques allow for combined ECG and respiratory triggering.[2] Spin echo (SE) sequences provide detailed morphologic information of the heart, the great vessels, and the adjacent structures.[3] For T1-weighted sequences, the echo time (TE) is usually 20 to 30 ms, and the repetition time (TR) is dependent on the R-R interval. A longer TR is used for T2-weighted sequences and the TE is typically 50 to 90 ms.[4] T1-weighted images provide a better signal-to-noise ratio (SNR) and excellent soft tissue contrast between epicardial fat, myocardium, and rapidly flowing blood.[3] T2-weighted images have increased image contrast for water-laden tissues with inflammation or necrosis or fluid-filled cysts. However, T2-weighted images in general have worse SNR (Table 38.1).

The fast or turbo spin echo (TSE) technique combines the acquisition of multiple profiles per excitation with the multislice mode, resulting in a marked reduction in imaging time. The contrast of those images is similar to that of SE images with the same TR and an equivalent TE. Fat is usually brighter with TSE than regular SE pulse sequences. TSE permits acquisition of T1- and T2-weighted scans in a fraction of time compared with the conventional spin echo sequence. Furthermore, this technique has a reduced susceptibility to motion artifacts and is insensitive to field inhomogeneity. The combination with inversion recovery and breath-hold techniques has led to improved image quality and tissue characterization.[5] When combined with an inversion recovery (IR) technique, the signal from fat can be suppressed by using a short inversion time before the SE pulse. Most tissues have a T1 relaxation time longer than that of fat, resulting in a signal increase on T1- and T2-weighted images. This leads to better contrast in these images. Applications of the IR technique are the distinct recognition of fatty tissues and the improved visualization of structures that are surrounded by fatty tissue, which often makes image analysis complicated.

For evaluation of cardiac function and tumor mobility, gradient recalled echo (GRE) techniques (TE 4–12 ms) are recommended.[6,7] GRE images are generally T1 weighted and are characterized by bright signal intensity (SI) from rapidly flowing blood, which is useful for the differentiation of thrombus or the assessment of turbulent flow in case of valvular regurgitation or intracardiac shunts. Because of the low soft tissue contrast, visualization of cardiac masses is not as adequate as with SE techniques, unless they are intraluminal. Steady-state free precession (SSFP) is a type of GRE optimized for assessment of cardiac function, offering the highest SNR per unit of time of all imaging sequences.[8] The resulting weighting relies on a T2/T1 ratio, where both fat and water return high signal as opposed to low signal from the myocardium. Because of the intrinsic homogeneous contrast between the blood pool and the heart during the cardiac cycle, along with an excellent spatial and temporal resolution, SSFP is the sequence of choice to assess the dynamic relationship of masses with the heart and vessels.

Unlike two-dimensional (2D) echocardiography, CMR has the potential to some extent for tissue characterization by comparing the T1 and T2 values of the mass to a reference tissue:[9] that is based on the observation that significant differences exist in T1 and T2 relaxation times. Previous studies have tried to determine specific T1 and T2 relaxation times of different tissues[10]; however, precise etiologic diagnoses are not possible.[11,12] T1 and T2 mapping CMR is a novel parametric approach to tissue characterization and has shown promising results for the assessment of cardiac thrombus and may have a potential role in overcoming some of the limitations.[13]

CONTRAST AGENTS

The most commonly used CMR contrast agent uses the paramagnetic element gadolinium in a complex with chelating molecules (e.g., with diethylenetriaminepentaacetic acid [DTPA][14]) to reduce toxicity. A number of agents are available. The distribution of nearly all currently available intravenous contrast agents is extracellular and contrast is enhanced on T1-weighted images. The normal concentration is 0.1 mmol/kg body weight.[15] Gadolinium provides a better delineation of the mass by different enhancement of myocardium and tumor tissue because of variation of tissue vascularity.[16]

BENIGN TUMORS OF THE HEART

Primary tumors of the heart are very rare, with an estimated incidence between 0.002% and 0.2% in unselected patients at autopsy. Three-quarters of the tumors are benign and nearly half of them are myxomas and about 10% are lipomas.[17–19] Fibroelastomas, rhabdomyomas, fibromas, hemangiomas, teratomas, and mesotheliomas are found

TABLE 38.1 Typical Technical Parameters at 1.5 T for Evaluation of Cardiac or Paracardiac Masses

Sequence	Technical Features	Indication	Advantages/Disadvantages
T1-weighted spin echo	8–12 slices, thickness: 6–10 mm, NSA = 2, TE: 20–25 ms, TR: shortest, time 4–6 min, axial, sagittal, and coronal orientation	Defining anatomic structures, delineation of the mass to the adjacent tissue, visualization of vascular walls	A: Excellent soft tissue contrast D: Respiratory and flow artifacts
T2-weighted spin echo, double echo	8–12 slices, thickness: 6–10 mm, NSA = 2, TE: 50, 90 ms, TR: every 2nd or 3rd heartbeat, time: 5–8 min, axial orientation	Detecting the nature of cardiac masses by abnormal T2 values.	A: Better tissue contrast, demonstration of fluid components D: Very long examination time, lower SNR, and increased motion artifacts
T1- and T2-weighted fast spin echo	Examination time: 2–4 min, also breath-hold technique		A: Shorter imaging times, reduced motion artifacts D: Less SNR
Short inversion recovery	Inversion pulse, combination with spin echo or TSE	Suppression of fatty tissue	A: Eliminating artifacts from fat signal
T1-weighted spin echo with contrast agent administration	Axial orientation, antecubital Gd-DTPA administration (dose: 0, 1 mmol/kg)	Signal intensity behavior of suspected masses, assessment of the degree of vascularity	To assess invasive and infiltrative components of a tumor
Cine gradient echo with flow compensation	1–3 slices, thickness 8–10 mm, TE: 9 ms, TR: shortest, 16 phases NSA = 2, time: 1–3 min	Imaging the hemodynamic effects of a mass, i.e., mobility, transvalvular flow, differentiation between blood flow and thrombus, identify turbulent flow regions	A: Functional information D: Low soft tissue contrast
Cine gradient echo EPI	Breath-hold technique, 1–3 slices, thickness, 8–10 mm, TE: shortest, TR: shortest, time: 10–40 s	Equal to conventional gradient echo	A: Shorter acquisition time, reduced motion artifacts D: Less SNR

EPI, Echo planar imaging; *Gd-DTPA,* gadolinium-DTPA; *NSA,* numbers of signal averaged; *SNR,* signal-to-noise ratio; *TE,* echo time; *TSE,* turbo spin echo; *TR,* repetition time.
Modified from Hoffman U, Globits S, Frank H. Cardiac and paracardiac masses: current opinion on diagnostic evaluation by magnetic resonance imaging. *Eur Heart J.* 1998;19:553–563.

less frequently. Granular cell tumors, neurofibromas, and lymphangiomas are very rare.[20]

Myxoma

Myxomas comprise 30% to 50% of all primary cardiac tumors, occur frequently between the third and sixth decade of life, and have a slight female predominance.[21] In about 75%, myxomas originate from the left atrium, and in 15% to 20% from the right atrium. They usually develop from the interatrial septum close to the fossa ovalis. Only a few myxomas are located in the ventricles.[22] Myxomas are generally sporadic, but may occur in multiple and unusual locations, usually as part of the autosomal dominant syndrome known as Carney complex, which is present in about 7% of cases, and also includes lentiginosis and endocrine overactivity.[23] Rare aneurysmatic formations of part of the septum secundum can lead to a gallbladder-like cystic structure and can mimic an atrial myxoma by CMR.[24] The histologic structure shows a typical matrix of myxoma cells, large blood vessels at the base, and variable areas of hemorrhage, calcification, or even ossification.[25] They are generally polypoid, often pedunculated, round or oval with a smooth surface, often covered with thrombi, and are between 1 and 15 cm in diameter.[26] Clinical symptoms appear as a consequence of embolism or intracardiac obstruction and are determined by size, location, and mobility of the myxoma.[27,28]

On CMR, myxomas (Fig. 38.1) are mainly diagnosed by the typically pedunculated, jellylike, and prolapsing appearance and certain signal characteristics.[29] Therefore cine display should be obtained to show the mobility of the tumor.[30] Due to the endocardial origin, myxomas are characterized by an intermediate, but variable signal on SE images, similar to that of the myocardium. On SSFP images, myxomas tend to be isointense or slightly hyperintense relative to the myocardium but hypointense relative to the blood pool. Therefore the tumor can always be distinguished from the higher signal of the surrounding slowly flowing blood.[31,32] Intratumorous areas of subacute or chronic hemorrhage are typically characterized by high SI on both short and long TE.[33] Myxomas show a moderately high and heterogeneous contrast enhancement after intravenous injection of gadolinium, typically at the core, which appears to be the result of relatively high vascularity.[15,31] However, organizing thrombus may occur in the tumor, which will be responsible for areas of low SI on gadolinium imaging.

Lipoma

Cardiac lipomas (Fig. 38.2) are relatively common and account for about 10% of all primary tumors of the heart.[34] True lipomas are encapsulated, contain neoplastic fat cells, and occur in young age.[35,36] About 50% arise subendocardially, 25% subepicardially, and 25% from the myocardium.[37] Subepicardial lipomas may become quite large and may alter cardiac function, resulting in dyspnea or fatigue,[38] and involvement of the coronary arteries has also been reported.[39] Endocardial lipomas commonly arise from the interatrial septum and are located in the right atrium. Arrhythmias due to myocardial infiltration have been reported.[40] Lipomatous hypertrophy of the atrial septum (Fig. 38.3) is histologically characterized by infiltration of lipomatous cells between atrial muscle fibers. Unlike true lipomas they are unencapsulated and contain lipoblasts as well as mature fat cells.[41] This condition has been described in older, overweight patients who frequently have atrial fibrillation.[42]

On CMR, lipomas are characterized by bright signal on T1-weighted images and a slight decrease in signal on T2-weighted images similar to subcutaneous fat.[43] Injection of gadolinium is not needed because

from the ventricular myocardium at multiple locations as opposed to chronic renal disease and abnormalities of calcium phosphate metabolism.

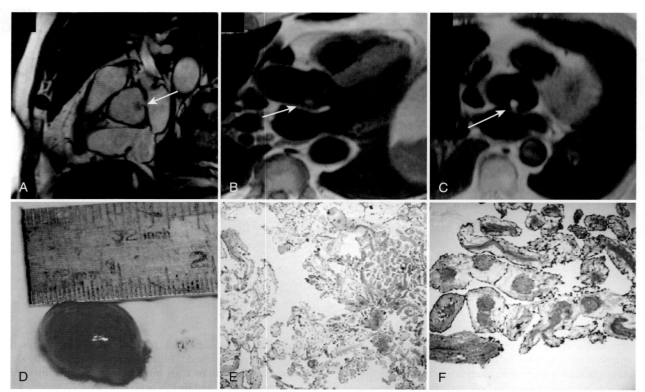

FIG. 38.4 Papillary fibroelastoma of the aortic valve. Steady-state free precession image (A) demonstrating a solid, intraluminal mass *(arrow)* attached to the commissure of the left coronary and noncoronary aortic valve leaflet. T1-weighted (B) and T2-weighted (C) spin echo images showing a solid lesion *(arrows)* with intermediate signal intensity. The macroscopic specimen (D) appeared as a translucent, gelatinous mass. The histologic specimen in the hematoxylin and eosin stain shows a benign lesion with multiple papillary fronds (E). The papillary fronds consist of three layers, comprising a collagenous core with low elastin content, an amorphous intermediate layer, and a delicate coat of single-layer endothelium (F), as demonstrated with the elastica–van Gieson stain.

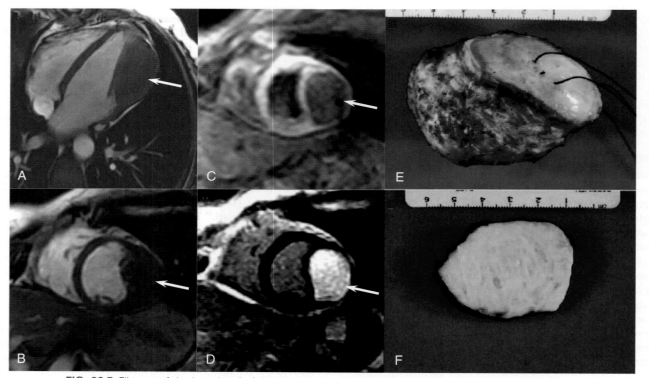

FIG. 38.5 Fibroma of the lateral wall of the left ventricle. Steady-state free precession four-chamber (A) and short-axis (B) images showing a slightly hypointense mass in the lateral wall of the left ventricle *(arrows)*. First-pass perfusion image in the short-axis plane (C) showing hypoperfusion of the mass surrounded by the normally perfused myocardium, which is suggestive of low tumor vascularity *(arrow)*. Late myocardial enhancement image (D) demonstrating high signal intensity of the mass *(arrow)* compared with the nulled normal myocardium. Gross pathology of the resected left ventricular mass (E). The cut section (F) showed an off-white whorled surface with foci of calcification. The lesion extended to the inked surgical margin. There was no hemorrhage or necrosis.

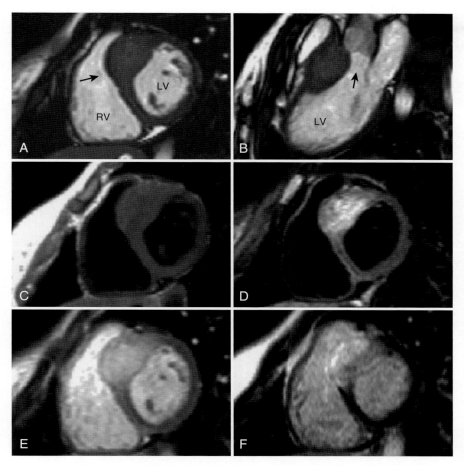

FIG. 38.6 Rhabdomyoma of the interventricular septum. Short-axis image from a steady-state free precession (SSFP) image obtained through the proximal septum (A) showing a markedly thickened septum *(arrow)* that appears to be homogeneous with the rest of the myocardium. SSFP image of the left ventricular outflow tract (B, *arrow*). T1-weighted turbo spin echo image (C) demonstrating that the signal from the markedly thickened septum is isointense compared with the rest of the myocardium. T2-weighted image with fat suppression (D) demonstrating high signal within the thickened septum, suggesting a different structure from the surrounding myocardium. Early after gadolinium injection (E), there is enhancement of the left ventricular and right ventricular cavities, as well as the myocardium, including the thickened septum. Late after gadolinium injection (F), the normal myocardium appears black. There is marked abnormal late enhancement throughout the entire segment of the thickened septum. *LV,* Left ventricle; *RV,* right ventricle.

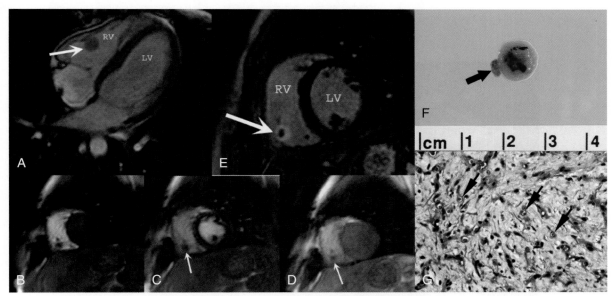

FIG. 38.7 Hemangioma of the right ventricle. Four-chamber steady-state free precession image (A) demonstrates a hypointense, spherical, and pedunculated mass within the mid right ventricle, which is attached to the free wall of the right ventricle via a short stalk *(arrow)*. Short-axis perfusion imaging demonstrates first-pass contrast arrival in the right ventricle (B), and peripheral contrast enhancement of the mass (C, *arrow*), with subsequent complete filling of the tumor on the second-pass arrival of the contrast in the right ventricle (D, *arrow*), which indicate vascularity of the lesion. Short-axis view of a 10-minute late gadolinium enhancement (E) demonstrates peripheral enhancement of the right ventricular *(RV)* mass *(arrow)*. Presence of this finding favors the diagnosis of cardiac hemangioma. Gross photograph of the resected tumor specimen (F) exhibits a polypoid, tan, gelatinous, and focally hemorrhagic lesion with a small stalk *(arrow)*. High-power photomicrograph (G) demonstrates a marked proliferation of capillary-sized blood vessels *(short black arrows)* within a slightly blue acid mucopolysaccharide ground substance. Features are consistent with capillary-type cardiac hemangioma. *LV,* Left ventricle.

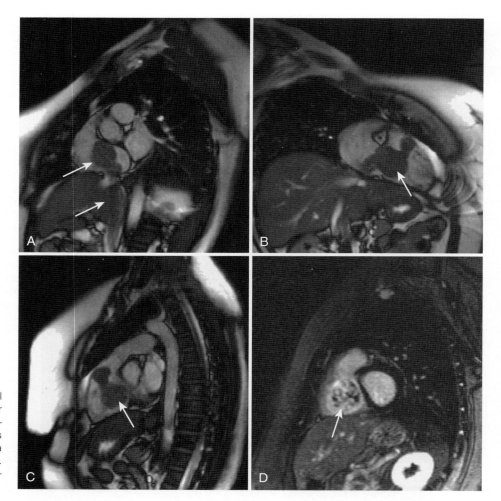

FIG. 38.8 Intravenous leiomyomatosis. Atrial short-axis (A), right ventricular two-chamber (B), and right ventricular outflow tract (C) steady-state free precession showing transvenous extension of tumor from the inferior vena cava to the right atrium and right ventricle *(arrows)*. The mass enhances late after gadolinium injection (D, *arrow*).

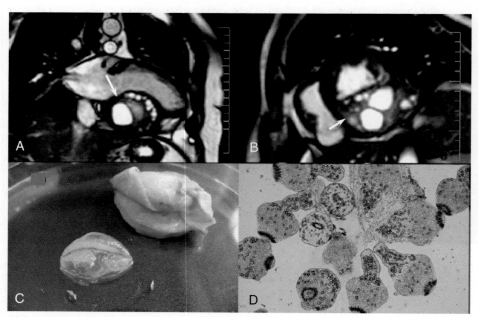

FIG. 38.9 Hydatid cyst. Two-chamber (A) and short-axis (B) steady-state free precession images showing a large multilocular cystic mass *(arrows)* involving the inferior wall and producing severe thinning of adjacent myocardium. Macroscopic image (C) of the excised hydatid material. Microscopic image of *Echinococcus granulosus* (D).

It presents as an immobile mass in the basal posterior mitral valve and adjacent ventricular myocardium, although in more severe cases it can extend circumferentially to involve the whole annulus. It is characterized by a low signal on GRE, T1- and T2-weighted sequences. After intravenous gadolinium administration, there is no enhancement at the core as opposed to a peripheral rim of circumferential enhancement, in keeping with a calcified core surrounded by a fibrotic envelope.[60] Caseous calcification of the mitral valve is a rare variant of MAC, in which the mass undergoes liquefaction necrosis. The core is a mixture of fatty acids, cholesterol, and amorphous eosinophilic material encased by a rim of fibrosis, calcification, and inflammatory cell infiltration. As a result, the fatty proteinaceous material in the core can generate high signal on T1-weighted images (and on T2-weighted images as well), as opposed to the low signal in MAC.[61] Another differentiating sign will be the central enhancement in both early and late phases after gadolinium injection.[62] These entities are believed to be benign because they are usually asymptomatic and discovered as incidental findings. However, complications such as mitral stenosis or regurgitation, embolization, and infective endocarditis have been described, all of which may prompt surgical intervention.

MALIGNANT TUMORS OF THE HEART

Nearly 25% of all primary cardiac tumors are malignant tumors. Metastases are 20 to 40 times more common than primary malignant tumors and appear in 6% of postmortems in malignant diseases. The most common primary malignant cardiac tumors are various types of sarcomas and lymphomas.[63,64]

Because of the small number of studied cardiac malignancies, and the differences in tumor age and vascularity, and a widespread variability in water content, a reliable tissue differentiation of cardiac malignancies is often not possible.[65,66] Distinct features of malignant tumors are the presence of necrosis, calcification, a high degree of vascularity, infiltration of the adjacent tissues, inhomogeneous appearance, and peritumorous edema.[67,68]

Sarcoma

Sarcomas of the heart or the great vessels comprise the largest group, accounting for 75% of all primary malignant cardiac tumors in adults.[69] There are various histologic types of sarcoma, such as angiosarcomas, leiomyosarcomas, fibrosarcomas, synovial sarcomas, rhabdomyosarcomas, undifferentiated pleomorphic sarcomas, and liposarcomas.[20,64,70] Angiosarcoma (Fig. 38.10) is the most frequent primary malignant cardiac tumor.[20] It is located within the right atrium near the atrioventricular groove in 80% of cases.[71] They appear preferentially between the third and fifth decade of life, with a male-to-female ratio of about 2:1.[72] In contrast, other types of sarcoma often occur in the left side of the heart, where they are often clinically mistaken for myxoma. Morphologically, angiosarcomas are usually hemorrhagic, often with poorly defined borders. They frequently invade contiguous structures such as the venae cavae and tricuspid valve, and are characterized by irregular anastomosing sinusoidal structures with papillary intraluminal tufting.[72] On CMR, angiosarcomas have a polymorphic appearance, with a central region of hyperintensity consistent with necrosis, and moderate SI in peripheral regions in T1- and T2-weighted images.[32] Because of the high degree of vascularity, signal enhancement is seen after intravenous injection of gadolinium. The typical appearance of angiosarcoma on CMR is a "cauliflower" aspect on black-blood images and an avid enhancement with "sunray" aspect after administration of contrast agent.[73]

Primary leiomyosarcomas are rare, highly aggressive, locally invasive tumors with a frequency of 0.25%. They arise in 75% from the inferior vena cava, but also have been reported with an origin of the superior vena cava or in the pulmonary veins.[70,74] This neoplasm demonstrates a SI on T1-weighted SE images slightly higher than liver parenchyma,

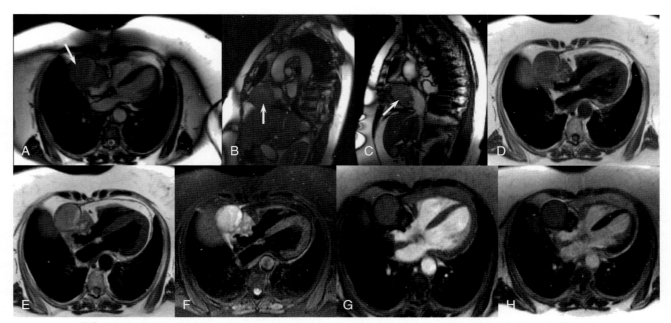

FIG. 38.10 Comprehensive evaluation of a right atrial mass. Four-chamber (A) and atrial short-axis (B and C) steady-state free precession images showing a large mass in the right atrial free wall invading the right atrial cavity *(arrows)*. The tumor has intermediate signal on T1-weighted (D) and high signal on T2-weighted images (E), which persisted after fat suppression (F). The presence of a large, heterogeneous, and invasive mass in the right heart associated with pericardial effusion suggests malignancy. There is significant enhancement early after gadolinium injection, suggesting vascularity (G). The enhancement pattern persists in the late phase (H). A biopsy was performed, and the diagnosis of angiosarcoma was made.

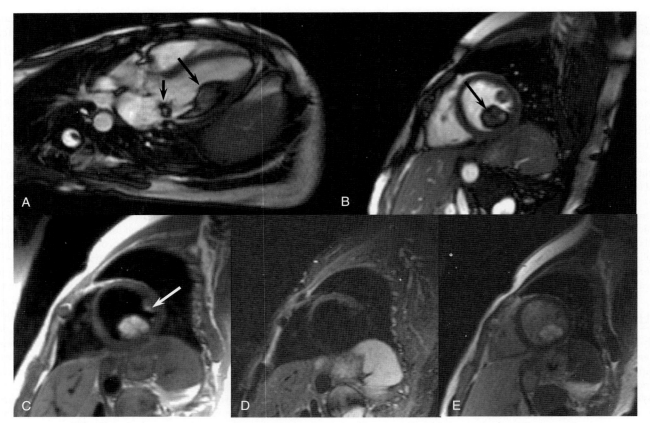

FIG. 38.11 Left ventricular liposarcoma. Left ventricular outflow tract (A) and short axis at papillary muscle level (B) steady-state free precession images showing abnormal tissue enlarging the posteromedial papillary muscle. Some abnormal tissue can also be seen in the mitral valve leaflets (black arrows). On a T1-weighted turbo spin echo image at the papillary level (C), there is a high signal not only in the posteromedial papillary muscle but also in part of the anterolateral papillary muscle (white arrow). There is signal drop-out on the same plane after fat suppression (D), suggesting fatty infiltration. Increased signal intensity is seen in the late phase after gadolinium injection (E). Surgical resection of the tumoral masses was performed, and the diagnosis of low-grade liposarcoma was made on histology.

but not as bright as the adjacent mediastinal fat. The SI is high on T2. After injection of gadolinium, a slight contrast enhancement of the tumor can be detected.[70] The advantage of CMR is the ability to assess intravascular tumor extension into the superior vena cava, the pulmonary veins, and the heart chambers.[75]

Liposarcomas (Fig. 38.11) are very rare and not represented in most surgical series of tumors. Grossly, they are bulky tumors as large as 10 cm.[72] Liposarcomas often have a pericardial origin and CMR is able to detect this pericardial mass with heterogeneous high signal on T1-weighted images and epicardial infiltration. After injection of gadolinium, liposarcomas may show a slight signal enhancement.[76]

Rhabdomyosarcomas are the most common primary cardiac malignancy in children. They arise from any location in the heart and always involve the myocardium and frequently also the valves.[77] Patients often present with congestive heart failure. On T1-weighted images, rhabdomyosarcomas are isointense to the myocardium. After administration of gadolinium, a homogeneous enhancement will be found, unless the tumor has necrotic areas, which will then show little or no enhancement.[78]

Undifferentiated sarcomas are mostly found in the left atrium (80%) and have no specific histologic markers.[78] CMR shows an irregularly shaped mass, with heterogeneous signal on T1-weighted images, high-intermediate signal on T2-weighted images, and heterogeneous enhancement after contrast administration.[79]

Lymphoma

Primary cardiac lymphomas (Fig. 38.12) are rare, usually non-Hodgkin in origin, with B-cell lymphoma being the most common type.[80] Postmortem studies in lymphoma patients have shown cardiac involvement in up to 25% of diagnoses. As a result, the diagnosis of primary cardiac lymphoma is made in the absence of extracardiac involvement. New data suggest that primary cardiac lymphoma is more often diagnosed premortem, maybe because of the awareness of the higher incidence of lymphoproliferative disorders related to Epstein-Barr virus (EBV) in patients with AIDS and in patients who have had transplantation.[72] The mean age at presentation for cardiac lymphoma is 38 years, with a slight predominance in men. Involvement of the right heart is much more common than of the left heart. On T1- and T2-weighted SE images, lymphomas appear isointense or hypointense to cardiac muscle. After injection of gadolinium, lymphomas appear heterogeneous with less-enhancing central regions consisting of necrosis.[66]

METASTATIC TUMORS OF THE HEART

The incidence of cardiac metastases has been described as between 10% and 14%. Primary tumors that metastasize to the heart can be divided into three categories of incidence: uncommon primary tumors that

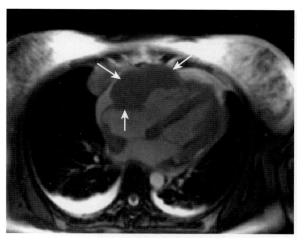

FIG. 38.12 Involvement of the heart by an aggressive large B-cell lymphoma *(arrows)*. Horizontal long-axis steady-state free precession image showing a homogeneous mass involving the lateral aspect of the right ventricle and extending superiorly to the right atrium.

have a high rate of metastasis to the heart (malignant melanoma, thyroid carcinoma, extracardiac sarcomas, lymphomas, malignant germ cell neoplasm, malignant thymoma, renal cell carcinomas); common tumors that have an intermediate rate of cardiac metastasis but account for the greatest number of cardiac metastases (carcinoma of the stomach, liver, ovary, colon, and rectum); and common tumors with rare metastases to the heart.[72] The most common epithelial malignancies to metastasize to the heart are carcinomas of the breast and of the lung.[71] The tumor burden in the heart is the highest with melanoma as compared with any other malignancy. There are four ways noncardiac tumors may invade the heart: (1) direct mediastinal infiltration of heart tissue in the case of lung cancer (see Fig. 38.9), breast cancer, or mediastinal lymphomas; (2) hematogenous spread by systemic tumors such as malignant melanoma, lymphoma, leukemia, and sarcoma; (3) transvenous spreading from the inferior vena cava in the case of renal or hepatic tumors and transvenous spreading from the pulmonary vein in the case of lung cancer; and (4) lymphatic spread.[20,38] Metastatic cardiac involvement can be localized or diffuse. Nodular formations can arise at discrete locations in the myocardium or diffusely encased in the epicardial surface. In most cases there is pericardial involvement, with superficial myocardial infiltration. In metastatic melanoma, the myocardium is involved in virtually every patient, with less frequent infiltration of epicardium and endocardium.[71]

CARDIAC THROMBUS

Intracardiac thrombus formation is often located in the left atrium in the case of dilatation and chronic atrial fibrillation, or in the left ventricle in the case of contractile dysfunction seen in cardiomyopathy (Fig. 38.13) or after myocardial infarction.[81] Tumor thrombus in the inferior vena cava and the right atrium can be seen in renal carcinomas and can mimic a solid cardiac mass.[82,83] The diagnosis of cardiac thrombus is clinically important to identify because patients are at risk of systemic or pulmonary embolization.[84,85] However, in most cases the diagnosis of cardiac thrombi is coincidental and patients are asymptomatic. Despite the fact that 2D echocardiography is the method of choice for diagnosis, false-positive rates as high as 28% in detection of left ventricular thrombi and 59% in detection of left atrial thrombi have been reported.[86,87]

On CMR images, fresh thrombi on T1-weighted SE images have often a higher signal than myocardium, and the contrast is further accentuated on T2-weighted SE images consistent with a high amount of hemoglobin.[81] However, depending on the age of the thrombus, other signal intensities are possible. After 1 or 2 weeks, the paramagnetic effect in the organizing thrombus because of deoxyhemoglobin and methemoglobin causes T1 and T2 shortening, which may result in increased SI in T1-weighted images and decreased SI in T2-weighted images.[88] Chronic organized thrombi are of low SI because of loss of water and protons. A problem concerning differentiation between thrombus and slow-flowing blood occurs especially in laminated or immobile thrombi on SE images.[89] Compared with thrombus formation, slow-flowing blood shows increased signal on T2-weighted images.[49,90] On GRE images, thrombi have the lowest SI compared with other cardiac structures, whereas blood appears brightest.[88] If thrombi contain calcification, they appear more heterogeneous.[33] T1 and T2 mapping sequences have not shown significant diagnostic capability compared with postgadolinium sequences, which remain the gold standard in thrombus imaging.[13] To differentiate thrombus from tumor, intravenous injection of contrast agents will be helpful. Thrombi usually do not show signal enhancement after intravenous injection of gadolinium, unless they are already organized.[15] Compared with other diagnostic procedures, CMR and computed tomography (CT) offer a high sensitivity of about 90%, with a slightly better specificity when compared with 2D echocardiography.[89]

PERICARDIAL LESIONS

Magnetic resonance evaluation of pericardial neoplasms in most cases involves identification of abnormal anatomic structures and boundaries rather than characterization of relative tissue intensities. A few exceptions to this are included in the differential diagnosis of mediastinal masses, such as fibroma, lipoma, and pericardial cysts. The value of CMR for evaluation of potential neoplasm lies largely in treatment planning, particularly preoperative assessment. The loss of normal anatomic boundaries is an important sign of neoplasm. Neoplastic involvement of the pericardium results in focal or diffuse obliteration of the normal pericardial signal. In the case of malignancy adjacent to cardiac structures, visualization of the pericardial line is an indication that pericardial invasion has not occurred.

Tumors

Of the patients with primary cardiac tumors, only 7% to 13% arise primarily from the pericardium.[91] The most common benign tumors of the pericardium are lipomas, teratomas, fibromas, hemangiomas, and neuromas. Lipomas and hemangiomas are often incidental findings without symptoms. On T1-weighted images, lipomas show high SI, whereas on T2-weighted images, a decrease in SI similar to subcutaneous fat is characteristic. Lipomas do not enhance after administration of contrast agent. Hemangiomas are characteristically hyperintense during and after administration of contrast agent because of their significant vascular content.[92] Fibroma is a typical pediatric tumor, but it might also be found in adults. Low SI on T2-weighted images and hypoisointense SI on T1-weighted images are typical findings for fibromas. Late gadolinium enhancement (LGE) imaging often reveals no or very little enhancement.[91,92] The rare primary malignancies of the pericardium include mesotheliomas, bronchial pheochromocytomas, lymphomas, thymomas, fibrosarcomas, and angiosarcomas.[93,94] Hemorrhagic effusions result from erosion into the intrapericardiac vessels or myocardial wall, with development of acute or subacute tamponade.

Mesothelioma is the most common primary malignant neoplasm of the pericardium,[95] originating from the mesothelial cells of parietal

APPROACH TO CARDIOVASCULAR MAGNETIC RESONANCE INTERPRETATION OF CARDIAC MASSES

When interpreting a study for a suspected cardiac mass, the first step is to confirm the presence of the mass and exclude potential confounders such as aneurysmal interatrial septum, hiatus hernia, aortic aneurysm, or prominent pericardial fat, all of which can mimic and be misinterpreted as a cardiac tumor. When single or multiple masses are confirmed, the next step is to provide basic morphologic details such as location, size, and extension of the mass. It is also worth describing whether the mass is homogeneous or heterogeneous, and whether the contours are regular and well-defined or irregular and ill-defined. A third step is to detail the relationship of the mass with adjacent structures, and describe if there are signs of compression, erosion, displacement, or invasion. Using cine and flow imaging, mobility and influence on cardiac contractility and valvular function can be assessed. For intravascular masses, it should be described whether there is partial or complete obstruction to flow, collateralization, or diversion of flow to other vascular systems (such as azygous dilatation in obstruction of the vena cavae). The fifth step is tissue characterization, with description of the SI relative to the myocardium on different GRE and TSE sequences. When gadolinium is administrated, presence of first-pass perfusion and degree of gadolinium enhancement in earlier and later stages should be documented.

Morphologic CMR features can predict the type of cardiac and paracardiac masses (Table 38.2). Large tumoral size (usually >5 cm), right-sided cardiac location, tissue inhomogeneity, ill-defined borders, tumor displacement or infiltration of adjacent structures, pleural/pericardial effusion, positive first-pass perfusion and LGE are all suspicious for malignancy, whereas the absence of these signs will suggest a benign mass. The following algorithm is suggested:

1. Exclusion of the most common benign cardiac tumors by their typical and often pathognomonic appearance. Typical features can be observed in myxoma (septal atrial origin, hypointense SI, moderate contrast enhancement, no effusion or infiltration), fibromas (left-sided, homogenous, hypointense SI, no contrast enhancement, infiltration in up to 50%), lipomas (hyperintense SI on T1-weighted SE images, hypointense in fat-suppressed images), and thrombi (typically in enlarged left atria in atrial fibrillation or left ventricular aneurysms, hypointense SI on GRE and SSFP, no contrast enhancement).

2. Features specific of malignant tumors such as an intracardiac lesion with pericardial effusion (especially with high SI on T1-weighted images suggesting a high proteinaceous or hemorrhagic component), a paracardiac lesion with inhomogeneous tissue composition or a mass that infiltrates adjacent tissue but is not an inflammatory pseudotumor.

3. With the exception of a myxoma, lesions of the right heart are always suspicious for malignancy/metastasis.[105]

In summary, CMR has proven to be a valuable tool in differentiating benign from malignant tumors of the heart and neoplasms from pseudotumors and should therefore be used for the assessment of cardiac masses.[105–108]

TABLE 38.2	Magnetic Resonance Imaging Features of the Most Common Cardiac Tumors			
	T1-Weighted SE	**T2-Weighted SE**	**GRE**	**Enhancement After Administration of Gd-DTPA**
Myxoma	Intermediate varying SI, calcified areas: hypointense and hemorrhage: increased SI	Low SI, especially in iron-containing myxomas	Very low SI compared with the surrounding blood pool	Hyperintense
Lipoma/lipomatous hypertrophy	Brightest SI similar to subcutaneous fat, using fat presaturation technique: reduced SI	Intermediate SI parallel to subcutaneous fat	Nonspecific	Nonspecific
Papillary fibroelastoma	Intermediate SI	Intermediate to high SI	Low SI compared with the surrounding blood pool	Hyperintense
Fibroma	Intermediate to slightly hyperintense SI compared with myocardium, when calcification (hypointense) and hemorrhage (hyperintense) are present: heterogeneous	Decrease in SI compared with TI	Nonspecific	Slight and heterogeneous
Rhabdomyoma	Homogeneous, slightly lower SI than myocardium	Strong increased SI	Very low compared with myocardium	Nonspecific
Hemangioma	Intermediate SI	Increased SI (because of slow-flowing blood in the tumor vessels), higher than myocardium	Nonspecific	Significant increasing SI, heterogeneous
Intravenous leiomyomatosis	Similar to myocardium	Similar to myocardium	Nonspecific	Nonspecific
Pericardial cysts (simple fluid) (proteinaceous fluid)	Lowest SI, flow void Low SI, but higher than in normal fluid, no flow void	Highest SI High SI	Nonspecific	Signal enhancement, visualization of intracystic septae
Angiosarcoma	Central hyperintense spot (blood vessels, hemorrhage, or necrosis), surrounded by intermediate SI regions	No change	Nonspecific	Strong

TABLE 38.2 Magnetic Resonance Imaging Features of the Most Common Cardiac Tumors—Cont'd

	T1-Weighted SE	T2-Weighted SE	GRE	Enhancement After Administration of Gd-DTPA
Lymphoma	Isointense to hypointense to cardiac muscle	Isointense to myocardium	Nonspecific	Heterogeneous with less-enhancing central regions
Liposarcoma	Bright SI equal to subcutaneous fat, but heterogeneous: decrease in SI, when fat presaturation is used	Not published	Not published	Not published
Leiomyosarcoma	High SI, slightly higher than liver parenchyma, but not as high as subcutaneous fat homogeneous, commonly connected with proteinaceous pericardial effusion	Not published	Not published	Not published
Thrombus	Intermediate, often slightly higher SI than myocardium, slightly higher than blood	Surrounding slow-flowing blood becomes higher SI than thrombus, contrast between thrombus and myocardium is further accentuated	Thrombus has the lowest SI	No signal enhancement, unless the thrombus is organized
Fresh	High SI (oxyhemoglobin)	Decreased SI		
Chronic (older than 2 weeks)	Higher SI (deoxyhemoglobin)			

Gd, Gadolinium; *GRE*, gradient recalled echo; *SE*, spin echo; *SI*, signal intensity.
Modified from Hoffman U, Globits S, Frank H. Cardiac and paracardiac masses: current opinion on diagnostic evaluation by magnetic resonance imaging. *Eur Heart J.* 1998;19:553–563.

PROGNOSIS OF CARDIAC TUMORS

Prognosis after surgery is usually excellent in the case of benign tumors. Local recurrence of myxoma is uncommon but could be related to inadequate resection, multicentricity, origin in a chamber other than the left atrium or familial tumors. Nearly all malignant cardiac tumors are rapidly fatal. Sarcomas of the heart have a better prognosis if they arise in the left atrium, have no necrotic regions, and have not metastasized at the time of diagnosis.[72] Achievement of remission is unusual and can be achieved with chemotherapy in lymphomas.[109]

CONCLUSION

CMR techniques have contributed significantly to the ability to detect cardiac and paracardiac masses and play an important role in the diagnostic evaluation, which is complementary to echocardiography.[110] Because of its larger field of view, CMR adds diagnostic information by assessing extracardiac components of a mass, such as mediastinal involvement and extension into large pulmonary vessels. CMR allows the exclusion of conditions that can mimic cardiac tumors. The findings will also be helpful in characterizing paracardiac masses and in guiding therapeutic strategies. Comprehensive CMR evaluation of cardiac mass morphology, tissue composition, and perfusion in conjunction with information on tumor spread and operability allows diagnosis of patients with cardiac mass.[107,111] As compared with other image modalities, multiparametric CMR provides a better global cardiac assessment, including tumor tissue characterization, which has been proven to be likely predictive of the pathologic diagnosis.[106,112] Nevertheless, histologic confirmation is required in most cases, especially when there is a suspicion of malignancy.

REFERENCES

A full reference list is available online at ExpertConsult.com

39

Cardiovascular Magnetic Resonance Assessment of Right Ventricular Anatomy and Function

Alicia M. Maceira and Dudley J. Pennell

Accurate noninvasive assessment of right ventricular (RV) mass and systolic function is important in several pathologies, such as grown-up congenital heart disease,[1,2] pulmonary hypertension,[3,4] interstitial lung disease,[5] valvular heart disease,[6] and arrhythmogenic RV cardiomyopathy.[7] Right ventricular function is also a prognostic factor in coronary artery disease[8,9] and heart failure,[10,11] even after cardiac resynchronization therapy.[12] This chapter aims to summarize the features of the normal right ventricle, briefly describe cardiovascular magnetic resonance (CMR) techniques for assessing RV dimensions and function, and give reference values for the assessment of the right ventricle.

NORMAL RIGHT VENTRICULAR ANATOMY

The right ventricle is a thin, highly trabeculated structure that is triangular in form and, on gross inspection, appears to be wrapped around the left ventricle. It has three well-differentiated components with specific structure and function. The inlet portion extends from the tricuspid valve to the insertions of the papillary muscles on the ventricular wall, the trabecular portion involves the RV body and apex and is the main pumping component, and the outlet portion or infundibulum extends up to the pulmonary valve and has a thin, nontrabeculated wall (Fig. 39.1). The anterosuperior wall of the right ventricle is rounded and convex, its inferior surface is flattened and forms a small part of the diaphragmatic surface of the heart, and its posterior wall is formed by the ventricular septum, which bulges into the right ventricle, owing to the much greater left ventricular (LV) systolic pressure,[13] so a transverse section of the cavity presents a semilunar outline. The right ventricle has a continuum of muscle bands that rotate by approximately 160 degrees from the epicardium to the endocardium.[14] The principal axis of these fibers is oblique to the long axis of the right ventricle. RV contraction is then more dependent on longitudinal shortening than that of the LV. In the normal adult, the total RV free wall mass is 21 ± 13 g/m^2.[15]

The right ventricle has several distinctive features. In its upper left portion, there is a conical pouch called the conus arteriosus or infundibulum, from which the pulmonary artery arises. A tendinous band connects the posterior surface of the conus arteriosus to the aorta. Also, as a subpulmonary ventricle, the RV has a lower ejection fraction and

thinner walls than the left ventricle. RV wall thickness is usually 3 to 5 mm, the proportion between right ventricle and left ventricle being as 1 to 3[16]; it is thickest at the base and gradually becomes thinner toward the apex. The whole inner surface except the conus arteriosus is covered by more or less prominent muscular columns called trabeculae carneae and from some of them (papillary muscles), the chordae tendineae connect the myocardium to the tricuspid valve, with its septal leaflet more apically placed than the septal leaflet of the mitral valve.[17] The anterior tricuspid valve leaflet is usually the largest and extends from the infundibular region anteriorly to the inferolateral wall posteriorly; the septal leaflet extends from the interventricular septum to the posterior ventricular border; the posterior leaflet attaches along the posterior margin of the annulus from the septum to the inferolateral wall.[18] Finally, a muscular band frequently extends from the base of the anterior papillary muscle to the ventricular septum. This band is considered to prevent overdistension of the ventricle and is called the moderator band.[19]

The depictions of the moderator band, the infundibulum, and the different levels of insertion of the tricuspid and mitral septal leaflets are important diagnostic features for identification of the right ventricle, which can be difficult in some congenital cardiomyopathies.

Importance of Assessing Right Ventricular Dimensions and Function

The measurement of RV dimensions, morphology, and function is important in several situations, such as congenital heart disease, LV heart failure, pulmonary hypertension, pulmonary embolism, valvular heart disease, lung disease, and arrhythmogenic RV cardiomyopathy.

RV failure may result from conditions that lead to impaired RV contractility, such as RV infarction, right-sided cardiomyopathies, valvular heart disease or severe sepsis; to RV pressure overload, including pulmonic stenosis, pulmonary primary hypertension, and pulmonary hypertension secondary to left heart disease, lung disease, or thromboembolic disease; and to RV volume overload, for instance, tricuspid or pulmonary regurgitation. Many disorders, such as corrected and uncorrected adult congenital heart disease and intracardiac shunts, may result in right ventricle failure through a combination of pathophysiologic mechanisms. Also, decompensated right ventricle (both acute

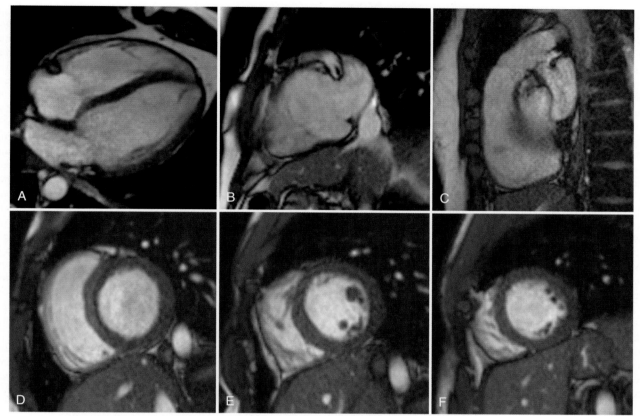

FIG. 39.1 Steady-state free precession cines in different views that allow the evaluation of the right ventricle. Top row depicts a four-chamber view (A), two-chamber view (B), and right ventricular outflow tract view (C). Bottom row shows three short-axis orientations at basal (D), mid (E), and apical (F) levels. The inlet portion extends from the tricuspid valve to the insertions of the papillary muscles on the ventricular wall and can be assessed in A and B, the trabecular portion involves the RV body and apex and is the main pumping component (A, D, E, F), and the outlet portion or infundibulum extends up to the pulmonary valve and has a thin, nontrabeculated wall (C). Note the rounded shape of the anterosuperior wall. In the short-axis sections the right ventricle presents a semilunar outline.

and acute-on-chronic) is increasing as the prevalence of predisposing conditions grows.

The prognostic value of RV function has been shown in several conditions such as LV heart failure,[20,21] valvular heart disease,[22] pulmonary hypertension,[23] congenital heart disease,[24] or myocardial infarction (MI).[25] Thus the early detection of RV dysfunction can have an impact on therapeutic decision making and on prognosis. Finally, improved understanding of the RV response to pressure and volume overload might lead to more optimal surgical and medical treatments.

Techniques for Assessing Right Ventricular Dimensions and Function

Global RV function has been traditionally difficult to assess, given its irregular shape, which cannot be assumed to any geometrical model. Several imaging techniques have been used in the past to assess RV dimensions and function. The chest radiograph is a simple method to assess RV size with the cardiothoracic ratio, but this may be misleading because an enlarged RV may compress the LV, resulting in a normal cardiothoracic ratio. Angiography used to be the gold standard for assessment of RV volumes and regional and global function. But this technique is invasive, involves ionizing radiation and the use of potentially nephrotoxic contrast, and is not as accurate as CMR.[26] Echocardiography and radionuclide ventriculography have been used for the

assessment of RV dimensions and function. More recently, "nongeometric" techniques such as three-dimensional (3D) echocardiography, CMR, and multidetector-row computed tomography (CT) permit accurate assessment of RV volumes, function, and mass.

Echocardiography

Echocardiography is the most frequently used technique for assessing the right ventricle; it is cheap, widely available, and can be used bedside in very ill patients. It provides information about RV morphology, dimensions, septum convexity, function, tricuspid regurgitation, and estimates of pulmonary arterial pressure and RV pressure. But the assessment of the right ventricle with echocardiography has several limitations. First, the location of the right ventricle behind the sternum restricts the window that can be accessed by the ultrasound beam. Second, the complex shape and thin walls of the right ventricle make it necessary to image the right ventricle from several projections, although the short-axis view is usually the most helpful. Third, the thick trabeculations in the chamber may be confused with a thrombus, a tumor, or hypertrophic cardiomyopathy. Finally, there is a lack of accurate mathematical models to quantify RV mass and volumes with M-mode or two-dimensional echocardiography (2DE) because quantitative measurements are based on geometric assumptions that do not apply to the right ventricle. A qualitative approach for RV volume assessment is usually applied, with the RV size being described as either normal or mildly, moderately, or severely enlarged. If the RV is the same size as the LV, it is usually characterized as moderately enlarged, and if larger than the LV, it is severely enlarged. Also, qualitative evaluation of RV function is usually applied with RV characterized as normal or mildly, moderately, or severely dysfunctional. An approximation to quantification has been introduced with M-mode measurement of the tricuspid annular plane systolic excursion (TAPSE).[27] This parameter provides a rough estimate of RV function but it is not angle independent: it only takes into account the longitudinal function of the RV, which is the predominant, but not unique, component of RV systolic function, and, because it is measured at the basal segment, the presence of regional wall motion abnormalities will affect its accuracy. The fractional area change in the four-chamber view has also been used but, again, this takes into account only the lateral free wall and the presence of regional wall motion abnormalities or RV dilatation might affect its accuracy (Fig. 39.2). Other indicators of RV function are flow Doppler-derived indices such as the myocardial performance index,[28] tissue Doppler measurements of myocardial tricuspid annular myocardial velocities and time intervals, and strain and strain rate measurements of contractility whether with tissue Doppler or speckle tracking imaging (STI). Tissue Doppler is an angle-dependent technique, and incorrect alignment with the ultrasound beam, poor signal-to-noise ratio (SNR) and variability because of placement of the region of interest may affect the results.[29] Speckle tracking imaging is a promising technique that has been applied to the right ventricle[30] to measure longitudinal strain in the six segments in which the right ventricle is classically divided.[31] This technique is useful for the diagnosis of various right heart diseases,

but it may have problems in the case of thin wall or poor image quality in the RV lateral wall, and there is variability across vendors. Doppler transesophageal echocardiography is another echocardiographic method of RV assessment, but it is semiinvasive, is not well suited for evaluation of anteriorly positioned right ventricles, and requires special skills. Three-dimensional echocardiography (3DE) has emerged as a more accurate and reproducible approach to ventricular quantitation, mainly by avoiding the use of geometric assumptions of the ventricular shape. Real-time 3DE is an online acquisition of a 3D dataset of the heart without the need for electrocardiographic and respiratory gating.[32] It calculates right ventricular ejection fraction (RVEF) using the volumetric semiautomated border detection method, which needs to be manually adjusted, and after acquisition and display of end-diastolic and end-systolic frame, long-axis, planes, and volumetric data of the right ventricle are analyzed offline. Eventually, curves of regional and global RVEF are produced and analyzed. However, there are practical problems, such as full cardiac visualization, good-quality endocardial border recognition for manual endocardial tracing, and time consumption. Also, these methods need a stable cardiac rhythm and constant cardiac function during image acquisition, although new single-beat 3DE techniques allow a fast acquisition in one short breath-hold. 3DE has been compared with CMR for the evaluation of RV function, and improved results in comparison with 2D echocardiography have been obtained, both with the usual technique[33,34] and with the new single-beat 3DE,[35] with consistent underestimation of RV volumes and ejection fraction with 3DE. Although 3DE has been used mainly for the left ventricle, assessment of the right ventricle with 3DE is feasible during routine standard echocardiography.

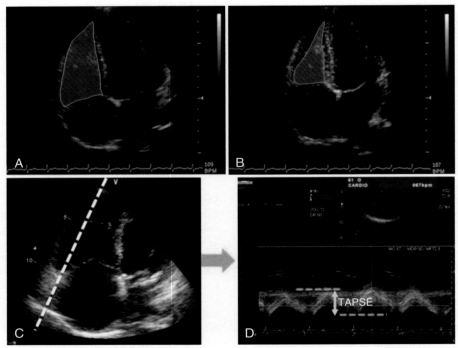

FIG. 39.2 M-mode and two dimensional echocardiographic methods for right ventricular (RV) function assessment. (A and B) RV planimetry in diastole (A) and systole (B) from which the fractional area change can be derived. (C and D) M-mode measurement of the tricuspid annular plane systolic excursion *(TAPSE)*. Both parameters provide a rough estimate of RV function with significant accuracy and reproducibility problems. TAPSE only takes into account the longitudinal function of the right ventricle, which is the predominant, but not unique, component of RV systolic function, and does not account for regional wall motion abnormalities. The fractional area change is measured in only one plane, so the presence of regional wall motion abnormalities or RV dilatation greatly affect its accuracy.

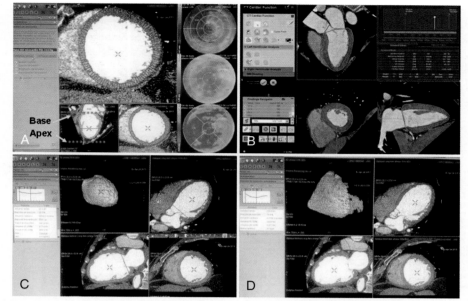

FIG. 39.3 Example of ventricular function analysis with computed tomography. (A and B) Analogous to cardiovascular magnetic resonance, they show myocardial analysis for left ventricular function quantification both with ejection fraction and with wall thickening. (C and D) The ventricular threshold method for measurement of both LV (C) and right ventricular (D) volumes.

Radionuclide Angiography

This technique provides a reliable quantitative measurement of ventricular function not based on geometric assumptions with good agreement with CMR.[36] Although echocardiography and CMR are the two most commonly used imaging techniques for noninvasive assessment of the right ventricle, nuclear imaging provides new opportunities for comprehensive evaluation of the right ventricle from a single study, because it can assess RV perfusion and metabolism as well as morphology and ejection fraction. Some years ago this technique did not work well for the right ventricle, owing to problems such as the limited count numbers in this chamber and the overlap of other cardiac chambers.[37,38] Currently, gated positron emission tomography (PET) has shown moderate-to-high correlation with CMR and CT in the assessments of RV volume and ejection fraction simultaneously with quantification of myocardial glucose metabolism in conditions such as pulmonary hypertension.[39] Gated blood-pool single-photon emission computed tomography (SPECT) appears a promising technique because it does not require geometric assumptions and provides both global and regional RV function quantification with good diagnostic accuracy compared with CMR.[40] Still, these techniques have disadvantages compared with other imaging modalities, such as poor resolution, the use of ionizing radiation, the need for an adequate bolus injection for first-pass studies and a regular rhythm, and the lack of clinical experience. Therefore they have been of limited use for the study of the right ventricle so far.

Multislice Computed Tomography

Multislice CT (MSCT), although not a first-line technique for RV function quantification, is emerging as an alternative tool, especially for patients with implantable devices (a contraindication for CMR). However, MSCT uses ionizing radiation and potentially nephrotoxic contrast, and requires a low and stable heart rate during acquisition.[41] The quantification of ventricular volumes throughout the cardiac cycle requires retrospective electrocardiogram (ECG)-gated helical acquisition, which increases the radiation significantly. Postprocessing is with either a volume threshold approach or, similar to CMR, myocardial analysis is automated but most

times requires manual adjustment (Fig. 39.3). In a study that compared accuracy and reproducibility of MSCT with CMR in the quantification of RV function, spiral MSCT with reconstruction at 5% intervals had good agreement with CMR for RVEF and volumes, with good accuracy and reproducibility,[42] but at the expense of an average radiation dose of 12 to 18 mSv. Another study that compared volumetric quantification of RV-shaped phantoms with CMR, MSCT, and real-time 3DE showed that CMR images yielded the most accurate measurements, whereas MSCT measurements showed slight but consistent overestimation; and 3DE showed small underestimation.[43]

Cardiovascular Magnetic Resonance

CMR has some important advantages over other imaging techniques, which have led to the growing enthusiasm for its use. CMR offers accurate and reproducible tomographic, static, or cine images of high spatial and temporal resolution in any desired plane without exposure to contrast agents or ionizing radiation. It allows the acquisition of true RV short-axis images encompassing the entire right ventricle with high spatial and temporal resolution, thereby providing highly accurate and reproducible quantitative RV mass and functional data regardless of its position in the thorax.[44,45] Nowadays, this technique is considered the gold standard for quantitative assessment of RV volume, mass, and function.

Imaging Strategies for Cardiovascular Magnetic Resonance of the Right Ventricle

Before the study begins, it is essential to obtain an accurate ECG gating with minimal ectopy and to instruct the patient in breath-holding. Sometimes oxygen may be applied to improve breath-hold length. Ventricular ectopy can be a problem, mainly in patients with congenital heart disease or with suspicion of arrhythmogenic RV cardiomyopathy (ARVC). If this condition is present, pretreatment with an antiarrhythmic agent should be considered or, if this is unavailable or unsuccessful, prospective triggering with acquisition window limited to systole can diminish artifacts.

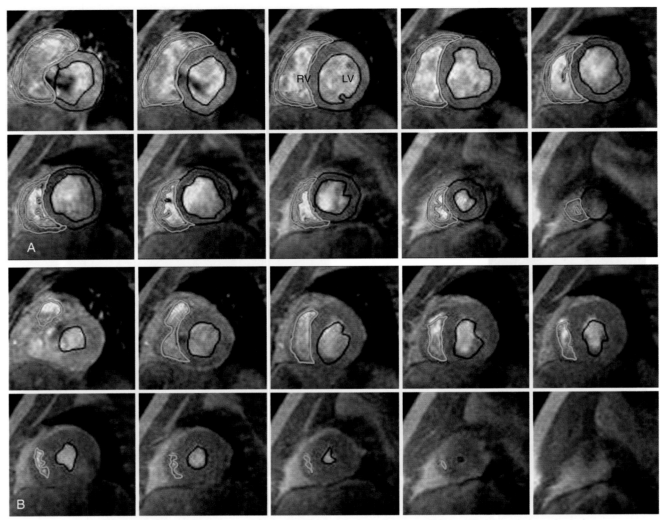

FIG. 39.9 Summation of discs is used to quantify ventricular volumes and mass. The ventricular volume is equal to the sum of the endocardial areas multiplied by the distance between the centers of each slice, both for the end-diastolic volume (A) and the end-systolic volume (B). The ventricular mass is calculated as the sum of the epicardial minus the endocardial areas multiplied by the distance between the centers of each slice, as shown in A. *LV,* Left ventricle; *RV,* right ventricle.

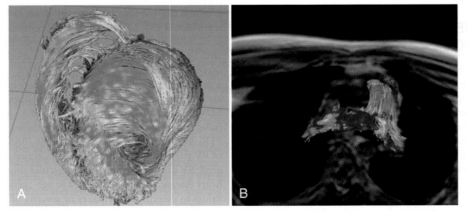

FIG. 39.10 Diffusion tensor imaging of the left ventricle/right ventricle (A) and four-dimensional flow assessment of the pulmonary artery and branches (B) of the right ventricle. Both techniques are promising for assessment of fiber geometry and flow dynamics, respectively.

TABLE 39.1 SSFP Right Ventricular Volumes, Systolic Function, and Mass (Absolute and Normalized to BSA) by Age Decile (Mean, 95% CI): Males

	20–29 Years	30–39 Years	40–49 Years	50–59 Years	60–69 Years	70–79 Years
Absolute Values						
EDV (mL) SD 25.4	177 (127–227)	171 (121–221)	166 (116–216)	160 (111–210)	155 (105–205)	150 (100–200)
ESV (mL) SD 15.2	68 (38–98)	64 (34–94)	59 (29–89)	55 (25–85)	50 (20–80)	46 (16–76)
SV (mL) SD 17.4	108 (74–143)	108 (74–142)	107 (73–141)	106 (72–140)	105 (71–139)	104 (70–138)
EF (%) SD 6.5	61 (48–74)	63 (50–76)	65 (52–77)	66 (53–79)	68 (55–81)	70 (57–83)
Mass (g) SD 14.4	70 (42–99)	69 (40–97)	67 (39–95)	65 (37–94)	63 (35–92)	62 (33–90)
Normalized to BSA						
EDV/BSA (mL/m²) SD 11.7	91 (68–114)	88 (65–111)	85 (62–108)	82 (59–105)	79 (56–101)	75 (52–98)
ESV/BSA (mL/m²) SD 7.4	35 (21–50)	33 (18–47)	30 (16–45)	28 (13–42)	25 (11–40)	23 (8–37)
SV/BSA (mL/m²) SD 8.2	56 (40–72)	55 (39–71)	55 (39–71)	54 (38–70)	53 (37–69)	52 (36–69)
EF/BSA (%/m²) SD 4	32 (24–40)	32 (25–40)	33 (25–41)	34 (26–42)	35 (27–42)	35 (27–43)
Mass/BSA (g/m²) SD 6.8	36 (23–50)	35 (22–49)	34 (21–48)	33 (20–46)	32 (19–45)	31 (18–44)

BSA, Body surface area; *CI*, confidence interval; *EDV*, end-diastolic volume; *EF*, ejection fraction; *ESV*, end-systolic volume; *SD*, standard deviation; *SSFP*, steady-state free precession; *SV*, stroke volume.

TABLE 39.2 SSFP Right Ventricular Volumes, Systolic Function and Mass (Absolute and Normalized to BSA) by Age Decile (Mean, 95% CI): Females

	20–29 Years	30–39 Years	40–49 Years	50–59 Years	60–69 Years	70–79 Years
Absolute Values						
EDV (mL) SD 21.6	142 (100–184)	136 (94–178)	130 (87–172)	124 (81–166)	117 (75–160)	111 (69–153)
ESV (mL) SD 13.3	55 (29–82)	51 (25–77)	46 (20–72)	42 (15–68)	37 (11–63)	32 (6–58)
SV (mL) SD 13.1	87 (61–112)	85 (59–111)	84 (58–109)	82 (56–108)	80 (55–106)	79 (53–105)
EF (%) SD 6	61 (49–73)	63 (51–75)	65 (53–77)	67 (55–79)	69 (57–81)	71 (59–83)
Mass (g) SD 10.6	54 (33–74)	51 (31–72)	49 (28–70)	47 (26–68)	45 (24–66)	43 (22–63)
Normalized to BSA						
EDV/BSA (mL/m²) SD 9.4	84 (65–102)	80 (61–98)	76 (57–94)	72 (53–90)	68 (49–86)	64 (45–82)
ESV/BSA (mL/m²) SD 6.6	32 (20–45)	30 (17–43)	27 (14–40)	24 (11–37)	21 (8–34)	19 (6–32)
SV/BSA (mL/m²) SD 6.1	51 (39–63)	50 (38–62)	49 (37–61)	48 (36–60)	46 (34–58)	45 (33–57)
EF/BSA (%/m²) SD 5.2	37 (27–47)	38 (27–48)	38 (28–49)	39 (29–49)	40 (30–50)	41 (31–51)
Mass/BSA (g/m²) SD 5.2	32 (22–42)	30 (20–40)	29 (19–39)	27 (17–37)	26 (16–36)	24 (14–35)

BSA, Body surface area; *CI*, confidence interval; *EDV*, end-diastolic volume; *EF*, ejection fraction; *ESV*, end-systolic volume; *SD*, standard deviation; *SSFP*, steady-state free precession; *SV*, stroke volume.

TABLE 39.3 SSFP Right Ventricular Diastolic Function and Atrioventricular Plane Descent (Absolute and Normalized Values) by Age Decile (Mean, 95% CI): Males

	20–29 Years	30–39 Years	40–49 Years	50–59 Years	60–69 Years	70–79 Years
Absolute Values						
PFR$_E$ (mL/s) SD 137	545 (277–814)	491 (223–760)	438 (169–706)	384 (116–652)	330 (62–599)	276 (8–545)
PFR$_A$ (mL/s) SD 175	366 (23–709)	413 (70–756)	461 (118–804)	508 (165–852)	556 (213–899)	604 (260–947)
PFR$_E$/PFR$_A$ SD* 0.49	1.6 (0.6–2.5)	1.2 (0.3–2.2)	1.0 (0.0–1.9)	0.7 (−0.2–1.7)	0.6 (−0.4–1.5)	0.5 (−0.5–1.4)
Septal AVPD (mm) SD 4.1	16 (8–24)	15 (7–24)	15 (7–23)	14 (6–22)	14 (6–22)	13 (5–21)
Lateral AVPD (mm) SD 4.4	23 (14–32)	23 (14–31)	22 (14–31)	22 (13–30)	21 (13–30)	21 (12–29)
Normalized Values						
PFR$_E$/BSA (mL/s/m²) SD 71	280 (142–419)	252 (114–390)	224 (85–362)	195 (57–334)	167 (29–306)	139 (1–277)
PFR$_E$/EDV (s⁻¹) SD 0.75	3.1 (1.6–4.6)	2.8 (1.4–4.3)	2.6 (1.1–4.1)	2.3 (0.9–3.8)	2.1 (0.6–3.6)	1.9 (0.4–3.3)
PFR$_A$/BSA (mL/s/m²) SD 94	190 (6–374)	213 (29–397)	236 (52–420)	259 (75–443)	283 (98–467)	306 (122–490)
PFR$_A$/EDV (s⁻¹) SD 1.07	2.1 (0.0–4.2)	2.5 (0.4–4.6)	2.9 (0.8–4.9)	3.2 (1.1–5.3)	3.6 (1.5–5.7)	4.0 (1.9–6.1)
Septal AVPD/long length (%) SD 4.5	18 (9–27)	18 (9–27)	17 (9–26)	17 (8–26)	17 (8–26)	16 (8–25)
Lateral AVPD/long length (%) SD 4.1	23 (15–31)	23 (15–31)	23 (15–31)	23 (15–31)	23 (15–31)	23 (15–31)

A, Active; *AVPD*, atrioventricular plane descent; *BSA*, body surface area; *CI*, confidence interval; *E*, early; *PFR*, peak filling rate; *SD*, standard deviation; *SD**, standard deviation of log transformed data; *SSFP*, steady-state free precession.

TABLE 39.4 SSFP Right Ventricular Diastolic Function and Atrioventricular Plane Descent (Absolute and Normalized Values) by Age Decile (Mean, 95% CI): Females

	20–29 Years	30–39 Years	40–49 Years	50–59 Years	60–69 Years	70–79 Years
Absolute Values						
PFR_E (mL/s) SD 117	471 (241–701)	419 (189–649)	368 (137–598)	316 (86–546)	264 (34–494)	213 (−17–443)
PFR_A (mL/s) SD 153	355 (54–656)	360 (59–660)	365 (64–665)	370 (69–670)	374 (74–675)	379 (79–680)
PFR_E/PFR_A SD* 0.46	1.6 (0.7–2.5)	1.3 (0.4–2.2)	1.0 (0.1–1.9)	0.8 (−0.1–1.7)	0.7 (−0.2–1.6)	0.5 (−0.4–1.4)
Septal AVPD (mm) SD 3.0	16 (10–22)	15 (9–20)	13 (7–19)	12 (6–18)	11 (5–17)	10 (4–16)
Lateral AVPD (mm) SD 3.5	22 (15–29)	21 (14–28)	21 (14–28)	20 (13–27)	20 (13–27)	19 (12–26)
Normalized Values						
PFR_E/BSA (mL/s/m²) SD 68	278 (145–411)	247 (114–380)	216 (83–349)	185 (52–318)	153 (20–286)	122 (−11–255)
PFR_E/EDV (s⁻¹) SD 0.85	3.4 (1.8–5.1)	3.1 (1.5–4.8)	2.8 (1.2–4.5)	2.5 (0.9–4.2)	2.2 (0.6–3.9)	1.9 (0.3–3.6)
PFR_A/BSA (mL/s/m²) SD 89	211 (36–386)	212 (37–388)	214 (39–389)	215 (40–390)	217 (42–392)	218 (43–393)
PFR_A/EDV (s⁻¹) SD 1.03	2.4 (0.4–4.4)	2.6 (0.6–4.6)	2.8 (0.8–4.8)	3.0 (1.0–5.0)	3.2 (1.2–5.2)	3.4 (1.4–5.4)
Septal AVPD/long length (%) SD 3.9	19 (11–27)	18 (11–26)	17 (10–25)	17 (9–24)	16 (8–23)	15 (7–22)
Lateral AVPD/long length (%) SD 4.0	24 (16–32)	24 (16–32)	24 (16–32)	24 (16–32)	24 (16–32)	24 (16–31)

A, active; *AVPD*, atrioventricular plane descent; *BSA*, body surface area; *CI*, confidence interval; *E*, early; *PFR*, peak filling rate; *SD*, standard deviation; *SD**, standard deviation of log transformed data; *SSFP*, steady-state free precession.

TABLE 39.5 SSFP Right Ventricular Summary Data for All Ages (Mean ± Standard Deviation, 95% CI)

	All	Males	Females
EDV (mL)	144 ± 23 (98–190)	163 ± 25 (113–213)	126 ± 21 (84–168)
EDV/BSA (mL/m²)	78 ± 11 (57–99)	83 ± 12 (60–106)	73 ± 9 (55–92)
ESV (mL)	50 ± 14 (22–78)	57 ± 15 (27–86)	43 ± 13 (17–69)
ESV/BSA (mL/m²)	27 ± 7 (13–41)	29 ± 7 (14–43)	25 ± 7 (12–38)
SV (mL)	94 ± 15 (64–124)	106 ± 17 (72–140)	83 ± 13 (57–108)
SV/BSA (mL/m²)	51 ± 7 (37–65)	54 ± 8 (38–70)	48 ± 6 (36–60)
EF (%)	66 ± 6 (54–78)	66 ± 6 (53–78)	66 ± 6 (54–78)
EF/BSA (%/m²)	36 ± 5 (27–45)	34 ± 4 (26–41)	39 ± 5 (29–49)
Mass (g)	48 ± 13 (23–73)	66 ± 14 (38–94)	48 ± 11 (27–69)
Mass/BSA (g/m²)	31 ± 6 (19–43)	34 ± 7 (20–47)	28 ± 5 (18–38)
PFR_E (mL/s)	371 ± 125 (126–615)	405 ± 137 (137–674)	337 ± 117 (107–567)
PFR_E/BSA (mL/m²)	202 ± 69 (67–337)	207 ± 70 (68–345)	197 ± 68 (64–330)
PFR_E/EDV (s⁻¹)	2.6 ± 0.8 (1.0–4.1)	2.4 ± 0.75 (1.0–3.9)	2.7 ± 0.85 (1.0–4.3)
PFR_A (mL/s)	429 ± 168 (99–759)	489 ± 175 (146–833)	368 ± 153 (67–668)
PFR_A/BSA (mL/m²)	233 ± 93 (50–415)	250 ± 94 (66–434)	215 ± 89 (40–390)
PFR_A/EDV (s⁻¹)	3.0 ± 1.0 (1.0–5.1)	3.1 ± 1.0 (1.0–5.2)	2.9 ± 1.0 (0.9–5.0)
PFR_E/PFR_A	0.9 ± 0.47 (−0.1–1.8)	0.8 ± 0.49 (−0.1–1.8)	0.9 ± 0.46 (0.0–1.8)
Septal AVPD (mm)	14 ± 3.6 (6–21)	15 ± 4.1 (6–23)	13 ± 3.0 (7–19)
Septal AVPD/long length (%)	17 ± 4.2 (9–25)	17 ± 4.5 (8–26)	17 ± 3.9 (9–25)
Lateral AVPD (mm)	21 ± 3.9 (13–29)	22 ± 4.4 (13–30)	21 ± 3.5 (14–27)
Lateral AVPD/long length (%)	23 ± 4.0 (15–31)	23 ± 4.1 (15–31)	24 ± 4.0 (16–32)

A, Active; *AVPD*, atrioventricular plane descent; *BSA*, body surface area; *CI*, confidence interval; *E*, early; *EDV*, end-diastolic volume; *EF*, ejection fraction; *ESV*, end-systolic volume; *PFR*, peak filling rate; *SSFP*, steady-state free precession; *SV*, stroke volume.

of prevalent cardiovascular and pulmonary disease have been published,[79] with slight differences in methodology.

Another CMR approach that may be particularly valuable for quantifying regional RV free wall systolic function is myocardial tagging,[80,81] a technique that enables the clinician to assess the complex mechanism of myocardial contraction and to quantify myocardial strain. Klein and colleagues[82] analyzed the RV free wall motion and contraction in humans with CMR tagging. In this study, percent segmental shortening (PSS) was obtained to measure the amount of contraction, and a vector analysis was used to show the trajectory of the RV free wall in systole. PSS increased through time to an average of 12% across all segments (inferior, mid, and superior wall) at the base, 14% at the mid ventricle, and 16% at the apex, with a wave of motion toward the septum and outflow tract. Naito and colleagues[83] determined PSS only at the mid ventricle and found a PSS of 6.7% in the superior wall segment and 20% for the midwall segment. Fayad and colleagues[84] reported similar PSS values: 24.7% in the midwall segment of the midventricular slice and 28.7% in the midwall segment of the apical slice. A 3D reconstruction of RV

FEMALES

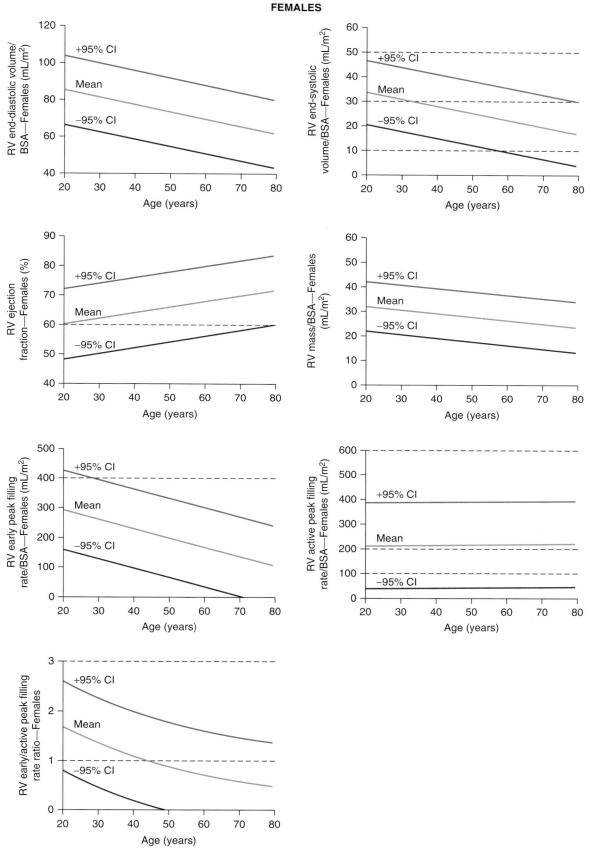

FIG. 39.11 Normal values for right ventricular *(RV)* end-diastolic volume, end-systolic volume, mass, and parameters of diastolic function for females normalized to body surface area *(BSA)*. *CI,* Confidence interval.

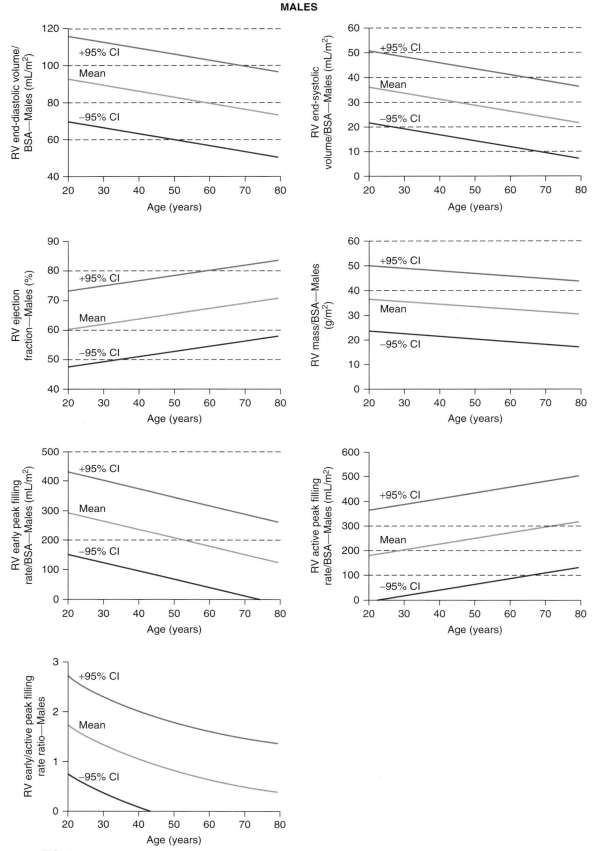

FIG. 39.12 Normal values for right ventricular *(RV)* end-diastolic volume, end-systolic volume, mass, and parameters of diastolic function for males normalized to body surface area *(BSA). CI,* Confidence interval.

contraction with CMR tagging[85] shows a primary contraction of the RV tangential to its own surface plane and a circumferential contraction as the RV moves apically, with a twisting motion similar to that described by Klein and colleagues.[86] Still, although CMR tagging seems a promising method for the assessment of regional function, especially with stress techniques in ischemic heart disease, it remains to be seen whether it provides clinically relevant information beyond that provided by standard cine CMR. Further studies are needed to better define the clinical role of CMR tagging. Myocardial phase contrast has also been used in small studies with promising results, but at the time of this writing, this technique is at a very initial stage and far from clinical use.[87] Equally, CMR feature tracking (CMR-FT) assessment of RV strain shows acceptable levels of agreement with 2DE and has been used to objectively quantify global and regional RV dysfunction and dyssynchrony in patients with ARVC and other conditions, with incremental value over conventional CMR imaging.[88] CMR-FT is promising, although further work is needed to standardize the acquisition and analysis processes, to define normal values, and to assess its use in disease populations with RV dysfunction.

CARDIOVASCULAR MAGNETIC RESONANCE ASSESSMENT OF RIGHT VENTRICULAR ANATOMY AND FUNCTION IN DISEASE

Right Ventricular Assessment in Heart Failure

In left heart failure, atrial pressure rises, forcing open a number of pulmonary capillaries. When all reserve capillaries are open, the increase in pulmonary pressure leads to an increased load on the RV. Therefore the function of the RV during exercise in heart failure is important.[89] The prognostic value of RV function in advanced heart failure of various causes is being increasingly recognized[90,91]; therefore the estimation of RV function is now warranted in the standard evaluation of patients with heart failure, because it is helpful in the clinical assessment and prognostic stratification of such patients. RV dysfunction is also present in one-third of patients with heart failure with preserved ejection fraction, usually associated with an advanced stage and poor outcomes.[92]

Di Salvo and colleagues[93] studied 67 patients with heart failure who had been referred for cardiac transplantation with ischemic (46%) or dilated (54%) cardiomyopathy. An RVEF of 35% or more at rest and with exercise predicted overall survival. Maximal oxygen consumption was also predictive of survival, with a modest correlation between RVEF and maximal oxygen consumption. Also, in patients with moderate heart failure, de Groote and colleagues[94] showed that three variables, NYHA classification, percent of maximal predicted VO₂, and RVEF, were independent predictors of both survival and event-free cardiac survival. Left ventricular EF and peak VO₂ normalized to body weight had no predictive value. The event-free survival rates from cardiovascular mortality and urgent transplantation at 1 year were 80%, 90%, and 95% in patients with an RVEF less than 25%, with an RVEF of 25% or more and less than 35% and with an RVEF of 35% or more, respectively. At 2 years, survival rates were 59%, 77%, and 93%, respectively, in the same subgroups. Throughout the years, a number of papers have shown similar results. More recently, it has been shown that increased (>2 SD beyond the mean) RV volumes at a CMR study predict mortality in heart failure patients.[95] Another study including 250 patients with dilated cardiomyopathy studied with CMR showed that a RV ejection fraction lower than 45% was an independent predictor of death or cardiac transplantation during a median follow-up period of 6.8 years.[96] Therefore CMR quantitative RV volumetric assessment should be measured on all studies that are performed on patients with heart failure.

Right Ventricular Assessment in Ischemic Heart Disease

Isolated RV infarction is relatively rare, but concurrent RV infarction in the setting of an inferior infarction because of proximal right coronary occlusion[97] occurs in up to half of LV infarctions.[98] RV infarction can be detected and evaluated in extent by using late gadolinium enhancement (LGE) CMR. RV necrosis causes a loss of contractile mass, and if the inferior interventricular septum is involved, there is also a loss of septal augmentation of RV function. The existence of RV dysfunction in patients with inferior MI is associated with high rates of morbidity and mortality.[99,100] Cardiogenic shock is more frequent if the RV is involved in inferior infarctions,[101] whereas reperfusion of acute RV infarcts by primary angioplasty has been shown to greatly improve RV function.[102] It has been shown that RVEF quantified late after MI is an important predictor of prognosis adjusted for patient age, LV infarct size, and LVEF.[103] Accordingly, evaluation of RVEF with CMR is important in the setting of acute infarction, not only for RV mass and function quantification but also for detection and quantification of necrosis with late gadolinium techniques that can improve risk stratification and potentially refine patient management after MI.

Right Ventricular Assessment in Arrhythmogenic Right Ventricular Cardiomyopathy

In ARVC, normal myocardium is replaced by fibrofatty tissue, and electrical instability develops. This disorder usually involves the right ventricle, but the left ventricle and septum may also be affected.[104] After hypertrophic heart disease, ARVC is the number one cause of sudden cardiac death in young people, especially athletes. Evident forms of the disease are straightforward to diagnose on the basis of a series of diagnostic criteria proposed by the International Task Force for Cardiomyopathy[7]; however, the diagnosis of early and mild forms of the disease is often difficult. CMR is regarded as the best imaging technique for detecting RV structural and functional abnormalities.[106] The main advantage of CMR is the possibility of planning any desired view so that regions such as the outflow tract, which are hard to visualize with other techniques, can be assessed with great precision.

The most common findings in ARVC are RV wall motion abnormalities, mainly in the subtricuspid region, systolic dysfunction, and dilatation,[107] and these features are the only CMR-derived parameters included in the current diagnostic criteria, which try to be very specific in the general population and very sensitive in individuals who have a high likelihood of inherited/genetic disease. CMR can also detect fatty infiltration; however, this alone does not allow a definitive diagnosis of ARVC because fatty infiltration occurs in a high proportion of healthy people, particularly elderly subjects. It is normally present in areas of the heart such as the atrioventricular groove, around the coronaries, and in the epicardium, and there is a high interobserver variability in its detection.[108] LGE may show myocardial fibrosis in the right ventricle or in the left ventricle of these patients, but LGE is not incorporated in the current diagnostic criteria because of several limitations such as the difficulty of detecting LGE in the thin RV wall and of distinguishing fibrosis from fat, low specificity of LV LGE, and high variability of detection between centers. Importantly, diagnosis of ARVC should always be made according to the criteria proposed by the Task Force and never according to findings from a single test such as CMR.

Congenital Heart Disease

A comprehensive summary of the role of CMR in congenital heart disease is detailed in Chapters 40 and 41. Assessment of RV size, location, and connections as well as of function and pulmonary flow are important.[109] In congenital heart disease, the right ventricle may support the pulmonary (subpulmonary right ventricle) or the systemic circulation (systemic right ventricle). In many of these patients, RV dysfunction develops and leads to considerable morbidity and mortality. Therefore RV function in certain conditions needs close surveillance and timely and appropriate intervention to optimize outcomes. Many of these patients have come into the adult age, and this has created a patient population in which the right ventricle is often the center of attention. Despite major progress being made, assessing the right ventricle in either the subpulmonary or the systemic circulation remains challenging, often requiring a multi-imaging approach. CMR is of use not only in the assessment of the anatomy and physiology of congenital heart disease but also, in some cases, in risk stratification.[110,111]

Pulmonary Hypertension and Lung Transplantation

The fact that CMR is a radiation-free, highly accurate, and reproducible technique for quantitative assessment of RV mass and volume makes it the most appropriate imaging modality for serial studies on the same patient. Cine CMR has been used to study pulmonary hypertension,[112] its response to therapy,[113,114] and the progression of RV failure in this condition.[115] CMR can accurately estimate mean pulmonary artery pressure in patients with suspected pulmonary hypertension and calculate pulmonary vascular resistance (PVR) by estimating all major pulmonary hemodynamic metrics measured at right heart catheterization.[116] CMR has been used to confirm the diagnosis of cor pulmonale through increased RV mass measurements above 60 g.[117] Pulmonary flow patterns are known to be abnormal in pulmonary hypertension,[118] and this may affect RV afterload, whereas diastolic function has also been found to be abnormal in pulmonary fibrosis by using tricuspid flow patterns.[119] More recently, it has been shown in a study including 58 patients with pulmonary hypertension that the presence of LGE in the RV insertion point in patients with pulmonary hypertension is a marker for more advanced disease and poor prognosis. In addition,

CMR-derived RVEF is an independent noninvasive imaging predictor of adverse outcomes in this patient population.[120] CMR has been used to determine the time course of changes in ventricular mass and function after lung transplantation.[121,122] Frist and colleagues[123] observed that RVEF normalized in the early post-lung transplantation period. Other early changes included a decrease in RV end-diastolic volume to below normal levels, with persistence at this level even in the late studies. RV mass also regressed early, but remained increased in comparison to healthy control subjects. The authors concluded that RV anatomic normalization occurred later than functional normalization, and RV mass remained increased. Fayad and colleagues[124] also studied RV tagging in patients with chronic pulmonary hypertension. Regional short-axis shortening was reduced in patients in comparison with healthy controls, and the greatest reductions in shortening were found in the outflow tract and basal septal region.

CONCLUSION

The role of the right ventricle in acquired and congenital heart disease is being increasingly recognized. CMR is a highly accurate, reproducible, and versatile technique that is considered the ideal imaging modality for the comprehensive evaluation of RV dimensions and global and regional function. Accurate quantitation of RV volumes and systolic function provides important diagnostic and prognostic information in a wide range of conditions. However, further clinical studies are needed to establish standards for the best use of CMR for predicting patient outcome and the role of serial evaluation in the case of known RV dysfunction.

REFERENCES

A full reference list is available online at ExpertConsult.com

40

Simple and Complex Congenital Heart Disease: Infants and Children

Andrew J. Powell and Tal Geva

The role of cardiovascular magnetic resonance (CMR) in the evaluation of infants and children with congenital heart disease is now widely accepted as a result of ongoing technologic advances and the growing realization of its clinical value. Improvements in CMR hardware and the development of new, highly efficient/faster imaging methods, have allowed for sufficient spatial and temporal resolution to comprehensively evaluate the complex cardiac anatomy and function in pediatric patients despite their small body size and rapid heart rate. Although transthoracic echocardiography (TTE) provides much of the necessary noninvasive diagnostic information for most patients in this age group, CMR offers an important alternative with added value in several circumstances: (1) when TTE fails to provide the required diagnostic information; (2) when clinical assessment and diagnostic tests are inconsistent; (3) as an alternative to diagnostic invasive x-ray cardiac catheterization with its associated higher risk and cost; and (4) to obtain diagnostic information for which CMR offers unique advantages (e.g., flow measurements, fibrosis, parametric mapping).

This chapter reviews the anatomy, clinical management, and CMR evaluation of common congenital heart disease lesions involving infants and children. Patient preparation, sedation, and monitoring strategies for children undergoing CMR are discussed in Chapter 12.

PRINCIPLES OF CARDIOVASCULAR MAGNETIC RESONANCE EVALUATION IN CONGENITAL HEART DISEASE

Preexamination planning is crucial given the wide array of CMR imaging sequences available and the often-complex nature of the clinical, anatomic, and functional issues in patients with congenital heart disease. It is essential to perform a careful review of the patient's medical history, including details of all prior cardiovascular surgical procedures, interventional catheterizations, diagnostic test results, and current clinical status. As with TTE and invasive cardiac catheterization, CMR examination of congenital heart disease is a dynamic diagnostic procedure that is optimally performed with continuous review and interpretation of the data by the supervising physician. Unexpected findings or suboptimal image quality often require adjustment of the examination protocol, imaging planes, techniques, and sequence parameters. Reliance on standardized protocols and postexamination review alone in these patients may result in incomplete or even erroneous interpretation, or the need to repeat the CMR examination.

One of the strengths of CMR is its ability to accurately and precisely measure ventricular and vascular structures. Care must be taken, however, when determining whether these measurements fall within the normal range because adjustment for the variation in body size remains challenging. Simply dividing by body surface area (BSA) is inadequate for most parameters, particularly in infants and children but also in unusually large or small adults.[1] Several investigators have demonstrated that linear dimensions (e.g., ascending aorta diameter) are best adjusted to the square root of BSA, area measurements to BSA, and volumetric measurements to BSA raised to the 1.3 to 1.4 power.[2,3] Thus for example, one cannot simply apply to children a normative range for ventricular volume indexed to BSA that was derived in adults. CMR-based normative data from healthy children are available, although they are often limited by a smaller than ideal sample size, particularly in the youngest age range.[4–12] Furthermore, it is essential to apply the same measurement technique (e.g., whether to include papillary muscles or myocardial trabeculations in the blood pool) as that which was used to derive the normative data.

ATRIAL SEPTAL DEFECTS AND OTHER INTERATRIAL COMMUNICATIONS

Anatomically, five different defects can result in an interatrial shunt (Fig. 40.1):

1. A patent foramen ovale is bordered on the left by septum primum and by the superior limbic band of the fossa ovalis (septum secundum) on the right. A patent foramen ovale is seen in almost all newborns and decreases in frequency with age.
2. A secundum atrial septal defect (ASD) (Fig. 40.2) is the most common cause of an atrial level shunt after patent foramen ovale. Usually the defect is caused by deficiency of septum primum, but rarely, it results from a deficiency of septum secundum.
3. A primum ASD is a variant of incomplete common atrioventricular canal and is the third most common interatrial communication. This defect involves the septum of the atrioventricular canal and is almost always associated with a cleft anterior mitral valve leaflet. Any associated defect within the fossa ovalis (e.g., secundum ASD) is regarded as a separate abnormality.
4. A sinus venosus septal defect results from deficiency of the sinus venosus septum, which separates the pulmonary veins from the systemic veins and the sinus venosus component of the right atrium (RA) (Fig. 40.3). Most commonly, a sinus venosus defect is between the right upper pulmonary vein and the cardiac end of the superior vena cava. Rarely, the defect involves the right lower and/or middle pulmonary veins and the inferior aspect of the RA near its junction with the inferior vena cava. From an anatomic standpoint, a sinus venosus defect is not an ASD because it does not allow direct communication between the left and right atria. Instead, the interatrial flow travels between the left atrium (LA), one or more of the pulmonary veins, the sinus venosus septal defect, the superior (or inferior) vena cava, and the RA. The defect usually allows

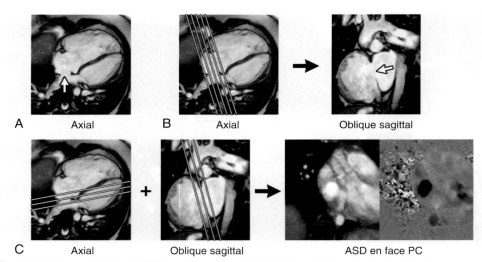

FIG. 40.4 Atrial septal defect *(ASD)* imaging protocol. (A) Axial cine balanced steady-state free precession (bSSFP) image showing a large secundum ASD *(white arrow)*. (B) The axial bSSFP image is used to plan a stack of oblique sagittal cine bSSFP images to visualize the ASD and the superior and inferior defect margins. (C) The axial and oblique sagittal images are used together to plan a stack of velocity-encoded phase contrast *(PC)* cine images to visualize the ASD flow en face. This provides insight into the oval shape of the defect and may demonstrate additional ASDs. (From Fratz S, Chung T, Greil GF, et al. Guidelines and protocols for cardiovascular magnetic resonance in children and adults with congenital heart disease: SCMR expert consensus group on congenital heart disease. *J Cardiovasc Magn Reson.* 2013;15:51.)

- Contrast-enhanced three-dimensional (3D) magnetic resonance angiography (MRA) and/or electrocardiogram (ECG) and respiratory navigator-gated 3D bSSFP imaging of the thorax.
- Blood flow measurements: ascending aorta (Qs) and main pulmonary artery (Qp); optional, superior vena cava and descending aorta at the diaphragm (Qs), and left and right pulmonary arteries (Qp).

After Closure

The CMR examination goals after ASD closure are similar to the preprocedure ones. Additional aims in patients who have undergone transcatheter device closure of an ASD include excluding device malposition, device interference with the atrioventricular valves and venous blood flow, and thrombus formation. Patients who have undergone a repair of a sinus venosus defect are at risk for superior vena cava and right pulmonary vein obstruction. Mitral regurgitation from a residual mitral valve cleft is common after primum ASD repair, and should be assessed quantitatively. All of these aims can be accomplished using the imaging protocol above before closure.

VENTRICULAR SEPTAL DEFECTS

A ventricular septal defect (VSD) is a communication between the RV and LV through an opening in the interventricular septum. Several VSD anatomic classification systems are in use. Fig. 40.5 shows one such system modified from Van Praagh et al.,[27] which includes the following: (1) defects at the junction between the conal septum and the muscular septum bordering the membranous septum (referred to as membranous defects) or associated with malalignment of the conal septum (conoventricular defects) (Fig. 40.6); (2) defects in the muscular septum (called muscular or trabecular defects) (Fig. 40.7); (3) defects in the inlet septum (known as atrioventricular canal-type or inlet defects); and (4) defects in the outlet septum (variably called outlet, doubly committed subarterial, subpulmonary, conal septal, or supracristal defects).

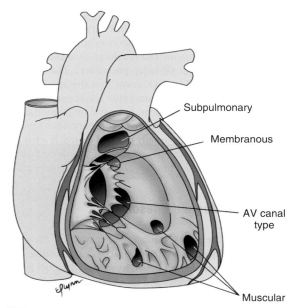

FIG. 40.5 Anatomic types of ventricular septal defects (see text for details). *AV*, Atrioventricular.

The natural history of a VSD relates to the size and location of the defect. Defects in the membranous or muscular septum often become smaller over time and may spontaneously close. In contrast, malalignment conoventricular defects, outlet septum defects, and atrioventricular canal-type defects are usually large and rarely spontaneously close. Consequently, these patients often undergo surgical closure in infancy. Venturi effects associated with VSDs in the membranous or outlet septum may cause aortic valve leaflets (usually the right coronary leaflet) to prolapse through the defect. Although the leaflet prolapse typically

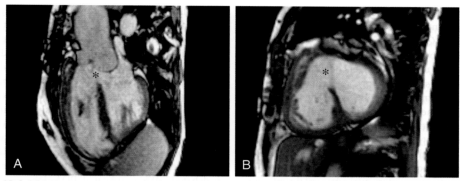

FIG. 40.6 Malalignment conoventricular septal defect *(*)* imaged with cine balanced steady-state free precession in ventricular long-axis (A) and short-axis (B). (From Wald RM, Powell AJ. Congenital heart disease. In: Kwong R, ed. *Cardiovascular Magnetic Resonance Imaging.* Totowa, NJ: Humana Press; 2008:537–568.)

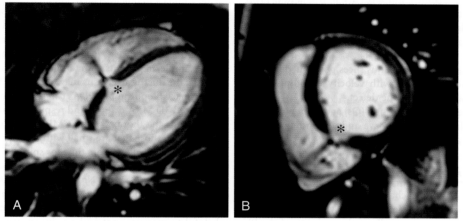

FIG. 40.7 Muscular ventricular septal defect *(*)* imaged with cine balanced steady-state free precession in ventricular long-axis (A) and short-axis (B) views. Note the turbulent flow jet seen in the right ventricle.

reduces the effective orifice size of the defect, it may also lead to aortic regurgitation. VSDs, particularly those associated with turbulent flow jets, also predispose patients to the development of endocarditis.

Symptoms are predominantly determined by the size of the shunt through the VSD, which, in turn, is related to the defect size and the relative resistances of the pulmonary and the systemic vascular beds. In most situations, pulmonary resistance is lower than systemic resistance, and there is a left-to-right shunt. The resulting increased blood flow to the lungs and left heart may lead to dilation of the pulmonary arteries, pulmonary veins, LA, and LV. Because most of the shunt flow passes through the VSD into the RV during systole, RV dilation is usually not present. If the shunt is small and the patient is asymptomatic, an intervention to close the defect is not warranted. When the shunt is large, symptoms from pulmonary overcirculation (e.g., tachypnea, diaphoresis, poor feeding, and slow weight gain) may develop in the first few months of life. If the defect is unlikely to become small over time or if these symptoms cannot be managed medically, surgical closure in infancy is recommended. Untreated, patients with VSDs and large left-to-right shunts may develop irreversible pulmonary artery hypertension from elevated pulmonary vascular resistance. In such cases, the flow through the defect will become increasingly right-to-left, resulting in cyanosis (Eisenmenger syndrome).

A surgical approach is by far the most common technique used to close VSDs and carries a low mortality risk even when performed in the first few months of life. Typically, the surgeon works through the tricuspid valve and applies a patch to cover the defect. In selected patients, such as those with apical defects, a limited right ventriculotomy may be required for effective closure. Experience with transcatheter delivery of occlusion devices is growing, and this approach may be appropriate in selected circumstances.

Cardiovascular Magnetic Resonance

As mentioned, TTE is the primary clinical diagnostic imaging modality in patients with suspected or known VSD, and is usually adequate. Occasionally, in larger patients, acoustic windows may be insufficient and CMR is indicated to define the defect size and location as well as identify associated conditions such as aortic valve prolapse. CMR may also be of use when the hemodynamic burden of a defect is uncertain by providing reliable quantitative data on the Qp:Qs ratio, and on ventricular volumes and function. Moreover, CMR has been shown to be an important, noninvasive test in the diagnosis and management of defects in the outlet septum when TTE assessment of this region is inadequate.[28]

VSD location and size can be demonstrated by cine gradient recalled echo (GRE) or spin echo sequences.[29,30] Very small defects may be difficult to resolve; however, the associated turbulent flow can be made conspicuous on GRE sequences provided the echo time (TE) is long enough to allow for sufficient spin dephasing (see Fig. 40.7). It is useful to assess the ventricular septum using stacks of images oriented in at least two planes. The four-chamber plane provides base-to-apex localization, whereas the short-axis plane shows the location in the superior-to-inferior axis (see Figs. 40.6 and 40.7). Also, as described in the section

The goals of the CMR examination include (1) delineating pulmonary venous drainage, (2) measuring the Qp:Qs ratio and pulmonary artery flow distribution, (3) estimating the RV systolic pressure by evaluating the interventricular septal configuration, and (4) calculating biventricular volumes, mass, and EF. These goals can be achieved by the following protocol:

- Cine bSSFP: axial stack from the mid liver to the top of the aortic arch for pulmonary venous and arterial anatomy
- Cine bSSFP: ventricular long-axis planes and a short-axis stack from base-to-apex for quantitative assessment of biventricular volumes and EF
- Contrast-enhanced 3D MRA and/or ECG and respiratory navigator-gated 3D bSSFP imaging of the thorax
- Blood flow measurements: ascending aorta (Qs) and main pulmonary artery (Qp); left and right pulmonary arteries (Qp) and anomalous vein

Postoperative

The goals of a postoperative assessment include those of the preoperative assessment along with the need to carefully assess for obstruction and defects along the surgically created pulmonary venous drainage pathway. All of these aims can be accomplished using the preoperative imaging protocol above and tailored cine bSSFP imaging planes to visualize the pulmonary venous connection to the LA.

COARCTATION OF THE AORTA

Coarctation of the aorta is a discrete narrowing most commonly located just distal to the left subclavian artery, at the ductus arteriosus insertion site (Fig. 40.10). Hypoplasia and elongation of the distal transverse arch is a frequent association. Coarctation may be present alone or in combination with other heart lesions, including bicuspid aortic valve, subvalvar and valvar aortic stenosis, mitral valve abnormalities, ASD, VSD, persistent PDA, and conotruncal anomalies.

Infants tend to present with symptoms of heart failure and systemic hypoperfusion as the ductus arteriosus closes; if untreated, they may progress to shock or death. Older children and adults typically have isolated coarctation and may have minimal symptoms. Even in asymptomatic patients, relief of the aortic obstruction is indicated for hemodynamically significant lesions because of the high rate of late complications, including heart failure, systemic hypertension, premature coronary artery disease, ruptured aortic or cerebral aneurysms, stroke, aortic dissection, infective endarteritis, and premature death.[41]

Therapeutic options for coarctation include surgical repair and percutaneous balloon angioplasty and stent placement. Currently, resection of the coarctation with an end-to-end anastomosis and augmentation of the transverse arch, if needed, is the most widely practiced surgical repair and has the lowest incidence of recurrent obstruction. Other approaches have included subclavian flap aortoplasty, patch augmentation, and conduit interposition. Coarctation in infants is treated surgically in the majority of centers because of the lower risk of residual obstruction, recurrence, and technique-related complications compared with percutaneous interventions.[42] In the event of recurrent coarctation following surgical repair, balloon angioplasty with or without stent placement is often the preferred approach. Coarctation in older children or adults is increasingly being treated primarily by percutaneous interventions. Regardless of the initial treatment, subsequent surveillance for restenosis, aneurysm formation, and dissection is warranted.[43]

Cardiovascular Magnetic Resonance Preintervention and Postintervention

TTE is usually the only diagnostic imaging needed for evaluation of young children with suspected coarctation or following intervention for coarctation. With increasing age, acoustic windows typically deteriorate, leading to an incomplete assessment by TTE. In these circumstances, CMR is able to provide high-quality anatomic imaging of the aortic arch in its entirety (Fig. 40.10), an assessment of the hemodynamic severity of the obstruction, and an evaluation of LV mass, volumes, and function. In a retrospective study of 84 adult patients following intervention for coarctation of the aorta, Therrien et al.[44] showed that the combination of clinical assessment and CMR on every patient was more "cost-effective" for detecting complications than combinations that relied on TTE or chest radiography as imaging modalities. Other studies have shown the utility of CMR in infants and children with

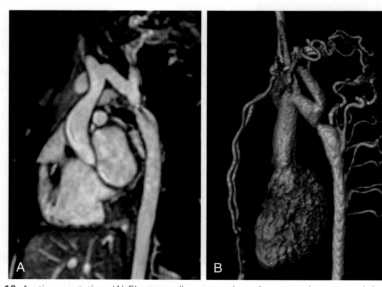

FIG. 40.10 Aortic coarctation. (A) Electrocardiogram and respiratory navigator-gated three-dimensional (3D) balanced steady-state free precession oblique sagittal reformat showing severe discrete narrowing at the aortic isthmus with an associated turbulent flow jet. (B) Volume rendered contrast-enhanced 3D magnetic resonance angiography revealing several tortuous collateral vessels and dilated internal mammary arteries.

coarctation and other anomalies of the aortic arch.[45–47] Computed tomography (CT) can also provide excellent anatomic imaging of the aorta but has the disadvantage of ionizing radiation exposure and the need for iodinated contrast make it a less attractive modality for serial follow-up.

With regard to aortic anatomy, careful attention should be given to the transverse aortic arch and isthmus, brachiocephalic vessels, collateral vessels that may bypass the obstruction, and possible aneurysms or dissections at the repair sites. Regions of vessel narrowing should ideally be measured in cross section as elliptical lesions are common. If a coarctation is present, its diameter, length, and distance to neighboring vessels should be reported, as this may influence decisions regarding percutaneous intervention. Given the association of a bicuspid aortic valve with coarctation, the aortic valve morphology should be noted as well as the dimensions of the aortic root and ascending aorta, as they may be dilated.

Blood velocity and flow measurements with CMR have been used to gain insight into the functional significance of a coarctation. One approach has been to assess the flow pattern in the descending aorta distal to the coarctation, preferably at the level of the diaphragm (see Fig. 40.11). Characteristics suggestive of a hemodynamically significant coarctation include decreased peak flow, decreased time-averaged flow, delayed onset of descending aorta flow compared with the onset of flow in the ascending aorta, decreased acceleration rate, and prolonged deceleration with increased antegrade diastolic flow.[48–51] Another approach to assessing coarctation severity is to measure the peak coarctation jet velocity and estimate a pressure gradient using the modified Bernoulli equation.[52–55] Note, however, that such measurements may be technically difficult in a long, tortuous coarctation segment and that the pressure estimates may not be indicative of anatomic severity because of collateral flow. Finally, CMR has been used to quantify collateral flow entering the descending aorta distal to the obstruction via retrograde flow from the intercostal arteries or vessels arising off the aortic arch and arch branches.[49,56–58] With this technique, proximal flow is measured just proximal or distal to the site of obstruction, and distal flow in the descending aorta at the level of the diaphragm. A greater distal-to-proximal flow ratio is seen with increased collateral flow and suggests more severe obstruction. If little collateral flow is found, the surgeon may elect to perform a left heart bypass to the descending aorta during the repair to reduce the risk of spinal cord ischemic injury when correction requires interruption of aortic flow.

CMR evaluation of coarctation should also include calculation of LV volumes, EF, mass, and mass-to-volume ratio. These data are clinically relevant because systemic hypertension is often present and may lead to LV hypertrophy and dysfunction. Upper body hypertension may be caused by aortic arch obstruction but systemic hypertension is also prevalent following coarctation repair even without residual coarctation, particularly in patients who had relief of obstruction at an older age. It is good practice to measure both upper arms and lower extremity cuff blood pressures at the time of the CMR examination to help identify patients with systemic hypertension and estimate the pressure gradient across any aortic obstruction. Note that there may be little upper-to-lower extremity blood pressure differential even with important aortic obstruction when there is a significant collateral circulation bypassing the obstruction.

The goals of the CMR examination include (1) assessing the aortic arch anatomy and degree of obstruction; (2) calculating LV volumes, mass, and EF; and (3) evaluating aortic valve morphology and function. These goals can be achieved by the following protocol[26]:

- Cine bSSFP: stack of contiguous thin slices in an oblique sagittal plane oriented in long axis (parallel) to the aortic arch for evaluation of arch anatomy.
- Black-blood spin echo (optional): stack of contiguous thin slices in an oblique sagittal plane oriented in long axis (parallel) to the aortic arch for evaluation of arch anatomy. This is particularly valuable following endovascular stent placement because there is less metallic susceptibility artifact than with cine sequences.
- Cine bSSFP: ventricular long-axis planes and a short-axis stack from base-to-apex for quantitative assessment of LV cavity volume, mass, and EF.
- Contrast-enhanced 3D MRA and/or ECG and respiratory navigator-gated 3D bSSFP imaging of the thorax (see Fig. 40.10).
- Blood flow measurements: ascending aorta, main pulmonary artery, descending aorta at the level of the diaphragm for assessment of the descending aorta flow profile (see Fig. 40.11) and aortic valve function.
- Blood flow measurements (optional): just distal to the coarctation in long axis and cross section for measurement of the peak velocity and/or for quantitation of collateral flow.

TETRALOGY OF FALLOT

TOF is the most common type of cyanotic congenital heart disease.[59] Although TOF involves several anatomic components, the anomaly is thought to result from a single developmental anomaly—underdevelopment of the subpulmonary infundibulum (conus).[60] The resulting pathology is notable for anterior, superior, and leftward deviation of the infundibular (conal) septum, causing subpulmonary stenosis;

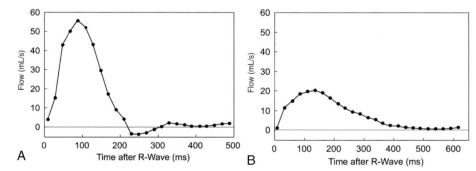

FIG. 40.11 Evaluation of coarctation severity based on the flow pattern in the descending aorta at the level of the diaphragm. (A) Descending aorta flow pattern in a patient with repaired coarctation and no residual obstruction. Note the sharp upstroke and short deceleration phase. (B) Descending aorta flow pattern in a patient with severe coarctation. Note the blunted upstroke and prolonged deceleration.

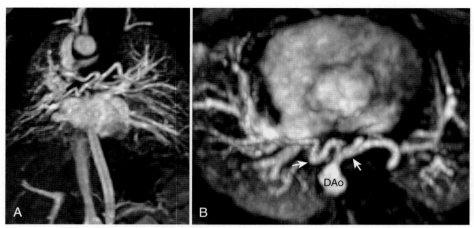

FIG. 40.12 Multiple aortopulmonary collateral (APC) vessels in a newborn with tetralogy of Fallot and pulmonary atresia evaluated by contrast-enhanced three-dimensional magnetic resonance angiography. (A) Subvolume maximum intensity projection (MIP) image in the coronal plane showing multiple APCs arising from the descending aorta. (B) Subvolume MIP image in the transverse plane showing APCs arising from the descending aorta *(DAo)* and splitting into two large branches, one to the left lung and one to the right lung *(arrows).*

pulmonary valve stenosis from annular hypoplasia, thickened leaflets, and abnormal commissures; a large conoventricular septal defect; and overriding of the aortic valve above the interventricular septum. The degree of RV outflow tract (RVOT) obstruction varies from mild to complete obstruction (i.e., TOF with pulmonary atresia). The mediastinal pulmonary arteries are often small, and may even be discontinuous or absent. In patients with pulmonary atresia or absent branch pulmonary arteries, pulmonary blood flow comes from a PDA and/or collateral vessels arising from the aorta and its branches. Approximately 5% to 6% of patients with TOF have a major coronary artery crossing the anterior aspect of the RVOT.[61] Most commonly, it is the left anterior descending coronary artery which arises from the right coronary artery and traverses the infundibular free wall to reach the anterior interventricular groove. Preoperative identification of a major coronary artery crossing the RVOT is important to avoid inadvertent damage to the coronary artery during surgical relief of RVOT obstruction. Finally, approximately 25% of patients have a right aortic arch.

Although the clinical presentation and course of patients with TOF varies, most patients develop cyanosis during the first year of life. Surgical repair is usually performed before the age of 6 months. A typical repair includes patch closure of the VSD and RVOT obstruction relief using a combination of resection of obstructive muscle bundles and an overlay patch. When the pulmonary valve annulus is moderately or severely hypoplastic, the RVOT patch is extended across the pulmonary valve annulus into the main pulmonary artery, destroying the valve mechanism and leading to pulmonary regurgitation. In patients with TOF and pulmonary atresia, or when a major coronary artery crosses the RVOT, a conduit—either a homograft or a prosthetic tube—is placed between the RVOT and the pulmonary arteries.

Patients undergoing surgical repair of TOF as young children have excellent short-term survival[62]; however, they experience significant morbidity and mortality related to biventricular dysfunction and arrhythmia in their adult years.[63–65] These sequelae are believed to be at least in part related to chronic pulmonary regurgitation caused by efforts to relieve pulmonary valve stenosis with the initial TOF repair. Thus pulmonary valve replacement is often performed subsequently to improve the long-term outcome.[66,67] Other common concerns in repaired TOF patients include RVOT tract or pulmonary arterial obstruction, tricuspid regurgitation, and residual ASDs and VSDs.

Cardiovascular Magnetic Resonance
Preoperative
For most infants, TTE provides all of the necessary diagnostic information for surgical repair; however, when the pulmonary arteries are hypoplastic and aortopulmonary collateral vessels are suspected, other modalities are often needed to adequately delineate these structures. Contrast-enhanced MRA is well suited for this task (Fig. 40.12). Compared with conventional x-ray angiography, MRA has been shown to be highly accurate in depicting all sources of pulmonary blood supply in patients with complex pulmonary stenosis or atresia, including infants with multiple small aortopulmonary collaterals.[33,38]

Postoperative
CMR provides a comprehensive imaging assessment of postoperative TOF patients and its use is recommended by a number of expert guideline statements.[35,68–70] Information derived from CMR on pulmonary regurgitation, biventricular size and function, RVOT aneurysm (Fig. 40.13), and pulmonary artery stenosis often dictates clinical care. In particular, CMR parameters are a key component to determine whether patients should undergo pulmonary valve replacement.[71] Moreover, in an effort to improve risk stratification, a growing number of studies have linked CMR data to adverse outcomes. A report from the International Multicenter TOF Registry (INDICATOR) showed that RV hypertrophy and decreased CMR LV and RV EF are associated with death or sustained ventricular tachycardia.[72] Focal fibrosis, as identified by late gadolinium enhancement (LGE), is common after TOF repair, and a greater extent of RV involvement is associated with older age, worse symptoms, exercise intolerance, RV dysfunction, and clinical arrhythmia.[73] The utility of diffuse fibrosis assessment using T1 measurement techniques is now being explored.[74,75]

The goals of the CMR examination include (1) quantitative assessment of biventricular volume, mass, stroke volume, and EF; (2) imaging the RVOT, pulmonary arteries, aorta, and aortopulmonary collaterals; (3) quantification of pulmonary regurgitation, tricuspid regurgitation, cardiac output, and Qp:Qs ratio; and (4) assessment of myocardial fibrosis. These objectives can be achieved with the following protocol[26]:
- Cine bSSFP: ventricular long-axis planes and a short-axis stack from base-to-apex for quantitative assessment of biventricular volumes, mass, and EF.

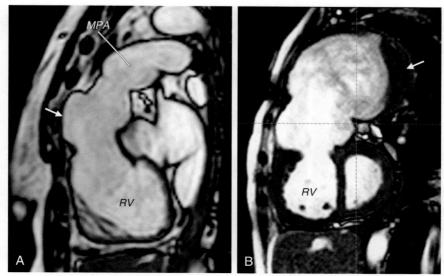

FIG. 40.13 Right ventricular *(RV)* outflow tract aneurysm following repair of tetralogy of Fallot. (A) Cine balanced steady-state free precession (bSSFP) image showing a thin, dyskinetic anterior wall *(arrow)* of the right ventricle, at least in part related to placement of an RV outflow tract patch. (B) Cine bSSFP image demonstrating a massive aneurysm of the RV outflow tract and main pulmonary artery *(MPA)*. Note the mural thrombus in the MPA *(arrow)*.

- Cine bSSFP: stack parallel to the RVOT.
- Cine bSSFP: axial plane to image the branch pulmonary arteries.
- Contrast-enhanced 3D MRA and/or ECG and respiratory navigator-gated 3D bSSFP imaging of the thorax.
- Blood flow measurements: main and branch pulmonary arteries, ascending aorta, and atrioventricular valves.
- LGE: ventricular long-axis and short-axis planes.

TRANSPOSITION OF THE GREAT ARTERIES

Transposition of the great arteries (TGA) is defined as discordant alignments between the ventricles and the great arteries; the aorta arises from the RV and the pulmonary artery arises from the LV. The most common type of TGA and the focus of the subsequent discussion is with visceroatrial situs solitus (S), ventricular D-loop (D), and dextro malposition of the aortic valve relative to the pulmonary valve (D). This anatomical arrangement can be summarized as {S,D,D} TGA. Associated cardiac anomalies with their approximate prevalence include VSDs in 45% of patients, coarctation or interrupted aortic arch in 12%, pulmonary stenosis in 5%, RV hypoplasia in 4%, and juxtaposition of the atrial appendages in 2%.[76] The principal physiologic abnormality is that desaturated systemic venous blood flows to the RA, RV, and the aorta, and oxygenated pulmonary venous blood flows to the LA and LV, and then back to the lungs. These parallel systemic and pulmonary circulations result in profound hypoxemia. Consequently, survival depends on the presence of an ASD, VSD, and/or PDA that allows mixing of blood between the systemic and pulmonary circulations.

Surgical management of D-loop TGA in the 1960s and 1970s consisted mostly of an atrial switch procedure—the Senning or Mustard operations. In both procedures, the systemic and pulmonary venous blood is redirected within the atria so that the pulmonary venous blood reaches the tricuspid valve, RV, and aorta, whereas the systemic venous blood reaches the mitral valve, LV, and pulmonary arteries (Fig. 40.14). The main technical difference between these two procedures is that in the Mustard operation, pericardium is used to redirect the blood flow

and in the Senning operation native atrial tissue is used. The most common sequelae following atrial switch operations are RV (systemic ventricle) dysfunction, tricuspid regurgitation, sinus node dysfunction, atrial arrhythmias, obstruction of the atrial baffle pathways, and atrial baffle leaks. During the 1980s, the arterial switch operation largely replaced the atrial switch procedures. In this operation, the ascending aorta and main pulmonary artery are transected and then connected to the concordant semilunar valve root, and the coronary arteries are transferred to the new aortic valve. The advantages of the arterial switch operation over the atrial switch procedures include the establishment of the LV (rather than the RV) as the systemic ventricle, and the avoidance of extensive suture lines in the atria, which contribute to arrhythmia. Recent data on long-term outcomes of the arterial switch operation continue to show excellent overall survival with low morbidity.[77,78] The most common postoperative complications include stenosis of the main and branch pulmonary arteries (Fig. 40.15), dilatation of the neoaortic root, aortic valve regurgitation, and coronary artery stenosis.[79] The Rastelli operation is another surgical option for TGA patients with an associated subvalvar and valvar pulmonary stenosis and a VSD. It consists of patch closure of the VSD so that the LV outflow is directed to the aortic valve, and placement of a conduit from the RV to the pulmonary arteries. More recently, this anatomic variant has also been treated with complete removal of the native pulmonary root and valve, translocation of the entire aortic root and coronary arteries to the LV outflow tract, and placement of a homograft between the RVOT and the pulmonary arteries.

Cardiovascular Magnetic Resonance
Preoperative
CMR is seldom requested for preoperative assessment of infants with D-loop TGA because TTE usually provides all of the necessary diagnostic information.[76]

Postoperative Atrial Switch Operation
CMR has a central role in the noninvasive imaging surveillance of patients who have undergone an atrial switch operation.[69,80] Assessment

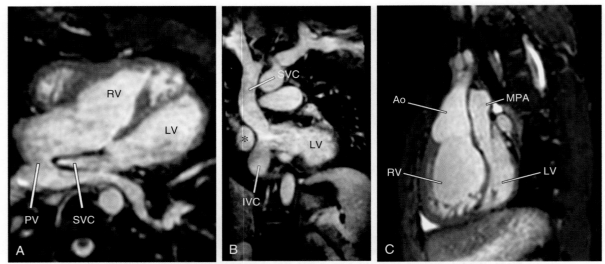

FIG. 40.14 Mustard palliation for transposition of the great arteries. Electrocardiogram and respiratory navigator-gated three-dimensional balanced steady-state free precession data was reformatted offline in multiple user-defined planes. (A) Transverse plane showing the pulmonary venous *(PV)* pathway to the right ventricle *(RV)* and superior vena cava *(SVC)* pathway to the left ventricle *(LV)*. (B) Oblique sagittal plane depicting the SVC and inferior vena cava *(IVC)* pathways to the LV, and the PV pathway *(*)* in cross-section. (C) Oblique sagittal plane showing the LV outflow tract connecting to the main pulmonary artery *(MPA)* and the RV outflow tract connecting to the aorta *(Ao)*.

of the systemic RV, a key concern in this patient group, can be difficult by TTE because of its substernal position and complex shape. CMR, however, routinely provides complete tomographic imaging of the RV, which allows for accurate and reproducible measurements of volume, mass, and EF.[81,82] CMR is also useful for evaluating the systemic and pulmonary venous baffle pathways for obstruction and leaks.[83,84] The physiologic impact of baffle leaks can be gauged by measuring blood flow in the main pulmonary artery and ascending aorta to calculate the Qp:Qs ratio. Note, however, that a Qp:Qs ratio close to 1 can be seen even in large baffle leaks when there is bidirectional flow; thus, anatomic imaging information and the systemic oxygen saturation must also be considered.

Studies in patients who have undergone an atrial switch operation have found RV LGE indicative of focal myocardial fibrosis, although the reported prevalence of this finding varies.[85–88] In cross-sectional studies, the presence and extent of LGE have been associated with greater age, RV dysfunction, reduced peak oxygen uptake, electrophysiologic parameters, arrhythmia, and adverse clinical events. The best evidence establishing the prognostic value of LGE comes from a longitudinal study of 55 atrial switch operation patients which showed that RV LGE was independently associated with a composite endpoint primarily composed of atrial tachyarrhythmia.[87]

The goals of the CMR evaluation include (1) quantitative assessment of the systemic RV volume, mass, and EF; (2) imaging of the systemic and pulmonary venous pathways for obstruction and baffle leaks; (3) quantitation of tricuspid valve regurgitation; (4) evaluation of the LV and RV outflow tracts for obstruction; and (5) assessment of myocardial fibrosis. These goals can be achieved with the following protocol[26]:

- Cine bSSFP: axial stack from the mid-liver through the top of the aortic arch for dynamic imaging of the venous pathways, atrioventricular valve regurgitation, and the great arteries.
- Cine bSSFP: oblique planes to image the superior and inferior limbs of the systemic venous pathway in long axis.
- Cine bSSFP: ventricular long-axis planes to assess biventricular function and the outflow tracts.

- Cine bSSFP: ventricular short-axis stack from base-to-apex for quantitative assessment of biventricular volumes, mass, and EF.
- Contrast-enhanced 3D MRA and/or ECG and respiratory navigator-gated 3D bSSFP imaging of the chest (see Fig. 40.14).
- Blood flow measurements: main pulmonary artery, ascending aorta, tricuspid valve, and mitral valve.
- LGE: ventricular long- and short-axis planes.

Postoperative Arterial Switch Operation

Studies have shown that detection of pulmonary artery stenosis in arterial switch operation patients by CMR is accurate and superior to the information obtained by TTE (see Fig. 40.15).[89–91] CMR can also provide high-resolution imaging of the proximal coronary arteries and define their relationship to the surrounding structures such as the aorta and main pulmonary artery.[92–94] The largest report consisted of 84 CMR examinations and yielded diagnostic image quality of the proximal coronary arteries in 95% and showed stenosis in 11%.[94] There are two principal CMR techniques to diagnose inducible myocardial ischemia: (1) evaluation for perfusion defects using vasodilator stress agents (e.g., adenosine or dipyridamole); and (2) evaluation of wall motion, most commonly using dobutamine stress. In addition, the LGE technique is highly sensitive for detecting myocardial infarction and focal fibrosis. In two reports describing a total of 55 asymptomatic arterial switch operation patients who underwent stress perfusion CMR, no defects at stress were detected.[93,95] Moreover, the LGE technique has identified prior myocardial infarction in only a small proportion of patients after arterial switch operation.[93,95,96] Thus based on these studies, both CMR stress imaging and LGE appear to have a low positive yield in asymptomatic arterial switch operation patients. Larger studies that include symptomatic patients and have longer-term follow-up are needed to better define the indications and prognostic value of these CMR techniques.

The goals of the CMR evaluation include (1) quantitative assessment of biventricular volumes and function; (2) imaging the LV and RV outflow tracts for obstruction; (3) imaging the aorta, main pulmonary artery, and branch pulmonary arteries for obstruction; (4) measurement

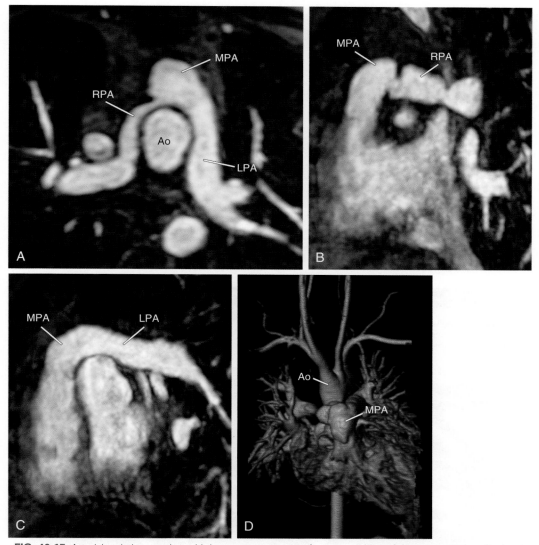

FIG. 40.15 Arterial switch operation with Lecompte maneuver for transposition of the great arteries. Contrast-enhanced three-dimensional magnetic resonance angiography with subvolume maximum intensity projection (A–C) and volume rendering (D) showing the main pulmonary artery *(MPA)* bifurcation positioned anterior to the ascending aorta *(Ao)*, right pulmonary artery *(RPA)* stenosis, and an unobstructed left pulmonary artery *(LPA)*.

of aortic root size; (5) quantitation of aortic and pulmonary valve regurgitation; (6) identification of residual atrial and ventricular septal defects, and calculation of the Qp:Qs ratio; and (7) description of the proximal coronary origins, course, and degree of obstruction. These goals can be achieved with the following protocol[26]:

- Cine bSSFP: ventricular long-axis planes and a short-axis stack from base-to-apex for quantitative assessment of biventricular dimensions and EF.
- Cine bSSFP: axial stack to assess for branch pulmonary artery obstruction.
- Cine bSSFP: stack in short axis to the aortic root to assess the degree of dilation and visualize any regurgitation jet.
- Cine bSSFP: ascending aorta long-axis plane to assess for obstruction.
- Contrast-enhanced 3D MRA (see Fig. 40.15).
- ECG and respiratory navigator-gated 3D bSSFP imaging of the coronary arteries.
- Blood flow measurements: main and branch pulmonary arteries and ascending aorta.

- If there is a concern for inducible myocardial ischemia, a vasodilator or dobutamine stress protocol and myocardial LGE imaging should be considered.

SINGLE VENTRICLE

The normal human heart is composed of three chambers at the ventricular level (between the atrioventricular valves and the semilunar valves): the LV sinus, the RV sinus, and the infundibulum. From an anatomic standpoint, a single ventricle heart is present when one of the two ventricular sinuses is absent. The infundibulum is always present and has a variety of names such as infundibular outlet chamber, rudimentary or hypoplastic RV, and rudimentary chamber. There are two types of single ventricle:

1. Single LV (Fig. 40.16) in which there is an absence of the RV sinus and the presence of an LV and an infundibulum. The communication between the LV and the infundibulum is termed the bulboventricular foramen.

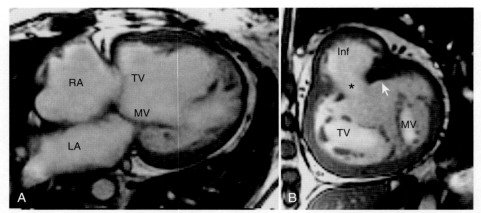

FIG. 40.16 Double-inlet single left ventricle. Cine balanced steady-state free precession images in horizontal long-axis (A) and short-axis (B) planes. Note that both mitral valve *(MV)* and the tricuspid valve *(TV)* enter the left ventricle, which is characterized by a smooth septal surface *(arrow)*. The bulboventricular foramen *(*)* provides an exit from the left ventricle to the infundibulum *(Inf)*. *LA*, Left atrium; *RA*, right atrium.

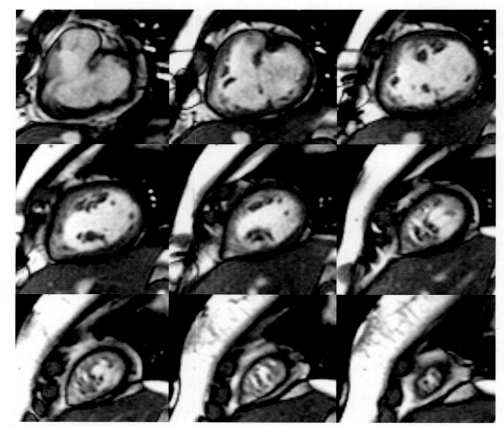

FIG. 40.17 Double-inlet single right ventricle. Stack of cine steady-state free precession images in a short-axis plane. Note the absence of a ventricular septum.

2. Single RV (Fig. 40.17) in which the ventricular mass consists of the RV sinus and the infundibulum, together forming a common chamber. The septal band is present, indicating the location of a ventricular septum, but there is no macroscopically recognizable LV sinus on the other side of the septum.

There are other congenital cardiac anomalies that do not have a single ventricle from a strict anatomic standpoint but whose anatomy precludes the establishment of a normal two-ventricle circulation. These conditions are often grouped under the term "functional single ventricle" or "functional univentricular hearts," and are managed similarly to single ventricle hearts. Examples include tricuspid atresia, mitral atresia, severely unbalanced common atrioventricular canal defect, and hypoplastic left heart syndrome.

Single ventricle physiology is characterized by complete mixing of the systemic and pulmonary venous return flows. The proportion of the ventricular output distributed to the pulmonary versus systemic circulations is determined by the relative resistance to flow in the two circuits and heavily influences the systemic oxygen saturation. Management is

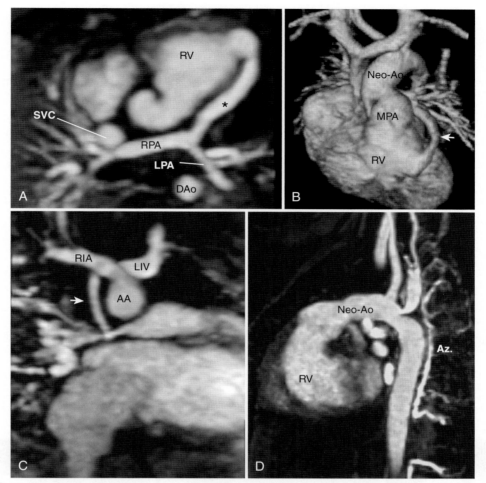

FIG. 40.18 Hypoplastic left heart syndrome. Contrast-enhanced three-dimensional (3D) magnetic resonance angiography in infants before bidirectional Glenn shunt. (A) Subvolume maximum intensity projection (MIP) in an oblique transverse plane showing a conduit (*) from the right ventricle (RV) to the pulmonary arteries. (B) 3D volume rendering in the same patient showing the conduit (arrow) as well as the anastomosis between the main pulmonary artery and the reconstructed neo-aorta (Neo-Ao). (C) Oblique coronal subvolume MIP in a patient with a modified right Blalock-Taussig shunt. The shunt (arrow) extends from the right innominate artery (RIA) to the right pulmonary artery, and there is pulmonary artery stenosis at the insertion site. (D) Oblique sagittal subvolume MIP showing a reconstructed Neo-Ao. AA, Ascending aorta; Az., azygos vein; DAo, descending aorta; LIV, left innominate vein; LPA, left pulmonary artery; MPA, main pulmonary artery; RPA, right pulmonary artery; SVC, superior vena cava.

typically directed toward a series of surgeries culminating in the Fontan operation. The first surgery is often performed in the first week or two of life. Its goals are to establish an appropriate amount of pulmonary blood flow to avoid overcirculation to the lungs, yet adequate systemic saturation, and to provide unobstructed flow to the systemic circulation. A variety of surgical procedures may be performed, depending on the specific patient details and institutional preference. Examples include the stage I procedure, Blalock-Taussig shunt, and pulmonary artery band placement (Fig. 40.18). The next surgery is typically a superior cavopulmonary anastomosis (bidirectional Glenn) operation, performed at 4 to 6 months of age. As a result of this procedure, the superior vena cava supplies pulmonary flow, and the inferior vena cava blood skips the lungs and is directed to the ventricle and then out to the systemic circulation. The third and often final surgery is the Fontan operation, performed between 18 months and 3 years of age. With this procedure, inferior vena cava blood is also directed to the pulmonary arteries. Thus the systemic and pulmonary circulations are separated with inferior

and superior vena cava flow passively draining to the lungs, and pulmonary venous return actively pumped by the single ventricle out to the body. This largely eliminates hypoxemia. Since it was first described in 1971,[97] the Fontan operation has undergone multiple modifications (Fig. 40.19), including direct anastomosis of the right atrial appendage to the main pulmonary artery (called an atriopulmonary anastomosis), RA-to-RV conduit, lateral tunnel between the inferior vena cava and the undersurface of the ipsilateral branch pulmonary artery (Fig. 40.20), fenestration of the lateral tunnel baffle, and an extracardiac conduit between the inferior vena cava and the ipsilateral branch pulmonary artery.

With refinement of patient selection criteria, medical therapy, and surgical techniques, the results of this stage surgical management approach to single ventricle heart disease have improved. Nevertheless, this patient population continues to be at risk for complications such as ventricular systolic and diastolic dysfunction; valve regurgitation; aortic arch, Fontan pathway, and pulmonary artery obstruction; pulmonary vein

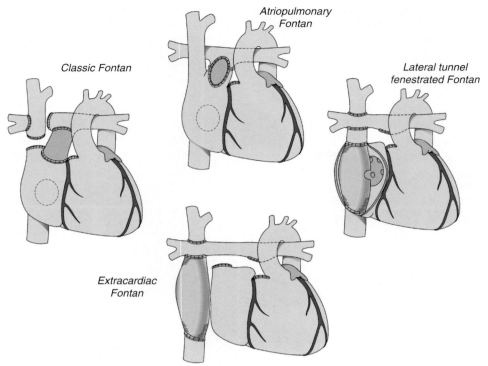

Classic Fontan

Atriopulmonary
Fontan

Lateral tunnel
fenestrated Fontan

Extracardiac
Fontan

FIG. 40.19 Diagrams of four variations of the Fontan operation.

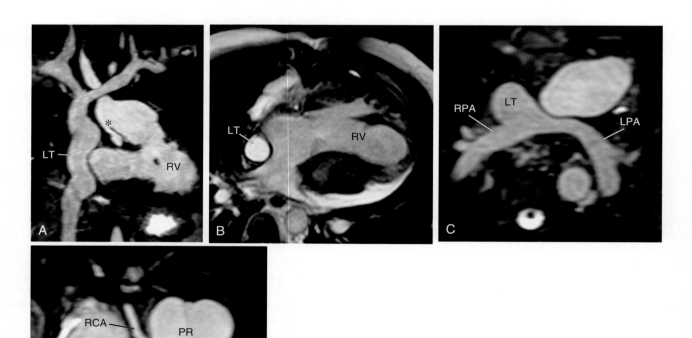

FIG. 40.20 Lateral tunnel Fontan operation in a patient with hypoplastic left heart syndrome. Reformatted electrocardiogram and respiratory navigator-gated three-dimensional balanced steady-state free precession angiogram. (A) Coronal plane demonstrating the lateral tunnel *(LT)* and aorto-pulmonary anastomosis *(*)*. (B) Axial plane to show the LT in cross section. (C) Axial plane to show the connection of the LT to the right pulmonary artery *(RPA)* and left pulmonary artery *(LPA)*. (D) Oblique axial plan to highlight the hypoplastic native aortic root *(AoR)*, right coronary artery *(RCA)*, left coronary artery *(LCA)*, and native pulmonary root *(PR)*. *RV,* Right ventricle.

compression; thromboembolism; protein-losing enteropathy; plastic bronchitis; hepatic and renal dysfunction; arrhythmias; and premature death. Such adverse developments are usually poorly tolerated; thus prompt detection with diagnostic imaging is an important element in caring for these patients.

Cardiovascular Magnetic Resonance
Before the First Operation

CMR is seldom requested before the first palliative operation because TTE usually provides all of the necessary diagnostic information.

Before the Superior Cavopulmonary Anastomosis Operation

Traditionally, the superior cavopulmonary anastomosis operation is preceded by invasive cardiac catheterization for assessment and planning. However, in a prospective randomized clinical trial, CMR was shown to be a safe, effective, and less costly alternative to routine catheterization in selected patients.[98,99]

The goals of the CMR examination include (1) measuring ventricular mass, volume, and function; (2) quantifying significant valve regurgitation; (3) evaluating the pulmonary arteries, pulmonary veins, atrial septum, and aortic arch for obstruction; and (4) assessing aortopulmonary and venovenous collateral vessels.[100,101] These goals can be achieved by the following protocol:
- Cine bSSFP: axial stack from the mid-liver through the top of the aortic arch for dynamic imaging of the heart and vasculature.
- Cine bSSFP: ventricular long-axis planes and a ventricular short-axis stack from base-to-apex for quantitative assessment of ventricular volumes and EF.
- Cine bSSFP: aortic arch long-axis plane.
- Fast (turbo) spin echo with blood suppression (optional): axial plane to image the branch pulmonary arteries and aortic arch in long axis.
- Contrast-enhanced 3D MRA and/or ECG and respiratory navigator-gated 3D bSSFP imaging of the chest (see Fig. 40.18).
- Blood flow measurements: main and branch pulmonary arteries, ascending aorta, descending aorta at the diaphragm; superior vena cava, inferior vena cava, pulmonary veins, and atrioventricular valves.
- LGE: ventricular long- and short-axis planes.

Before the Fontan Operation

Several reports have critically examined the necessity of invasive cardiac catheterization before the Fontan operation.[102–104] One retrospective study showed that single ventricle patients who did not require a catheterization-based intervention and had a pre-Fontan CMR and TTE but not a catheterization had similar short-term outcomes as those who underwent an invasive catheterization.[105] The CMR examination goals and imaging protocol are the same as those before the superior cavopulmonary anastomosis operation noted earlier.

After the Fontan Operation

The utility of TTE in patients after a Fontan operation is often limited by increasing body size, acoustic interference from scar tissue, and incomplete visualization of the Fontan pathway and aorta. CMR is not subject to these drawbacks (see Fig. 40.20) and provides a more reliable quantitative assessment of ventricular size and function[106] and blood flow. It has thus become an important clinical tool in these fragile patients, with a growing body of research to support its use.[35,69] One study showed that a larger CMR-derived end-diastolic volume (EDV) was independently associated with an increased risk of death and transplant, and the addition of EDV to clinical variables led to improved risk stratification for transplant-free survival.[107] In another report, LGE was seen in 28% of Fontan patients, and a greater extent of LGE was associated with lower EF, increased EDV, increased mass, and a higher frequency of nonsustained ventricular tachycardia.[108] Studies using CMR blood flow measurements have also revealed new information about the importance of aortopulmonary collateral vessels,[100,101,109–113] energy losses in the Fontan connection,[114–116] and the value of computational fluid dynamics in surgical planning.[117]

The goals of the CMR examination include (1) assessing the systemic veins, Fontan baffle, and pulmonary arteries for obstruction and thrombus; (2) detecting Fontan baffle fenestrations or leaks; (3) evaluating the pulmonary veins for compression; (4) quantifying ventricular volumes, mass, and function; (5) detecting ventricular outflow tract obstruction; (6) quantifying significant valve regurgitation; (7) imaging the aorta for obstruction or aneurysm; and (8) assessing aortopulmonary and venovenous collateral vessels. These goals can be achieved by the following protocol[26]:
- Cine bSSFP: axial stack from the mid-liver through the top of the aortic arch for dynamic imaging of the heart and vasculature.
- Cine bSSFP: ventricular long-axis planes and a ventricular short-axis stack from base-to-apex for quantitative assessment of ventricular volumes and EF.
- Cine bSSFP: aortic arch long-axis plane.
- Contrast-enhanced 3D MRA.
- ECG and respiratory navigator-gated 3D bSSFP imaging of the thorax (see Fig. 40.20).
- Blood flow measurements: superior vena cava, Fontan baffle above and below any fenestration or baffle leak, branch pulmonary arteries, pulmonary veins, ascending aorta, descending aorta at the diaphragm, atrioventricular valves.
- LGE: ventricular long-axis and short-axis planes.

CONCLUSION

As outlined in this chapter, CMR provides unique information in the infant and child with simple and complex congenital heart disease population—both for guiding management and for monitoring patients after mechanical intervention. As these children often require many decades of monitoring, the non-ionizing radiation attribute of CMR is a particular advantage.

ACKNOWLEDGMENT

We thank the physicians, technologists, nurses, and support personnel in the CMR Unit at Boston Children's Hospital for their help. Parts of the text and figures of this chapter have been included in other chapters recently written by the authors on the CMR evaluation of congenital heart disease.

REFERENCES

A full reference list is available online at ExpertConsult.com

41

Simple and Complex Congenital Heart Disease: Adults

Eric V. Krieger, Sara L. Partington, and Anne Marie Valente

The number of adults with congenital heart disease living in the United States is estimated to be at least 1.4 million, and at least 300,000 of these people have complex forms of congenital heart disease.[1] The majority of these patients have undergone surgical repairs in childhood, and lifelong follow-up is recommended. Many adults with congenital heart disease do not recognize subtle changes in exercise capacity and serial imaging of adults with congenital heart disease is important to monitor for hemodynamic and anatomic sequelae. Cardiovascular magnetic resonance (CMR) imaging has become an attractive imaging modality for surveillance of the long-term cardiac complications in this population because of its excellent tissue border delineation, tissue characterization, and quantification of biventricular volumes and valvular regurgitation. CMR allows for serial comparisons without the need for ionizing radiation or iodinated contrast. The objective of this chapter is to review select congenital heart disease diagnoses that are referred for CMR imaging. For each congenital heart disease condition, we will present a suggested CMR protocol with the acknowledgement that a there is considerable anatomic variability and individualization of protocols is often required. Knowledge of the patient's anatomy, surgical interventions, and prior imaging is critical to focus the protocol so that the essential information is obtained within a reasonable amount of time, as many of these adults will undergo serial examinations.

EBSTEIN ANOMALY

Anatomy and Natural History

Ebstein anomaly is a malformation of the tricuspid valve and right ventricle, which encompasses a large spectrum of disease severity. There is failure of delamination of the septal and posterior tricuspid valve leaflets from the myocardium, resulting in apical displacement of the tricuspid valve (≥ 0.8 cm/m² relative to the anterior mitral leaflet insertion site). The portion of the right ventricle proximal to the functional tricuspid valve becomes "atrialized." The anterior leaflet of the tricuspid valve is large and redundant, and often has fenestrations and tethering attachments to the right ventricular (RV) free wall. The posterior leaflet is often dysplastic and atrially displaced.

The etiology of Ebstein anomaly is not known; however, in rare cases, genetic factors such as mutations in the transcription factor NKX2.5,10p13–p14 deletion, or 1p34.3–p36.11 deletion have been described. The most severe cases of Ebstein anomaly result in fetal hydrops and fetal demise. Patients with Ebstein anomaly often develop progressive right heart failure and exercise intolerance. However, some individuals with mild forms of this disease can be asymptomatic into adulthood.

Surgical Repairs

When possible, the surgical intervention for Ebstein anomaly involves tricuspid valve repair. In the current era, the repair generally involves a right atrial (RA) reduction, plication of the atrialized right ventricle and a tricuspid valve repair involving the creation of a monocusp tricuspid valve using the redundant anterior tricuspid valve leaflet with a posterior annuloplasty (cone procedure).[2] In patients who are unsuitable for tricuspid valve repair, a bioprosthetic tricuspid valve replacement is generally performed. Evaluation of the patient after Ebstein repair involves assessing the degree of residual tricuspid regurgitation or stenosis, assessing RA size and the RV size and function. The right coronary artery lies in close proximity to the repaired tricuspid valve annulus site and it is important to assess for evidence of late gadolinium enhancement (LGE) following surgery for Ebstein anomaly.

Cardiovascular Magnetic Resonance Evaluation of Ebstein Anomaly

Tricuspid Valve Anatomy and Tricuspid Regurgitation Fraction

An accurate assessment of the tricuspid valve anatomy, including assessing the leaflet sizes, the subvalvar apparatus, the presence of tethering attachments of the anterior leaflet to the RV free wall, and the location of the tricuspid valve functional annulus, is important for planning repair. Understanding the amount and structure of the tricuspid leaflet tissue provides the surgeon information on whether enough leaflet tissue is accessible to repair, rather than replace, the tricuspid valve.

Balanced steady-state free precession (bSSFP) cine imaging of the tricuspid valve can be performed in the four-chamber view and the RV two-chamber view. It is important to determine the orientation of the tricuspid valve inflow because it may be oriented toward the right ventricular outflow tract (RVOT) or directed at the RV apex; therefore off-axis views are often required. Determining the severity of tricuspid regurgitation may be challenging in patients with Ebstein anomaly but may be quantified with phase contrast CMR (PCMR).[3]

Right Atrial and Right Ventricular Size and Function

Progressive tricuspid regurgitation and abnormal RV myocardium lead to right heart dilation. Measurements of RA and RV volumes are typically performed in axial or short-axis orientation with endocardial contours drawn in end systole and end diastole.[4] When contouring the right ventricle, it can be useful to assess the functional RV size that excludes the atrialized right ventricle and only includes the RV volume distal to the functional tricuspid valve annulus and coaptation point. Many centers will report both the functional RV size and function and the anatomic RV size and function (using the anatomic tricuspid annulus as a landmark). The ability to accurately and reproducibly measure RV volume is important because RV size has been associated with clinical outcomes in patients with Ebstein anomaly.[5] Additionally, mismeasurement of RV stroke volume can result in errors when calculating tricuspid regurgitation severity.

Progressive RV dilation or dysfunction in the setting of severe tricuspid regurgitation is imaging criteria for tricuspid valve surgical intervention. The index of right-sided to left-sided heart volumes derived from CMR has been shown to correlate well with other established markers of heart failure.[6] Contouring the end-diastolic volume measurements of the right ventricle, RA, left ventricle, and left atrium (LA) can provide a total right/left-volume index (Fig. 41.1):

Total right/left-volume index
= (right atrium + atrialized right ventricle
+ functional right ventricle)/(LA + left ventricle)   **Eq. 41.1**

Indexes such as these may eventually be used to help guide timing of tricuspid valve intervention.

Associated Cardiac Abnormalities

Patients with Ebstein anomaly commonly have atrial septal defects (ASDs), and may occasionally have RVOT obstruction, or myocardial noncompaction. CMR can be used to assess the morphology of the interatrial septum and to calculate the Qp:Qs ratio by performing PCMR across the aorta and pulmonary artery.[7]

A suggested CMR protocol for adults with Ebstein anomaly is presented in Box 41.1.

COARCTATION OF THE AORTA

Anatomy and Natural History

Coarctation of the aorta is typically a fibrous ridge in the aortic isthmus, just distal to the insertion of the left subclavian artery. Although often discrete, aortic coarctation can also be long segment or associated with a diffusely hypoplastic transverse aorta. Aortic coarctation is associated with a diffuse vascular abnormality and is associated with aortic aneurysm, cerebral aneurysms, or endothelial dysfunction.[8] Awareness of these abnormalities is important because the entire aorta and cerebral vessels should be imaged in patients with aortic coarctation.

Aortic coarctation sometimes presents in adulthood as difficult-to-manage systemic hypertension and the diagnosis may be suspected from a murmur, diminished lower extremity pulses, or arm–arm or arm–leg blood pressure discrepancy. Those who had an aortic coarctation repair early in life have up to a 5% risk of re-coarctation in adulthood and present similarly.[9]

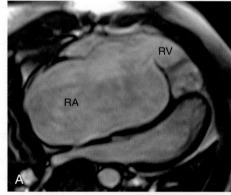
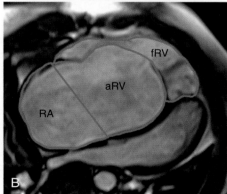

FIG. 41.1 Balanced steady-state free precession four-chamber view of a patient with Ebstein anomaly (A) demonstrating the severely dilated right atrium *(RA)* and the relatively smaller right ventricle. End-diastolic contours (B) outlining the RA, the atrialized right ventricle (*aRV*, the portion of the right ventricle distal to the anatomic tricuspid valve annulus but proximal to the coaptation point of the tricuspid valve) and the functional right ventricle (*fRV;* the portion of the right ventricle distal to the coaptation of the tricuspid valve).

BOX 41.1   Cardiovascular Magnetic Resonance Protocol for Ebstein Anomaly

Localizers
Electrocardiogram-gated cine balanced steady-state free precession
- Axial stack through the heart and branch pulmonary arteries
- Three-chamber right ventricular stack, two-chamber left, four-chamber views
- Ventricular short-axis stack from the base to the apex
- Right ventricular outflow tract view parallel to the right ventricular outflow tract
- Right ventricular two-chamber view
- Oblique planes to image tricuspid valve inflow orientation
- Oblique sagittal plane to image the atrial septum

Contrast-enhanced three-dimensional magnetic resonance angiogram[a]
Electrocardiogram-gated phase contrast through-plane flow in the main pulmonary artery, aorta, tricuspid and mitral valves[b]
Late gadolinium enhancement to assess for myocardial fibrosis[c]

These protocols were adapted from Boston Children's Hospital Cardiac Magnetic Resonance Imaging Program.
[a]In general, our practice is to obtain a gadolinium-enhanced three-dimensional magnetic resonance angiogram with the first cardiovascular magnetic resonance (CMR) examination, and then optional for subsequent examinations.
[b]In cases where Qp:Qs ratio is of interest, flow across the branch pulmonary arteries, superior vena cava, and inferior vena cava/descending thoracic aorta may be assessed to improve level of confidence.
[c]In general, our practice is to obtain late gadolinium enhancement (LGE) imaging to assess for myocardial fibrosis with the first CMR examination, and the frequency of repeating this technique in subsequent examinations is dependent on the initial findings and specific condition. For example, some CMR laboratories repeat LGE imaging every 3 years in patients with conotruncal anomalies (tetralogy of Fallot, transposition of the great arteries, double outlet right ventricle).

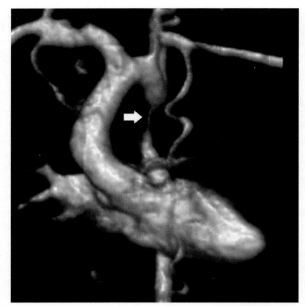

FIG. 41.2 Three-dimensional volume-rendered magnetic resonance angiogram in a patient with an aortic coarctation *(arrow)*. Note the large left internal thoracic artery that functions as a bridging collateral and is a sign of hemodynamically significant coarctation.

Surgical Repairs

There are several types of surgical repairs for native aortic coarctation, and they are dictated by the anatomy. For patients with a discrete coarctation, an end-to-end anastomosis is performed. If there is associated transverse aortic arch hypoplasia, an extended end-to-end procedure may be required.

Some patients with complex aortic coarctation have undergone interposition graft repairs, and those with Dacron material are particularly susceptible to aneurysm formation. The subclavian flap procedure was performed in the early surgical experience, and involved transecting the left subclavian artery and placing it over the narrowed portion of the descending aorta. Patients who have undergone this procedure will no longer have the left subclavian artery attached to the transverse arch.

Cardiovascular Magnetic Resonance Evaluation of Aortic Coarctation
Aortic Arch

CMR imaging of native and re-coarctation will be discussed together. The anatomic features of aortic coarctation can be seen with bright-blood cine or double-inversion black-blood spin echo images in the oblique sagittal plane. Gadolinium-enhanced magnetic resonance angiography (MRA) also demonstrates the coarctation (Fig. 41.2) and double oblique reformats can be used to measure the minimal luminal diameter and the reference vessel size.[10,11] If collateral vessels are seen on contrast-enhanced (CE) MRA or PCMR demonstrates flow augmentation in the descending aorta, the obstruction is probably hemodynamically important.[12,13] A prolonged deceleration time of the systolic flow in the distal descending thoracic aorta also indicates hemodynamically significant aortic coarctation.[11,14]

Four-dimensional velocity mapping is not widely available but is an emerging technique to show turbulence at the coarctation site, and characterize altered aortic velocity profiles, providing insight into which patients may be at higher risk for aortic wall complications, such as dissection.[15,16]

BOX 41.2 **Cardiovascular Magnetic Resonance Protocol for Aortic Coarctation**

Localizers
Electrocardiogram-gated cine balanced steady-state free precession
- Four-chamber view, left ventricular two-chamber and, left ventricular long-axis view to the aorta
- Ventricular short-axis stack from the base to the apex
- Oblique sagittal view of the aortic arch ("candy-cane" view)

Consider double-inversion recovery black-blood images in the oblique sagittal plane if artifact on balanced steady-state free precession imaging
Contrast-enhanced three-dimensional magnetic resonance angiogram in sagittal orientation with first acquisition timed to the aorta[a]
Electrocardiogram-gated phase contrast through-plane flow in the main pulmonary artery, aorta and consider proximal descending aorta proximal to the coarctation (distal to left subclavian artery) and descending aorta at the level of the diaphragm
Late gadolinium enhancement to assess for myocardial fibrosis[b]

These protocols were adapted from Boston Children's Hospital Cardiac Magnetic Resonance Imaging Program.
[a]In general, our practice is to obtain a gadolinium-enhanced three-dimensional magnetic resonance angiogram with the first cardiovascular magnetic resonance (CMR) examination, and then optional for subsequent examinations.
[b]In general, our practice is to obtain late gadolinium enhancement (LGE) imaging to assess for myocardial fibrosis with the first CMR examination, and the frequency of repeating this technique in subsequent examinations is dependent on the initial findings and specific condition. For example, some CMR laboratories repeat LGE imaging every 3 years in patients with conotruncal anomalies (tetralogy of Fallot, transposition of the great arteries, double outlet right ventricle).

Patients with aortic coarctation are prone to aneurysms in the ascending aorta, cerebral vasculature, and at the site of surgical repair. Aneurysms at the site of previous Dacron patch repair are particularly prone to rupture and should be managed aggressively.[17–19] Screening for cerebral aneurysms is recommended, although neither optimal management nor frequency of surveillance is well defined.[20]

Left Ventricular Cavity Size and Function

Patients with native or re-coarctation are predisposed to systemic hypertension, particularly exercise-induced hypertension. Therefore standard measurements of left ventricular (LV) mass and function should be performed.[21]

Associated Cardiac Lesions

Over 50% of those with aortic coarctation have a bicommissural aortic valve and these patients are at greater risk for ascending aortic aneurysms.[17] Patients may also have subaortic stenosis, mitral valve abnormalities (e.g., parachute mitral valve and/or mitral stenosis) or ventricular septal defect (VSD).

A suggested CMR protocol for adults with aortic coarctation is presented in Box 41.2.

TETRALOGY OF FALLOT

Anatomy and Natural History

Evaluation of patients with repaired tetralogy of Fallot (TOF) is one of the most common adult congenital heart disease diagnoses referred for CMR. TOF represents the most common form of cyanotic congenital heart disease affecting up to 0.5 per 1000 live births.[22] Survival following TOF repair is excellent, but there is a 3-fold increase in mortality beginning in the third postoperative decade of life,[23] and 14% of patients develop markedly impaired functional status late after surgical repair, highlighting the importance of regular surveillance of these patients.[24] This congenital anomaly results from the anterior deviation of the conal septum, resulting in varying degrees of RVOT obstruction, VSD, an overriding aorta, and RV hypertrophy. Importantly, the degree of RVOT obstruction can range from only mild subpulmonary stenosis to the most severe form involving complete absence of the main pulmonary artery (TOF/pulmonary atresia), which occurs in approximately 15% of patients with TOF.

Surgical Repairs

In the current era, the majority of patients undergo surgical repair in infancy or childhood, although older adults may have first undergone a palliative shunt (Blalock-Taussig, Waterston, or Potts shunt) as a young child and then undergone a complete repair at an older age. Strategies to repair TOF have evolved over time. The early experience involved placing a transannular patch to eliminate the RVOT obstruction; however, current strategies have been modified to alleviate most of the RVOT obstruction while trying to preserve some of the integrity of the pulmonary valve. Patients with TOF/pulmonary atresia and those with anomalous left coronary artery from the right sinus may undergo an RV-to-pulmonary artery (RV-PA) conduit. Knowledge of the patient's surgical history before CMR is ideal because it will determine the specific CMR protocol to employ, focusing on the potential residual lesions.

Many patients with repaired TOF undergo a pulmonary valve replacement in adulthood. CMR is increasingly being used to aid in the decision making of timing of these interventions. Box 41.3 lists suggested imaging criteria for consideration of pulmonary valve replacement in asymptomatic patients with severe pulmonary regurgitation (PR).

Cardiovascular Magnetic Resonance Evaluation of Tetralogy of Fallot Repair
Right Ventricular Outflow Tract Obstruction and Pulmonary Arteries

A goal of TOF surgery is to relieve the RVOT obstruction, yet many patients are left with varying degrees of obstruction that may be located in the subpulmonary area, at the level of the pulmonary valve, or more distally in the main or branch pulmonary arteries (PA). Transannular patch repairs can result in RVOT regional wall motion abnormalities and aneurysms (Fig. 41.3). RVOT aneurysms are not only associated with decreased RV ejection fraction (EF) but are also associated with unfavorable ventricular interactions, resulting in a reduced LVEF.[25]

Visualization of the entire RVOT is important using specific RVOT long-axis (Fig. 41.4A) and two-chamber RV cine views (Fig. 41.4B). The RV two-chamber view allows visualization of the right atrium, tricuspid valve, RV, and main pulmonary artery all in one plane. Assessing for downstream stenosis in the branch pulmonary arteries can be performed with either a bSSFP stack in an axial plane or an MRA.

Newer catheter-based pulmonary valves are promising developments for patients with congenital heart disease affecting the right heart. At the current time, most percutaneous valves are placed inside existing RV-PA conduits or dysfunctional bioprosthetic valves. CMR is useful to determine the geometry of the RVOT and identify potential candidates for percutaneous pulmonary valve placement. Delineation of the coronary artery course is essential before any RVOT intervention because 5% to 7% of patients with TOF have an anomalous left coronary artery that may course across the RVOT which can complicate both surgical or transcatheter pulmonic valve implantation. Cardiac and respiratory-gated MRA images have sufficient spatial resolution to assess the origins and proximal coronary artery courses.

Pulmonary Regurgitation

Pulmonary regurgitation is the most common sequelae of TOF repair and is often associated with RV dilation (Fig. 41.5), predisposing to RV dysfunction, arrhythmias, and death. PCMR sequences assess antegrade

---

BOX 41.3 Imaging Criteria for Pulmonary Valve Replacement in Asymptomatic Patients With Repaired Tetralogy of Fallot With Severe Pulmonary Regurgitation

- Right ventricular end-diastolic volume index >150 mL/m² or Z-score >4. In patients whose body surface area falls outside published normal data: right ventricle/left ventricle end-diastolic volume ratio >2
- Right ventricular end-systolic volume index >80 mL/m²
- Right ventricular ejection fraction <47%
- Left ventricle ejection fraction <55%
- Large right ventricular outflow tract aneurysm
- Other significant hemodynamic abnormalities:
  - Right ventricular outflow tract obstruction with right ventricular systolic pressure >2/3 systemic
  - Severe branch pulmonary artery stenosis (<30% flow to affected lung)
  - More than moderate tricuspid regurgitation
- Left-to-right shunt from residual ventricular or atrial septal defect with pulmonary to aortic flow ratio >1.5
- Severe aortic regurgitation
- Severe aortic root dilation (>5 cm)

Data from Geva T. Repaired tetralogy of Fallot: the roles of cardiovascular magnetic resonance in evaluating pathophysiology and for pulmonary valve replacement decision support. *J Cardiovasc Magn Reson.* 2011;13:9.

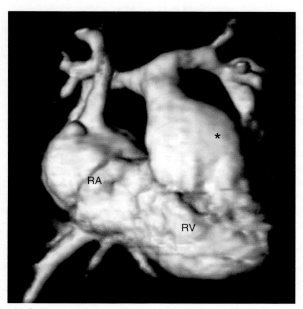

FIG. 41.3 Three-dimensional volume-rendered magnetic resonance angiogram in a patient with a transannular patch repair for tetralogy of Fallot with a right ventricular outflow tract aneurysm (*). *RA,* Right atrium; *RV,* right ventricle.

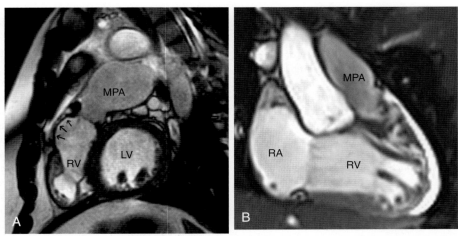

FIG. 41.4 Cine balanced steady-state free precession with right ventricular views for evaluating patients with tetralogy of Fallot. (A) Right ventricular outflow tract view demonstrates the right ventricle *(RV)* and pulmonary valve and delineates right ventricular outflow tract. (B) Right ventricular two-chamber view demonstrates the RV, tricuspid and pulmonary valve in a single plane. Arrows denote right ventricular outflow tract aneurysm. *LV,* Left ventricle; *MPA,* main pulmonary artery; *RA,* right atrium.

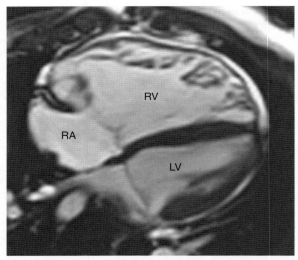

FIG. 41.5 Balanced steady-state free precession imaging of the four-chamber view in a patient with tetralogy of Fallot demonstrating right ventricular dilation secondary to long-standing pulmonary regurgitation. When planning the short-axis stack, it is important to include the basal lateral portion of the right ventricle that often extends well beyond the mitral annular plane. *LV,* Left ventricle; *RA,* right atrium; *RV,* right ventricle.

and retrograde flow across the main pulmonary artery (Fig. 41.6), and studies demonstrate this to be a highly reproducible technique for quantifying pulmonary regurgitation volume.[26] Pulmonary regurgitation fraction is calculated as retrograde flow volume divided by antegrade flow volume and, in our laboratory, a pulmonary regurgitation fraction greater than 40% is considered severe.

Right Ventricular Size and Function

Accurate quantification of RV size, function, and mass is particularly important in repaired TOF patients because RV dilatation, dysfunction, and hypertrophy are associated with adverse outcomes in this group.[27,28] Pulmonary valve replacement usually eliminates significant pulmonary regurgitation; however, optimal timing of pulmonic valve replacement to prevent the adverse sequelae of RV dilation and dysfunction remains unclear.[29] Pulmonic valve replacement usually results

in dramatic decreases in RV volumes and improvement in functional status,[30] but studies have demonstrated that RV systolic function generally remains unchanged.[31,32]

CMR is the gold standard for quantifying RV size and function in patients with repaired TOF and results in significantly better interobserver variability than transthoracic echocardiography (TTE).[33,34] LV dysfunction is present in >20% of adults with TOF repair, particularly those who were repaired later in life, had prior palliative shunts, or concomitant RV dysfunction. LV dysfunction has been associated with sudden cardiac death in this patient population.[28,35]

Tricuspid Regurgitation

There are several mechanisms that lead to tricuspid regurgitation in repaired TOF patients, including annular dilation, structural valve abnormalities, or as a consequence of valve disruption during prior TOF repair.[36] CMR allows for quantification of tricuspid regurgitation, and significant tricuspid regurgitation should be considered in surgical plans at the time of pulmonic valve replacement.

Ascending Aorta

Ascending aortic dilation is common in adults with repaired TOF. However, despite large aortic dimensions, aortic dissection is exceedingly rare. In fact, up to 25% of adults with repaired TOF have an aortic root diameter >4 cm; however, only 2.3% have an aortic diameter >5 cm.[37] Some patients develop progressive dilation of the aortic root that can lead to significant aortic regurgitation.[38]

Myocardial Fibrosis

LGE occurs commonly in locations of prior surgery (RVOT, VSD patch). Repaired TOF patients with greater degrees of LGE are at a higher risk of sustained symptomatic arrhythmia; however, it is unclear if LGE is associated with increased mortality in this patient population. LGE in the area of the VSD patch, RVOT patch, or septal insertion sites are not associated with worse outcomes.[39] Novel techniques such as T1 mapping (see Chapter 2), which acts as a marker for diffuse fibrosis, may also prove to act as prognostic indicators in patients with TOF; however, T1 mapping in the RV can be difficult, and definitive studies are lacking.[40,41]

A suggested CMR protocol for adults after TOF repair is presented in Box 41.4.

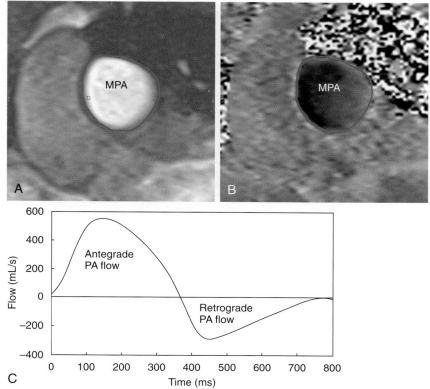

FIG. 41.6 Phase contrast cardiovascular magnetic resonance of the pulmonary valve to assess pulmonary regurgitation volume and regurgitation fraction. (A) Magnitude imaging of the main pulmonary artery *(MPA)*. (B) Phase contrast imaging of the MPA. (C) Flow profile demonstrating the antegrade flow, representing the area under the curve above the horizontal axis, and the retrograde flow, representing area under the curve below the horizontal axis. There is severe pulmonary regurgitation with a regurgitation fraction of 47%. *PA,* Pulmonary artery.

BOX 41.4 **Cardiovascular Magnetic Resonance Protocol for Repaired Tetralogy of Fallot**

Localizers
Electrocardiogram-gated cine balanced steady-state free precession
- Four-chamber view and two-chamber left ventricular, right ventricular views
- Ventricular short-axis stack from the base to the apex
- Right ventricular outflow tract outflow view parallel to the right ventricular outflow tract, then a second view orthogonal to the first right ventricular outflow tract view, right ventricular outflow tract short-axis view
- Axial stack to assess for branch pulmonary arteries and outflow tracts

Three-dimensional contrast-enhanced magnetic resonance angiogram[a]
Electrocardiogram-gated phase contrast through-plane flow in the main pulmonary artery, aorta, atrioventricular valves[b]
Late gadolinium enhancement to assess for myocardial fibrosis[c]
Consider coronary artery imaging with electrocardiogram and respiratory navigator gated three-dimensional balanced steady-state free precession
Consider T1 mapping to assess for diffuse fibrosis

These protocols were adapted from Boston Children's Hospital Cardiac Magnetic Resonance Imaging Program.
[a]In general, our practice is to obtain a gadolinium-enhanced three-dimensional magnetic resonance angiogram with the first cardiovascular magnetic resonance (CMR) examination, and then optional for subsequent examinations.
[b]In cases where Qp:Qs ratio is of interest, flow across the branch pulmonary arteries, superior vena cava, and inferior vena cava/descending thoracic aorta may be assessed to improve level of confidence.
[c]In general, our practice is to obtain late gadolinium enhancement (LGE) imaging to assess for myocardial fibrosis with the first CMR examination, and the frequency of repeating this technique in subsequent examinations is dependent on the initial findings and specific condition. For example, some CMR laboratories repeat LGE imaging every 3 years in patients with conotruncal anomalies (tetralogy of Fallot, transposition of the great arteries, double outlet right ventricle).

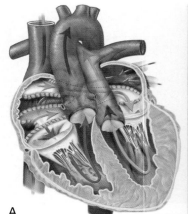

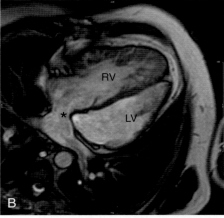

A

B

FIG. 41.7 (A) The atrial switch procedure (Mustard or Senning) for D-loop transposition of the great arteries. The atrial switch procedure uses intra-atrial baffles to redirect systemic venous return to the subpulmonic left ventricle and pulmonary venous return to the systemic right ventricle. (B) Balanced steady-state free precession image in a four-chamber orientation. Note the thin-walled subpulmonic left ventricle *(LV)* and the hypertrophied systemic right ventricle *(RV)*. Asterisk denotes the pulmonary venous pathway. (A, From Otto C, ed. *The Practice of Clinical Echocardiography.* 5th ed. Philadelphia: Elsevier; 2017:951.)

D-LOOP TRANSPOSITION OF THE GREAT ARTERIES

Anatomy and Natural History

D-loop transposition of the great arteries (TGA) is characterized by atrioventricular concordance and ventriculoarterial discordance. This results in parallel circulations, which sends oxygenated blood from the LA to the left ventricle to the pulmonary artery, while deoxygenated blood flows from the RA to the right ventricle to the aorta. It is a common form of cyanotic congenital heart disease and occurs in 3 out of 10,000 live births, accounting for 5% to 7% of all congenital heart disease defects. Without intervention, the mortality rate is >90% in the first year of life.[42] Approximately 50% those with D-loop TGA have an associated cardiac anomaly. Common lesions include VSD (40%), LV outflow tract (LVOT) obstruction (25%), or aortic coarctation (5%). The coronary artery pattern is also variable, with a high frequency of anomalous and interarterial coronary courses.[43–45]

Surgical Repairs

From the late 1950s until the early 1990s the atrial switch procedure was used to treat D-loop TGA and is often described by the eponyms the Mustard or Senning procedures (Fig. 41.7).[46,47] Even though the atrial switch has been largely abandoned (see later), there is a large population of adults previously treated with the atrial switch who are referred for CMR. During the atrial switch, systemic venous (deoxygenated) blood is rerouted leftward through the atrium to the mitral valve and left ventricle by intraatrial baffles. Pulmonary venous blood is redirected rightwards to the tricuspid valve and right ventricle. Following the atrial switch, the right ventricle is the systemic ventricle and the left ventricle is the subpulmonic ventricle. Common complications after the atrial switch include venous pathway stenosis, baffle leak, systemic right ventricular systolic dysfunction, tricuspid regurgitation, and LVOT obstruction.[48–50]

In the 1990s the arterial switch operation succeeded the atrial switch as the preferred treatment for D-loop TGA (Fig. 41.8). With the arterial switch operation, the great arteries are transected above the sinuses, the aorta is brought posteriorly to align with the left ventricle while the pulmonary arteries are brought anteriorly where

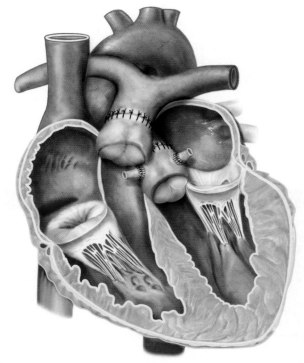

FIG. 41.8 The arterial switch procedure. This provides for a systemic left ventricle and a subpulmonic right ventricle but requires a neonatal coronary transfer. (From Otto C, ed. *The Practice of Clinical Echocardiography.* 5th ed. Philadelphia: Elsevier; 2017:951.)

they straddle the aorta to come into alignment with the RV. A coronary artery translocation is performed. Late complications after the arterial switch operation include neoaortic dilation and regurgitation, supravalvar pulmonic stenosis, branch pulmonary artery stenosis, and coronary artery obstruction.[51–53]

The Rastelli operation is performed for those with a VSD and pulmonic stenosis. In the Rastelli operation, a VSD patch is fashioned to baffle oxygenated blood across the VSD to the anterior aorta. The pulmonic artery is oversewn and an RV to pulmonary artery conduit is inserted. Late complications include dysfunction of the RV to pulmonary artery conduit, residual VSD, or LVOT obstruction.[54]

Cardiovascular Magnetic Resonance Evaluation of the Atrial Switch Operation

Baffle Complications

Baffle complications are the most frequent indication for re-intervention late after the atrial switch operation.[43] Narrowing typically occurs in the superior vena cava pathway and is particularly common in those with transvenous pacing or defibrillator leads. Few patients are symptomatic and most are managed conservatively. Inferior vena caval and pulmonary venous obstruction are less common. CMR evaluation of stenosis within the venous pathways requires careful planning to align imaging planes. Sagittal planes can identify the systemic and pulmonary venous pathways. Imaging planes are obtained through the superior vena cava, inferior vena cava, and pulmonary venous pathways (Fig. 41.9). The use of orthogonal planes can overcome artifact caused by partial volume averaging.[55] Black-blood imaging can be performed in areas of suspected pathway obstruction for additional anatomic definition. CE-MRA is sensitive in detecting hemodynamically important venous pathway obstruction but may miss milder narrowings.[56] Although CMR is generally safe in patients with pacemakers (see Chapter 11), local susceptibility artifact from pacemaker leads (and especially defibrillator leads) reduces the diagnostic accuracy of detecting pathway obstruction so computed tomography (CT) angiography should be considered.

Many patients with hemodynamically important superior vena cava obstruction will decompress down the azygous vein. Axial through-plane PCMR should normally confirm azygous flow directed cranially. If flow is reversed (the descending aorta can be used for reference), superior vena caval obstruction is likely.

Baffle leaks allows communication between the systemic and pulmonary venous pathways. These are often small but can be seen using thin-slice no-gap bSSFP orthogonal stacks through the atria. Dephasing jets can sometimes be seen. If comparison of flow by PCMR through the aorta and pulmonary suggests a shunt, a baffle leak should be suspected.

Systemic Right Ventricle and Tricuspid Valve

RV systolic dysfunction is nearly universal in the adult with an atrial switch operation and is associated with poor outcomes.[43,57] Detailed discussion of CMR evaluation of the systemic RV is discussed in detail in the section on L-loop TGA. Either a short-axis or axial stack should be contoured in end diastole and end systole for measures of RV volumes and function. Reference values for normal RV volumes are not established for this population.[55,58,59] Myocardial fibrosis, detected by LGE in the systemic right ventricle, has been associated with adverse outcomes, mostly atrial arrhythmias.[60]

Tricuspid (systemic atrioventricular) valve regurgitation is common and often functional, secondary to annular dilation rather than primary leaflet disease (in contrast to L-loop TGA). Tricuspid regurgitation volume can be calculated by comparing RV stroke volume to flow measured across the aortic valve.

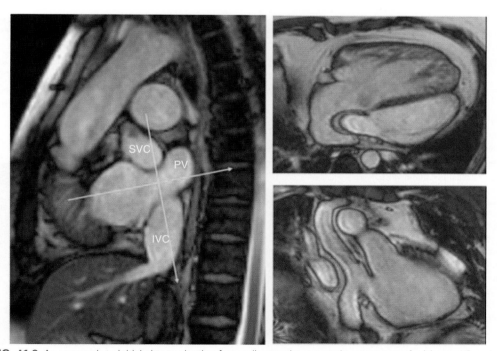

FIG. 41.9 An approach to initial plane selection for cardiovascular magnetic resonance of a Mustard/Senning patient. In sagittal projections the superior vena cava *(SVC)* and inferior vena cava *(IVC)* are identified at the point where the pulmonary venous *(PV)* pathway transects them. Using these landmarks provides horizontal and vertical long-axis views *(smaller panels at right)* that can be used for additional imaging, starting with a short-axis scout stack. Red denotes the location of the baffle. (From Broberg CS. Cardiac magnetic imaging of the patient with an atrial switch palliation for transposition of the great arteries. *Prog Pediat Cardiol.* 2014;38:49–55.)

Left Ventricular Outflow Tract Obstruction

After the atrial switch, LVOT obstruction acts as subpulmonic stenosis. Obstruction can be caused by a discrete subpulmonic ridge, posterior malalignment VSD, or systolic anterior motion of the mitral valve. Cine bSSFP images aligned to the LVOT will elucidate the mechanism of obstruction.[55] Subpulmonic obstruction is not always undesirable because pressure loading the subpulmonic left ventricle may produce a more favorable position of the interventricular septum.[48]

With these potential complications in mind, a suggested CMR protocol for adults after an atrial switch is presented in Box 41.5.

Cardiovascular Magnetic Resonance Evaluation of the Arterial Switch Operation

Outcomes after the arterial switch operation are better than the outcomes after an atrial switch operation, with less arrhythmia, less heart failure, and improved functional status.[61]

Supravalvar Pulmonic Stenosis and Branch Pulmonary Artery Stenosis

Supravalvar pulmonic stenosis can occur at the anastomotic site or where the pulmonary arteries are draped over the aorta as part of the Lecompte maneuver. Obstruction in the main pulmonary artery is less common but can occur if large coronary artery buttons had been harvested from the neopulmonic root. Cine bSSFP images can show the area of obstruction.

Branch pulmonary artery stenosis is best shown with CE-MRA (Fig. 41.10). Narrowing is often eccentric leading to an oval lumen. Double-oblique measurements should be performed. PCMR in the main, right and left pulmonary arteries allow for calculation of differential pulmonary blood flow.

Neoaortic Dilation and Regurgitation

The neoaortic root is native pulmonary artery tissue and often dilates after the arterial switch operation. Dilation is typically slowly progressive (<0.5 mm/year) and dissection is rare.[52,62] Electrocardiogram-gated respiratory navigated three-dimensional (3D) isotropic sequences are ideal for measuring the neoaortic sinuses because they minimize blurring from cardiac motion. Neoaortic valve regurgitation is often secondary to annular dilation and can be severe. PCMR in the ascending aorta can measure regurgitation volume. Slice location affects the degree of regurgitation detected, so consistency is important.[63]

Coronary Arteries

Coronary artery occlusion or ostial stenosis occurs after the coronary translocation in ~5% after the arterial switch operation.[64,65] Wall motion abnormalities or LGE should raise suspicion for coronary injury. Stress perfusion CMR and coronary imaging using free-breathing navigated 3D bSSFP sequences triggered in diastole can be used to evaluate for proximal coronary occlusions, but invasive coronary angiography is often needed for confirmation.[66,67]

A suggested CMR protocol for imaging adults after the arterial switch operation is presented in Box 41.6.

L-LOOP TRANSPOSITION OF THE GREAT ARTERIES

Anatomy and Natural History

L-loop transposition of the great arteries (also known as "physiologically corrected" or "congenitally corrected" TGA) is characterized by atrioventricular discordance and ventriculoarterial discordance (Fig. 41.11). Most patients have atrial situs solitus with ventricular inversion

---

BOX 41.5 Cardiovascular Magnetic Resonance Protocol for Transposition of the Great Arteries With Atrial Switch Operation

Localizers
Electrocardiogram-gated cine balanced steady-state free precession
- Superior and inferior vena cava baffles
- Pulmonary venous baffle
- Four-chamber view
- Ventricular short-axis stack from the base to the apex
- Right ventricular long-axis view to the aorta, two orthogonal views
- Left ventricular long-axis view to the pulmonary artery, two orthogonal views
- Branch pulmonary artery axial stack to assess for pulmonary artery stenosis

Three-dimensional contrast-enhanced magnetic resonance angiogram or electrocardiogram and respiratory navigator gated three-dimensional balanced steady-state free precession[a]
Electrocardiogram-gated phase contrast through-plane flow in the main pulmonary artery, aorta, tricuspid and mitral valves[b]
Late gadolinium enhancement to assess for myocardial fibrosis[c]

These protocols were adapted from Boston Children's Hospital Cardiac Magnetic Resonance Imaging Program.

[a]In general, our practice is to obtain a gadolinium-enhanced three-dimensional magnetic resonance angiogram with the first cardiovascular magnetic resonance (CMR) examination, and then optional for subsequent examinations.

[b]In cases where Qp:Qs ratio is of interest, flow across the branch pulmonary arteries, superior vena cava, and inferior vena cava/descending thoracic aorta may be assessed to improve level of confidence.

[c]In general, our practice is to obtain late gadolinium enhancement (LGE) imaging to assess for myocardial fibrosis with the first CMR examination, and the frequency of repeating this technique in subsequent examinations is dependent on the initial findings and specific condition. For example, some CMR laboratories repeat LGE imaging every 3 years in patients with conotruncal anomalies (tetralogy of Fallot, transposition of the great arteries, double outlet right ventricle).

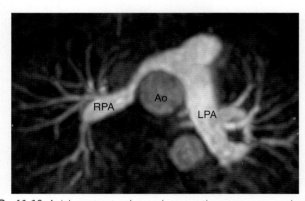

FIG. 41.10 Axial contrast-enhanced magnetic resonance angiogram demonstrating the relationship of the pulmonary arteries and ascending aorta after an arterial switch operation. Branch pulmonary artery stenosis often occurs where the pulmonary arteries are draped over the ascending aorta. Quantifying differential pulmonary blood flow gives clues to the hemodynamic significance of narrowing. *Ao,* Aorta; *LPA,* left pulmonary artery; *RPA,* right pulmonary artery.

BOX 41.6 Cardiovascular Magnetic Resonance Protocol for Transposition of the Great Arteries With the Arterial Switch Operation

Localizers
Electrocardiogram-gated cine balanced steady-state free precession
- Four-chamber view, left ventricular two-chamber, and left ventricular long-axis view to the neoaortic valve
- Ventricular short-axis stack from the base to the apex
Electrocardiogram and respiratory navigator gated three-dimensional balanced steady-state free precession for coronary artery imaging
Three-dimensional contrast-enhanced magnetic resonance angiogram timed to the pulmonary arteries[a]
Electrocardiogram-gated phase contrast through-plane flow in the main pulmonary artery and aorta[b]
Late gadolinium enhancement to assess for myocardial fibrosis[c]

These protocols were adapted from Boston Children's Hospital Cardiac Magnetic Resonance Imaging Program.
[a]In general, our practice is to obtain a gadolinium-enhanced three-dimensional magnetic resonance angiogram with the first cardiovascular magnetic resonance (CMR) examination, and then optional for subsequent examinations.
[b]In cases where Qp:Qs ratio is of interest, flow across the branch pulmonary arteries, superior vena cava, and inferior vena cava/descending thoracic aorta may be assessed to improve level of confidence.
[c]In general, our practice is to obtain late gadolinium enhancement (LGE) imaging to assess for myocardial fibrosis with the first CMR examination, and the frequency of repeating this technique in subsequent examinations is dependent on the initial findings and specific condition. For example, some CMR laboratories repeat LGE imaging every 3 years in patients with conotruncal anomalies (tetralogy of Fallot, transposition of the great arteries, double outlet right ventricle).

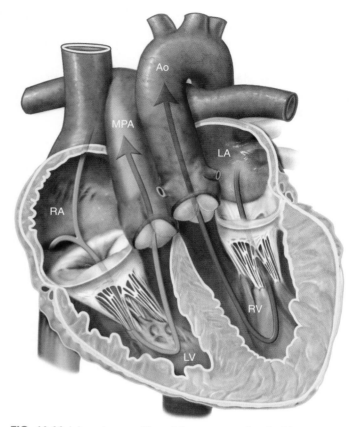

FIG. 41.11 L-loop transposition of the great arteries. In this rare acyanotic congenital heart defect there is ventricular inversion and transposed great arteries. The right ventricle *(RV)* pumps oxygenated blood to the aorta *(Ao)*, while the left ventricle *(LV)* pumps deoxygenated blood to the pulmonary artery. *LA,* Left atrium; *MPA,* main pulmonary artery; *RA,* right atrium. (From Otto C, ed. *The Practice of Clinical Echocardiography.* 5th ed. Philadelphia: Elsevier; 2017.)

and an aorta which is anterior and leftward. In this configuration the right ventricle will lie posterior and leftward. Approximately 10% of patients have mirror-image dextrocardia. The right ventricle can be identified by the moderator band and trabeculated septal surface (Fig. 41.12). L-loop TGA is rare, accounting for <1% of congenital heart disease. In isolation, patients with isolated L-loop TGA are acyanotic, although the majority of patients have associated defects (VSD 70%, abnormal tricuspid valve >50%, and pulmonary outflow obstruction in 40%). Patients with isolated L-loop TGA, without associated defects and normal tricuspid (systemic atrioventricular) valves, have a good prognosis. However, this is a minority of patients and those with additional anatomic abnormalities have a worse prognosis. Progressive tricuspid regurgitation is common and is associated with heart failure and death.[68,69]

Surgical Repairs

Patients with L-loop TGA and no associated defects often do not require surgery. For those who do require intervention, options include a physiologic repair in which the associated anatomic defects are corrected but the right ventricle remains the systemic ventricle. Alternatively, an anatomic repair (the double-switch) can be performed in young patients, which requires an atrial switch procedure and either an arterial switch or Rastelli. Evaluation of patients after the double-switch procedure requires evaluation of both the atrial switch and the arterial switch

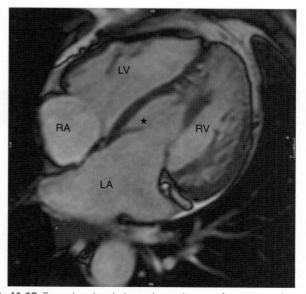

FIG. 41.12 Four-chamber balanced steady-state free precession cine image showing the anatomy of L-loop transposition of the great arteries. Asterisk denotes the septal leaflet of the tricuspid valve. *LA,* Left atrium; *LV,* left ventricle; *RA,* right atrium; *RV,* right ventricle.

portions. Refer to the text on evaluation of the patient with D-loop TGA for details.[50] The atrioventricular node and His bundles are abnormally located and complete heart block occurs at a rate of approximately 2% per year in adults.

Cardiovascular Magnetic Resonance Evaluation of L-Loop Transposition of the Great Arteries Following Physiologic Repair

Systemic Right Ventricle

The right ventricle is not optimally suited to support the systemic circulation and up to 50% of patients with L-loop TGA will have heart failure by age 50 years.[50,70] TTE evaluation of systemic RV function is difficult, with poor reproducibility, and CMR is the clinical gold standard for evaluation of systemic RV volumes and systolic function.[71] Nonetheless, there is wide variability in how different CMR laboratories process and contour RV images. The right ventricle can be contoured from either short-axis stacks perpendicular to the interventricular septum or axial stacks. Axial stacks allow easier tracking of the tricuspid valve plane but partial volume averaging can make the diaphragmatic surface difficult to contour and volumes and EF are different from those acquired in short axis.[59,72] The systemic right ventricle also has prominent trabeculations and there is variability as to whether trabeculations are included in the blood pool or in the myocardial mass. When included in the blood pool, postprocessing is faster, ventricular volumes are larger, and EF is smaller. Centers should develop internal consistency to allow comparison of individual patient's ventricular contours with prior studies.[55,73]

Tricuspid Valve

In L-loop TGA the tricuspid valve (systemic atrioventricular valve) is usually morphologically abnormal, demonstrating apical displacement, a dysplastic septal leaflet, and is often described as Ebstein-like. Regurgitation volume can be calculated by comparing RV stroke volume and anterograde aortic flow using PCMR or by comparing RV and LV stoke volumes, assuming no shunt. Tricuspid regurgitation places a volume load on an already pressure-loaded right ventricle and is associated with heart failure. Tricuspid valve repair is typically ineffective and early valve replacement improves outcomes.[70,74,75]

A suggested CMR protocol for imaging adults with L-loop TGA is presented in Box 41.7.

DOUBLE OUTLET RIGHT VENTRICLE

Anatomy and Natural History

Double outlet right ventricle (DORV) is a conotruncal anomaly in which both great arteries are completely or nearly completely aligned with the right ventricle. Rather than a single congenital abnormality, DORV encompasses a variety of configurations with very different presentations and types of surgical repair. In DORV, the VSD is the only source of egress from the left ventricle. The VSD size, relationship of the VSD to the great arteries, conal morphology, presence of outflow tract obstruction, and associated cardiovascular defects primarily determine the physiology as well as the treatment strategy.

Surgical Repairs

There are several physiologic variations of DORV that dictate the clinical presentation and approach to surgical repair:

1. TOF physiology: DORV with subaortic VSD and pulmonic stenosis. In the most common form of DORV (subaortic VSD), the surgical goal is to establish left ventricle-to-aortic continuity by patching the VSD to the aorta. If the VSD is aligned beneath the aorta, the pulmonary stenosis is present and the physiology is very similar to TOF. The left ventricle will eject blood across the VSD to stream out the aorta and the degree of right-to-left shunt depends on the amount of pulmonic stenosis. This configuration is repaired similarly to TOF. The subpulmonic obstruction is resected and a VSD patch is angled to baffle oxygenated blood from the left ventricle to the aorta. However, in DORV the pathway from the left ventricle to the aorta can be longer and more complex than is typical in TOF. The aortic valve is not just anatomically displaced from the left ventricle but also structurally separated from it with loss of normal mitral-aortic continuity. Subaortic stenosis is therefore a common cause of re-intervention.[76]

2. VSD physiology: DORV with large subaortic VSD and no pulmonic stenosis. With a subaortic VSD and no pulmonic stenosis, the physiology and repair will mirror a VSD. Unlike a simple VSD patch, however, the aorta is remote from the mitral valve so the pathway from the left ventricle to the aorta may become obstructed, as above.

3. TGA physiology: DORV with subpulmonary VSD ± aortic obstruction. DORV with subpulmonary VSD, bilateral conus, and side-by-side semilunar valves is known as the "Taussig-Bing" anomaly. With

---

BOX 41.7 Cardiovascular Magnetic Resonance Protocol for L-Loop Transposition of the Great Arteries

Localizers

Electrocardiogram-gated cine balanced steady-state free precession
- Four-chamber view and left ventricular two-chamber view
- Ventricular short-axis stack from the base to the apex
- Right ventricular two-chamber view to assess right ventricle and tricuspid valve

- Right ventricular long-axis view to the aortic valve
- Left ventricular long-axis view to the pulmonary valve

Three-dimensional contrast-enhanced magnetic resonance angiogram[a]

Electrocardiogram-gated phase contrast through-plane flow in the main pulmonary artery, aorta, tricuspid and mitral valves[b]

Late gadolinium enhancement to assess for myocardial fibrosis[c]

These protocols were adapted from Boston Children's Hospital Cardiac Magnetic Resonance Imaging Program.

[a]In general, our practice is to obtain a gadolinium-enhanced three-dimensional magnetic resonance angiogram with the first cardiovascular magnetic resonance (CMR) examination, and then optional for subsequent examinations.

[b]In cases where Qp:Qs ratio is of interest, flow across the branch pulmonary arteries, superior vena cava, and inferior vena cava/descending thoracic aorta may be assessed to improve level of confidence.

[c]In general, our practice is to obtain late gadolinium enhancement (LGE) imaging to assess for myocardial fibrosis with the first CMR examination, and the frequency of repeating this technique in subsequent examinations is dependent on the initial findings and specific condition. For example, some CMR laboratories repeat LGE imaging every 3 years in patients with conotruncal anomalies (tetralogy of Fallot, transposition of the great arteries, double outlet right ventricle).

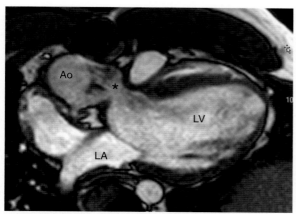

FIG. 41.13 Balanced steady-state free precession cine image oriented to the left ventricular outflow tract in a patient with double outlet right ventricle. Note that the aortic valve is remote from the mitral valve and the long complex pathway from the left ventricle *(LV)* to the anteriorly malposed aorta *(Ao)*, which is frequently narrowed. Asterisk denotes ventricular septal defect through which LV flow has been redirected and a common site of obstruction. *LA,* Left atrium.

a subpulmonic VSD, LV flow will stream out the pulmonary artery and the physiology and repair strategies will be similar to D-loop TGA and is typically repaired with the arterial switch operation (see earlier).

Cardiovascular Magnetic Resonance Evaluation of Double Outlet Right Ventricle

CMR imaging planes must be planned to align the LVOT with the aorta, which is more remote than in TOF (Fig. 41.13). Associated cardiac defects such as anomalous pulmonary or systemic veins are also common in DORV and can be seen on MRA.[77]

CMR imaging of patients with DORV and subpulmonary VSD can be equally as challenging. Subaortic stenosis is common and LVOT planes must take into account the long pathway from the left ventricle to the neoaorta. Aortic coarctation is common in this configuration, so arch imaging with MRA and oblique sagittal "candy-cane" bSSFP images can assess arch patency. The coronary transfer can be more challenging in DORV than D-loop TGA, so careful assessment for myocardial ischemia with LGE imaging and evaluation for segmental wall motion abnormalities is warranted.[64,78]

A suggested CMR protocol for imaging adults with repaired DORV is presented in Box 41.8.

SINGLE VENTRICLE (FONTAN PROCEDURE)

Anatomy and Natural History

Patients with Fontan repairs represent a broad spectrum of rare and complex cardiac abnormalities in which usually only one well-formed ventricle exists and cardiac repair resulting in two functional ventricles is not feasible. This may be due to a severely hypoplastic ventricle, hypoplastic atrioventricular valve, or in some cases, a common atrioventricular valve in the setting of a large VSD. The unoperated survival of patients with single ventricle physiology depends of the cardiac anatomy, the presence of adequate systemic outflow, and on the presence of adequate, but not excessive, pulmonary blood flow. Patients with some types of single ventricle cardiac anatomy, such as hypoplastic left heart syndrome, do not generally survive beyond the first few weeks of life without intervention.

BOX 41.8 Cardiovascular Magnetic Resonance Protocol for Double Outlet Right Ventricle

Localizers
Electrocardiogram-gated cine balanced steady-state free precession
- Four-chamber view and left ventricular two-chamber view
- Left ventricular long-axis view to the aortic valve with careful orientation to align the left ventricle, ventricular septal defect, and the anteriorly displaced aorta
- Ventricular short-axis stack from the base to the apex
- Right ventricular outflow tract outflow view parallel to the right ventricular outflow tract

Three-dimensional contrast-enhanced magnetic resonance angiogram timed to the pulmonary arteries[a]
Electrocardiogram-gated phase contrast through-plane flow in the main pulmonary artery, aorta, tricuspid and mitral valves[b]
Late gadolinium enhancement to assess for myocardial fibrosis[c]

These protocols were adapted from Boston Children's Hospital Cardiac Magnetic Resonance Imaging Program.
[a]In general, our practice is to obtain a gadolinium-enhanced three-dimensional magnetic resonance angiogram with the first cardiovascular magnetic resonance (CMR) examination, and then optional for subsequent examinations.
[b]In cases where Qp:Qs ratio is of interest, flow across the branch pulmonary arteries, superior vena cava, and inferior vena cava/descending thoracic aorta may be assessed to improve level of confidence.
[c]In general, our practice is to obtain late gadolinium enhancement (LGE) imaging to assess for myocardial fibrosis with the first CMR examination, and the frequency of repeating this technique in subsequent examinations is dependent on the initial findings and specific condition. For example, some CMR laboratories repeat LGE imaging every 3 years in patients with conotruncal anomalies (tetralogy of Fallot, transposition of the great arteries, double outlet right ventricle).

Surgical Repairs

The Fontan palliation generally involves a series of cardiac surgeries with the goal to separate the pulmonary and systemic circulations to decrease mixing of oxygenated and deoxygenated blood. This series of surgeries generally culminates in connecting the superior and inferior vena cava to the pulmonary arteries without a ventricular pumping chamber ejecting to the pulmonary arteries. In the current era, there is generally a direct anastomosis made between the superior vena cava and a branch pulmonary artery, creating a superior caval-pulmonary anastomosis (Glenn procedure). A baffle is created either within the right atrium (lateral tunnel Fontan) or outside the heart involving a tube graft (extracardiac Fontan) to connect the inferior vena cava to the pulmonary artery (Fig. 41.14). The one functional ventricular pumping chamber ejects oxygenated blood through the aorta to the systemic circulation.

Cardiovascular Magnetic Resonance Evaluation of the Patient After Fontan Repair
Fontan Baffle, Branch Pulmonary Arteries, and Pulmonary Veins

The baffles or conduits that are used to create the Fontan may become obstructed, particularly at the caval-pulmonary anastomosis site. The

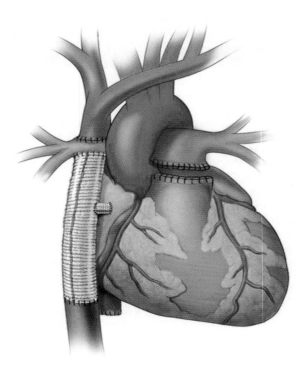

FIG. 41.14 The completed extracardiac Fontan circulation. The superior vena cava has been directly anastomosed to the right pulmonary artery and the inferior vena cava has been brought to the undersurface of the right pulmonary artery using an interposition graft. There is a small fenestration between the inferior limb of the Fontan and the pulmonary venous atrium. (From Kutty S, Rathod RH, Danford DA, et al. Role of imaging in the evaluation of single ventricle with the Fontan palliation. *Heart.* 2016;102:174–183.)

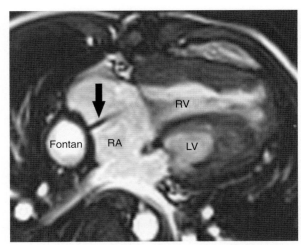

FIG. 41.15 Balanced steady-state free precession cine image of the four-chamber view of a patient with hypoplastic left heart with a fenestrated extracardiac Fontan demonstrating the Fontan baffle with a dephasing jet passing across a patent fenestration *(arrow)*. *LV*, Hypoplastic left ventricle; *RA*, right atrium; *RV*, right ventricle.

branch pulmonary arteries may be of small caliber and should be evaluated for any discrete stenosis. Small gradients within these connections can have significant impact in the hemodynamics because there is no ventricular pump to the pulmonary circulation and pulmonary flow depends solely on the systemic venous pressure. Fontan baffles can develop leaks, which result in shunting from the Fontan pathway to the systemic circulation, resulting in the right-to-left shunt and cyanosis. Many patients also have a fenestration within their Fontan baffle created at the time of Fontan surgery to act as a "pop-off" to allow ventricular filling in the setting of elevated Fontan pressures (Fig. 41.15), at the expense of mild arterial desaturation. Blood flow is often sluggish in the Fontan pathway and evaluation for thrombus is warranted.

An axial bSSFP stack from the mid liver to aortic arch is often used to assess cardiac and vascular anatomy. Narrowing within the Fontan baffle, branch pulmonary arteries, and Fontan baffle leaks or fenestrations can be identified on cine images. Pulmonary venous obstruction can also occur, particularly if there is atrial dilation resulting in pulmonary venous compression. MRA complements cine images in defining this anatomy. PCMR across the pulmonary arteries assesses for physiologic consequences of branch pulmonary artery stenosis or preferential flow to one lung. Fontan thrombus may be seen on cine images or be identified as a filling defect on MRA. If there is concern for thrombus, LGE with a long TI time (~ 600 ms) may be useful to delineate thrombus from native cardiac tissue.

Ventricular Size and Function

Heart failure remains the leading cause of death for patients with only one well-formed ventricle following Fontan surgery.[79] Ventricular size and systolic function should be quantified and the values are generally reported as combined ventricular volumes and EF. It is important to remember that in cases where there is a VSD and two ventricles both ejecting to the aorta, ventricular contours of both the right ventricle and left ventricle should be performed in the same end-systolic and end-diastolic phases.

Ventricular Outflow Tract Obstruction

Patients with a hypoplastic left ventricle frequently have hypoplastic aortas and usually undergo reconstruction of the ascending aorta with pulmonary artery tissue (Damus-Kaye-Stansel or Norwood procedure) as well as relief of any aortic arch narrowing or coarctation. Cine bSSFP of the LVOT and oblique sagittal views of the aortic arch compliment MRA images to assess these features.

Systemic Venous to Pulmonary Venous Collaterals

Patients with Fontan physiology are prone to develop systemic venous collateral vessels from the cavae to the pulmonary veins to offload the elevated caval pressures. These collaterals act as right-to-left shunts and result in arterial desaturation. Occluding the collaterals can be performed percutaneously in the catheterization laboratory and results in increased saturations but may worsen hemodynamics. The presence of coils is not a safety concern, but stainless-steel coils lead to significant image degradation.[80] Collaterals can also occur between the aorta and the pulmonary arteries in the setting of cyanosis and these collaterals result in volume loading of the ventricle and may require occluding if the ventricular volume load is significant. Collateral flow can be calculated with PCMR measuring flow in multiple vessels (see Chapter 5).

Fontan patients, particularly those who underwent a classic Glenn procedure, are at risk for pulmonary arterial venous malformations which are frequently too small to be seen by MRA but may be appreciated by rapid transit time from pulmonary artery flow to the pulmonary veins by time-resolved MRA.

BOX 41.9   Cardiovascular Magnetic Resonance Protocol for Fontan

Localizers

Electrocardiogram-gated cine balanced steady-state free precession
- Axial stack mid-liver to aortic arch, including visualization of the branch pulmonary arteries
- Ventricular two- and four-chamber views
- Ventricular short-axis stack from the base to the apex
- Ventricular outflow tract view

Consider double-inversion recovery black-blood images if artifact on balanced steady-state free precession imaging

Three-dimensional contrast-enhanced magnetic resonance angiogram[a]

Electrocardiogram-gated phase contrast images: superior vena cava, inferior vena cava, branch pulmonary arteries, ascending and descending aorta, pulmonary veins, Fontan baffle just below caval pulmonary anastomosis, Fontan baffle just above hepatic vein insertion to assess fenestration of Fontan baffle leak flow

Late gadolinium-enhanced to assess for myocardial fibrosis[b]

Consider postcontrast late gadolinium-enhanced with long inversion time if concern for thrombus within the Fontan pathway

---

These protocols were adapted from Boston Children's Hospital Cardiac Magnetic Resonance Imaging Program.

[a]In general, our practice is to obtain a gadolinium-enhanced three-dimensional magnetic resonance angiogram with the first cardiovascular magnetic resonance (CMR) examination, and then optional for subsequent examinations.

[b]In general, our practice is to obtain late gadolinium-enhanced (LGE) imaging to assess for myocardial fibrosis with the first CMR examination, and the frequency of repeating this technique in subsequent examinations is dependent on the initial findings and specific condition. For example, some CMR laboratories repeat LGE imaging every 3 years in patients with conotruncal anomalies (tetralogy of Fallot, transposition of the great arteries, double outlet right ventricle).

A suggested CMR protocol for adults after Fontan palliation is presented in Box 41.9.

CONCLUSION

In conclusion, an increasing number of adults with congenital heart disease are undergoing CMR imaging. Knowledge of the congenital heart anatomy, prior surgical interventions, and incorporating an imaging protocol for each individual patient is crucial to perform a successful CMR examination. The information provided by the CMR may identify prognostic information regarding future risk for adverse outcomes in this unique set of patients.

REFERENCES

A full reference list is available online at ExpertConsult.com

42

Pulmonary Vein and Left Atrial Imaging

Thomas H. Hauser and Dana C. Peters

The development of radiofrequency ablation for the treatment of atrial fibrillation has led to an increased interest in the accurate determination of pulmonary vein anatomy and left atrial fibrosis assessment to help plan the procedure and to monitor for postablation pulmonary vein stenosis. Contrast-enhanced magnetic resonance angiography (CE-MRA) readily demonstrates the pulmonary veins and is the method of choice for these imaging studies. In this chapter, we review the methods used to image the pulmonary veins and normal and anomalous pulmonary venous anatomy. We also describe how late gadolinium enhancement (LGE) imaging is used to identify atrial fibrosis and scar. The utility of cardiovascular magnetic resonance (CMR) before and after atrial fibrillation ablation is described.

IMAGING METHODS: PULMONARY VEINS

The pulmonary veins can be identified by using standard anatomic and functional CMR imaging sequences. Although these methods are sufficient for identifying the anatomic relationship of the pulmonary veins to the heart and the other major vascular structures, CE-MRA is usually used for a volumetric three-dimensional (3D) understanding of the intricate pulmonary venous anatomy. A 3D spoiled gradient echo sequence is acquired during the first pass of gadolinium (Gd) contrast.[1] Clinical protocols vary but have mainly common elements.[2–10] The technique uses short repetition times (TR; 2–5 ms), a high flip angle (25–60 degrees), and fractional echoes, all of which provide T1 weighting and minimal flow artifacts. The spatial resolution varies from 1–2 × 1–2 mm in-plane with 2 to 4 mm slices, before interpolation. A single 3D volume requires a 10 to 20 second breath-hold to suppress ventilatory motion, but scan time can be shortened using smaller fields of view, shorter TRs, partial Fourier, lower spatial resolution, parallel imaging, or compressed sensing.[11] Electrocardiogram (ECG) triggering is not employed, although it is recognized that the position and shape of the pulmonary veins changes throughout the cardiac cycle.[7,12] Images obtained with this method reflect the pulmonary veins at their maximal size.[13] Axial or coronal slabs are usually acquired, using either sequential or centric *k*-space filling. For the pulmonary vasculature, the arterial-venous transit time is very short (4–7 seconds)[14] and therefore artery-vein separation is highly challenging and generally not targeted. Contrast is injected with a gadolinium dose of 0.1 to 0.2 mmol/kg at a rate of 1 to 2 mL/s, followed by a saline flush. A precontrast mask can be acquired, although mask subtraction is not essential for pulmonary venography because the background lung signal is very low. Often a second time frame is acquired immediately after the first-pass image to ensure acquisition during peak contrast. Timing of the acquisition to the first pass of contrast through the pulmonary veins is critical, and is achieved using either a bolus timing scan[15] or with fluoroscopic triggering.[16] For either method, imaging is timed to begin with the appearance of contrast in the left atrium (LA). Time-resolved imaging using view-sharing methods[17,18] is also valuable, providing multiple 3D volumes during the passage of contrast.

More intravascular contrast agents (gadobenate dimeglumine, gadofosveset trisodium, or ferumoxytol)[19–21] are available to extend the duration of shortened blood T1, and improve quality, but they may reduce the contrast between blood and scar/fibrosis, if LGE CMR is acquired.

Image Display

Once the 3D MRA dataset is obtained, the images can be transferred to a workstation for further manipulation and analysis (Fig. 42.1). The simplest and often most informative is to dynamically view two-dimensional (2D) slices within the 3D dataset in the axial, coronal, and sagittal planes. The axial images usually provide a good overview of the pulmonary veins and their relationship to the LA, but the coronal and sagittal images are frequently required to determine specific anatomic findings, such as a left common or anomalous pulmonary vein.

Although 2D slices are very useful for viewing the individual pulmonary veins, it is difficult to produce a single summary image of the anatomy. Maximal intensity projection (MIP) and 3D reconstructions displayed as shaded surface or volume-rendered images take full advantage of the 3D dataset and provide very good summary images. By convention, the LA and pulmonary veins are viewed in the posterior-anterior orientation. These 3D views are most useful when the displayed volume is limited to the LA and pulmonary veins. Because the aorta is directly posterior to the left-sided pulmonary vein, it frequently obscures them from view in the MIP images. Three-dimensional reconstructed images are frequently preferred because the aorta can be excluded from the displayed volume. Three-dimensional rendered images can also be rotated, to better appreciate the anatomy. Software is also available for generating an endovascular reconstruction, simulating the view of the pulmonary vein ostia from "inside" the LA. Direct anatomic measurements should not be obtained from these postprocessed images but from the 2D slices instead.

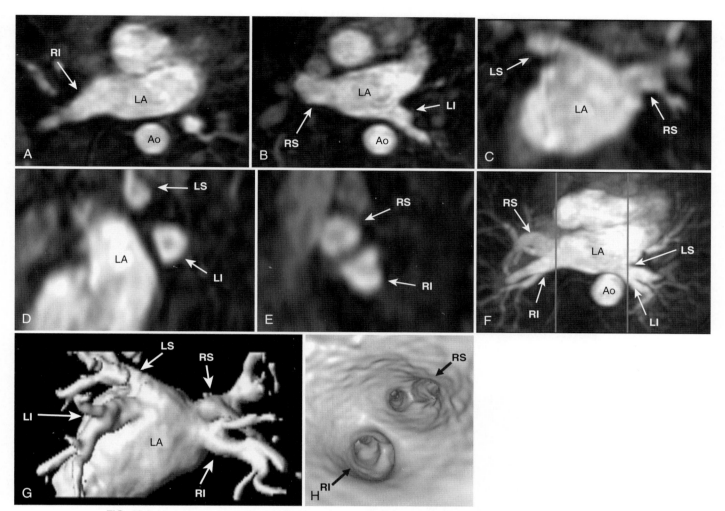

FIG. 42.1 Normal anatomy and quantification of pulmonary vein size. These images show the normal comple-ment of four pulmonary veins, along with left atrium *(LA)* and descending aorta *(Ao)*. The right inferior *(RI)*, right superior *(RS)*, and left inferior *(LI)* pulmonary veins are shown in the axial plane (A and B). The left superior *(LS)* and right superior pulmonary veins are shown in the coronal plane from the posterior-anterior orientation (C). The left-sided (D) and right-sided (E) pulmonary veins are shown in the sagittal plane (anterior to the left). All of the pulmonary veins are shown in the axial maximal intensity projection (F) and posterior-anterior volume-rendered (G) images. The ostia of the right-sided pulmonary veins can be identified in the endovascular reconstruction (H).

PULMONARY VEIN EMBRYOLOGY

A clear understanding of pulmonary vein embryology is important for understanding both normal pulmonary vein anatomy, nonpathologic variations from the normal anatomy, and congenital anomalies. The pulmonary veins and associated apical LA are derived from the primi-tive common pulmonary vein. The primitive pulmonary venous system initially has no connection with the heart and drains into the cardinal veins and the umbilico vitelline system. At approximately the fourth week of gestation, the pulmonary venous drainage coalesces into a single vessel.[22] At the same time, an outgrowth of the primitive LA extends toward the pulmonary venous system to meet this vessel to form the primitive common pulmonary vein and the venous connec-tions to the cardinal veins and the umbilic vitelline system degenerate. The common pulmonary vein then expands to form the smooth-walled body of the LA, whereas the primitive LA forms the trabeculated left atrial appendage.[23] The branches of the primitive common pulmonary vein form the adult pulmonary veins. The development of the LA and

pulmonary veins is asymmetrical, with the two right-sided pulmonary veins developing first whereas the left-sided pulmonary venous drainage enters the LA through a single trunk that eventually bifurcates to form two veins.[24]

Normal and Variant Pulmonary Venous Anatomy

Most commonly, there are four pulmonary veins that enter the LA: right superior, right inferior, left superior, and left inferior (see Fig. 42.1). Each of the veins is directed laterally, with the inferior veins directed posteriorly and the superior veins directed anteriorly. The left superior pulmonary vein frequently has a cranial angulation and may appear to arise from the superior portion of the LA.

Variant, nonpathologic pulmonary vein anatomy is very common, present in approximately 40% of patients.[2,25] Although numerous varia-tions have been described, the most common variations in the usual anatomy are a single left common pulmonary vein or an additional right middle pulmonary vein (Fig. 42.2).[3] These variations occur because of more or less incorporation of the primitive common pulmonary

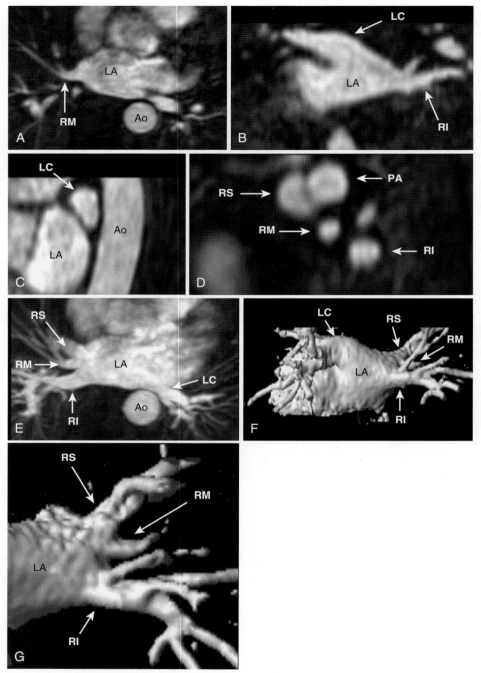

FIG. 42.2 Variant pulmonary venous anatomy. These images were obtained from a patient with right middle and left common pulmonary veins. The right middle *(RM)* pulmonary vein is shown in the axial plane (A). The left common *(LC)* pulmonary vein is shown in the coronal plane from the posterior-anterior orientation (B). The single left common (C) and all three right pulmonary veins (D) are shown in the sagittal plane (anterior to the left) along with the pulmonary artery *(PA)* immediately adjacent to the right superior pulmonary vein. All of the pulmonary veins are shown in the axial maximal intensity projection (E) and posterior-anterior volume-rendered (F) images. The aorta has been removed from the volume-rendered image. The right middle pulmonary vein is obscured by the right inferior pulmonary vein and is best seen with cranial angulation (G). It is frequently necessary to manipulate the point of view to see all of the pulmonary veins. *Ao,* Aorta; *LA,* left atrium; *RI,* right inferior pulmonary vein; *RS,* right superior pulmonary vein.

vein into the LA. Less incorporation leads to apparent fusion of pulmonary veins before entering the LA, whereas more incorporation results in additional pulmonary veins (Fig. 42.3).[26] Because the right-sided pulmonary veins form first and have more developmental time to be incorporated into the LA, it is more common to have additional veins on the right. Conversely, the left-sided pulmonary veins form later and are more likely to have a common trunk. These variations in pulmonary venous anatomy have not yet been identified as a cause of pathology.

CONGENITAL PULMONARY VENOUS ANOMALIES

Congenital pulmonary venous anomalies account for up to 3% of all congenital heart disease and approximately 2% of all deaths from congenital heart disease in the first year of life.[27] The congenital anomalies that affect pulmonary veins are atresia, stenosis, and anomalous connections, which can be total or partial. These conditions occur when the normal connections of the primitive pulmonary venous system form abnormally or if embryologic connections to the cardinal vein or umbilic vitelline systems persist, and are frequently associated with other major congenital cardiac anomalies.[28]

Anomalous pulmonary venous connections are the most common congenital anomaly.[27] In total anomalous pulmonary venous connection, there is no connection of the pulmonary veins to the LA such that all of the pulmonary venous drainage enters the right atrium directly or via a systemic vein. This anomaly is necessarily associated with an atrial right-to-left shunt. Pulmonary venous hypertension is common because of twists in the artery or compression from adjacent vascular structures,[29] whereas small atrial septal defects (ASDs) restrict systemic blood flow.[30] These conditions results in cyanosis and heart failure. Although the mortality rate for symptomatic infants is 80% at 1 year,[27] surgical repair is usually feasible and reduces the mortality rate to less than 25%.[31] In partial anomalous pulmonary venous return, one or more pulmonary veins but not all enter the right atrium or a systemic vein. There is usually an associated ASD, frequently of the sinus venosus type with the right superior or right middle pulmonary veins draining into the superior vena cava.[27] The physiology of this anomaly is similar to that of an ASD and depends on the magnitude of the left-to-right shunt and the presence of increased pulmonary vascular resistance.[28] Patients are often asymptomatic if the shunt is relatively small and the pulmonary vascular resistance is normal. As a result, the diagnosis may not be made until adulthood. The scimitar syndrome, named after the characteristic chest radiograph finding, is a specific form of partial anomalous pulmonary venous connection in which all of the venous drainage from the right lung enters the inferior vena cava (Fig. 42.4). This rare syndrome is also associated with anomalous arterial supply of the right lower lobe from the aorta, dextroposition of the heart, and hypoplasia of the right lung.[32]

Congenital pulmonary vein atresia is defined as the absence of any connection of the pulmonary veins to either the LA or any other vascular structure. This is a very rare condition that is not compatible with

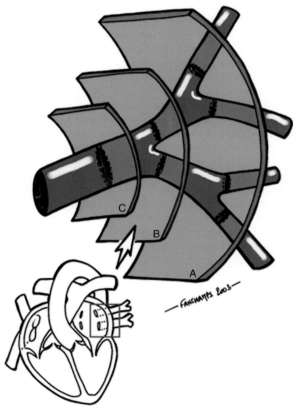

FIG. 42.3 Incorporation of the primitive common pulmonary vein into the left atrium. The incorporation of the primitive common pulmonary vein is variable and results in nonpathologic variations in the normal anatomy. This figure shows the results of variable incorporation of the left-sided pulmonary veins. The most common pattern is two left-sided pulmonary veins *(plane B)*. With less incorporation of the common pulmonary vein into the left atrium, there is only a single left common pulmonary vein *(plane C)*. With more incorporation, there are additional pulmonary veins *(plane A)*. (From Ghaye B, Szapiro D, Dacher JN, et al. Percutaneous ablation for atrial fibrillation: the role of cross-sectional imaging. *Radiographics*. 2003;23 Spec No:S19–33; discussion S48–S50.)

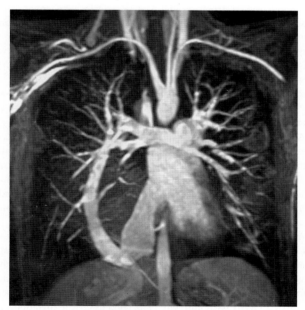

FIG. 42.4 Coronal thoracic cardiovascular magnetic resonance image in a patient with scimitar syndrome. This coronal maximal intensity projection image in the anterior-posterior orientation shows the typical findings of the scimitar syndrome. The single right pulmonary vein enters the inferior vena cava. The right atrium and descending aorta are also shown. (From Greil GF, Powell AJ, Gildein HP, et al. Gadolinium-enhanced three-dimensional magnetic resonance angiography of pulmonary and systemic venous anomalies. *J Am Coll Cardiol*. 2002;39:335–341.)

life, although infants may survive for a short period of time because of small connections between the pulmonary veins and esophageal or brachial veins.[28]

Congenital pulmonary vein stenosis can involve a focal segment of one or more pulmonary veins or more diffusely involve an entire pulmonary vein and is usually associated with other congenital cardiac malformations. Severe stenosis frequently results in cyanosis, heart failure, and death, although surgical repair is possible if only focal stenosis is present.[28]

Imaging patients with congenital anomalies using CE-MRA is a valuable method for determining the pulmonary venous anatomy. It is generally able to identify all pulmonary venous anomalies, providing new information in 75% and identifying previously unsuspected anomalies in 30%.[33]

PULMONARY VEINS AND THE PATHOPHYSIOLOGY OF ATRIAL FIBRILLATION

Atrial fibrillation is the most common sustained cardiac arrhythmia, affecting more than 5 million people in the United States,[34,35] and is a major cause of morbidity and mortality. It accounts for more than 400,000 hospitalizations each year[36] and increasing the risk of death by 50% for men and 90% for women.[37] Atrial fibrillation quintuples the risk of stroke[38] and is the attributed cause for 15% of all strokes.[36] The costs associated with the treatment of atrial fibrillation are estimated at US$6 billion.[39] Although several antiarrhythmic drugs are available for the treatment of atrial fibrillation, maintenance of sinus rhythm is frequently suboptimal[40–42] and all these drugs are associated with significant side effects or adverse events.[43]

Increasingly, evidence has shown that the pulmonary veins play a critical role in the pathophysiology of atrial fibrillation. As noted, the pulmonary veins and LA are both derived from the primitive common pulmonary vein[23] and therefore have many anatomic similarities. Both are smooth-walled structures that have electrically active myocardium. Approximately 90% of pulmonary veins contain atrial myocardium.[44] Although the myocardium in the LA is uniform, myocardium in the pulmonary veins is frequently discontinuous and fibrotic. Patients with a history of atrial fibrillation uniformly have myocardium in the pulmonary veins and an increased rate of structural abnormalities. These structural abnormalities result in abnormal electrical activation, with slow and anisotropic conduction. Proarrhythmic re-entrant beats and sustained focal activity can be easily induced.[45]

A landmark study demonstrated that the proarrhythmic electrical activity in pulmonary veins is directly responsible for the generation of atrial fibrillation in many patients.[46] Among those with paroxysmal atrial fibrillation, 94% were found to have ectopic foci in the pulmonary veins that were responsible for the induction of atrial fibrillation. Radiofrequency ablation of these foci resulted in complete suppression of atrial fibrillation in a majority of patients.

Although these studies are suggestive that re-entry may be important in the initiation of atrial fibrillation, the mechanisms that sustain atrial fibrillation are still not known. Proposed mechanisms include triggers and an abnormal LA substrate. Triggers potentially include regions with ectopic electrical activity or atrial rotors. The presence of a dilated LA, by itself and with associated electrical, metabolic, and structural remodeling,[47,48] is the abnormal substrate that may sustain atrial fibrillation.

Based on these findings, several related procedures were developed for the treatment of atrial fibrillation.[46,49–52] Each of these procedures uses radiofrequency ablation to electrically isolate the pulmonary veins from the LA, with or without additional ablation in the body of the LA. Short-term success rates range from 65% to 85% in patients with paroxysmal atrial fibrillation, with a reduction in morbidity and improved quality of life.[53]

IMAGING BEFORE AND AFTER ATRIAL FIBRILLATION ABLATION

Imaging is usually performed before atrial fibrillation ablation to determine the pulmonary vein anatomy (size and number/orientation of the pulmonary veins). In addition, CE-MRA may be performed after the ablation if the patient has signs/symptoms suggestive of pulmonary vein stenosis (see later). The accurate determination of pulmonary vein anatomy is critical for the planning and execution of atrial fibrillation ablation. To achieve success, the operator must place a series of radiofrequency lesions that encircle the pulmonary veins and electrically isolate them from the LA.[54] This necessarily requires that the pulmonary vein anatomy be determined before the procedure. In the initial development of the procedure the pulmonary veins were identified using invasive contrast venography.[55] Although this can be done successfully, it greatly increases the procedure time and only provides projection images of the pulmonary veins. Most centers now use CE-MRA, noncontrast MRA, or computed tomography (CT) angiography to determine the pulmonary vein anatomy before the procedure. Either technique provides high-resolution 3D tomographic images of the pulmonary veins and other mediastinal structures. These images can also be imported into the 3D electrophysiologic mapping systems that are an integral part of the procedure to combine anatomic and functional information during the procedure to form an integrated image.[56] Routine utilization of image integration has been associated with shorter procedure times and improved outcome after ablation for atrial fibrillation.[57,58]

It is also important to identify the relationship of the pulmonary veins to other mediastinal structures to avoid complications during the procedure. The formation of an atrial-esophageal fistula is a rare but catastrophic complication caused by excessive heating of the posterior LA wall and the adjacent esophagus.[59–63] The esophagus and its relationship to the LA can be readily identified on standard anatomic CMR sequences and on LGE (Fig. 42.5). The esophagus almost always directly abuts the posterior LA and is usually closer to the left-sided pulmonary veins, but the location is highly variable.[64–66] The esophagus is frequently within 5 mm of the pulmonary veins at a location that probably increases the risk for the formation of an atrial-esophageal fistula.[67,68] Indeed, the esophagus often appears enhanced on postablation LGE.[69] The risk of causing an atrial-esophageal fistula may be reduced by avoiding ablation in the region of the LA closest to the esophagus, but this may be difficult because the esophagus is mobile and may move during the course of the procedure.[70]

The pulmonary veins are sometimes imaged after the procedure if there is a suspicion for pulmonary vein stenosis. Pulmonary vein stenosis is an uncommon but severe complication of atrial fibrillation ablation (Fig. 42.6).[2,25,55,71–77] The application of radiofrequency energy to the pulmonary veins causes intimal proliferation and myocardial necrosis that can result in stenosis or occlusion.[78] Severe stenosis occurs in up to 3% of patients after the procedure and results in pulmonary hypertension and decreased perfusion of the affected lung segments.[79–81] Patients frequently present with cough or dyspnea, but a significant proportion are asymptomatic.[73] Stenosis is most likely to occur in smaller pulmonary veins in which the ablation lesions were placed further into the pulmonary vein trunk and with greater extent of ablation.[76,77] If stenosis does occur, pulmonary vein angioplasty is usually successful in restoring normal flow and alleviating symptoms.[82] Techniques that have emphasized placing ablation lesions within the body of the LA under intracardiac echocardiographic guidance have dramatically reduced the rate of pulmonary vein stenosis[72] such that screening for

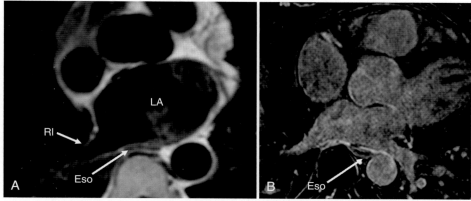

FIG. 42.5 Anatomic relationship of the esophagus to the pulmonary veins and the left atrium *(LA)*. (A) This axial T1-weighted fast spin echo image shows the esophagus immediately posterior to the LA and adjacent to the right inferior *(RI)* pulmonary vein. The esophagus is compressed between the enlarged left atrium and the spinal column. (B) In a different subject, postablation late gadolinium enhancement image also shows the esophagus *(Eso)*, adjacent to a region of ablation.

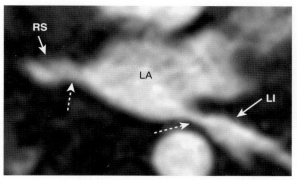

FIG. 42.6 Contrast-enhanced magnetic resonance angiography in a patient with pulmonary vein stenosis 6 months following pulmonary vein isolation. There is severe stenosis of the left inferior *(LI)* pulmonary vein and moderate stenosis of the right superior *(RS)* pulmonary vein, indicated by the dashed arrows. There is prestenotic dilation of the LI pulmonary vein. *LA*, Left atrium.

pulmonary vein stenosis after the procedure is no longer routinely performed.

Quantification of Pulmonary Vein Size Before and After Ablation

The accurate measurement of pulmonary vein size is essential for serial assessment of pulmonary vein stenosis and to further investigate the role of pulmonary veins in the initiation and maintenance of atrial fibrillation. Most investigators have measured pulmonary vein diameters in a specified plane, usually at the ostia.[2,55,77] These measurements tend to have poor reproducibility for several reasons (Fig. 42.7). Identification of the true ostia is very difficult because the pulmonary veins and LA are embryologically related with no clear anatomic border between them. The pulmonary vein ostia are not round, such that measurements taken at the same location vary significantly with the plane of measurement.[2,3] A further complication is that most measurements are derived from nongated images, although the pulmonary vein size varies significantly over the cardiac cycle.[7,83] These difficulties were highlighted in a study comparing pulmonary

vein diameter measurements performed using CT, intracardiac echocardiography, transesophageal echocardiography, and x-ray venography in the same patients.[84] Each of these methods identified different numbers and positions of pulmonary veins, with a poor correlation between diameter measurements obtained with each imaging modality.

Tomographic imaging of the pulmonary veins using CMR has several advantages. All of the anatomic information is obtained in a single 3D dataset that can be manipulated in numerous ways. This allows for anatomic measurements in any desired plane, including determination of the perimeter and cross-sectional area that may be more meaningful measures of pulmonary vein size. A simple method for determining pulmonary vein size in the sagittal plane is highly reproducible and provides these additional measures.[3] The maximal diameter, perimeter, and cross-sectional area are measured at the location in the sagittal plane at which the pulmonary veins separate from the LA and from each other (see Fig. 42.1). This is easily determined by scrolling through a reconstruction of the 3D dataset in the sagittal plane. Because the measurements are made in a standard plane and location, reproducibility is greatly improved compared with standard diameter measurements.[3] This allows for more accurate determination of interstudy differences in pulmonary vein size and increased statistical power in research studies. Even in the absence of severe stenosis, this method can identify small changes in pulmonary vein size after atrial fibrillation ablation that may be due to hemodynamic changes related to the restoration of sinus rhythm.[4] The determination of the perimeter and cross-sectional area is also advantageous. Patients with larger summed total pulmonary vein cross-sectional area are more likely to have recurrent atrial fibrillation after ablation independent of the type of atrial fibrillation or LA size.[85] Diameter measurements do not have predictive value.[53]

Left Atrial and Left Atrial Appendage Morphology

Increased LA "sphericity" (how closely the LA shape resembles a sphere) has been demonstrated to be a marker of poor prognosis,[86] related to atrial fibrillation recurrence after ablation, and more predictive than LA volume. Additionally, the LA appendage morphology may help risk stratify patients for thromboembolic event,[87] with "chicken wing" morphologies predicting fewer events.

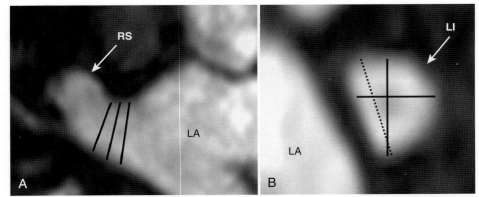

FIG. 42.7 Difficulty in measurement of pulmonary vein diameters. These images show a right superior *(RS)* pulmonary vein in the axial plane (A) and a left inferior *(LI)* pulmonary vein in the sagittal plane (B). There is no clear anatomic border between the RS pulmonary vein and the left atrium *(LA)* (A) such that several potential diameter measurements are possible *(solid lines)*. The left inferior pulmonary vein is oval (B). The diameters measured in the axial plane *(horizontal line)* and coronal plane *(vertical line)* differ from each other and from the true maximal diameter *(dashed line)*.

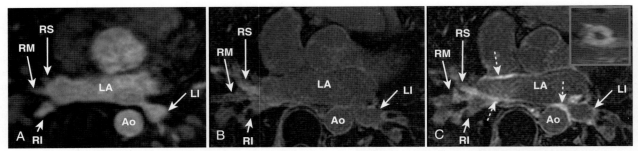

FIG. 42.8 Late gadolinium enhancement (LGE) imaging. These images show the pulmonary vein anatomy (A) in a patient who underwent LGE imaging before (B) and 6 weeks after (C) atrial fibrillation ablation. There is variant anatomy with an additional right middle *(RM)* pulmonary vein (A). Before ablation (B), there is no enhancement of the pulmonary veins. There is increased signal in the right superior *(RS)* and RM pulmonary veins due to artifact from the ventilatory compensation technique. After ablation (C) there is evidence of LGE/pulmonary vein scar *(dashed arrows)*. The inset shows a reformatted image of the left inferior *(LI)* pulmonary vein that shows circumferential scar. *Ao,* Aorta; *LA,* left atrium; *RI,* right inferior pulmonary vein.

Late Gadolinium Enhancement of the Left Atrium and Pulmonary Veins

Scar and fibrosis imaging using LGE has the potential to noninvasively assess both the extent of LA remodeling (fibrosis) associated with atrial fibrillation and the completeness of ablation lines after pulmonary vein isolation. LGE may have applications in both risk stratifying patients for ablation and in periprocedural or real-time guidance of an ablation, to ensure minimal gaps. The LGE technique used for atrial imaging[88] is a T1-weighted inversion recovery gradient echo (GRE) sequence, with imaging acquired >15 to 20 minutes after the injection of gadolinium contrast.[89,89a] Gadolinium contrast remains concentrated in the regions of scar/fibrosis, compared with muscle or blood, because of reduced clearance and the large contrast distribution volume in fibrotic regions.[90] To detect LA wall scar, the standard LGE method is modified to include fat suppression and to achieve higher spatial resolution (1.3 × 1.3 × 3–5 mm^3) by acquiring a 3D volume during free breathing with ventilatory motion compensated imaging (Fig. 42.8).[91] Fig. 42.9 describes potential pitfalls in atrial LGE imaging, including the importance of fat suppression, TI choice, phase-encoding direction choice, and the appearance of artifacts because of poor fat suppression and arrhythmia.

It also demonstrates the effects of timing of the 3D volume after contrast injection.

As with left ventricular thrombus imaging,[91a] long inversion time LGE has been shown to be superior for the identification of left atrial appendage thrombus.[91b] This offers the opportunity to combine pulmonary vein CE-MRA with long inversion time LGE to both assess pulmonary vein anatomy and exclude LA appendage thrombus.[91c]

Scar and Fibrosis Measurement

Similar to LGE in the left ventricle, scar can be segmented by carefully drawn regions of interest and thresholding (Fig. 42.10). First, a blood-pool region of interest and an LA wall region of interest are constructed, from which scar is segmented using a threshold. The threshold for atrial fibrosis and scar depends on the image contrast, but generally signal >3 SDs (measured in the blood) above blood pool signal is identified as scar.[92,93] Fibrosis extent is measured by segmenting the enhanced atrial myocardium (volume), and normalizing it by the total atrial myocardial volume, which is approximately equal to the atrial wall surface area × 2 mm (mean atrial wall thickness).[94] Such segmentations can be visualized in 3D, and the percentage of the wall which is enhanced can be quantified. However, this type of analysis is time-intensive and

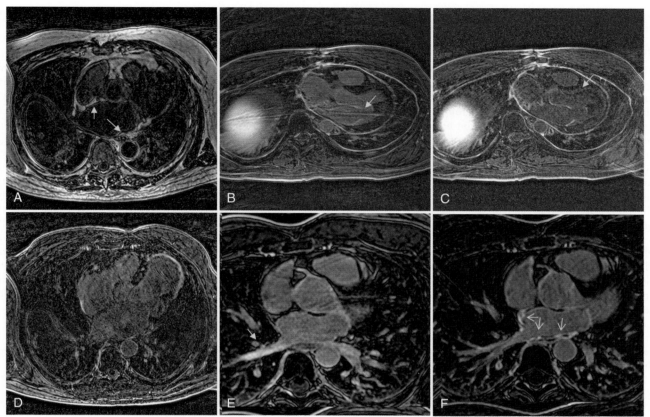

FIG. 42.9 Pitfalls in late gadolinium enhancement (LGE) imaging of atrial fibrosis and scar. (A–E) Preablation LGE. (A) Poor fat suppression *(arrows),* with poor TI choice which nulls blood. The fat which surrounds the left atrium is visible. (B) Phase-encoding direction should right–left. Arrows show respiratory motion artifact. (C) The same subject and slice as in B, except phase-encoding direction is right–left; the TI was too short. (D) Patient with arrhythmia, showing ghosted, poor-quality images. (E) Good-quality image, with inflow artifact in the right pulmonary vein *(arrow).* This can be reduced using a navigator pulse at the end of the data acquisition. (F). Excellent quality postablation image, with evident scar *(arrows).*

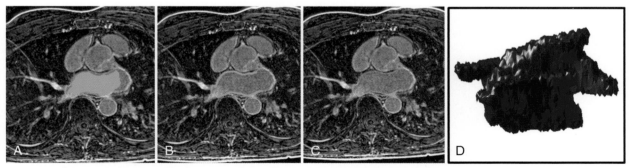

FIG. 42.10 (A–C) Axial late gadolinium enhancement images in a patient following pulmonary vein isolation demonstrating left atrial scar/hyperenhancement. (A) Segmentation of the left atrial cavity in one slice. (B) The left atrial wall can be considered to extend about 2 mm outward from the left atrial cavity. (C) The enhanced signal, based on thresholding, within the left atrial wall is identified as fibrosis or scar. (D) After segmenting the left atrial wall and scar/fibrosis in each slice, the percentage of the atrial wall that is enhanced can be measured and displayed. Images were obtained from a preablation patient with atrial fibrillation.

has moderate reproducibility.[93] Automated and semiquantitative methods are in development.

Postablation Assessments of Atrial Scar

Radiofrequency ablation for the treatment of atrial fibrillation results in scarring of the pulmonary vein and LA.[78] Several studies have found increased ablation scar or an increased number of fully ablated veins in subjects without recurrence.[95–97] Other groups have worked toward the goal of identifying gaps in the ablation lines around individual pulmonary veins using LGE, with mixed success. In studies of patients undergoing repeat ablations, some studies found no correlation between sites of electrical reconnection and minimal LGE,[98,99] whereas others found a relationship.[100] Probably, improved LGE quality and interpretation is required before LGE is able to guide reablation. CMR to guide ablations in real time has employed both T2-weighted images, T1-weighted images, and LGE.[96,101–104]

Atrial Fibrosis by Late Gadolinium Enhancement to Predict Atrial Fibrillation Recurrence Postablation

A series of studies[48,105–108] have developed evidence for the hypothesis that patients with more significant atrial fibrosis before ablation are more prone to atrial fibrillation recurrence after ablation. The largest and most recent multicenter study[109] used frequent monitoring of recurrence post-pulmonary vein isolation (PVI) procedure. Fibrosis extent indicates the percent of atrial wall tissue that is enhanced/fibrotic. Fibrosis extent (Utah stages) corresponded to: I, 0% to 10% fibrosis; II, 10% to 20%;

III, 20% to 30%; and IV, >30%. Some 260 patients were enrolled and monitored over a mean of 213 days of follow-up. Few (15%) of stage I patients and many (51%) of stage IV patients had atrial fibrillation recurrence, although Utah IV patients represent a small minority of the total population. In this study no other variable except for mitral valve disease (hazard ratio 3.45) predicted recurrence. LGE evidence of complete pulmonary vein encirclement was rarely achieved, though the lack of complete encirclement at 90 days did not predict atrial arrhythmia recurrence.[108]

Most of these studies are from a single group, and it is critical to note that atrial fibrosis imaging by LGE has not yet been correlated with pathology because of a lack of animal models of atrial fibrosis. However, effort has been made to correlate LA voltage mapping with fibrosis, with the goal of establishing one-to-one correspondence between low voltage and LA enhancement, as a surrogate validation. These studies find decreased bipolar voltage in regions of LGE enhancement,[92,98,110] with optimal cutoffs for low voltage corresponding to contrast-to-noise ratio >3 or enhancement ratio (LA wall to blood) >1.6. These studies range from strong to moderate to weak voltage to LGE correlations, and were mainly in mixed pre-PVI and post-PVI populations. Finally, patients with other cardiovascular diseases (i.e., heart failure without atrial fibrillation) also exhibit atrial fibrosis.[111,112]

REFERENCES

A full reference list is available online at ExpertConsult.com

43

Thoracic Aortic Disease

Christoph A. Nienaber

The anatomic and functional characteristics of the aorta, which may at first glance appear relatively straightforward, are now recognized to be complex. Recent insights from both modern imaging technology and better understanding of the hydraulic principles associated with the variety of aortic diseases have helped the medical community to realize the multiple facets of in vivo aortic pathology, as well as its varied clinical presentation.

Diagnostic modalities such as transesophageal echocardiography (TEE), cardiovascular magnetic resonance (CMR), and spiral computed tomography (CT) have all been shown to be useful to interrogate the aorta, both in chronic disease and in acute aortic syndromes. X-ray contrast angiography, the former gold standard in acute and chronic aortic syndromes, has been relegated to a secondary role after the emergence of the noninvasive techniques, most importantly CMR, with their high sensitivity, specificity, and practical advantages.[1-5] However, none of the diagnostic modalities listed above is ideal for all patients, and for a given individual, knowledge of both accuracy and limitations in the presenting clinical scenario are required.[4-7] Although the information content of CMR may greatly overlap with established methods such as echocardiography, CT, or angiography, the technique is more comprehensive and offers more options including four-dimensional (4D) functional imaging.

Besides images with high soft tissue contrast without any radiation, CMR can demonstrate and quantify functional parameters beyond anatomic depiction. Combining anatomical and functional information in a single acquisition means that CMR can potentially provide a more comprehensive evaluation of thoracic aortic disease, including aortic valve morphology and function. CMR is an ideal imaging modality for surveillance in a relatively young patient population requiring long-term or even lifelong follow-up care.[8-10] Although the cost-effectiveness of CMR has not been proven in all areas,[11] CMR is the preferred modality in both aortic disease, including aneurysm and dissection, and its precursors, and in congenital and inherited heart diseases. This chapter focuses on emerging advantages of CMR with respect to a spectrum of aortic pathologies.

PRINCIPLES OF CARDIOVASCULAR MAGNETIC RESONANCE IN AORTIC IMAGING

Spin Echo Cardiovascular Magnetic Resonance

Spin echo T1-weighted imaging provides the anatomic detail of the aortic wall and pathologic conditions such as atheromatous plaques, intimal flaps, or intramural hemorrhage and is still the basis of any aortic study, whereas T2-weighted images (repetition time: 2/3 RR; echo time: 80 to 100 ms) can be used in tissue characterization of the aortic wall or blood components. Electrocardiogram (ECG) triggering is essential in minimizing motion and pulsatility artifacts. Slice thickness of 3 to 8 mm and an echo time (TE) of 20 to 30 ms are standard,

whereas repetition time (TR) is determined from the RR interval of the ECG. A shorter acquisition time can be achieved with fast spin echo pulse sequences whereby a long train of echoes is acquired by using a series of 180-degree radiofrequency (RF) pulses; washout effects are even more substantial than in conventional spin echo techniques. A superior black-blood effect is achieved by using preparatory pulses[12] (such as presaturation, dephasing gradients, and preinversion) with one or more additional RF pulses outside the plane to suppress the signal intensity of in-flowing blood and nullify the blood signal (Fig. 43.1). Therefore "black-blood" fast T1-weighted and T2-weighted spin echo sequences have improved image quality, and constitute the method of choice for morphologic assessment of the thoracic aorta. Images are acquired in axial and additional planes, depending on the anatomy and diagnostic problems, to define the extent of the disease in three-dimensional (3D) space.

Gradient Echo Cardiovascular Magnetic Resonance and Flow Mapping

Gradient echo techniques provide dynamic and functional information, although with fewer details of the vessel wall. The bright signal of the blood pool on gradient echo images results from flow-related enhancement obtained by applying RF pulses to saturate a volume of tissue. With a short TR (4 to 8 ms) and low flip angle (20 to 30 degrees), maximal signal is emitted by blood flowing in the voxel and ECG-gated acquisition provides a high degree of temporal resolution throughout the cardiac cycle (up to 20 to 25 frames) to be displayed in cine format. Flow-related enhancement is produced by inflow of unsaturated blood exposed to only one RF pulse. As result, the laminar moving blood displays a bright signal in contrast to stationary tissues. The signal can be reduced if the flow is low, as in aortic aneurysms. Mural thrombi can be identified by persistent low-signal intensity in different phases of the cardiac cycle. Turbulent flow produces rapid spin dephasing and results in a signal void, providing additional information in many pathologic conditions such as coarctation, aortic valve insufficiency, aortic aneurysm, and dissection.[13] Particularly in aortic dissection, the detection of entry and reentry sites is a special capability of functional CMR that can be helpful in planning both surgical and endovascular therapy. Accurate quantitative information on blood flow is obtained from modified gradient echo sequences with parameter reconstruction from the phase rather than the amplitude of the magnetic resonance (MR) signal; this is also known as flow mapping or phase contrast or velocity-encoded cine CMR[14] (Fig. 43.2). In each pixel of velocity images, the phase of the signal is related to the velocity component in the direction of a bipolar velocity phase-encoding gradient. In the phase image, the velocity of blood flow can be determined for any site of the vascular system. Flow velocity is calculated by using a formula in which velocity is proportional to change in the phase angle of protons in motion. MR maps of flow velocity are obtained two-dimensionally, which is particularly important in profiles of nonuniform flow, such as in the great vessels. Quantitative data on flow velocity and flow volume are obtained from the velocity maps through a region of interest. The mean blood flow is estimated by multiplying the spatial mean velocity and the cross-sectional area of the vessel. Vector mapping has been used to describe flow patterns in different aortic diseases (e.g., hypertension, aneurysms, dissection, Marfan syndrome, coarctation).[15,16]

Magnetic Resonance Angiography

A variety of magnetic resonance angiography (MRA) techniques, including various pulse sequences, methods of data acquisition, and postprocessing, have been developed, but first-pass 3D contrast-enhanced MRA constitutes the method of choice for the evaluation of the aorta.[8,17,18] The technique relies on the contrast-induced T1-shortening effects of the gadolinium (Gd) contrast agent, whereby saturation problems with

slow flow or turbulence-induced signal voids are avoided. During the short intravascular phase, the paramagnetic contrast agent provides a precise signal in the arterial or venous system, enhancing the vessel-to-background contrast-to-noise ratio, irrespective of flow patterns and velocity and not only delineates the dissection lamella, but also filling of critical side branches. Intravenous bolus timing is necessary to ensure peak enhancement during the middle of CMR acquisition and not exceeding the acquisition time.[19] Improved gradient systems allow a considerable reduction of the minimum TRs and TEs and the acquisition of complex 3D datasets within a breath-hold interval of under 30 seconds. With the support of maximum intensity projection (MIP) images and the 3D multiplanar reformation, this technique delineates all the morphologic details of the aorta and its side branches in any plane in a 3D format (Fig. 43.3). Some caution has to be exercised in patients with poor renal function because this agent has been associated with the development of nephrogenic systemic fibrosis. From a technical point of view, blood pool imaging can be acquired without the use of a contrast agent using an ECG-gated and respiratory-navigated balanced steady-state free precession (SSFP) acquisition. After an intervention, first-pass contrast-enhanced angiography is instrumental in assessing the success of a procedure and in quantifying false lumen thrombosis, a well-established prognostic indicator. The image acquisition is timed according to the arrival of the contrast bolus in the proximal unaffected aorta and thrombosis is assumed to be present when there is no contrast agent in the false lumen. However, recent studies have shown that the flow rates in the false lumen are highly variable and often very slow.[20–22] The use of a new CMR technique with gadofosveset trisodium blood pool agent in equilibrium state is encouraging.[20,21]

Finally, phase contrast sequences may be used to assess blood flow and velocity in both lumens of a dissection. This imaging technique does not play a major role in the context of diagnostic imaging; however, it appears to be an interesting research tool and potentially provides parameters for a prognostic assessment of a given patient. These sequences can also be used to acquire 3D velocity information (Vx, Vy, Vz) for each voxel, within a 3D volume, over time (frequently called 4D phase contrast-CMR) (Fig. 43.4). This acquisition offers the potential to study aortic hemodynamics, flow patterns, and derived vessel wall parameters, such as wall shear stress. This technique can help to identify entry tears between the true and false lumens and to stratify patients according to their risk of aneurysm formation.[21,23]

Four-dimensional time-resolved angiography with keyhole (TRAK) is a contrast-enhanced MR angiography technique that can acquire multiple time-resolved 3D volumes over time using image acceleration

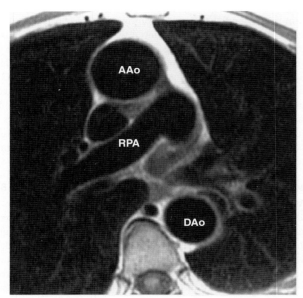

FIG. 43.1 Black-blood vascular imaging of the aorta obtained with cardiac gating and breath holding. Axial image shows the ascending *(AAo)* and descending *(DAo)* aorta at the level of the right pulmonary artery *(RPA)*. Note the excellent suppression of the luminal blood signal and demonstration of the vessel wall.

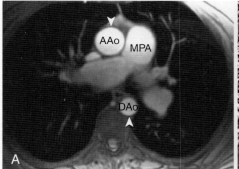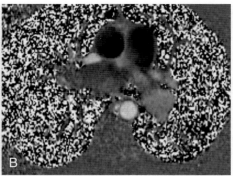

FIG. 43.2 Phase-contrast imaging of the aorta. Magnitude (A) and phase (B) axial images show the ascending *(AAo)* and descending *(DAo)* aorta at the level of the main pulmonary artery *(MPA)*. Flow encoding was superior to inferior. On the phase image (B), the ascending aorta and main pulmonary artery appear black, and the descending aorta appears white, owing to the opposite directions of flow in these arteries.

techniques.[24] It can be used to acquire several phases of contrast distribution, including, but not limited to, the arterial and venous phases. This technique can be used clinically to characterize flow-related phenomena, such as false lumen thrombus distribution and endoleak.[21,24]

DISSECTION OF THE THORACIC AORTA

Acute aortic dissection is a life-threatening medical emergency requiring prompt diagnosis and treatment. The 14-day period after onset has been designated as an acute phase because the rates of morbidity and mortality are highest during this period.[26,27] The two most frequently used classifications (DeBakey and Stanford) are based on the anatomic location and extension of intimal flap (Fig. 43.5). DeBakey's nomenclature is based on the anatomic site of the intimal tear and the extent of the resulting dissection. In a type I dissection, the intimal tear

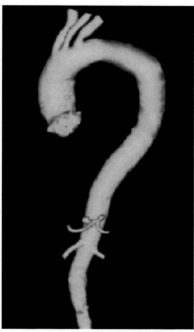

FIG. 43.3 Gadolinium-enhanced three-dimensional magnetic resonance angiography of the thoracic aorta (surface-shaded display algorithm).

originates in the ascending aorta, and the dissecting hematoma extends past the origin of the left subclavian artery, whereas type II dissections are confined to the ascending aorta. Type III dissections begin after the origin of the left subclavian artery and extend distally. The Stanford classification is conceptually founded on prognostic grounds, where type A involves the ascending aorta (Fig. 43.6), regardless of the site of the entry tear, and type B dissections spare the ascending aorta and often imply a better prognosis.[25] In general, acute dissections of the ascending aorta require emergency surgery, whereas descending aortic dissections may be managed with medical therapy and stent-grafting; in any case rapid diagnosis of the dissecting process and a delineation of its anatomic details are critical for successful management.[28,29] The primary imaging goal is not only to establish the diagnosis of dissection, but also detection of entry and reentry sites, presence and degree of aortic insufficiency, and the flow pattern in the true and false lumen as well as in critical aortic branches.[5] The latter is crucial for patient selection for transcatheter endovascular repair of type B acute and chronic aortic dissection as an alternative to open surgery.[30,31] For diagnostic purposes the true lumen can be differentiated from the false lumen by the anatomic and functional (flow-related) features. In addition, the visualization of remnants of the dissected media as cobwebs adjacent to the outer wall of the lumen may help to identify the false lumen. The leakage of blood from the descending aorta into the periaortic space, which can appear with high signal intensity and can result in a left-sided pleural effusion, is usually better visualized on axial images. A high signal intensity of a pericardial effusion indicates a bloody component and is considered to be a sign of impending rupture of the ascending aorta into the pericardial space. A detailed anatomic map of aortic dissection must indicate the type and extension of dissection and distinguish the origin and perfusion of branch vessels from the true or false channels. In stable patients, adjunctive gradient echo sequences or phase contrast images can be instrumental in identifying aortic insufficiency and entry or reentry sites, as well as in differentiating slow flow from thrombus in the false lumen.[20,32] The third step in the diagnosis of aortic dissection and definition of its anatomic detail relies on the use of Gd-enhanced 3D MRA. Because 3D MRA is rapidly acquired without any need of ECG triggering and Gd has minimal toxicity in patients with good renal function, this technique may even be used with severely ill patients.[33] With spin echo sequences, artifacts caused by imperfect ECG gating, respiratory motion, or slow blood pool can result in intraluminal signal, simulating or obscuring an intimal flap. In Gd-enhanced 3D MRA, the intimal flap is easily detected, and the

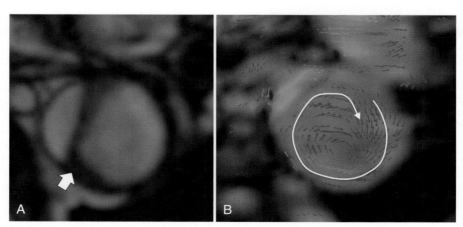

FIG. 43.4 Transverse images of type B aortic dissection (A and B) acquired using four-dimensional phase contrast magnetic resonance imaging. These images demonstrate the velocity of blood flow in the heart and aorta. High-velocity blood flow is shown in turquoise and low velocity in blue.

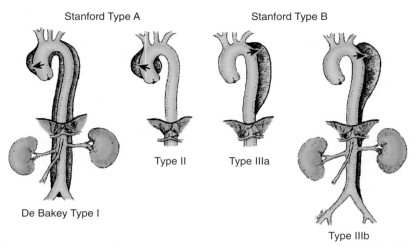

Stanford Type A   Stanford Type B

De Bakey Type I

Type II   Type IIIa

Type IIIb

FIG. 43.5 Commonly used classification systems for aortic dissection. Although the DeBakey classification (I, II, IIIa, IIIb) focuses on the anatomic extent, the Stanford classification (A, B) highlights the involvement of the ascending aorta and the prognostic aspects of dissection.

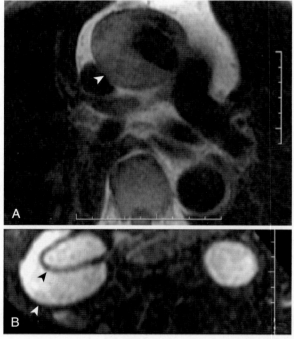

FIG. 43.6 Stanford type A aortic dissection. (A) Axial T1-weighted black-blood image shows nearly circumferential compression of the true aortic lumen by a false lumen (arrowhead). High signal intensity in the false lumen makes it difficult to differentiate thrombosis from flowing blood. (B) Axial reformatted image from contrast-enhanced magnetic resonance angiography shows an intimal flap (black arrowhead) with flow in the false lumen (white arrowhead).

relationship with aortic vessels is clearly depicted. Entry and reentry sites appear as a segmental interruption of the linear intimal flap on axial or sagittal images. The analysis of MRA images should not be limited to viewing MIP images or surface-shaded display; it should also include a complete evaluation of reformatted images in all three planes to confirm or improve spin echo information and exclude artifacts. Combining the spin echo with MRA images completes the diagnosis and anatomic

definition.[34] At present, CMR is one of the most accurate tools in the detection of aortic dissection. A high degree of spatial resolution and contrast, and the capability for multiplanar acquisition provide excellent sensitivity and specificity rating at approximately 100% in the published series.[34–35]

In selecting the diagnostic modality of choice, begin by considering what diagnostic information needs to be obtained. First, any chosen study must confirm or refute the diagnosis of dissection. Second, the study must determine whether the dissection involves the ascending aorta (type A) or is confined to the descending aorta (type B). Third, a number of anatomic features of the dissection should be identified, including its extent, the sites of entry and reentry, the presence of thrombus in the false lumen, the extent of branch vessel involvement, the presence and severity of aortic insufficiency, the presence of a pericardial effusion, and the presence of coronary artery involvement. It is also important to consider the accuracy of the diagnostic information obtained because a false-negative diagnosis may result in avoidable death, whereas a false-positive diagnosis might lead to unnecessary surgery.

According to the present information, CMR and TEE are the most sensitive modalities, with both performing better than aortography. The sensitivities of aortography, CT, and CMR are all quite high, whereas the specificity of TEE may be comparable only when a strict definition of a positive study is applied. Finally, availability, speed, safety, and cost should be taken into consideration in comparing various modalities. Aortography is rarely immediately available, requires transport of the patient, is a lengthy study, has the associated risks of both an invasive study and intravenous contrast, and is the most expensive. Yet it may be necessary in selected patients who are being considered for combined surgical treatment, especially those with a high likelihood of coronary artery disease or evidence of involvement of major arterial trunks arising from the aorta. CT scanning has the advantage that it is more easily obtained in less time and is noninvasive, but it is overall less accurate than the other techniques. CMR is usually less available in most hospitals, requires transportation of the patient, and is considered undesirable for unstable patients or those requiring very close monitoring. Meanwhile, TEE is readily obtained, quick to complete at the bedside and thus ideal for unstable patients, and is the least costly of the four imaging techniques. These options render angiography obsolete in the diagnostic workup of aortic dissection. Thus detecting dissection of the thoracic aorta should be a noninvasive strategy using CT or CMR in hemodynamically stable patients and TEE in patients who are too unstable for transportation. Comprehensive and detailed evaluation can thus be reduced to a single noninvasive imaging modality in the evaluation of suspected aortic dissection.

Although CMR may be less practical than CT and TEE to evaluate patients presenting with suspected aortic dissection, it is well suited for patients with stable chronic dissections. The extraordinary accuracy of CMR and the optional functional images may render CMR the gold standard for defining aortic anatomy and risk of rupture in dissection patients; for surveillance of dissection, CMR has already been widely accepted regardless of medical treatment, surgical repair, or endovascular management.

CMR can be used to custom design an individual stent graft for lesions such as aneurysms, aortic dissections, and localized aortic ulcers. With customized aortic endoprosthesis, such entities are becoming more frequently an ideal target for interventional treatment rather than surgical approaches that have high mortality and morbidity[36] (Fig. 43.7).

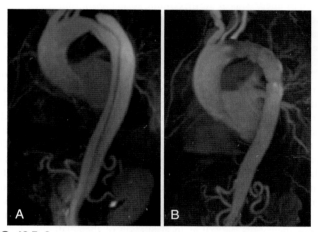

FIG. 43.7 Contrast-enhanced magnetic resonance angiography (MRA) of chronic type B dissection originating from the aortic arch region. (A) Follow-up MRA at 7 days after stent-graft placement shows a completely sealed proximal entry to the thrombosed false lumen. (B) The diameter of the true lumen is normalized, and the descending aorta is reconstructed.

AORTIC INTRAMURAL HEMATOMA

An important differential diagnosis of aortic dissection is intramural hematoma (IMH), which usually presents with the same clinical picture and risk profile as overt aortic dissection.[37] Tomographic modalities such as CMR may be used to identify IMH with no luminal component, which is considered an imminent precursor of aortic dissection.[38,39] With high-resolution tomographic imaging, the imaging diagnosis of IMH is now feasible, suggesting IMH as a precursor of dissection, with a 30% progression to overt dissection.[39,40] Because of these findings in vivo before death, IMH appears more likely to be a variant of dissection than a separate entity.[41,42] Typical epiphenomena of dissection such as aortic insufficiency, pericardial or pleural effusion may also occur in IMH. Spontaneous rupture of aortic vasa vasorum, especially of nutrient vessels to the media layer, has been suggested to initiate the process of aortic disintegration without an intimal tear. With a pathogenesis that explains the high rate of progression to overt aortic dissection and a prognosis and survival that are similar to those in aortic dissection, urgent diagnosis of IMH is very important.

The diagnosis of IMH relies on the visualization of intramural blood and/or evidence of localized increased wall thickness.[43] CMR techniques, however, not only visualize the blood in the wall, but also allow an assessment of the age of the hematoma based on signal changes caused by the formation of methemoglobin (Fig. 43.8). Acute IMH (early stage) is well imaged on T2-weighted spin echo images because of high initial signal intensity of blood, whereas blood of 1 to 5 days of age has lower signal intensity on T2 images. High signal intensity within the aortic wall on T1 spin echo images suggests subacute IMH, whereas acute IMH may be determined on T1 images from the isodense appearance of blood and aortic wall.[41,43] Although TEE has an excellent sensitivity to detect aortic dissection, the definite distinction between IMH and normal findings may require a second tomographic modality such as CT or CMR, because a false-negative result (or false exclusion of IMH) is more likely to be avoided with independent morphologic information. In conclusion, as a precursor of dissection, IMH requires diagnostic attention by use of high-resolution tomographic imaging; owing to its physical properties, CMR may play a prominent role not only to diagnose IMH, but also to assess its age and to differentiate IMH from mural thrombosis; angiography certainly is not diagnostic in the setting of IMH.

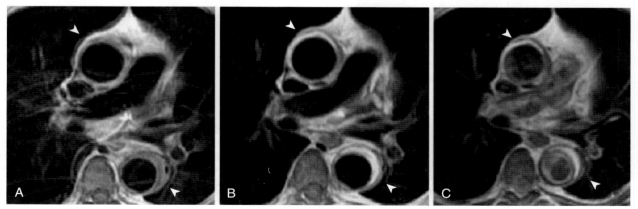

FIG. 43.8 T1-weighted spin echo axial image of intramural hematoma of the ascending and descending aorta. The abnormal wall thickening *(arrowheads)* present intermediate signal intensity in panel A (oxyhemoglobin, acute phase) and high signal intensity in panel B (methemoglobin, subacute phase). (C) T2-weighted spin echo image signal intensity is high in the acute phase (recent hemorrhage).

However, false aneurysm or occlusion of the side of rupture may permit temporary survival. A long examination time and difficult access to the polytraumatized patient have been considered to be the main limitations of CMR in acute aortic pathology. The development of fast CMR techniques has shortened the examination time to a few minutes; therefore MRI can be used even in critically ill patients. The value of CMR in detecting traumatic aortic rupture in comparison with angiography and conventional CT was reported in a series of 24 consecutive patients.[59] The potential for CMR to detect the hemorrhagic component of a lesion by its high signal intensity is beneficial in traumatized patients. On spin echo images in the sagittal plane, a longitudinal visualization of the thoracic aorta makes it possible to distinguish a partial lesion from a lesion encompassing the entire aortic circumference. This discrimination is of prognostic significance because a circumferential lesion may be more likely to rupture.[59] The presence of periadventitial hematoma and/or pleural and mediastinal hemorrhagic effusion may also be considered a sign of instability. In the same sequence used to evaluate the aortic lesion, without the need of any additional time, the wide field of view of CMR provides a comprehensive evaluation of chest trauma such as lung contusion and edema and pleural effusion and rib fractures. MR angiography does not add any diagnostic value to spin echo CMR, and it cannot supply information on parietal lesions and hemorrhagic fluids outside the aortic vessel. Recently, the development of endovascular technique has provided additional opportunities in the treatment of acute onset and chronic traumatic aortic disease (see Fig. 43.12).[60–62]

Aortic Coarctation

Coarctation is a common congenital anomaly, with an incidence of 20 to 60 per 100,000 live births, and represents 5% to 8% of all congenital cardiovascular disorders. The obstructive lesion results from an abnormality in the aortic media and refers to an enfolding of the posterolateral aortic wall in the region of the ligamentum or ductus arteriosus. This is usually a discrete phenomenon occurring just distal to the ductus and is also labeled postductal coarctation. Because it is usually asymptomatic in the neonatal period, it is also referred to as adult coarctation versus preductal or infantile coarctation, which is less common than adult coarctation and usually associated with hypoplasia of the arch. There is usually a dilation of the descending aorta distal to the coarctation. As a result of the obstruction caused by the coarctation, collateral vessels develop to increase flow into the descending aorta. Increased flow through intercostal arteries results in their dilation, and notching along the inferior aspect of the ribs, which usually takes 8 to 10 years to become significant enough to be observed on a chest radiograph.

With its multiplanar image acquisition, large field of view, and dynamic quantitative flow imaging capacity, CMR appears the modality of choice for evaluation of coarctation (Fig. 43.13). The left oblique sagittal view centered on the middle of the ascending and descending aortas is an ideal orientation that may also demonstrate associated aortic stenosis, left ventricular hypertrophy, and ventricular septal defects. This is important because there is a high association of bicuspid aortic valve and ventricular septal defects with coarctation. The severity of the stenosis can be expressed as the ratio of the diameters or cross-sectional areas measured at the coarcted segment and above the diaphragm.[63] However, although the anatomic narrowing of the aorta establishes the diagnosis of coarctation, an assessment of its clinical significance depends on determining its hemodynamic effects. Cine CMR has been applied to evaluate flow turbulence across the coarctation; the severity of coarctation is quantified on the basis of the length of flow void.[64] Further functional information can be provided by CMR flow mapping, which can define the severity of the stenosis by measuring velocity jets at the level of coarctation and mean flow deceleration in the descending aorta.[65] With this technique, it is possible to predict

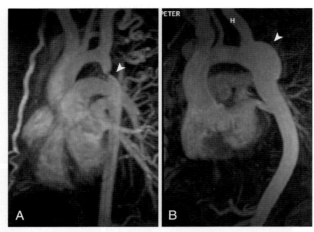

FIG. 43.13 (A) Magnetic resonance angiography of aortic coarctation depicts focal stenotic segment *(arrowhead)* at the isthmic zone and multiple intercostal collateral arteries joining the descending aorta. (B) Medium-sized Dacron patch aneurysm *(arrowhead)* diagnosed 30 years after coarctation surgery.

the coarctation severity with good sensitivity and specificity (95% and 82%, respectively) compared with catheter angiography. Flow mapping is also able to quantify the flow pattern and volume of collateral flow in the descending aorta, which are other important parameters of the severity of coarctation, and this information may be crucial in the choice of surgical strategy. Collateral flow is present if distal aortic flow is greater than proximal flow and it is possible to quantify collateral circulation by subtracting flow volume in the proximal descending aorta from that in the distal portion. The presence of collateral flow indicates a hemodynamically significant coarctation. Furthermore, a pressure gradient calculated with flow mapping CMR by use of the modified Bernoulli equation ($P = 4V^2$)[66] can be used to determine the need for surgical/endovascular repair (a pressure gradient greater than 15 mm Hg is considered an indication for intervention). However, this threshold is arbitrary and therefore it may be more appropriate to use the measurement of collateral flow.

Several therapeutic strategies are available for the treatment of aortic coarctation, depending on the morphology of the affected aorta as well as the age and clinical condition of the patient.[67,68] Surgery for aortic coarctation is recommended at an early age because long-term results seem to be better. Recently, interventional procedures and balloon angioplasty have come into wide use and provide good results, especially in mild or moderate cases.[69,70] An accurate selection of favorable anatomy by high-resolution imaging modalities is particularly important in interventional procedure to ensure a low rate of complications and restenosis.[71] An increased risk for aneurysm formation at the site of repair has been reported after both synthetic patch aortoplasty and subclavian-flap arterioplasty (see Fig. 43.13).[72–74] Moreover, restenosis, aortic dissection, and pseudoaneurysms have been reported after surgery or balloon angioplasty in up to 42% of patients.[75] Therefore routine follow-up is recommended for patients who underwent repair of an aortic coarctation, independently of surgical technique used and timing of the repair. New interventional techniques, such as endovascular stent-grafting, have currently been applied to the treatment of postsurgical patch aneurysms with excellent results, avoiding the need for further surgical intervention.[76,77]

Aortitis

Although there are many causes of aortitis, Takayasu arteritis is the type most often studied with CMR because of the diffuse stenotic nature

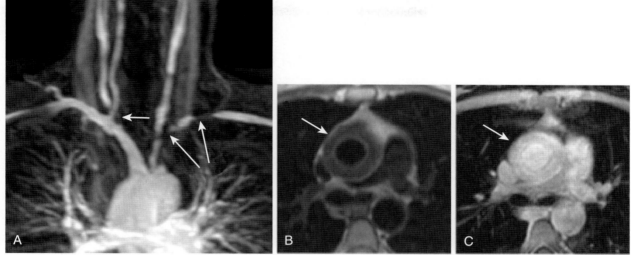

FIG. 43.14 Takayasu arteritis. (A) Coronal maximum intensity projection three-dimensional magnetic resonance angiography shows significant stenosis of right common carotid artery at its origin *(small arrow)*. The left subclavian artery has two stenotic segments *(large arrows)* with a small area of poststenotic dilatation in between. There are also some luminal irregularities of the left common carotid artery. Axial unenhanced (B) and gadolinium (Gd)-enhanced (C) T1-weighted cardiovascular magnetic resonance shows wall thickening of the ascending aorta *(arrow)*, which is enhanced on the Gd-enhanced image.

of the disease, which often makes vascular access impossible by catheterization.[78] In Takayasu disease, the aortic arch vessels are primarily affected, but thoracic and abdominal aorta may also be involved (Fig. 43.14). Active inflammatory disease demonstrates diffuse thickening of the aortic wall, typically enhanced after Gd administration in T1-weighted images. The chronic stage, however, is characterized by extensive perivascular fibrosis without postcontrast enhancement.[79] MRA is the preferred imaging modality for the study of branch vessels stenosis and has replaced invasive angiography, which carries a risk of pseudoaneurysm formation at the site of arterial puncture. Recently, the capability of F-18 fluorodeoxyglucose hybrid camera positron emission tomography (PET) combined with CMR to detect early stages of Takayasu arteritis has been demonstrated.[80]

INTERVENTIONAL CARDIOVASCULAR MAGNETIC RESONANCE

CMR guidance of vascular interventional procedures offers several potential advantages over fluoroscopy-guided techniques, including image acquisition in any desired orientation, superior 3D soft tissue contrast with simultaneous visualization of the interventional device and 4D functional imaging, and absence of ionizing radiation. The feasibility of real-time CMR-guided interventions has been demonstrated for a wide range of vascular interventional procedures in animals and patients.[81–84] In terms of endovascular aortic stent-graft placement, CMR appears to be particularly useful because it can provide preinterventional evaluation of aortic pathology, real-time interventional image guidance, and immediate evaluation of treatment success or procedure-related complications, as well as follow-up examinations.[85] Passive device tracking using material-induced susceptibility artifacts of the interventional

instrument for CMR visualization requires no hardware or instrument modifications and appears to be promising in terms of potential clinical applications. However, CMR-compatible instruments with satisfactory susceptibility artifacts are required, as well as CMR-compatible guide wires with adequate mechanical support. To date, the limitations of interventional CMR are long procedure times, lack of true real-time monitoring, and stent artifacts, which necessitate further modifications before they can be recommended for clinical use.[86,87] However, CMR-guided interventions are feasible and may become an important advance in the near future.

CONCLUSION

With recent advances in the understanding of aortic diseases, both power and versatility have put magnetic resonance imaging in the focus of diagnostic workup and surveillance of all aortic pathology. Technical refinements, from classic anatomic imaging, 3D Gd-enhanced MRA and tissue characterization to 4D functional imaging, have rendered CMR ideal for assessment of acquired disease, such as aortic dissection, intramural hematoma, and aneurysm, along with postoperative follow-up evaluation, with better diagnostic reliability and prognostic information than other imaging modalities. The guidance of vascular interventional procedures by CMR offers potential advantages over fluoroscopy-guided techniques and will continue to advance in the near future.

REFERENCES

A full reference list is available online at ExpertConsult.com

44

Cardiovascular Magnetic Resonance Angiography: Carotids, Aorta, and Peripheral Vessels

Harrie van den Bosch, Jos J.M. Westenberg, and Albert de Roos

Magnetic resonance angiography (MRA) is an important imaging modality for the diagnosis, clinical workup, and treatment planning in patients suspected of a wide range of vascular pathology. The aim of MRA is to visualize the arterial and/or venous system by creating high contrast between the blood flow and its surrounding stationary tissue. To fulfill this aim, several techniques may be used in clinical practice. Depending on its demands and the conditions required to optimally visualize specific vessels of interest, imaging techniques are chosen. In the first part of this chapter, techniques will be addressed that are currently available and applied for MRA. Contrast-enhanced MRA (CE-MRA) is probably the most widely used MRA technique. CE-MRA is applied either by fast imaging of the first pass of an intravenously injected bolus of a gadolinium (Gd) chelate agent or by a prolonged imaging approach with a blood-pool contrast agent. The latter approach is applied when imaging requires a time window that surpasses the first arterial pass. Because of the reported adverse events, such as nephrogenic systemic fibrosis (NSF) (see Chapter 3), accumulation of Gd in the brain, kidneys, and bone tissue associated with Gd-based contrast agents, an increasing interest in non–CE-MRA techniques is currently observed. Black-blood and bright-blood non–CE-MRA techniques will be discussed. Finally, flow imaging by time-resolved three-dimensional (3D) phase contrast (i.e., four-dimensional [4D] flow magnetic resonance imaging [MRI]), with the aid of newly developed visualization tools, is a relatively new technique that may be used to visualize complex flow structures and add quantitative hemodynamic information.

In the second part of this chapter, we will address the anatomical regions imaged by MRA and discuss the state of the art. Special focus will be on the carotid arteries, thoracic and abdominal aorta, renal arteries, mesenteric artery, and the peripheral arteries.

CONTRAST-ENHANCED MAGNETIC RESONANCE ANGIOGRAPHY: TECHNICAL APPROACH

In CE-MRA, vessels in the field of view of interest are imaged during the arterial first pass of intravenously injected paramagnetic contrast material.[1] These contrast agents have a short T1 relaxation time and will produce high signal on T1-weighted images. In clinical practice, Gd-bound chelates, for example diethylenetriamine pentaacetic acid (DTPA), are used as the paramagnetic contrast agents. The Gd ion is a rare-earth element, and toxic to humans when unbound. Therefore in MRA, Gd contrast is based on chelates to control the distribution of Gd within the body and to overcome toxicity while maintaining their contrast enhancement capacity. A very important property of these

chelates is their chemical stability, which depends on the chemical structure and ionicity of the complex.[2] A stable chelate has less tendency to release free Gd ions in the human body. Gd chelates can be distinguished in two structural categories: macrocyclic and linear Gd chelates. In macrocyclic structures, the Gd chelate is more stable and therefore the chance of free Gd ions in the body is reduced. Breaking of the bond between Gd and the chelate (transmetallation) is more likely to occur with linear agents than with macrocyclic agents. However, even though the macrocyclic agents are more resistant to transmetallation, development of NSF is described in patients with advanced renal failure (effective glomerular infiltration rate <20 mL/min/1.74 m^2, acute deterioration of renal function or on dialysis) before Gd contrast administrations.[3] Most reported cases of NSF fibrosis are linked with linear Gd-chelates. Awareness of this association has given rise to effective screening of patient with possible renal failure using the Choyke questionnaire,[4] use of more stable Gd-chelates, and international recommendations for the use of Gd-based contrast agents in daily practice.[5–7] Somewhat concerning are anecdotal reports of NSF-like symptoms following Gd administration but in the absence of renal dysfunction.[7a]

Gd-chelates create intravascular signal by shortening the T1 relaxation time of blood in proportion to the concentration of contrast material. At 1.5 T, T1 of blood is 1200 ms. The T1 relaxation time is shortened by Gd according to Eq. 44.1[8]:

$$1/T1 = 1/1200\,\text{ms} + R_1[\text{Gd}] \qquad \textbf{Eq. 44.1}$$

where R_1 = T1 relaxivity of gadolinium, and [Gd] = gadolinium concentration in blood.

Gd CE-MRA is insensitive to blood flow, in contrast to non-CE-MRA techniques as time-of-flight (TOF) and phase-contrast (PCA) MRA. Consequently, in CE-MRA, image quality is not degraded by flow disturbances.

Gd contrast agents can be classified depending on their distribution in tissue after intravenous administration, that is, extracellular or intravascular. Most of the Gd chelates used in clinical routine are extracellular agents. After intravascular administration they diffuse rapidly through the capillary walls into the extravascular space. In CE-MRA, arteries are preferably imaged during the initial passage of contrast. Timing of starting the image acquisition is essential to reduce signal from Gd diffused to the extracellular space and to overcome venous enhancement, which can lead to artifacts and image degradation.

The application of CE-MRA was improved by the introduction of Gd-chelates that have the capability to bind to larger molecules in the blood such as albumin and thus remain relatively intravascular. These contrast agents (e.g., gadobenate dimeglumine) provide a prolonged imaging time window because of a decreased decay time of contrast in blood. The use of such agents enables imaging beyond the initial passage of contrast bolus, which may be a benefit when acquisition needs to be gated to cardiac or respiratory motion, or when high resolution is required in small vessels such as the coronary arteries.[9] When compared with an extravascular Gd-chelate, blood pool agents show an improved conspicuity of small vessels.[10] Further development of macromolecular blood pool agents in the near future may play an important role in CE-MRA.

Three-Dimensional Contrast-Enhanced Magnetic Resonance Angiography Pulse Sequences

The CMR sequence used in CE-MRA needs to fulfill the following: T1-weighting is required, as well as the obtaining of a large 3D volume with sufficient spatial resolution, preferably fast within the first pass of contrast and within a breath-hold to suppress respiratory motion. Therefore fast T1-weighted 3D spoiled gradient-echo (GRE) sequences are used for image acquisition. In clinical routine, 3D CE-MRA preferentially is performed on a 1.5 T or 3 T system with strong gradient systems to reduce scan time, such that 3D datasets can be acquired during breath-holding. Typically, a short repetition time (TR) and echo time (TE) is used, 3 to 8 ms and 1 to 3 ms, respectively. Flip angle is 20 to 40 degrees to achieve optimized T1 weighting.

Furthermore, subsampling imaging techniques such as parallel imaging are implemented to reduce total scan time.[11] Advanced k-space sampling techniques (spiral, keyhole, echo planar imaging [EPI]) may also be used to speed up acquisition.

At postprocessing, the 3D nature of the dataset allows viewing of the data from any desired angle, that is by creating multiplanar reformats (MPR) or rotational maximum intensity projection (MIP). This results in multiple images in various anatomic orientations. Thin (i.e., <3 mm thick) slices are required to provide a useful evaluation of these images. In some situations, it may be useful to use thicker slices (e.g., 10 mm) to reduce the number of slices and allow faster scanning. Although the ability to rotate the MIP is lost with such thick slices, scan times can be as short as 1 second.

Bolus Timing

Precise bolus timing is essential for first-pass CE-MRA. Arterial imaging is performed in the time window between arterial and venous enhancement and this time window depends on the rate of contrast agent injection, and will be patient specific.[12] The transit time of contrast from the injection site (usually in the veins in the arm) to the field of view with the vessels of interest depends on several factors, for example, injection rate, injection site, heart rate, and stroke volume.

The Gd contrast concentration in the arterial blood is proportional to the injection rate and inversely proportional to the cardiac output:

$$[Gd]_{arterial} = \text{injection rate (mol/s)/cardiac output (L/s)} \qquad \textbf{Eq. 44.2}$$

T1 for blood is related to the injection rate and cardiac output by combining Eq. 44.1 and Eq. 44.2.[13]

Maximum arterial signal intensity is achieved when the start of the acquisition and the contrast infusion are synchronized such that peak arterial Gd concentration coincides with the acquisition of the central portion of k-space.[14] The center of k-space contributes most to overall image contrast, whereas the periphery of k-space provides image information of details and contributes to spatial resolution. Therefore for improved arterial/venous differentiation, central k-lines have to be sampled before venous return. In CE-MRA, different types of k-space

filling can be used in the available 3D pulse sequences. It is important to adjust bolus timing to the order of k-space filling used.

In linear ordering, lines of k-space can be acquired in any order (high k-space lines first, low k-space lines first, or at random). Linear ordering can be used in a CE-MRA protocol when precise timing of the contrast bolus is difficult or arrival time may be prolonged.

For most CE-MRA examinations, elliptical-centric ordering is the preferred k-space sampling method used. Typically, the center of k-space is acquired first and the periphery later (e.g., elliptic-centric Contrast-ENhanced Timing Robust Angiography [CENTRA],[15] Differential Rate K-space Sampling [DRKS], or PEak Arterial K-Space filling [PEAKS]).

To determine the delay between the start of the venous contrast injection and the start of the acquisition, either a small test bolus or fluoroscopic real-time imaging can be used. The timing method by using a test bolus (1 to 2 mL) is robust and easy to perform. However, it will lengthen the procedure by a few minutes and requires an additional administration of contrast. In fluoroscopic real-time imaging, the inflow of contrast is imaged in the field of view with the vessels of interest. At the moment of contrast arrival, the acquisition is started automatically; however, the short delay of a few seconds, which is needed to switch from the fluoroscopic real-time imaging to the actual start of CE-MRA acquisition, can be a disadvantage.

CONTRAST-ENHANCED VERSUS NON–CONTRAST-ENHANCED MAGNETIC RESONANCE ANGIOGRAPHY

The association between CE-MRA and NSF[16,17] in patients with severe renal dysfunction and linear Gd-chelates[5] has been appreciated for over a decade.

Moreover, Gd accumulation in tissue in patients without renal impairment has been reported in several studies. Kanda et al. reported residual Gd concentrations in the brain, particularly in the dentate nucleus and globus pallidus, of patients without severe renal dysfunction[18] and foci of hyperintensity on unenhanced T1-weighted magnetic resonance (MR) images associated with previous administration of linear Gd-chelates, and which may be associated with the total number of previous Gd-based contrast material administrations.[19] Deposition of Gd has also been demonstrated in bone, skin, and liver.[20,21] Currently, previous administration of macrocyclic Gd-chelates shows no association with Gd accumulation in tissue[22,23]; however, these macrocyclic contrast chelates have been in use in clinical practice for a shorter time than the linear chelates. Nevertheless, the application of CE-MRA and the amount of administered Gd contrast is of clinical importance, especially in patients with impaired renal function, and issues of long-term retention may be of particular concern in children/young adults. Awareness of NSF-related incidents associated with CE-MRA and reports on accumulation of Gd in various tissues have also led to a renewed interest in non–CE-MRA. Improvements in CMR hardware and software, including the widespread availability of parallel imaging have helped to reduce acquisition times and have made some non–CE-MRA methods clinically practical. Non–CE-MRA methods may be classified into three categories: black-blood, bright-blood, and 4D flow visualization.

Black-Blood Imaging

Black-blood imaging of blood vessels uses double-inversion recovery to null the signal of flowing blood.[24] This technique is flow-sensitive. Two 180 degree inversion recovery prepulses are applied to null the signal of flowing blood: the first prepulse is nonslice selective and inverts the longitudinal magnetization vector in the entire body, whereas the second inversion prepulse is slice selective and inverts the magnetization in the imaging slice back to its original orientation. Signal of blood

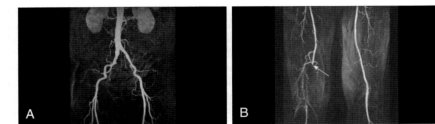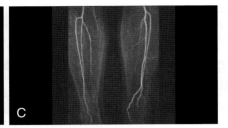

FIG. 44.6. (A) Contrast-enhanced magnetic resonance angiography of the distal aorta and common iliac arteries. (B) Peripheral arteries show an occlusion of the right superficial femoral artery *(arrow)*. (C) Run-off arteries.

To cover the whole region of the distal abdominal aorta and the run-off vessels, two methods are clinically used: the single-injection 3-station moving-table (bolus-chase) technique and the multistation/multiinjection method. In both methods, imaging is performed in a coronal orientation, usually with three stations with overlapping fields of view, covering the complete anatomic region. Typically, the first station covers the distal abdominal aorta and pelvic region, the second station the upper legs, and the third station lower legs. The quadrature body coil or phased-array surface coils are used for signal transmission and reception. In both techniques, 3D volumes are planned on acquired 2D time of flight survey images. Thereafter, precontrast mask images are acquired in all stations. Subtraction of the precontrast mask images from the contrast-enhanced images will suppress surrounding tissue.[152]

In the bolus-chase technique, a biphasic contrast material injection protocol is typically used. The first half of the contrast bolus is administered at a flow rate of 1.0 to 1.2 mL/s and the remaining half at 0.5 to 0.6 mL/s. Contrast injection is followed by a saline flush at 0.5 to 0.6 mL/s. Modern commercially available 1.5 T and 3 T CMR scanners allow acquisition of CE-MRA of the run-off vessels with a bolus-chase technique with excellent diagnostic performance.[153]

In the multistation/multiinjection approach, the three regions of the legs stations are acquired sequentially with two or three separate bolus injections of contrast medium.[154] Gd-contrast is injected at a rate of 1 to 1.5 mL/s, resulting in high signal intensity in the arteries. A disadvantage of this approach is that it is more time consuming, when compared with the bolus-chase technique. However, in patients with multiple risk factors, adequate arterial enhancement with minimal venous enhancement can be obtained with this technique.[155] The first station covering the distal abdominal aorta and pelvic region is acquired during breath-holding and the acquired resolution is of the first two stations is 1.3 mm × 1.3 mm with a slice thickness of 3 mm, typically. The third station covering the lower leg scan be acquired with a submillimeter voxel size, allowing accurate diagnostic evaluation.[156]

Acquired high-resolution image data can be postprocessed using multiplanar reconstructions or MIPs; however, for obtaining an adequate diagnosis, evaluation of 2D source images is essential. Furthermore, the role of CE-MRA in the evaluation of possible restenosis in (metallic) stents is limited because of dephasing of CMR signal, causing signal void. New developments in CMR imaging technology provide large homogeneous field of view at 3T, revealing robust CE-MRA of the complete vascular tree of the run-off vessels and allowing accurate clinical evaluation of patient on high field 3T scanners.[153] Moreover, two-point Dixon fat suppression allows subtractionless CE-MRA, avoiding possible misregistration artifacts between precontrast mask dataset and contrast-enhanced images.[157] Furthermore, new techniques, such as three-station bolus-chase MRA with real-time fluoroscopic tracking and precise triggering of table motion can provide high-resolution imaging of the run-off vessels. These new developments potentially can reduce contrast material dose and examination time.[158]

REFERENCES

A full reference list is available online at ExpertConsult.com

45

Pulmonary Artery

Csilla Celeng, R. Nils Planken, David A. Bluemke, and Tim Leiner

Pathologies involving the pulmonary arterial system include pulmonary embolus (PE), pulmonary arterial hypertension (PAH), congenital anomalies, and pulmonary artery tumors. These diseases present a unique clinical diagnostic challenge often requiring multiple diagnostic examinations spanning the entire radiologic armamentarium. Initially, cardiovascular magnetic resonance (CMR) played only a minor role in evaluation of the pulmonary arterial system. However, with the advent of improved, high-performance gradients and bolus gadolinium, contrast-enhanced cardiovascular magnetic resonance (CE-CMR) is now well suited for this challenge. It not only provides precise, three-dimensional (3D) anatomic information, but also provides functional data critical to a complete evaluation of the pulmonary arterial system. Beyond the basic flow parameters, four-dimensional (4D)-CMR is able to assess information about more advanced parameters (e.g., wall shear stress); however this technique requires standardization before routine clinical application. Further developments are expected in the field of molecular imaging by using target-specific contrast agents in humans, allowing the interaction and detection of pathological mechanisms. CMR is noninvasive and requires neither iodinated contrast nor ionizing radiation, and consistently demonstrates anatomic accuracy comparable with that of computed tomography (CT) while providing reproducible functional data previously only available by catheter based pulmonary angiography.

PULMONARY EMBOLISM

Venous thromboembolism (VTE) incorporates deep venous thrombosis (DVT) and PE. VTE is one of the major contributors to global disease burden: the incidence ranges from 100 to 200 per 100,000 persons per year with an increased incidence from 200 to 700 per 100,000 in those ≥70 years.[1] The risk for the disease doubles in each decade after the age of 40 years.[2] PE represents the most serious and potentially life-threatening condition related to VTE. It often occurs as a consequence of DVT when a blood clot breaks off, migrates, and eventually obstructs the pulmonary arteries. An estimation model based on data from six countries of the European Union showed that 317,000 deaths could be attributable to VTE.[3] Approximately one-third of patients suffered from sudden death caused by PE, 59% died as a result of existing but undiagnosed PE, and only 7% of patients who died were appropriately identified with PE. Because the presenting signs and symptoms are nonspecific and overlap in a wide variety of common ailments, diagnosing PE is challenging and relies on a multidimensional prognostic model. Risk stratification of patients into high-risk, intermediate-risk, and low-risk categories is based on the additive value of clinical scores, imaging tests, and laboratory markers.[4] Therefore the current workup typically includes two or more of the following tests: blood assays, computed tomography angiography (CTA) or ventilation/perfusion (V̇/Q̇) scintigraphy, compression venous ultrasonography (CUS) of the deep venous system, and occasionally the reference standard, catheter-based pulmonary angiography. From the resulting array of diagnostic information, the clinician must then assess the patient's likelihood of having PE and initiate treatment. The most extensively used clinical score in acute PE is the pulmonary embolism severity index (PESI) or its simplified version (sPESI), which is helpful in the prognostic assessment of 30-day mortality. For hemodynamically stable patients, pretest probability relies on the revised Geneva score and/or Wells rule, which both aim to stratify patients into three-level (low, intermediate, and high risk) or two-level (PE unlikely and PE likely) schemes based on information that is easy to obtain.[4] Elevated plasma levels of D-dimer as well as markers of myocardial injury (cardiac troponin I or T) and/or ventricular dysfunction (brain natriuretic peptide-BNP and N-terminal-pro BNP) support the diagnosis of PE. However, the relatively low positive predictive values of laboratory biomarkers do not allow reliable exclusion of PE. The suspicion of PE is therefore a common indication for imaging.

CTA is the most used noninvasive imaging method for detection of PE. A negative CTA in patients with low/intermediate risk allows for safely ruling out PE, although in patients with negative CTA, but high probability of PE, further investigations are required.[4] The high spatial resolution of current CT scanners and the administration of contrast media allows for the identification of PE at least to the segmental level. However, potential pitfalls can occur, especially at distal levels of the pulmonary arteries. A retrospective review of PE on CTA showed discordance between subspecialists in chest radiology and general radiologists in 26% of the cases. The disagreement was most frequent if the PE was adjudicated as solitary (46% of solitary PEs were later adjudicated as negative) or segmental/subsegmental (27% of segmental and 59% of subsegmental PE were later considered as negative).[6] Additionally, CTA exposes the patient to ionizing radiation and requires iodinated intravenous contrast, which is potentially nephrotoxic and can provoke allergic reactions. Radiation exposure is of particular concern in young adults and those who are referred for multiple CTA scans because of a history of prior PE.

V̇/Q̇ scintigraphy is a combined noninvasive procedure that uses nuclear radiotracers for diagnosing PE. The reported radiation exposure of the examination is significantly lower compared with CTA (1.1 mSv vs. 4 mSv) and might be a preferred alternative over CTA in younger patients, especially women, in whom radiation exposure of CTA is associated with higher risk of breast cancer.[4,7,8] However, V̇/Q̇ scans are frequently nondiagnostic, which raised concerns because of the need for further diagnostic tests. Diagnostic accuracy can be improved by incorporation of a single photon emission tomography (SPECT) to V̇/Q̇ scintigraphy.[9]

Catheter-based pulmonary angiography remains the reference standard technique for the exclusion of PE. The use of this method, however, is infrequent due to the good diagnostic accuracy provided by

46

The Pericardium: Anatomy and Spectrum of Disease

Jay S. Leb and Susie N. Hong

The pericardium is an important structure in the evaluation of patients with cardiovascular disease. Understanding pericardial anatomy and the complex hemodynamics associated with pericardial pathology is critical in assessing the pericardium and its impact on cardiovascular function. Unfortunately, clinical evaluation through history and physical examination, clinical laboratory tests, and electrocardiograms (ECG) may be nonspecific and overlap with other clinical syndromes in patients with pericardial disease. Advanced noninvasive imaging, including echocardiography, cardiac chest computed tomography (CT), and cardiovascular magnetic resonance (CMR), is vital in the evaluation and diagnosis of pericardial disease. When combined with a high degree of clinical suspicion, these modalities help advance our understanding pericardial pathophysiology and, ultimately, guide clinicians to optimal treatment and therapies.

IMAGING MODALITIES

Several noninvasive imaging modalities are available to assess the pericardium, with each modality having its strengths and limitations. As a result of the complex nature of the pericardium and its impact on cardiovascular hemodynamics, multimodality imaging is often required to completely evaluate the pericardium.

Chest X-Ray

Chest x-radiography is often the first imaging modality that may suggest pericardial disease and prompt further testing. An enlarged cardiac silhouette may suggest the presence of a pericardial effusion, although this finding has limited sensitivity and poor specificity.[1] Additionally, the chest x-ray (CXR) may detect pericardial calcifications and raise the possibility of constrictive pericarditis; however, calcification is not necessary for pericardial constriction and, in fact, is frequently absent in clinical presentations of constriction.[2–4]

Echocardiography

Direct visualization of the heart through transthoracic echocardiography (TTE) is the most common noninvasive cardiovascular imaging modality for the evaluation of the heart and pericardium. Two-dimensional (2D) TTE with Doppler examination is an excellent, readily available, portable tool for the identification and assessment of pericardial disease. Real-time TTE can detect abnormal cardiac function and hemodynamic compromise secondary to underlying pericardial disease, including pericardial effusions and tamponade physiology. However, patient body habitus, chest trauma, and/or poor acoustic windows attributed to underlying lung disease (e.g., emphysema) may result in suboptimal views and limit TTE in visualizing the entire pericardium.[5,6] Pericardial thickness is also not reliably assessed by TTE. Although transesophageal echocardiography (TEE) may be more accurate, it is moderately invasive, and the field of view remains limited to the available acoustic windows.[7]

Computed Tomography

Cardiac CT and CMR provide a larger field of view than echocardiography, enabling visualization of the entire pericardium and the surrounding structures, providing excellent anatomic definition without limitation to specific windows.[2,8,9] Although optimal imaging of the pericardium with CT and CMR requires ECG gating to minimize motion artifact, standard chest CT and nongated magnetic resonance imaging (MRI) performed for other indications often reveal most pericardial abnormalities, particularly pericardial effusions or calcifications.[3] Cardiac CT and CMR may be useful when TTE findings are nondiagnostic, particularly for assessment of pericardial thickness and evaluation of pericardial constriction, loculated pericardial effusions, hematomas, and/or pericardial masses.[5,9,10]

A specific advantage of CT (as compared with CMR) is its ability to identify pericardial calcification, a frequent, but not obligatory, finding in constrictive pericarditis.[8] Cardiac CT with multidetector scanners and ECG synchronized data acquisition is now widely available, offering the advantage of very short scan times with limited cardiac and respiratory motion artifact.[11,12] Additionally, CT provides excellent spatial resolution, as a result of the use of multidetector, high-resolution volumetric acquisition. Retrospective ECG-gated CT may also provide reasonable temporal resolution to assess interventricular septal motion in the evaluation of constrictive physiology, although this is better assessed by TTE or real-time CMR.[13]

Disadvantages of CT include use of ionizing radiation, the need for intravenous iodinated contrast for adequate blood–tissue contrast, and limited hemodynamic assessment. Additionally, CT images may not adequately discriminate pericardial fluid from thickened pericardial tissue.[8]

Cardiovascular Magnetic Resonance Imaging

CMR provides a comprehensive evaluation of the pericardium, both anatomically and hemodynamically, without ionizing radiation. CMR has the ability to obtain morphological, functional, and hemodynamic information in a single examination, which is frequently required when assessing pericardial disease and its impact on cardiovascular function. Balanced steady-state free precession (bSSFP) cine imaging is used to evaluate left ventricular (LV) and right ventricular (RV) motion and can assess the impact of pericardial disease on overall cardiac function. CMR also provides advantages over CT and echocardiography in its ability to characterize the contents of pericardial effusions and pericardial masses through the use of T1-weighted and T2-weighted imaging, first-pass perfusion, and late gadolinium enhancement (LGE).[6,14] Additionally, real-time imaging by CMR may give vital hemodynamic assessments regarding cardiac motion and inflow patterns while the patient is free-breathing, allowing for the identification of constrictive and/or tamponade physiology. Multiplanar and multisequence CMR can be used to characterize the extent and composition of pericardial abnormalities and real-time CMR sequences allow for functional assessment, including chamber compression caused by ventricular interdependence and interventricular septal motion.[2,15,16] Administration of conventional extracellular gadolinium (Gd)-based contrast agents may assist in detecting of pericardial inflammation or enhancing masses.

NORMAL PERICARDIAL ANATOMY

The pericardium is an elastic dual-layered fibroserous membrane that surrounds nearly the entire heart and extends superiorly to the origins of the great vessels.[17] It consists of an outer fibrous component and a dual-layered inner serous sac. The tough fibrous outer pericardium is loosely attached to the sternum and costal cartilage (anteriorly) and the proximal great vessels (superiorly), and is more firmly attached to the central tendon of the diaphragm (inferiorly).[18,19] The serous pericardium consists of an outer parietal layer, which is intimately adherent to the inside of the fibrous pericardium, and commonly referred to as the pericardium. The inner visceral serosal layer is adjacent to the heart (but not directly attached), covers the epicardial fat and vessels, and typically referred to as the epicardium. A film of clear pericardial fluid (~15–50 mL) normally separates the two serosal surfaces.[3,19] The small amount of fluid minimizes the friction between the two layers as the heart expands and contracts. The serosal layers, consisting of the visceral and parietal pericardium, merge at two complex lines of reflection: one at the base of the aorta and pulmonary trunk, and the other at the insertions of the superior and inferior vena cavae and the four pulmonary veins.[17] The entire pericardium generally lies between variable amounts of epicardial and pericardial adipose tissue.[8]

The pericardial cavity is a complex space consisting of the pericardial cavity proper and interconnecting cul-de-sacs known as sinuses, which are further subdivided and connected to multiple recesses.[13,20,21] Because of the merging of the serosal layers at two distinct points, the reflections of the serous pericardium become arranged as two complex tubes; one enclosing the base of the aorta and main pulmonary artery and the other enclosing the vena cavae and the four pulmonary veins.[22] The transverse sinus is the space between these two pericardial tubes and lies superior to the left atrium (LA) and posterior to the ascending aorta and main pulmonary artery. The transverse sinus connects to the following four recesses: superior aortic, inferior aortic, left pulmonic, and right pulmonic. The cul-de-sac delineated by the inferior border of the tube, surrounding the venous structures, is the oblique sinus. The oblique sinus is an inverted U-shaped space which lies posteriorly to the LA and includes the posterior pericardial recess. The pericardial cavity proper includes the postcaval, left pulmonary venous, and right pulmonary venous recesses.[13] The transverse sinus is the space between these two pericardial tubes and lies superior to the LA and posterior to the ascending aorta and main pulmonary artery. The transverse sinus connects to the following four recesses: superior aortic, inferior aortic, left pulmonic, and right pulmonic recesses. These recesses are usually linear in appearance and become more band-like and rounded as they accumulate with fluid. Appreciating the normal appearance of these sinuses and recesses is important because these spaces can be misinterpreted as adenopathy, dissection, or an abnormality of an adjacent mediastinal structure.[13,23–25]

Although the pericardium is not required for normal cardiac function, it has several homeostatic roles. These include (1) limitation of intrathoracic cardiac displacement; (2) maintenance of normal ventricular compliance; (3) balancing RV and LV output over several cardiac cycles through diastolic and systolic interactions; (4) buffering of changes in chamber filling and output; (5) assisting atrial filling via more negative pericardial pressure during ventricular ejection; (6) limitation of acute dilatation; (7) minimizing friction between cardiac chambers and surrounding structures; and (8) providing an anatomic and immunologic barrier to inflammation and infection from contiguous structures such as the lungs.[14,19] However, the presence of an intact pericardium may be detrimental in clinical situations in which fluid rapidly fills the pericardial space, resulting tamponade physiology.

Imaging Findings of Normal Anatomy

The normal pericardium is seen as a very thin linear density surrounding the heart. Discrimination of the pericardium from the myocardium by noninvasive imaging requires the presence of interposed epicardial fat or the presence of pericardial fluid with associated enlargement of the pericardial space.[18] The thickness of the epicardial fat is increased in patients with obesity and/or diabetes and has been found to increase the risk of coronary atherosclerosis.[26–28] The pericardium is best visualized over the right ventricle and, as a result of less epicardial and pericardial fat to provide adjacent tissue contrast, may not be well visualized around the left ventricle.[8] Technical factors, such as spatial and temporal resolution, may affect pericardial thickness measurements because the normal pericardium is a thin irregularly shaped sac that moves with cardiac and respiratory motion, affecting the pericardial recesses to varying degrees. The superior aortic and left pulmonic recesses are less impacted by cardiac motion, whereas the inferior aortic recess, left pulmonary venous recess, and right pulmonic recess border the LA or left ventricle, and are often blurred because of cardiac motion.[29]

The maximum normal pericardial thickness measured through advanced noninvasive imaging is typically 2 mm, which is slightly greater than normal cadaveric pericardial thickness, which measures up 1 mm.[30–32] This difference is primarily caused by the inherent limitations of spatial and temporal resolution of CT and CMR. A possible pitfall in determining pericardial thickness by CT is that trace pericardial effusions, as well as partial volume effects, may produce the appearance of focal thickening.[33] These imaging effects, along with normal intrinsic inhomogeneity in pericardial thickness, produce significant variations in pericardial thickness, and should not be mistaken for disease. The superior aortic recess of the transverse pericardial sinus, which surrounds the ascending aorta, may be mistaken for an aortic dissection or lymphadenopathy.[21,24] The oblique pericardial sinus, which is located behind the LA, may simulate abnormalities in the esophagus, descending thoracic aorta, and subcarinal and bronchopulmonary lymph nodes.[23,25] Recognizing the appearance of these normal structures is important to avoid mistaking them for mediastinal disease.[21,25]

CMR, with its superior tissue contrast, is an excellent modality to evaluate the heart and pericardium. It is able to differentiate between small amounts of pericardial fluid and actual thickening. With CMR, the normal pericardium appears as a linear low-intensity signal between the high-intensity mediastinal and sub-epicardial fat. It is best visualized during systole (Fig. 46.1).[32] bSSFP cine imaging is used to evaluate cardiac motion and can be helpful in detecting pericardial effusions. Black-blood T1-weighted spin echo sequences, such as double inversion recovery fast spin echo, are commonly performed to evaluate the pericardial anatomy thickness and morphology. T2-weighted spin echo sequences, usually with a short tau inversion recovery sequence to null the signal from fat (referred to as a triple inversion spin echo sequence), is used to depict difference between pericardial thickening and small amounts of fluid. Normal pericardium will demonstrate low signal on both T1-weighted and T2-weighted sequences, whereas pericardial fluid will be high signal on the T2-weighted imaging.[8,34] Pericardial

later (1 week to 2 months, known as postpericardiotomy syndrome). Infectious or postinfectious pericardial effusions often resolve spontaneously but may continue as chronic relapsing pericarditis or progress to constrictive pericarditis. Myopericarditis occurs when an infectious or inflammatory process involves both the pericardium and the myocardium simultaneously. Malignant effusions are more commonly caused by metastatic disease or local invasion rather than primary neoplastic disease of the pericardium.[50]

more proteinaceous fluid, as in malignancy, hemopericardium, purulent exudates, or myxedema.[10] On CMR, transudative effusions will demonstrate water characteristics and will demonstrate high signal intensity on T2-weighted imaging and low signal on T1-weighted imaging.[3,6,10] Transudative pericardial effusions are often even brighter than epicardial fat on gradient echo images.[18] More proteinaceous effusions will tend to show intermediate signal intensity on both T1-weighted and T2-weighted images and lower signal intensity than blood in the ventricular cavities

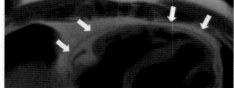
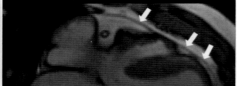

pericardial calcifications may be visualized as regions of low signal intensity by CMR.

A key finding in the diagnosis of pericardial constriction is the presence of early diastolic septal flattening giving the appearance of a "septal shutter," which occurs as a result of the differential timing of the opening and closing of the mitral and tricuspid valve with restricted right and left heart filling pressures. The diseased, noncompliant pericardium limits cardiac filling, causing rapid, high-velocity early diastolic filling with minimal mid-to-late diastolic filling, because of the imposed external volume limitation. Additionally, the cardiac volume constraint causes the function of one ventricle to be linked to the other, resulting in ventricular interdependence, resulting in a "shuttering" of the interventricular septum with opening and closing of the mitral and tricuspid valves. Additionally, rapid diastolic filling and ventricular interdependence leads to septal flattening or abnormal leftward bowing of the interventricular septum, rather than its normal rightward convexity. This is most pronounced during inspiration because the decline in intrathoracic pressure results in a decrease in pulmonary venous pressure and, therefore, less LA filling (the rigid pericardium limits transmission of intrathoracic pressures to the heart). Right atrial filling is not as impacted by changes in intrathoracic pressure, resulting in increased right-sided filling relative to the left. When encased in a rigid pericardium, the septum shifts leftward and flattens during inspiration because of the increase in RV filling, and rightward during expiration, resulting in pronounced septal shift (Fig. 46.5). Originally noted on TTE, both the septal shutter and septal shift with respiratory variation can be visualized on real-time midventricular short axis or four-chamber cine CMR and may be helpful in distinguishing constriction from restrictive cardiomyopathy.[34,71]

Constriction is often localized to the right side of the heart and may be localized to just the region of the right atrioventricular groove.[38,72] The use of contrast-enhanced CMR may suggest pericardial inflammation in effusive–constrictive pericarditis.[48] CMR tagging methods, such as spatial modulation of magnetization (SPAMM), may also be useful in diagnosing constriction. Tagging stripes laid down in end diastole are successively imaged during ventricular systole, where normal slippage between myocardium and pericardium results in the appearance of discontinuities or breaks in the stripes at the myocardium–pericardium interface among normal patients. In patients with constrictive pericarditis with adhesion of the parietal pericardium, this slippage is lost in the affected regions. Lines now appear "tethered" and the tag lines passing through the myocardium–pericardium interface maintain continuity during systolic deformation.[3,73]

Ventricular filling patterns can be assessed by CMR using flow velocity encoding (phase contrast) sequences. In constrictive pericarditis, an increased mitral level E-wave (early filling) may be observed as a consequence of increased diastolic pressure, whereas the A-wave (atrial filling) may be of reduced height owing to reduced late diastolic filling.[16]

PERICARDIAL TUMORS

Primary Pericardial Tumors

Primary pericardial tumors are uncommon, with most pericardial tumors a result of invasion (e.g., lung cancer), hematogenous seeding (e.g., melanoma), or lymphatic spread (e.g., breast cancer) of other primary pathologies. Primary pericardial tumors are more commonly malignant and include mesothelioma, angiosarcoma, lymphoma, or liposarcoma. Benign pericardial tumors include lipomas, teratomas, fibromas, neuromas, and hemangiomas, and are extremely rare.[9,19] Thymomas involving the pericardium may be either malignant or benign.

Imaging Findings of Primary Pericardial Tumors

An underlying pericardial neoplasm should be suspected if hemorrhagic pericardial effusions are found with diffuse or nodular pericardial thickening. When evaluating any suspected pericardial mass, CT and CMR imaging are often necessary to accurately assess the lesion characteristics and its relationship with the adjacent structures. Benign pericardial tumors found in children are often associated with large pericardial effusions.[19] Primary mesothelioma of the pericardium, the most common primary pericardial malignancy, usually presents with a hemorrhagic pericardial effusion or pericardial plaques and may lead to pericardial constriction.[19,74,75] Lymphoma, angiosarcoma, and liposarcoma typically appear as large irregular masses, often associated with pericardial effusions.[9]

Lipomas can be readily recognized by their typical signal characteristics with CMR or CT.[3] On CT, lipomas generally have low attenuation. On CMR, T1-weighted spin-echo images, lipomas have characteristic high-signal intensity that is not generally altered by contrast administration and may demonstrate an "India ink artifact," which is an out-of-phase, T1-weighted imaging related to peripheral signal drop out in voxels containing both fat and nonfat components.[9] Confirmation of the presence of fat signal is achieved by demonstrating signal loss on

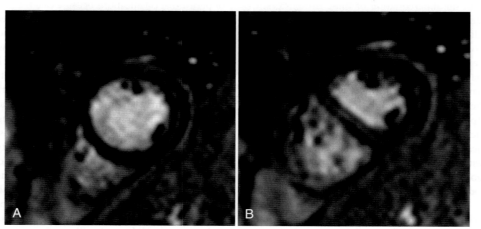

FIG. 46.5 Real-time free-breathing cardiovascular magnetic resonance sequence in a short axis view in a patient with acute pericarditis and constrictive physiology. (A) Normal filling during expiration with (B) septal flattening and phasic change in left and right ventricles during inspiration.

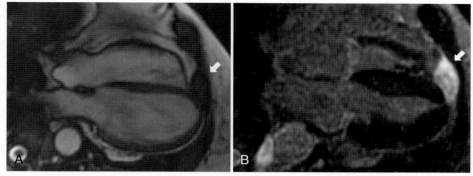

FIG. 46.6 Metastatic invasion of mediastinal liposarcoma with local invasion of the pericardium. (A) Steady-state free precession imaging of pericardial mass *(arrow)*. (B) Pericardial mass demonstrating late gadolinium enhancement, suggestive of underlying malignancy *(arrow)*.

fat-suppressed imaging.[39] Depiction of regions of calcium or fat in a pericardial mass on CT or CMR suggests a teratoma.[9] Fibromas more commonly arise from the pleura, but may arise from the pericardium as well. They are usually homogenous in appearance and appear isointense to hypointense, as compared with myocardium on T1-weighted images, and hypointense on T2-weighted images. Fibromas may or may not demonstrate contrast enhancement.[39,76,77] Hemangiomas are generally bright on T1-weighted and T2-weighted images because of their content of slow moving blood and demonstrate intense heterogeneous enhancement following contrast administration.[39]

Secondary Malignant Pericardial Tumors

Secondary malignant pericardial involvement is much more common than primary pericardial tumors and reported in approximately 10% to 12% of all patients dying with malignancy.[78,79] Among 110 patients with cardiac metastases, autopsy studies revealed the pericardium was involved in more than 70% of cases, yet a pericardial effusion was found in only one-third of those with pericardial involvement.[79] Malignant pericardial involvement is often clinically silent and may be found incidentally. However, it can also present with symptoms of pericarditis, tamponade, or constriction. Patients with large pericardial effusions who present with tamponade without clinical signs of pericarditis (e.g., chest pain, rub, fever, and ECG changes), may be more likely to have a malignant effusion than other patients with large pericardial effusions.[80] Pericardial effusions caused by either malignancy or treatment of malignancy are more likely than other effusions to require repeat pericardiocentesis or surgical management.[81] Malignant involvement of the pericardium may result from local invasion (lung, breast, esophagus, stomach, lymphoma, thymoma, and pleural mesothelioma) or metastatic spread (breast, lung, melanoma, renal, and others) (Fig. 46.6).[3,19,77,79] Malignancies most likely to metastasize to the pericardium are typically lung, breast, and esophageal cancer, melanoma, leukemia, and lymphoma.[50,78,79,81,82] Patients with symptomatic malignant pericardial effusion generally have a poor prognosis, although those with breast cancer, leukemia, or lymphoma may have a better prognosis than others.[82,83]

Imaging Findings of Metastatic Pericardial Tumors

Metastatic involvement of the pericardium may be suggested by the existence of a pericardial effusion with nodular pericardial thickening or pericardial mass, which can be visualized by TTE, CT, or CMR.[18]

However, pericardial effusions and pericardial thickening may also occur in patients with malignancy because radiation, drugs, and infections may also cause pericardial disease in this population.[77,81]

Hemorrhagic pericardial effusions are strongly suggestive of underlying malignancy/metastatic pericardial disease.[8,79] The other major cause of a hemorrhagic pericardial effusion is aortic dissection propagating proximally to involve the pericardium, although these patients often die before reaching the hospital. Acute hemorrhagic effusions may be identified by their high signal intensity on T1-weighted and T2-weighted spin echo images. Extension of local tumor to the pericardium may be confirmed by focal loss of the pericardial line with or without associated effusion (Fig. 46.6).[8,34] On the other hand, an intact pericardial line may be observed if an adjacent tumor extends up to the pericardium but not through it.[9] Cine gradient echo CMR may help determine if the tumor is adherent to the pericardium.[77]

Most malignant tumors enhance after contrast administration.[9,76] On noncontrast imaging, most neoplasms have low signal intensity on T1-weighted images and high signal intensity on T2-weighted images. However, metastatic melanoma may have high signal intensity on T1-weighted and T2-weighted images because of the paramagnetic metals bound by melanin.[84] Lymphomas appear isointense to hypointense to myocardium on T1-weighted and T2-weighted images.[39] They may show lesser contrast enhancement in central regions that may be necrotic.[9,85]

CONCLUSION

The pericardium is a complex and important structure in the evaluation of the cardiovascular system. Pericardial pathology can result in a spectrum of clinical presentations, ranging from little or no symptoms to severe hemodynamic compromise and collapse. Advanced noninvasive imaging modalities such as CMR have broadened our understanding of pericardial diseases and their impact on the cardiovascular system. When combined with a high degree of clinical suspicion, CMR can serve as an important tool to diagnose and guide clinical management and therapeutic strategies.

REFERENCES

A full reference list is available online at ExpertConsult.com

47

Interventional Cardiovascular Magnetic Resonance

Toby Rogers and Robert Lederman

An ideal imaging guidance system for cardiovascular, catheter-based interventional procedures would offer real-time, high-resolution, three-dimensional (3D) imaging of important anatomic tissues and chambers, irrespective of respiratory, cardiac, or patient motion alongside excellent visualization of catheters, guidewires, and other interventional devices. Such tools would quickly enable novel, minimally invasive alternatives to open surgical procedures.

X-ray fluoroscopy guides most contemporary catheter-based procedures. However, fluoroscopy has important limitations (Table 47.1). Iodinated radiocontrast, which provides the ability to outline chamber and vascular lumens, is injected only periodically. Tissue detail is minimal. Additionally, fluoroscopy provides only two-dimensional (2D) "projection" imaging, with limited depth perception. Iodinated radiocontrast is nephrotoxic in susceptible individuals. Ionizing radiation increases lifetime cancer risk, particularly in children.[1,2] Finally, operators and personnel risk disabling orthopedic injuries from the weight of protective lead apparel.[3]

Ultrasound is often used in combination with x-ray fluoroscopy procedures. For example, transesophageal echocardiography (TEE) provides adjunctive imaging during atrial septal defect closure or transcatheter aortic valve replacement, by assisting with device sizing, positioning, and postdeployment assessment. However, transthoracic echocardiography (TTE) offers limited acoustic windows, and suffers "shadowing" artifacts caused by devices.

Cardiovascular magnetic resonance (CMR) more closely approaches the idealized imaging guidance system described earlier. CMR offers superior tissue imaging, in any arbitrary orientation, without ionizing radiation or nephrotoxic contrast. Rapid imaging techniques and modified CMR visible devices now permit real-time CMR guided catheter applications. The ability to visualize both tissue and interventional devices may enable catheter-based procedures in the future that currently require open surgical exposure. In the meantime, CMR right heart catheterization provides superior hemodynamic characterization combining high fidelity flow, pressure, and function measurements.

INTERVENTIONAL CARDIOVASCULAR MAGNETIC RESONANCE LABORATORY CONFIGURATION

Early real-time magnetic resonance imaging (MRI) systems employed low field strength magnets (0.2–0.5 T), open or closed bore configurations,

and sometimes embedded x-ray fluoroscopy systems.[4,5] Major limitations included relatively low signal-to-noise ratio (SNR), inhomogeneous magnetic field interfering with rapid imaging, and limited patient access when employing long, closed bores. Newer, short-bore, 1.5 T systems with high performance gradients provide excellent field homogeneity and higher SNR. Newer scanners also include large arrayed radiofrequency (RF) receivers (≥32), intended for parallel imaging techniques to improve imaging speed. These additional receiver channels can also be used to attach "active" catheter devices to improve their visibility. By contrast, higher field 3 T systems disproportionately increase heating but do not notably enhance image quality using workhorse (balanced steady state free precession [bSSFP]) pulse sequences, and are therefore difficult to justify for interventional CMR (iCMR) applications.

In addition, commercial vendors now provide interactive scan user interfaces that increasingly resemble echocardiography. These interfaces drive sophisticated image reconstruction hardware and software that permit images to be acquired with ease and displayed to operators with minimal delay in multiple scan planes.

Combined x-ray and CMR catheterization laboratories, so-called XMR labs, now enable rapid and convenient CMR catheterization procedures, especially in pediatrics and heart failure (Fig. 47.1). In these laboratories, conventional x-ray fluoroscopy guidance is immediately available to perform interventions using CMR fusion imaging or for situations requiring emergency bailout. XMR laboratories are now commercially available. For example, the National Heart Lung and Blood Institute (NHLBI) laboratory at Children's National Medical Center in Washington, DC, combines a biplane x-ray fluoroscopy system with a 1.5 T cardiac scanner (Fig. 47.1). These systems are separated by RF-shielded doors and can be used independently or together for combined procedures.[6] An automated transport table moves patients seamlessly between the two modalities. Alternative designs include single-room layouts, in which both x-ray and CMR systems are located inside the RF shield.[7] Wave guides and penetration panels are strategically positioned in the room so that communication and patient monitoring hardware can be installed without disrupting the RF shield.

Communication, Monitoring and Image Display

Rapid CMR requires rapid gradient switching that causes substantial acoustic noise. This noise prevents verbal communications between operators, the patient, and staff. Wireless noise-cancelling headsets are

TABLE 47.1 Advantages and Disadvantages of Different Imaging Modalities to Guide Interventional Procedures

Imaging Modality	Advantages	Disadvantages
iCMR	• Excellent soft tissue imaging • Simultaneous display of multiple arbitrary imaging perspectives • Real-time device tracking in 3D • Image-based physiology assessment • No ionizing radiation • No lead aprons • No nephrotoxic contrast • Uninterrupted imaging to detect complications more efficiently	• Clinical devices currently unavailable and require hardware attachments • Acoustic noise • Claustrophobia • Rapid emergency response more difficult • ECG monitoring for cardiac procedures more difficult • Peripheral nerve stimulation from rapidly switching gradients • Imaging systems require large capital outlay
X-ray fluoroscopy	• Excellent temporal resolution • Widely available in most centers • Clinical devices available • ECG monitoring simple • Floating table permits remote imaging (i.e., groin site) • Greater physician/nurse access to patient	• Poor soft tissue imaging • 2D "projection" imaging offers limited depth perception • Cancer risk from ionizing radiation • Nephrotoxic contrast required • Chronic orthopedic injuries from lead apron apparel • Angiography interrupted during device deployment resulting in complication detection after contrast injection
Ultrasound	• Good soft tissue imaging • Excellent temporal resolution • Widely available • Imaging based physiology assessment (i.e., Doppler) • New x-ray + ultrasound fusion capability (CartoMerge, HeartNavigator, etc.)	• Limited acoustic windows • Device related "shadow" artifacts • No tip tracking capability • Transesophageal and intracardiac echo are invasive • Limited orientation-dependent imaging

2D, Two-dimensional; *3D*, three-dimensional; *ECG*, electrocardiogram; *iCMR*, interventional cardiovascular magnetic resonance.

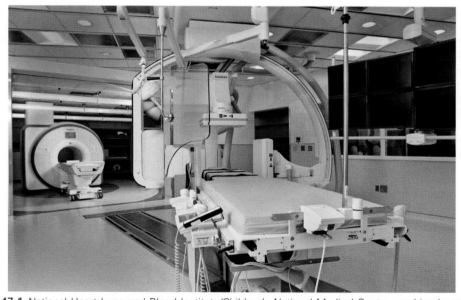

FIG. 47.1 National Heart Lung and Blood Institute/Children's National Medical Center combined x-ray and interventional cardiovascular magnetic resonance (iCMR) suite, Washington, DC. The iCMR suite combines a biplane x-ray system *(foreground)* and a 1.5 T CMR scanner *(background)*. The x-ray table docks with the CMR table to enable the patient to be easily transferred between the two modalities.

used at NHLBI (Fig. 47.2). This versatile system allows staff and patients to speak simultaneously on open microphones and allows separate and parallel conversations with patients and among staff.

Gradients, RF interference, and magnetohydrodynamic effects severely distort the electrocardiogram (ECG). Electronic filters enable heart rate monitoring; however, ECG waveform morphology is not readily interpretable for ST-segment monitoring of myocardial ischemia or injury.[8,9] Multichannel invasive pressure waveform monitoring, temperature monitoring, and oxygen saturation monitoring can use commercial systems, without modification from x-ray catheterization

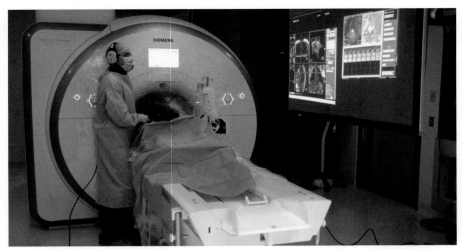

FIG. 47.2 Working inside the interventional cardiovascular magnetic resonance (iCMR) catheterization laboratory. The operator communicates with the patient and with staff inside and outside the iCMR room with sound-suppression microphones and headsets. Real-time CMR, scanner control interface and patient hemodynamics are displayed inside the room using video projectors.

laboratories. Several manufacturers are developing dedicated hardware that will interface with existing catheterization laboratory high-fidelity hemodynamic recording systems. In the meantime, open source kits for local assembly of suitable hemodynamics interfaces are available (http://nhlbi-mr.github.io/PRiME).

Interventional catheterization suites require continuous operator monitoring of multiple information streams, including hemodynamics, imaging control, and interventional images. This is similarly true during iCMR procedures, especially using active devices.[6,10] MRI-conditional liquid crystal display (LCD) video displays are available from most scanner manufacturers. We prefer two banks of less expensive LCD video projectors that project onto a fabric screen, which depict hemodynamics, scanner interface, and 3D-rendered images separately, one at each end of the CMR system (Fig. 47.2). The projectors are housed in RF-shielded boxes and video signals are passed into the room via fiber optic cables through the waveguide.

Interventional Cardiovascular Magnetic Resonance Real-Time Scanner Interface

The iCMR scanner user interface requires several key features not typical for diagnostic CMR. Commercial or investigational graphic user interface based scanning host computer systems are available from most systems vendors (Interactive Front End, Siemens[11]; MR Echo, General Electric; eXTernal Control, Philips Healthcare) and as standalone commercial (RT Hawk, Heart Vista) or open-source solutions (Vurtigo, Sunnybrook Health Sciences Center, http://www.vurtigo.ca).

One of the most useful features is the colorized display of individual receiver channels that are attached to "active" catheter receiver coil devices. This makes catheter devices readily apparent and has proven useful in vivo. Another is interactive "projection-mode" imaging wherein slice select is disabled and catheter devices are displayed as the operator is used to seeing them under conventional x-ray fluoroscopy. For tracking balloon catheters filled with dilute gadolinium (Gd) contrast during CMR catheterization, we find it helpful to interactively adjust slice thickness and saturation magnetization preparation, to help find the catheter tip should it move outside of the selected plane, and to interactively adjust temporal resolution for catheterization steps requiring fine motor control. Operationally, we find it useful to display multiple slices during interventional procedures, both separately and combined

in a 3D-rendered image (Fig. 47.3).[12] Other laboratories are experimenting with voice-control, automatic adjustment of slice location to correspond to catheter position, and automatic adaptation of imaging parameters to speed of catheter manipulation.

Safety Considerations

Patient care staff must undergo formal comprehensive training in CMR safety. For example, the hospital emergency medical response team is unlikely to be familiar with CMR operations and may unwittingly jeopardize themselves, their colleagues, or the patient by rushing into the room with a steel oxygen tank. Rapid patient evacuation from the CMR catheterization laboratory needs to be practiced repeatedly in mock drills. Ferromagnetic objects that cannot be removed from the room must be attached to the wall during CMR guided procedures. It is good practice for all devices on wheels in the x-ray section of the iCMR suite (e.g., anesthetic machine, intraaortic balloon pump, or defibrillator) to be tethered to the wall or floor. Oxygen, inhalational anesthetic, and vacuum for suction can be fed through RF-protective wall ports, eliminating in-room cylinders. At NHLBI, we drill emergency evacuation from the CMR room on a quarterly basis.[13] Swift evacuation relies on clear delineation of roles for all staff. In an emergency, we can start chest compressions within 10 seconds and move the patient back into the x-ray room for defibrillation in under 1 minute. In the near future, CMR-conditional external defibrillators should be commercially available so that arrhythmias can be managed without evacuating the patient from the scanner.

RF energy from CMR transmit coils will concentrate on long conductive devices causing local heating, potentially leading to burns.[14] Box 47.1 lists factors associated with heating, especially long conductive devices and cables. This complex problem is described later under "active" catheter devices. Interventionists must also take care that connections to intravascular coils as well as surface coils do not inadvertently form loops, which can cause patient burns.

REAL-TIME IMAGING

Rapid CMR is required for invasive procedures, for catheter visualization, and for imaging of anatomic structures.[15] Efficient image data sampling methods,[16–25] parallel imaging,[26–28] and coherent steady state

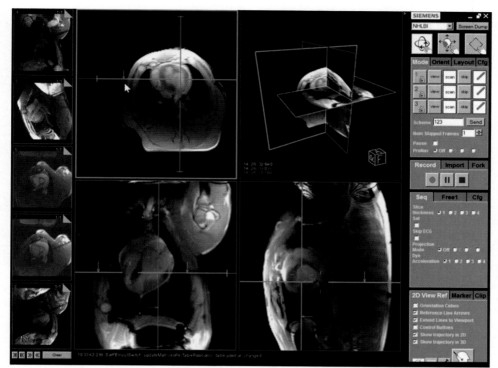

FIG. 47.3 Screenshot of a commercial interventional cardiovascular magnetic resonance (iCMR) user interface. The iCMR interface is designed to accommodate interleaved multislice real-time CMR image acquisition *(three panels on left),* a volume rendering of the slices indicating their three-dimensional relationship *(center panel),* "postage stamps" to store and recall important graphical slice prescriptions *(bottom row),* and interactive scanner parameter control *(right panels).*

BOX 47.1 Factors Influencing Heating-Related Injury by Cardiovascular Magnetic Resonance Interventional Devices

Interventional Device Factors
- Length of conductive elements
- Geometric shape
- Orientation in the magnet
- Distance from the radiofrequency transmitter
- Physical proximity to tissues
- Insulation

Patient Factors
- Body mass and surface area
- Convective cooling of intravascular devices by local blood flow
- General body temperature
- Implanted conductive devices
- Tissue thermosensitivity

Magnetic Resonance Imaging Scanner Factors
- Field strength
- Pulse sequence
- Flip angle
- Scanning duty cycle
- Position relative to bore isocenter[140] (closer is better)

---

techniques[29–33] have enabled real-time CMR without significant degradation in image quality in the field of interest. Frame rates as high as 10 to 15 images per second are now possible using multichannel ($\geq$32) coils that use parallel imaging techniques to achieve acceleration factors of three or more. In addition, interactive, real-time color flow imaging may supplement anatomic detail with critical physiologic detail, such as leaks or gradients, during therapeutic procedures and interventions.[34] Slice orientation can automatically follow the tip of catheter devices as they move, so-called adaptive imaging, so that catheter features are kept in view during manipulation. These methods also can be applied automatically to alter scanning parameters such as field-of-view and temporal resolution.[35]

INTERVENTIONAL CARDIOVASCULAR MAGNETIC RESONANCE CATHETER DEVICES

Interventional devices must be conspicuous and clearly distinguishable from tissue to conduct therapeutic procedures. Conventional x-ray devices are generally unsuitable, because most incorporate steel braids to increase x-ray attenuation for visibility and to enhance catheter performance characteristics such as steerability, pushability, and trackability. The steel causes severe blooming or susceptibility artifacts that destroy much of the CMR image (Fig. 47.4). Removing these ferrous components usually renders the catheter devices virtually invisible under CMR, and usually renders them floppy and mechanically unsuitable as catheters.

iCMR catheter devices are generally classified as passive or active. Passive devices have elements that cause discrete susceptibility imaging artifacts that darken images, or T1 shortening elements that brighten images. Alternatively, active devices have built-in micro-coils and

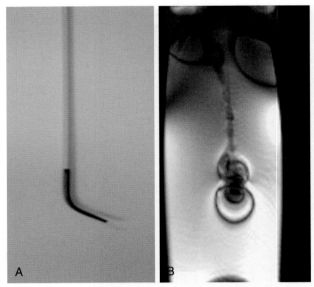

FIG. 47.4 Cardiovascular magnetic resonance (CMR) artifact caused by steel braiding in standard x-ray catheters. (A) Photograph of stainless steel braided Kumpe catheter. (B) In a water phantom, steel braiding causes severe 'blooming' signal void artifact rendering it useless for CMR guided interventional procedures.

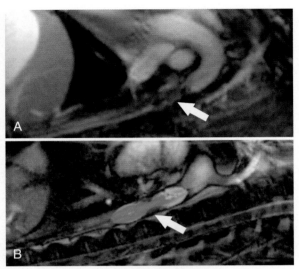

FIG. 47.5 Passive and active device imaging during aortic coarctation repair. (A) A dilute gadolinium partially filled balloon, delivered over a nitinol guidewire, is positioned across the coarctation (arrow). The wire and balloon catheter shaft are poorly visualized against the anatomic background. (B) The same balloon, delivered over an active guidewire from which the signal is colored in green, is clearly more conspicuous compared with solely passive catheter devices.

electrical circuitry that allow the device to act as a RF receiver and/or transmitter.

Passive Devices

Stents[36] and guidewires[37–40] made from copper, dysprosium, cobalt–chromium alloy, nitinol, titanium, and platinum suffer less severe susceptibility artifacts compared with iron-alloys. They can be coated to improve biocompatibility. Carbon dioxide creates a dark CMR signal by excluding proton spins; carbon dioxide gas has been injected in humans for selective CMR angiography and has been used to fill balloon catheters for diagnostic CMR-guided catheter tracking in patients.[41–43] Unfortunately, volume averaging makes it difficult to distinguish passive devices from neighboring anatomic features. Guidewires[44–46] have been made out of nonmetallic polymers, and clinical cardiovascular interventions have been conducted using polymer guidewires.[47] Polymer guidewires lack the trackability, torquability, and tactile responsiveness of metallic guidewires; a new segmented nitinol design overcomes these limitations.[48]

Devices that appear bright are less vulnerable to volume averaging effects and are more easily visualized against anatomic background. Dilute Gd chelates such as gadopentate dimeglumine (Gd-DTPA) have been used to fill[49] and coat catheters[50,51] and balloons,[52] offering bright device imaging. Ultimately, we have found this passive approach to be inferior in vivo compared with active catheter device visualization (Fig. 47.5). Investigational, off-resonance, chemical-selective visualization using F-19[53] or C-13[54] and other hyperpolarized agents have been proposed for catheter tracking. Off-resonance effects have been exploited to track metallic catheter and guidewire components.[55,56] Clinical diagnostic catheterization for hemodynamic studies can be conducted using dilute Gd-filled balloon catheters,[6] iron-contrast filled,[57] or CO_2-filled[58] catheters as an alternative.

Active Devices

Highly sensitive, ultrasmall receiver coils can be incorporated into devices to locate (catheter-tracking[59]) or to visualize them,[60–62] or both.

A minimum of two coils at the tip of a catheter is required to enable the computer to calculate the position of the catheter in 3D space and depict it on an image. This approach is particularly attractive to procedures that require high spatial location accuracy, for example electrophysiology mapping and ablation. Tracking also permits the user interface to store coordinates of key locations, for example ablation points.

Alternatively, devices incorporate conductive wires (or loop antenna) along the length of the device. Signals from these devices are displayed on top of previously acquired anatomic roadmaps (device localization only) or combined into the array of receivers used to update real-time CMR images. The device position or signal receiver can be color coded, to distinguish them from grey-scale background images of the anatomy. Devices displayed in this way are readily visible inside thick-slab projections resembling projection x-ray images showing devices in profile. Distinct signals can be imparted to the tip of devices so that it can be tracked in 3D, ideal for intracardiac applications. Alternatively, direct current applied to conductive elements along the device induce magnetic field inhomogeneities, disrupt local signal, and create dark impressions.[63]

Unfortunately, the long conductive transmission wires used to connect catheter coils to the CMR transmitter or receiver system are susceptible to RF heating, which may damage neighboring tissue. Multiple approaches to reduce heating can be combined to make catheter devices safe, such as attaching circuitry to decouple and detune the transmission lines, intermittent chokes and transformers in the transmission lines, and insulation.

Another hybrid approach is to incorporate closed-loop receiver coils into stents or catheter devices, without connecting via transmission lines to the CMR system. These "inductively-coupled" devices resonate at predetermined geometric shapes and thereby amplify local RF signal.[64,65] Unfortunately, inductively coupled catheter devices cannot easily be displayed in color during real-time CMR, as can other actively visualized catheter devices, and are best visualized at lower flip angles that compromise imaging.

The NHLBI active guidewire for cardiovascular applications incorporates a loop antenna for active visualization of the whole shaft and a separate active marker to distinguish the guidewire tip.[66] The device also incorporates a fiberoptic temperature probe for continuous monitoring of RF-induced heating. The device appears in color overlay on real-time CMR images (Fig. 47.6).

Finally, CMR pulse sequence techniques can reduce the energy deposited per image, and therefore heating, with an acceptable penalty in image quality.[15] Such techniques include radial sampling, spiral sampling, and echo planar imaging (EPI), which use fewer excitation pulses and longer repetition times, variable flip angle sequences[67] and parallel imaging. Techniques that reduce specific absorption rate at high fields, such as adaptive parallel transmission, may also prove helpful at lower fields to reduce device heating during CMR guided interventions.[68]

Device Solutions for Cardiovascular Applications

In our experience, it has been useful to use a combination of both active and passive devices during complex interventional procedures, albeit in animal models. Real-time, active visualization of the device tip in 3D is desirable during certain procedures such as atrial transseptal puncture or myocardial wall injection. Similarly, active approaches prove useful while surveying devices for common failure modes such as buckling, looping, or kinking. Passive approaches unencumbered by electrical hardware attachments are sufficient for simple procedures such as placing introducer sheaths that typically do not move once positioned. More importantly, combining passive devices (such as balloons filled with dilute Gd-DTPA) with active devices (such as an active guidewire) generates wonderful and useful images (Fig. 47.5).

Catheters for iCMR are usually manipulated manually by the operator in a similar fashion to a standard x-ray catheterization laboratory. However, by applying current to wire coils wound at the tip of a catheter, it is possible to remotely steer a catheter under real-time iCMR guidance.[69,70] Using this approach, Hetts et al. developed an endovascular catheter system and demonstrated comparable procedure times for navigation through a vascular phantom with MRI and conventional x-ray guidance.[71] The same group used these catheters to perform renal artery catheterization and embolization in swine.[72] However, it is questionable

whether remote-controlled catheters really decrease procedure time in experienced hands.[73]

APPLICATIONS

Extra-Anatomic Bypass

Advances in transcatheter therapy for many congenital cardiovascular conditions have reduced the need for invasive open surgery. As noted earlier, children may be particularly sensitive to the harmful effects of x-ray radiation. Children with complex congenital cardiovascular disease often undergo multiple x-ray procedures and have greater cumulative radiation exposure and greater lifetime risk of radiation-induced malignancy. Radiation-sparing procedural guidance with CMR is attractive and forms the basis for a number of real-time CMR guided research applications.

Full visualization of all anatomic structures and soft tissue may facilitate complex procedures that involve crossing anatomic boundaries and connecting remote vascular structures. Using a double-doughnut CMR configuration, Kee et al. conducted preclinical[74] and clinical[75] transjugular intrahepatic porto-systemic shunt (TIPS) procedures. Even in this proof-of-concept experiment, MRI reduced the number of transhepatic needle punctures compared with historical controls. Arepally et al. created an elegant catheter-based mesocaval shunt outside the liver capsule.[76]

Ratnayaka et al. developed the preclinical capability to use catheters instead of surgery for one of the three staged surgical repairs to palliate children with single ventricle physiology. They demonstrated real-time iCMR guided cavopulmonary shunt using active needles, Gd-filled balloon-mounted covered stents, and custom-built endografts (Fig. 47.7).[77] Although theoretically feasible using x-ray fluoroscopy and contrast angiography, CMR enables visualization of origin and destination vascular structures in orthogonal planes as well as all interposed tissues. Furthermore, CMR enables immediate identification of important complications, for example, pericardial effusion or vascular dissection. The ultimate goal is to develop percutaneous approaches to replace some of the open-chest surgeries that children with complex congenital heart disease will require over their lifetime.

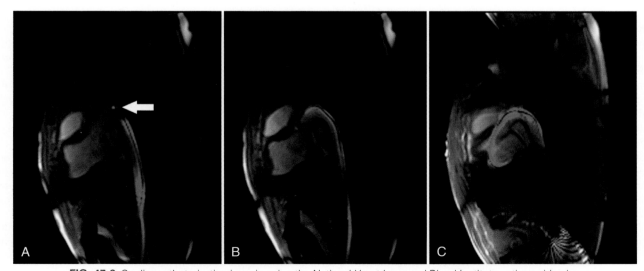

FIG. 47.6 Cardiac catheterization in a pig using the National Heart Lung and Blood Institute active guidewire. The full length of the guidewire is conspicuous and the tip has a separate and distinct signal *(arrow)*. During left heart catheterization, the guidewire is navigated to (A) the aortic arch, (B) the aortic valve, and (C) through the aortic valve into the left ventricle under real-time cardiovascular magnetic resonance guidance.

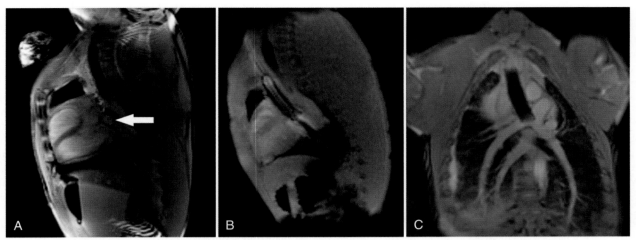

FIG. 47.7 Real-time cardiovascular magnetic resonance (CMR) guided percutaneous cavopulmonary shunt. Central venous access is obtained via the right internal jugular vein. (A) An active needle is used to puncture from the superior vena cava in to the right pulmonary artery under real-time CMR guidance *(arrow)*. (B) A covered endograft is then deployed from the superior vena cava into the right pulmonary artery. (C) The endograft now connects the superior vena cava and the right pulmonary artery.

Endomyocardial Biopsy

Endomyocardial biopsy remains the preferred diagnostic test in patients with unexplained cardiomyopathy and in heart transplant recipients with suspected rejection. Yet x-ray guided biopsy is essentially a blind procedure because neither important structures, such as valves or chordae, nor the target endocardium can be visualized. In pathologies affecting the heart in a nonuniform distribution, biopsy can often provide inconclusive results because a negative specimen may simply reflect that a nonaffected part of the heart was sampled. In contrast, CMR offers a number of tools for advanced tissue characterization that may help distinguish normal from abnormal myocardium, for example, late Gd enhancement (LGE) and T1 mapping. Real-time iCMR guided endomyocardial biopsy could potentially enhance diagnostic yield and safety by targeting abnormal myocardium and avoiding vulnerable structures. Both passive-visualization and active-visualization bioptomes have been developed for in vitro and preclinical testing.[78,79] We developed an animal model of focal myocardial pathology and demonstrated significantly higher diagnostic yield with iCMR versus x-ray guided biopsy (Fig. 47.8).[79]

Aortic Aneurysm, Dissection and Coarctation Stenting

Percutaneous endograft repair for thoracoabdominal aneurysms and aortic dissection are performed for patients with suitable anatomy, considered high risk for surgery. Aorta size, proximal and distal landing zones for stents and grafts, and vicinity to crucial arterial branches are vital measurements required for these procedures. These procedures are typically performed using x-ray fluoroscopy, with adjunctive intravascular ultrasound. Bulky stent/graft devices may distort the native anatomy, preventing operator confidence in preacquired fluoroscopic roadmaps. Ultrasound scatters within stents/endograft, offering limited external visualization. Real-time iCMR guided abdominal aortic aneurysm[80] and aortic dissection[81] endograft repair have been performed successfully in swine models using active and passive nitinol stents (Fig. 47.9). Post-procedure assessment using phase contrast flow within and adjacent to the endograft demonstrated the versatility of iCMR-guided endograft therapy. Real-time iCMR guided aortic coarctation stent repair has also successfully been performed in a swine coarctation model using commercially available clinical-grade devices[38] (see Fig. 47.5).

Atrial Transseptal Procedures

Atrial transseptal puncture is usually conducted as the first step in numerous cardiac procedures, such as pulmonary vein ablation. A needle is advanced from a vein, through the right atrium into left atrium (LA) across the interatrial septum. Currently, this procedure is conducted using subtle x-ray fluoroscopic visual cues and tactile feedback from sharp catheter devices, with or without adjunctive TEE or intracardiac echocardiography. Poor tissue visualization and limited acquisition windows, combined with unusual atrial anatomy, can lead to life-threatening perforation and pericardial tamponade in as many as 1% to 6% of procedures, even in experienced hands. Using custom active needles, real-time iCMR guided atrial transseptal puncture has been successfully performed in swine (Fig. 47.10).[82,83] Related therapeutic procedures, such as closure of atrial septal defects and patent foramen ovale, have been reported in swine using passively visualized nitinol devices delivered with catheters.[84,85]

Transthoracic Cardiac Access and Closure

Using active needles and guidewires, and passive sheaths and catheters, we have successfully performed real-time iCMR guided percutaneous transthoracic access to the left ventricle (LV) and the LA.[86–88] After delivery of large-bore sheaths, the access port was closed using off-the-shelf nitinol occluder devices or collagen vascular plugs. The delivery system for the nitinol occluders was modified to incorporate a loop antenna for active visualization.[66] Via closed-chest transthoracic approach, Ratnayaka et al. performed muscular ventricular septal defect (VSD) closure using nitinol occluders and the same modified delivery system (Fig. 47.11).[89] Alternative applications could include delivery of partial or full mitral or tricuspid prosthetic valves, which are large devices currently under investigation, and which are usually delivered via surgical transthoracic access to the heart.

The ability to manage complications in the CMR scanner is important. Using off-the-shelf titanium needles, Halabi et al. performed real-time iCMR guided pericardiocentesis in a swine model of pericardial effusion.[90] CMR-conditional nitinol or Inconel needles are available commercially but, although they are safe to use in the iCMR environment, they are practically invisible. Needles with passive or active markers are sorely needed.

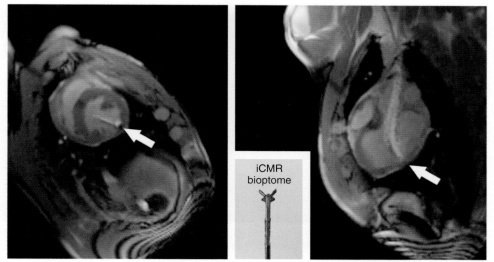

FIG. 47.8 Real-time interventional cardiovascular magnetic resonance *(iCMR)* guided endomyocardial biopsy. The active visualization CMR bioptome appears in color overlay on real-time CMR images. The arrows indicate the jaws of the bioptome. Orthogonal views ensure the bioptome is accurately directed to the desired endocardial surface. Inversion-recovery real-time CMR can be used to highlight areas of abnormal tissue after administration of systemic gadolinium contrast.

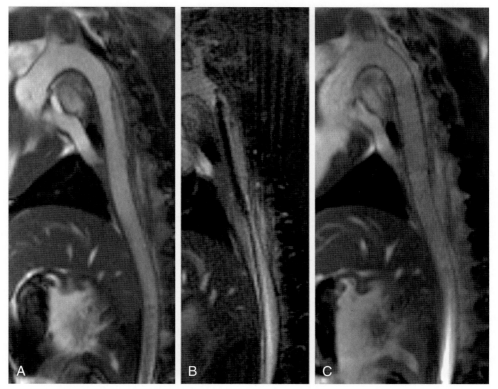

FIG. 47.9 Real-time interventional cardiovascular magnetic resonance (iCMR) guided aortic dissection repair in a swine model. (A) Baseline CMR showing dissection of the descending aorta. (B) Passively visualized stent positioned in the descending aorta at the level of the dissection. (C) Final CMR demonstrates successfully delivered stent and repair of the dissection. (Courtesy Holger Eggebrecht and Harold H. Quick, PhD, University Essen, Germany.)

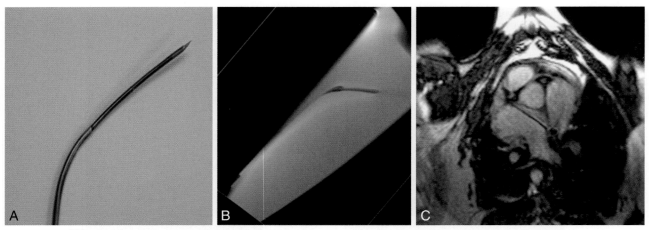

FIG. 47.10 Atrial transseptal puncture in a pig using an active needle. (A) Photograph of the active transseptal puncture needle. (B) Cardiovascular magnetic resonance of the needle in a water phantom and (C) in vivo across the interatrial septum.

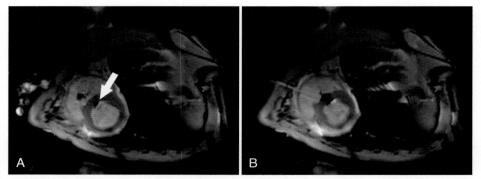

FIG. 47.11 Real-time interventional cardiovascular magnetic resonance (iCMR) guided direct transthoracic ventricular septal defect closure. The right ventricle is accessed directly through the chest wall using a CMR active needle under real-time iCMR guidance. The ventricular septal defect (VSD) is crossed antegradely and then closed using a nitinol muscular occluder device. The delivery cable for the occluder device is also active. (A) The left ventricular disk *(arrow)* is deployed and pulled back against the septum. (B) The right ventricular disk is deployed and pushed forward against the septum to close the VSD. The right ventricle free wall puncture is closed using an off-the-shelf vascular closure plug.

Invasive Coronary Artery Imaging

Percutaneous, real-time iCMR guided coronary selective angiography,[91] angioplasty,[92] and stent insertion[93] has been reported in healthy animals. Although these works are impressive, clinical translation of these coronary artery therapeutic procedures remains hindered by seemingly insurmountable obstacles. Currently x-ray fluoroscopy provides spatial resolution of 100 μm at a usual working temporal resolution of 66 ms, to manipulate guidewires that are 350 μm wide and stent devices that are 600 μm across. It seems unlikely—barring an unforeseen technical breakthrough—that real-time CMR can provide comparable spatial and temporal resolution currently required for safe guidewire and catheter manipulation through delicate diseased human coronary arteries. Similarly, very low profile, distinctly conspicuous CMR-compatible catheter devices would be required for clinical implementation, and such devices are not currently available.

Peripheral Vascular Disease

Several groups have shown the feasibility of iCMR guided balloon angioplasty in healthy animals,[94,95] animal models of arterial stenosis,[96–99] and humans with obstructive peripheral artery disease.[100] Dilute Gd-DTPA (bright signal), undiluted Gd-DTPA (dark signal), or carbon dioxide gas have been used to inflate balloons and provide balloon-tissue contrast ensuring full inflation. Active receiver coils, either embedded on the balloon catheter or inserted through the wire port of the balloon filled with dilute Gd-DTPA, provide added contrast to adjacent tissue by further enhancing the bright signal within the inflated balloon. Radio-opaque markers are typically added to balloon catheters to indicate the shoulder points of the balloon and assist with lesion length assessment before and during deployment. These markers act as small susceptibility markers to assist with positioning and balloon deployment under iCMR.

Both balloon-expandable and self-expanding stents are implanted to prevent arterial recoil, and to alleviate flow-limiting dissection. Both stent designs have been successfully deployed under iCMR guidance in animals[101–103] and humans.[104] Local susceptibility and shielding effects result in imaging voids within and adjacent to stents. Inductively coupled stents (described earlier) may ameliorate this problem.[64] Chronic total arterial occlusion recanalization is particularly challenging under x-ray fluoroscopy because only the patent inflow, occluded artery, and patent outflow distal artery beyond the obstruction can be visualized with conventional angiography. Guidewires and catheter traversal through the "invisible" occluded segment may cause perforation and hemorrhage. These procedures are often long, and require excessive nephrotoxic contrast. Successful real-time iCMR guided chronic total occlusion recanalization and subsequent balloon angioplasty was successfully performed in swine model of peripheral artery occlusion, using modified active chronic total occlusion wires and support catheters.[105]

X-Ray Fused With Magnetic Resonance Imaging

3D structures can be segmented from CMR datasets and coregistered with live x-ray fluoroscopy to provide anatomic context. XFM has been used successfully to enhance imaging guidance in a wide range of cardiovascular interventions, including pulmonary stenosis angioplasty, aortic coarctation stenting (Fig. 47.12), VSD closure, and for cardiac resynchronization therapy to optimally place the LV lead.[106] Because anatomy is clearer and frequent contrast angiography is not required, total fluoroscopy time and iodinated contrast volume can be substantially reduced with XFM.[107] To be useful, XFM requires accurate coregistration of both imaging modalities. A number of groups have developed techniques to improve coregistration and to incorporate respiratory and cardiac motion.[108,109]

Diagnostic Right Heart Catheterization

Using off-the-shelf nonbraided balloon catheters, it is feasible to perform diagnostic right-heart catheterization in patients.[41] Dilute Gd-filled balloons are conspicuous using real-time CMR (Fig. 47.13). Ratnayaka et al. performed both x-ray and iCMR-guided right-heart catheterization in 16 patients, demonstrating that CMR was useful to navigate through the right heart and selectively engage left and right pulmonary arteries.[6] iCMR-guided cardiac catheterization is now classified as a standard medical procedure at the National Institutes of Health for all patients requiring right-heart catheterization, unless there is a clear contraindication (e.g., a pacemaker or other MRI-unsafe metallic implant). As mentioned before, iCMR-guided catheterization is of particular value in pediatric patients for reducing exposure to ionizing radiation. At Children's National Medical Center, most routine right heart catheterizations for cardiac transplant patients are now performed under CMR guidance. Combining a full CMR study with invasive hemodynamics provides accurate measurement of key parameters, such as pulmonary vascular resistance[110] and right ventricular (RV) function. Additional scans can be easily added to the scanning protocol,

depending on the patient's clinical presentation; for example, lung perfusion to screen for chronic thromboembolic pulmonary artery disease.[111]

With procedural workflow optimization it is possible to repeat measurements at rest and under physiological provocation, such as exercise, inhaled nitric oxide or intravascular volume challenge, all within a reasonable timeframe.[112] Investigators from the University of Leuven in Belgium expertly applied this technology in patients with chronic thromboembolic pulmonary hypertension and in endurance athletes.[113,114] Subjects performed supine exercise in the CMR scanner with a pulmonary artery catheter in place for assessment of pulmonary vascular resistance and RV function during physiological stress. Hemodynamic parameters only measureable with exercise CMR catheterization, such as pulmonary vascular and RV reserve, may be valuable prognostic indicators in patients with little or no overt pathology at rest.[115]

Tissue Delivery and Ablation

Real-time iCMR guided endomyocardial cell delivery has achieved millimeter-scale precision using modified CMR needle-catheters in animal models for many years.[116–121] These technically impressive delivery systems await suitable cell preparations or interstitial tissue augmentation materials for applications to patients.

High intensity focused ultrasound is an alternative to RF energy for targeted tissue ablation. Preclinical CMR-conditional, high intensity focused ultrasound catheters have been developed and successfully used to ablate tissue such as renal parenchyma.[122] Importantly, histopathology demonstrated coagulation necrosis with comparable volumes to the lesions seen with contrast-enhanced CMR. However, just like RF ablation lesion visualization, high intensity focused ultrasound depends on administration of systemic Gd contrast for lesion conspicuity. Maximum safe dose of Gd contrast therefore precludes repeated ablation and imaging cycles. Although this may be acceptable for large solid tumor ablation, it is not helpful for more targeted and complex ablation procedures, such as arrhythmia ablation in the heart.

Minimally invasive procedures involving the myocardium are particularly amenable to CMR guidance because of the high contrast between myocardium and blood, and because of the readily obtained contrast between normal and pathologic myocardial tissue. Unfortunately, contemporary approaches to the use of CMR to treat rhythm disorders fail to address the key shortcoming of RF ablation, that without surgical exposure, there is no interactive visualization of irreversibly necrotic myocardium after ablation. Edema lesions take minutes to appear and

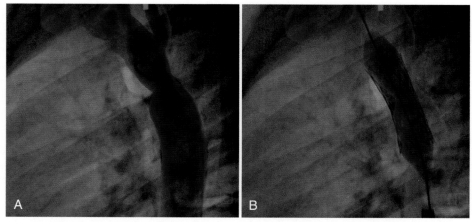

FIG. 47.12 Coarctation stent angioplasty in a 17-year-old patient. (A) X-ray fused with cardiovascular magnetic resonance (XFM) coregistration confirmation with contrast aortogram. (B) Coarctation stent angioplasty under XFM guidance allows for accurate stent positioning to avoid left subclavian artery occlusion. (Courtesy Elena Grant et al., Children's National Health System, Washington, DC.)

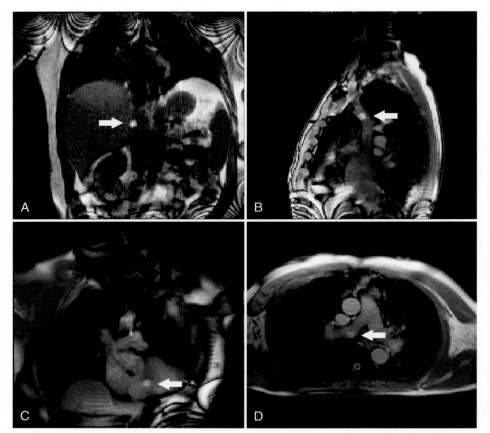

FIG. 47.13 Real-time interventional cardioavascular magnetic resonance (iCMR) guided right-heart catheterization using passive catheters. Nonbraided balloon wedge end-hole catheters are filled with dilute gadolinium. The balloon at the tip of the catheter appears as a white ball on real-time CMR *(arrow)*. Catheter in the inferior (A) and superior (B) vena cavae, right ventricle (C), and right pulmonary artery (D).

exaggerate the zone of irreversible conduction block.[123] As an alternative to RF energy, Kholmovsky and colleagues recently demonstrated cryoablation lesions during real-time iCMR.[124] Using active needle-tip catheters and passive visualization deflectable sheaths, originally designed for cell delivery, our laboratory demonstrated feasibility of real-time iCMR guided myocardial chemoablation using Gd-doped caustic agents such as ethanol or acetic acid.[125] iCMR enabled real-time visualization of chemoablation lesions as they were created; needle delivery of caustic agents into the thick ventricular myocardium created fully transmural lesions; and acetic acid caused immediate tissue necrosis with very homogenous and well-circumscribed lesions. Real-time iCMR guided chemoablation could improve the efficacy of ventricular tachycardia ablation by ensuring accurate targeting of pathological myocardial substrate with fully transmural and irreversible lesions.

Cardiac Electrophysiology

Therapeutic endomyocardial catheter ablation is widely performed using endomyocardial mapping systems and x-ray fluoroscopy to abolish atrial and ventricular tachyarrhythmia. In these procedures, a mapping catheter is advanced into the cardiac chambers, guided by endocardial electrogram patterns to localize the arrhythmia. Key targets are subjected to RF or cryoablation to create nonconductive zones to abolish the arrhythmia. Because available imaging modalities afford poor visualization of tissue and anatomic structures, these procedures can be challenging and time consuming. Roadmaps created using prior electromagnetic maps, CMR, or CT can be used to fuse with updated catheter images[126,127];

however, these roadmaps are subject to intrinsic registration errors, to nonperiodic cardiac and respiratory motion,[128] to alterations in volume as loading conditions change, and to catheter-induced geometric distortion. That said, electroanatomic mapping systems have become sufficiently sophisticated that near-zero fluoroscopy guided electrophysiology procedures are now widely attainable.[129,130]

Catheter treatment of atrial fibrillation is performed by creating lines of ablation to isolate all four pulmonary veins. Even in experienced hands, these procedures, guided by x-ray fluoroscopy and electromagnetic mapping, usually require hours of radiation exposure. Of note, "image-guided" treatment of atrial fibrillation, conducted under direct surgical exposure, can take minutes. It is tantalizing to speculate that comparable image-guided treatment of atrial fibrillation might be afforded by real-time iCMR guidance without surgical exposure. Real-time iCMR guidance systems using actively tracked catheters and filtered local electrograms have been developed.[131] Preclinical experiments have demonstrated close correlation between LGE and electroanatomic maps, and feasibility of performing electrophysiology studies with real-time CMR guidance.[132–135] Using an early generation iCMR-conditional ablation system and passively visualized catheters, ablation of simple atrial arrhythmias, such as atrial flutter, was successfully performed in patients in Europe (Fig. 47.14).[136,137] Newer generation systems provide more accurate catheter tracking through active visualization, combining 3D electroanatomic maps, LGE and real-time iCMR, which should permit electrophysiologists to target more complex arrhythmias such as atrial fibrillation or ventricular tachycardia (Fig. 47.15).[138,139] CMR

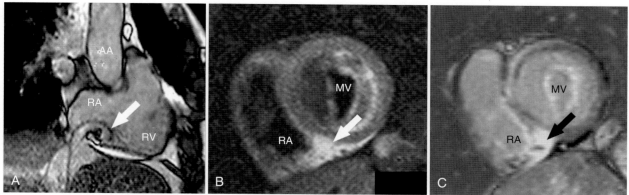

FIG. 47.14 Interventional cardiovascular magnetic resonance (iCMR) guided ablation using passive catheters. The catheter tip, positioned at the level of the cavo–tricuspid isthmus, contains a passive marker for CMR conspicuity *(arrow)*. The newly created ablation lesions *(arrows)* are visible using T2-weighted (B) and late gadolinium enhancement (C) images. *AA*, Ascending aorta; *MV*, mitral valve; *RA*, right atrium; *RV*, right ventricle. (Courtesy M. Grothoff, M. Gutberlet, and G. Hindricks, Departments of Radiology and Cardiology of the Heart Center Leipzig, University Leipzig.)

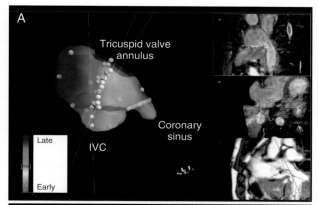

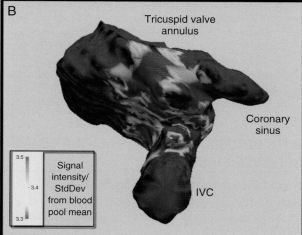

FIG. 47.15 Interventional cardiovascular magnetic resonance (iCMR)-guided ablation using active catheters. Screenshot of an iCMR-electrophysiology user interface showing an activation map acquired during coronary sinus pacing and before ablation. White dots are planned ablation points and red dots are delivered ablation sites. Catheters are depicted on the three-dimensional (3D) image of the right atrium with the pacing catheter in the coronary sinus and the ablation catheter in the inferior vena cava. Smaller panels on the right display CMR images in multiple planes that change automatically to follow the ablation catheter. (B) Maximum intensity projection 3D late gadolinium enhancement map of the right atrium 3 months postablation. Scar is thresholded approximately three standard deviations above the blood pool mean. *IVC,* Inferior vena cava.

electrophysiology is a fertile topic and much progress can be expected in the coming years.

CONCLUSION

Real-time CMR combined with CMR conspicuous devices may offer a complete imaging solution for therapeutic cardiovascular interventions. Superior tissue imaging, no ionizing radiation or nephrotoxic contrast, imaging based physiology assessment, and 3D perspective are among many advantages over existing guidance modalities. The requirement for conspicuous commercial-grade catheter devices remains a challenge. Nonetheless, minimally invasive and novel therapeutic interventions once considered impossible with traditional imaging may now be possible using this rapidly evolving technology.

REFERENCES

A full reference list is available online at ExpertConsult.com

48

Pediatric Interventional Cardiovascular Magnetic Resonance

Kuberan Pushparajah and Reza S. Razavi

The last two and a half decades have seen phenomenal advances made in the field of cardiovascular magnetic resonance (CMR), and these advances have supported research into interventional applications using CMR.[1-4] Conventional x-ray fluoroscopically guided cardiac catheterization and interventions are associated with the risk of exposure to ionizing radiation for both patients and staff. This is particularly relevant in younger patients, who are often required to undergo multiple procedures. The need for an imaging modality offering multiplanar imaging, superior structural delineation of complex cardiac anatomy, and additional physiologic information, without the risk of ionizing radiation, has brought CMR guidance of cardiac catheterization procedures to the fore. In the last 10 years, clinical programs using CMR-guided cardiac catheterization have developed and show promise.[5-8]

Since the first magnetic resonance (MR) images showing live human anatomy were produced,[9-11] this technique evolved to enable a variety of clinical applications of MR.[12,13] Over the years, improvements in signal detection, fast data handling, advanced understanding of spin systems, pulse sequences, and artifact suppression have resulted in much faster scan times and considerable improvements in image resolution.[14-22] These ultrafast imaging techniques form the basis of real-time imaging, used for CMR-guided cardiac catheterization. However, the first important step in making CMR cardiac catheterization a clinical reality is the design of a suitable interventional CMR system.[23-27]

INTERVENTIONAL CARDIOVASCULAR MAGNETIC RESONANCE SYSTEMS

In the design of an interventional CMR suite, it is important to retain the full capabilities of a state-of-the-art diagnostic scanner without encumbering the interventionalist or creating a risk of high radiofrequency (RF) or switched magnetic field exposure. Open-magnet designs allow easier access to the patient, but are not typically available in field strengths higher than 1 T. The cylindrical horizontal bore systems offer higher field strengths and gradient slew rates, allowing higher-resolution imaging, shorter scan times, higher signal-to-noise ratio (SNR), reduced image distortion, and improved functionality with real-time imaging, all of which are of paramount importance when endovascular interventions are considered.[28] A trade off with the traditional cylindrical magnet design is access to the patient. More recently, magnets with shorter bores and flared margins have been introduced and offer better patient access, especially for cardiovascular interventions, without compromising the advanced CMR features of diagnostic scanners. Rapid improvements in the processing power of computers, along with the use of powerful and intuitive software, have allowed researchers to develop novel strategies for image data acquisition and reconstruction. It is now possible to achieve frame rates of as high as 20 images per second with the aid of new parallel imaging techniques, while maintaining suitable spatial resolution for interventional applications.[29-34]

Despite the inherent potential and promise of CMR-guided interventions and operations, there are still obstacles associated with performing the complete procedure in the CMR scanner, particularly because of the lack of CMR-compatible catheters and devices. Therefore the initial work in interventional CMR exploited multimodality imaging, such as x-ray and CMR (XMR) or XMR and ultrasound. Such hybrid units already in existence allow the use of separate modalities or a combination of them when needed. Cross-modality image integration, with spatial and temporal information about the anatomy, pathology, and therapy devices, can be provided to the users of these systems. XMR systems, which combine x-ray and CMR by having both modalities in the same room with a tabletop design, allow patients to be moved from one modality to the other in less than 1 minute (Fig. 48.1).[35-38]

Image fusion modalities are now in existence as a commercial product for clinical use. The use of x-ray fused with CMR (XFM) uses previously acquired CMR images and overlays them onto x-ray fluoroscopic images in the cardiac catheterization laboratory. These can be aligned by means of external fiducial markers or internal anatomical structures,[39,40] with the ability to correct for cardiac and respiratory motion.[41] This has already been shown to reduce radiation exposure, screening time, and use of iodinated contrast agents in selected cases of cardiac catheterization in congenital heart disease.[42] Although not a form of solely CMR-guided catheterization, such technology allows the application of CMR technology in the cardiac catheter laboratory even in nonhybrid suites.

MERITS OF CARDIOVASCULAR MAGNETIC RESONANCE GUIDANCE

Improved Visualization of Cardiac Anatomy

A problem with x-ray-guided cardiac catheterization is the inherent poor contrast of soft tissues, such as the heart and great vessels. This makes it difficult for the cardiologist to manipulate or position guidewires, catheters, balloons, or interventional devices within the heart and surrounding vessels. A skilled operator usually relies on recognizing anatomic structures from previous experience or on contrast angiographic images acquired earlier in the procedure. The lack of adequate visualization increases the risk of perforating the heart or great vessels, especially when performing complex interventional procedures.

Certain interventional cardiac procedures involve selection of an appropriate cardiac device and its successful deployment within the heart, which requires accurate measurement of the size of defects and nearby anatomic structures. Such measurements are possible under x-ray fluoroscopy (XRF), but can be difficult.

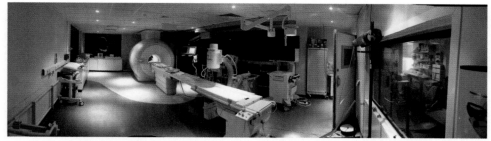

FIG. 48.1 Schematic room plan of a typical x-ray and magnetic resonance (XMR) suite. XMR room with the x-ray and magnetic resonance (MR) equipment joined by a movable tabletop. The C-arm of the x-ray unit is seen in the foreground, ceiling-mounted MR monitor and controls are seen in the distance, and the 5-gauss area is demarcated by a change in the floor coloring from the MR to the x-ray end of the room.

A successful interventional cardiac procedure therefore relies heavily on adequate visualization of the heart or vessel. This implies the need for superior imaging methods that provide excellent visualization without increasing the risk to the patient. CMR fits this role very well because it provides exceptional structural delineation of both the heart and its surrounding vasculature and therefore allows safe guidance of interventional procedures.

Reduced Ionizing Radiation

There is a strong case for pediatric cardiac catheterization procedures to be made safer, especially in terms of ionizing radiation. According to the UK National Radiation Protection Board, the mean risk that a solid tumor will develop as a result of a single cardiac catheterization procedure is approximately 1 in 2500 in adults. This risk increases to 1 in 1000 in children if exposure occurs at 5 years of age.[43–46] Also, the proportion of the body that is irradiated increases as the size of the patient decreases, and some procedures in patients with congenital heart disease often require much longer x-ray exposure. These risks are multiplied in children in particular, because they often undergo multiple cardiac catheter procedures.[47] In addition to the patients, there is also a significant risk from ionizing radiation to the staff in the catheter laboratory during these procedures, despite the use of protective shields.[48–51]

Physiologic Information

Conventional cardiac catheterization is used not only to provide anatomic information and perform intervention but also to obtain functional information. Invasive pressures and blood gases are commonly used to calculate systemic and pulmonary blood flow and resistance with the Fick principle. XRF angiography is also used to assess global ventricular function as well as regional wall motion abnormalities. The functional information obtained at cardiac catheterization is used alongside anatomic information to assess patient suitability for surgery or interventional cardiac catheterization or the need for long-term vasodilator therapy in patients with pulmonary vascular disease.

The Fick principle to quantify flow is dependent on multiple measurements (hemoglobin, aortic/pulmonary artery oxygen saturation, partial pressure, oxygen consumption), which can be a considerable source of inaccuracy. In addition, in patients with large intracardiac shunts and high pulmonary blood flow, accuracy is further reduced.[52–57] Therefore there is a need for a method of flow quantification that allows accurate and reproducible measurement of pulmonary vascular resistance (PVR). Velocity encoded phase contrast CMR enables noninvasive quantification of blood flow in major vessels. Cardiac output and the pulmonary-to-systemic flow ratio (Qp:Qs) measured using this technique have been shown to be accurate.[58–64] In addition, phase CMR has

been validated in numerous phantom experiments, allowing for a novel method of quantification of PVR in patients with pulmonary hypertension by using invasive pressure measurements and CMR flow data.[65–67] This method has since been used in a large clinical case series with good results and forms part of routine clinical practice in institutions where this is available.[8,68]

Assessment of global and regional ventricular function can also be carried out much more accurately with cine steady-state free precession (SSFP) CMR than with x-ray angiography. When using CMR for assessing global ventricular function, there is no need to make assumptions about cardiac geometry, unlike with XRF or even echocardiography. This is particularly important when assessing right ventricular (RV) function and regional wall motion in the normal or systemic ventricle in patients with functionally single ventricle physiology.

Finally, combining invasive pressure measurements with CMR-derived blood flow and ventricular volumes also opens up interesting new ways of looking at pathophysiology. It allows for the study of pulmonary vascular compliance, derived ventricular pressure–volume loops, and assessment of load-independent ventricular function.[69–72] Pharmacological stress studies have also been applied in CMR/XMR catheter studies to assess hemodynamic responses.[72–76]

MAGNETIC INSTRUMENTATION AND VISUALIZATION STRATEGIES

Crucial to the success of interventional CMR is real-time tracking and visualization of catheters, guidewires, and devices in the CMR environment. Several groups around the world are putting considerable effort into developing CMR-suitable catheters and devices. Device localization under CMR is made possible by a variety of approaches that can be broadly classified as either electrically passive or electrically active.[77]

Passive Catheter Tracking and Visualization

The passive tracking technique is commonly based on visualization of susceptibility artifacts or signal voids caused by the interventional device under CMR imaging. This is a well-studied technique and to date it is the most clinically feasible (Figs. 48.2 and 48.3).[78–82] Passive visualization often does not require any special hardware or software and therefore it can be performed on any commercial CMR system.

The ideal passive tracking catheter or guidewire must be made of a material that provides adequate physical properties such as torque and steerability, and allows tracking without obscuring the underlying anatomy. Ferromagnetic materials cause large susceptibility artifacts and therefore are not generally suitable for CMR-guided procedures. This rules out most metals used for making cardiac devices. However, certain alloys, such as nitinol (nickel and titanium), have magnetic

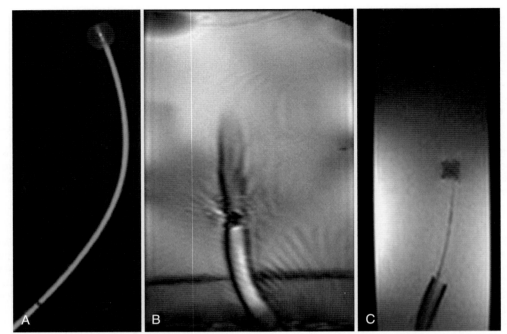

FIG. 48.2 Passive tracking. (A) Inflated balloon angiographic Bermann catheter filled with 0.8 mL CO_2. (B) CO_2-filled balloon catheter manipulated in a phantom. (C) Dysprosium catheter: a catheter impregnated with dysprosium oxide is manipulated in an in vitro set-up mimicking endovascular intervention. The catheter is clearly visualized along its full length, despite being orientated along B_0. (A, Courtesy Arrow International, Reading, PA.)

susceptibility close to that of tissue. Therefore they are best suited for making guidewires and braided catheters that are MR compatible but not necessarily CMR safe.

The polymeric materials used for making catheters typically have low magnetic susceptibility and therefore cannot be easily localized on CMR images.[83] This implies that, if materials with higher susceptibility can be incorporated into the wall of the catheters or sheaths or the lumen filled with a suitable contrast agent, then improved visualization can be achieved.

One approach to generating susceptibility artifacts is locally impregnating the catheter wall with gadolinium (Gd)-like compounds, such as dysprosium oxide, in the form of rings or along the length of the catheter during the extrusion process (see Fig. 48.2C).[82] Another approach is to use Gd contrast agents in varying concentrations within catheter lumens[84] or impregnated into catheter walls to create either a positive or negative signal on CMR imaging.[85]

Metallic devices and guidewires produce susceptibility artifacts, which aid visualization by way of the artifacts, but different metals behave differently under CMR. Titanium alloys produce narrower artifacts compared with ferromagnetic, or even certain other nonferromagnetic alloys such as nickel–chromium, which can produce large RF and susceptibility artifacts. However, commercial guidewires can heat up during CMR because of standing wave formation along the conductive parts longer than a quarter wavelength at the resonant frequency, which corresponds to approximately 12 cm in humans at 1.5 T,[86] which is relevant for cardiac catheterization where wires are inserted to at least that length and nearly always much further.

Guidewires with a fiberglass core and nonmetallic guidewires made of resin microparticle compound covered by polytetrafluoroethylene have been used for MR-guided interventions in animals.[87,88] More recent wire developments include the use of fiberglass MR safe guidewires, which were used in preclinical and clinical trials and led to successful interventions in congenital heart disease, but these were difficult to steer and proved to be fragile.[89,90] There continues to be a drive for the development of an optimal guidewire and techniques to measure heating risks in vivo have been employed.[91] Consequently, a newer nitinol based guidewire with iron oxide markers along the length to impart visibility has been developed with good preclinical results.[92]

In the case of balloon angiographic catheters, if the balloon is inflated with carbon dioxide, as is done conventionally with x-ray, then the inflated balloon creates a signal void in the CMR image, thus enabling visualization (see Fig. 48.2A and B). This method has been used successfully to guide catheters in patients under CMR (see Fig. 48.3).[5,93] Although this technique allows easy visualization of the tip, the length is impossible to visualize because the signal void from the catheter length is masked by volume averaging and dephasing effects of thicker slices.[94] A similar approach is to inflate the balloon of the angiographic catheter with a 1% concentration of Gd contrast agent[7] and the balloon appears as a white ball because of the signal from the contrast-filled balloon.

The success of passive visualization also relies on dedicated scan techniques. A dynamic gradient echo sequence, such as SSFP, has been shown to be ideal for passive catheter tracking, especially when signal voids or susceptibility artifacts are used for visualization.[93,95] Cardiac catheterization under XRF guidance is usually performed at imaging speeds of 25 to 30 frames per second. The frame rates available for CMR-guided interventions are not comparable because of the postprocessing of CMR images and their subsequent display, allowing a maximum of 10 to 14 frames routinely. Some of the proposed passive catheter tracking techniques require image subtraction or positive contrast to improve visualization of markers on the catheter, which means that, along with faster scan techniques, faster image processing algorithms are required.[81,96–99]

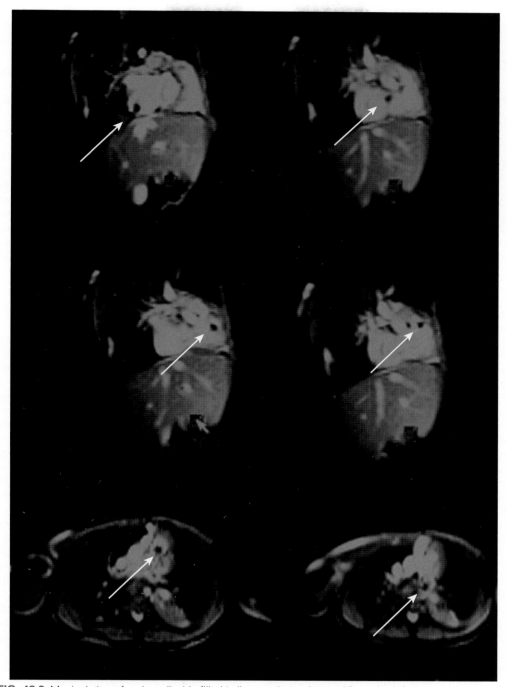

FIG. 48.3 Manipulation of carbon dioxide-filled balloon catheter *(arrows)* from the inferior vena cava to the right pulmonary artery using solely magnetic resonance guidance. Real-time interactive images: repetition time 2.9 ms, echo time 1.45 ms, flip angle 45 degrees, matrix 128 × 128, field of view 250 to 350, and temporal resolution 10 to 14 frames per second. Arrows show the signal void of the catheter tip as it traverses the inferior vena cava, right atrium, tricuspid valve, and right ventricular outflow tract and enters the pulmonary artery.

Active Catheter Tracking and Visualization

The active catheter tracking and visualization method uses an electrical connection to the CMR scanner, and localization or tracking of the device requires the device itself, along with any additional hardware or software that comes with it. Typically, the device is equipped with a coil or an antenna that functions in either receive-only mode or transmit/receive mode.

Active catheters used as receivers have a coil or an antenna that receives signal from tissue in its immediate vicinity.[100] These devices do not transmit signal into the patient but rely on the body coil to

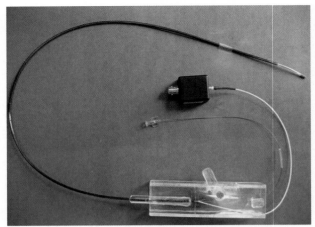

FIG. 48.4 Active catheter designed for intramyocardial injection. (Courtesy Dr. Parag Karmarkar, Johns Hopkins University, Baltimore, MD.)

transmit into the patient. The signal received by these coils can then be used to pinpoint their position, for imaging of local tissue, or both. There are two important types of active catheters: those based on small coils positioned, for example, at the end of a catheter, and those based on a loopless antenna that can run along a catheter or can be made into a guidewire (Fig. 48.4).[101–105] In addition, active designs in which signal voids along the catheter are created by electrically controlled magnetic field inhomogeneities have also been investigated.[106]

A small resonant coil at the tip of a catheter can be identified by a series of three one-dimensional (1D) projections along each axis.[100] This can be done quickly (in three repetition times) and so could be repeated for very fast update of the catheter position, allowing real-time tracking of the catheter. The position of the catheter could then be projected over a previously acquired road map. Similar techniques have been combined with fast/real-time sequences, imaging the heart or vessels using surface coils, and the combined (interleaved) sequence has allowed simultaneous localization of the catheter and imaging of the surrounding tissue. Further adaptation of these sequences has allowed automatic changing of the imaging plane to match the change in the position of the catheter. Another development of active catheter tracking by the group at the National Institutes of Health allows the visualization of two simultaneously acquired planes as well as visualization of the catheter or device positions in real time, thus reducing the major problem of the catheter moving through the plane when only one imaging plane is visualized.[107–110]

The great advantage of these active systems is that location of the catheter is unambiguous. Active visualization has great potential because it allows the whole length of the catheter or guidewire to be visualized and the imaging plane to be adapted to the moving catheter automatically. It may even allow high-resolution imaging of a small area of interest, such as a plaque in the vessel, when the coil or antenna is used in its imaging mode.[111] However, the main disadvantage is concerned with safety.[86,112–116] These devices use intravascular coils as RF antennas, and the connection to the external circuits via a long wire in the strong magnetic field makes induction of an electrical current and heating possible. There have been developments to overcome this risk, such as electrical decoupling of loopless antennas and the use of optical coupling and long fiber optic connections.[117] An innovative active catheter design that uses miniaturized transformers showed no significant RF heating and holds promise for a safe transmission line for interventional applications (Fig. 48.5).[118]

Another approach to device localization is what some authors refer to as semiactive catheter tracking, implying passive localization of an electrically isolated resonant coil.[77] These resonant coils locally enhance B_1 and signal reception so that, for very low global flip angles, the signal from the fiducial is prominent.[119–124] The resonant coils can be interrogated by gradient echo sequences, such as SSFP with low flip angles. Catheters with multiple resonant coils can be tracked easily compared with passive catheters and have a relatively better safety profile compared with some of the active catheter designs (Fig. 48.6).

Catheter visualization and localization using 19F CMR in conjunction with proton imaging appears to be a promising alternative to existing methods that either are associated with safety concerns if active markers are used or have insufficient direction-dependent contrast if passive visualization is used (Fig. 48.7).[125] Other multispectral CMR methods tried before include catheter tracking and angiography using hyperpolarized gases.[126,127] Catheter-tracking techniques using inductively coupled RF coils or hyperpolarized 13C and visualization strategies using novel *k*-space sampling also hold promise.[128–130]

SAFETY ISSUES

Bioeffects of Magnetic Fields

The patient undergoing a CMR scan typically is exposed to three forms of electromagnetic radiation: static magnetic field, gradient magnetic field, and RF electromagnetic field. These can cause bioeffects at significantly high exposure levels. A health care worker in such a setting can also be exposed to electromagnetic fields, although exposure is more chronic and intermittent. However, numerous studies have shown no substantial risks to patients from the electromagnetic fields used in clinical CMR scanners.[131–134] The risks to the health care worker, especially in a CMR setting, are fiercely debated, but the consensus is that more work needs to be carried out before occupational electromagnetic field exposure limits can be set.[135,136] Furthermore, the bioeffects specifically related to the use of interventional CMR have not yet been fully investigated.

Many reports in the literature regarding the bioeffects of static magnetic fields are conflicting. There is no strong evidence to suggest that there are any significant cardiac or neurologic effects from static magnetic fields of less than 2 T. In addition, several studies have shown that high static magnetic fields do not significantly alter skin and body temperature.[137–142]

Gradient magnetic fields can induce electrical fields and current in conductive media, including biologic tissue, according to Faraday law of induction. The thermal effects of switched magnetic fields are considered negligible and are not believed to be clinically significant. Electrical stimulation of the retina is believed to cause magnetophosphenes, which are completely reversible, with no known residual side effects. Some volunteers have also reported experiencing a metallic taste and vertigo while undergoing imaging within ultrahigh field magnets. These bioeffects caused by gradient fields are unusual in fields of less than 2 T.[143]

The exposure limits for RF radiation are set in terms of specific absorption rate in Wkg-1, which is the mass normalized rate at which RF power is coupled with biologic tissue. The main bioeffects associated with exposure to RF radiation relate to the generation of heat in tissues. Controversially, some researchers have reported that electromagnetic fields cause cancer and developmental abnormalities in animal models. However, the efficiency and absorption pattern of RF radiation is mainly determined by the physical dimensions of the tissue in relation to the incident wavelength, which implies that laboratory animal experiments cannot be simply scaled or extrapolated to humans.[144–146]

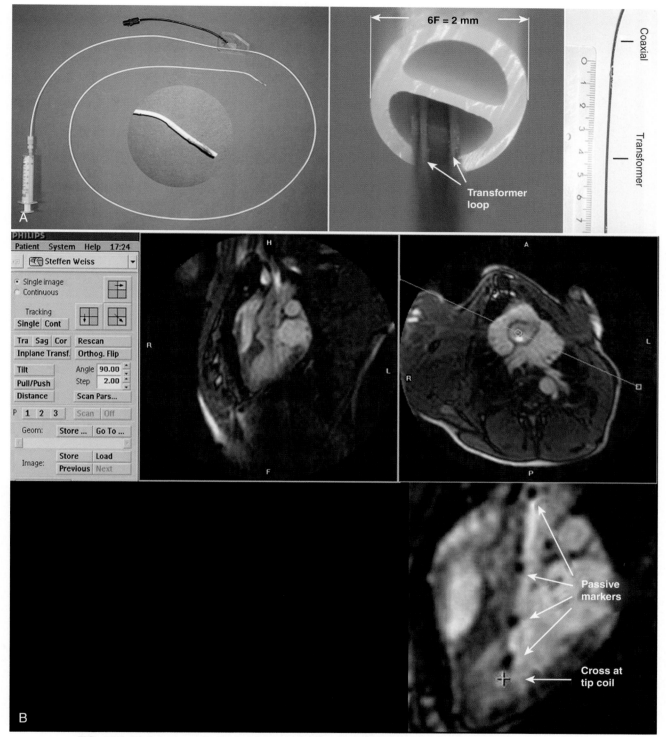

FIG. 48.5 (A) Safe transmission line for active catheter tracking created with integrated miniaturized transformers. (B) To evaluate the transformer concept for active tracking in vivo, a 6 Fr *(6F)* catheter was built for catheterization of the arterial and venous system of a swine. The catheter is seen being manipulated in the heart by the active tracking method. (Courtesy Dr. Steffen Weiss, Philips Research, Hamburg, Germany.)

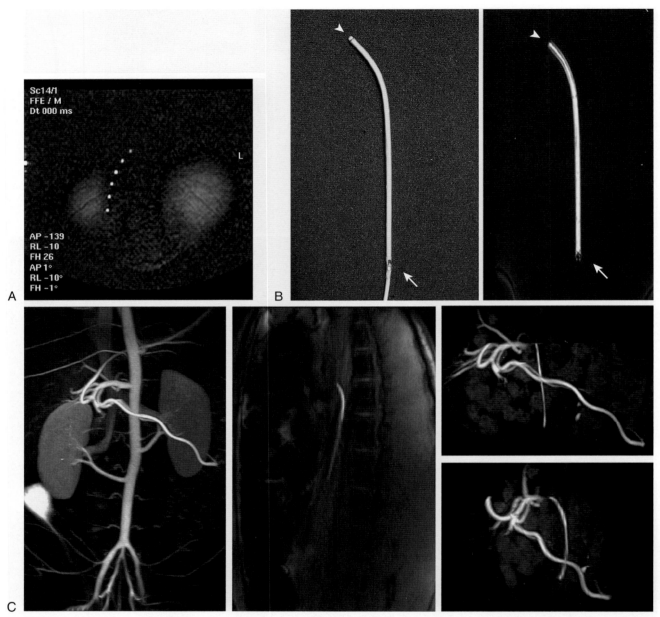

FIG. 48.6 (A) A 5 Fr balloon angiographic catheter with six prewound fiducial markers mounted onto the surface was manipulated in a 20 mm polyethylene tube taped to the chest of a volunteer. A real-time spoiled gradient echo sequence (fast field echo [FFE]: repetition time 2.3 ms, echo time 1.2 ms, flip angle 50 degrees, slice thickness 20 mm) followed by an interactive FFE sequence with interleaving of scans with flip angles of 2 degrees and 50 degrees and a frame rate of 4 frames per second was used. All six markers are visualized along the length of the catheter. (B) Distal end *(arrowhead)* of a 6 Fr catheter with an integrated self-resonant radiofrequency circuit *(arrow).* (C) The active wireless catheter is shown being guided with real-time projection reconstruction steady-state free procession imaging into the celiac trunk. (A, Courtesy Arrow International, Reading, PA. B and C, Courtesy Dr. Harald H. Quick, University of Essen, Germany.)

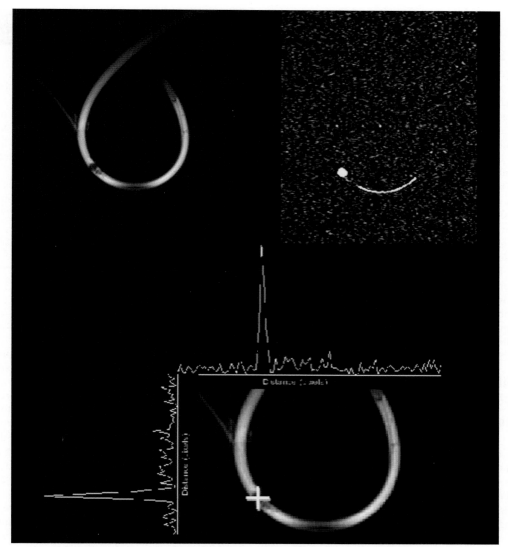

FIG. 48.7 Corresponding 1H *(top left)* and 19F *(top right)* images of a 7 Fr catheter containing perfluorooc-tylbromide. With a simple peak search algorithm in the image space, the catheter tip position was extracted and two orthogonal 19F projections were used to determine the position of the catheter tip *(+),* as shown. (From Kozerke S, Hedge S, Schaeffter T, et al. Catheter tracking and visualization using 19F nuclear magnetic resonance. *Magn Reson Med.* 2004;52:693–697.)

Heating and Electrical Safety of Interventional Equipment

The heating of wires, devices, implants, and other instruments is an important safety issue that is holding back the rapid advance of interventional CMR. Heating as a result of RF radiation occurs by three mechanisms, according to Maxwell's theory of electromagnetism.[112]

When a conductive device or instrument is moved through a magnetic field, small "rings" of current are induced called eddy currents and create internal magnetic fields opposing the change. The kinetic energy that goes into driving the eddy currents inside the metal will give off that energy as heat. Therefore intravascular guidewires or device delivery systems with a metal core are unsafe in the CMR environment, with documented heating up to 165°F of the tip.[112,113,147,148]

Electromagnetic induction heating has often been blamed for thermal injuries caused by monitoring cables used in CMR. RF electromagnetic fields and time-varying gradient magnetic fields can induce voltage in conductive media and cause current to flow. The circulating currents cause power loss by heating that is referred to as induction heating. A loop in a monitoring cable would increase the inductance of the circuit; therefore larger currents would be induced, resulting in greater heating of the cable.[86,149,150]

If a circuit is in a resonant state, then there is maximum current induction such that significant electromagnetic induction heating occurs. Lengths of wire, for example, can behave as RF antennas that capture electromagnetic waves to extract power from them. The electromagnetic waves entering the antennas have electrical charges and corresponding currents associated with them. When the antenna is approximately half a wavelength long, resonance occurs and the electrical energy remains confined to the immediate vicinity of a given antinode. Hence, the highest electrical field of the antennas is believed to be at the tip. The electrical properties of the media surrounding the antennas and the operating frequency also determine the wavelength.[115,116] Newer designs of wires and cables aimed at reducing heating are currently being investigated, along with novel RF shielding technologies.[151,152]

Magnetic Force and Torque

In addition to the bioeffects of CMR and heating and electrical safety of interventional devices, a significant risk to interventional procedures is magnetic force and torque exerted by the magnetic field on metallic devices.[153,154]

Conventional guidewires made of ferromagnetic materials, such as stainless steel, and catheters with metallic braiding, are inherently unsafe for use in the CMR environment. Interventional devices that are ferromagnetic will be subject to both deflection force (translational movement) and torque (rotational movement); therefore they cannot be used for procedures within a CMR scanner. Hence, all CMR imaging facilities must have safeguards to ensure that ferromagnetic objects are not brought into the vicinity of the magnet.

However, there are certain other metallic alloys, such as nitinol, that are CMR compatible. They produce minimal susceptibility artifacts and are not affected by the magnetic field in terms of deflection force and torque. This is an important consideration in developing suitable catheters and guidewires for use in interventional CMR procedures. It should be remembered however that any conducting wire including those made from nonferromagnetic materials such as nitinol can still be susceptible to heating and still be unsuitable for use in CMR procedures.

X-RAY AND CARDIOVASCULAR MAGNETIC RESONANCE GUIDANCE

X-Ray and Cardiovascular Magnetic Resonance Facility Design

The room design of a typical XMR facility is shown in Fig. 48.1. There are many design features that make this room different from standard CMR facilities. The design and clinical practice framework for our XMR facility is outlined in a paper by White et al.[25]

The XMR suite is designed so that half of the room is outside the 5-gauss line of the magnet, permitting the use of traditional instruments and devices as well as echocardiography and RF ablation equipment when required. A movable tabletop allows patients to be moved easily between modalities in less than 60 seconds. The paramount consideration in the design, construction, and operation of an XMR facility is safety, and a comprehensive safety protocol must be drawn up to minimize possible hazards (Box 48.1).

Traditionally, CMR scans are planned and conducted from the control room, away from the magnet and the patient. However, during CMR-guided cardiac catheterization, there is a need for real-time changes to the scanning plane and sequence parameters to follow catheter manipulation in the heart and great vessels. Also, the person carrying out the procedure needs to have a clear view of the CMR images while performing the cardiac catheter. Therefore it is useful to have a fully functional set of ceiling-mounted, movable screens and scanner controls within the CMR scanner room that can be placed at either end of the bore of the scanner, in close proximity to the patient. Some units also have the facility for image overlay with semiautomated whole heart segmentation tools[155] and these are now commercially available (examples include Interactive Front End, Siemens; RTHawk, HeartVista; Cleartrace, MRI Interventions; iSuite, Philips).

The XMR suite includes appropriate CMR-compatible anesthetic equipment and monitoring equipment for invasive pressure monitoring via the catheter. A great deal of thought has been given to the safety of patients under anesthesia, especially during the transfer between the x-ray and CMR tables. All of the anesthetic and monitoring tubing and

---

BOX 48.1 X-Ray and Cardiovascular Magnetic Resonance Facility: Safety Features

- Compulsory safety training of all CMR interventional staff
- Specially designed clothes without pockets
- Safety officer restricting entry to the main room during x-ray and CMR intervention
- Clear demarcation of ferromagnetic safe and unsafe areas within the room
- CMR-compatible anesthetic and monitoring equipment
- Noise-proof headphone systems for all staff within the room
- X-ray-shielded and radiofrequency-shielded scrub room
- Positive pressure air handling and filtration system
- Tethering of all ferromagnetic equipment to the wall or floor
- Safety checks whenever a patient is transferred between x-ray and CMR to ensure that metallic instruments used for catheterization are not taken across to the CMR end of the room
- Written log of all safety infringements and regular review of safety procedures

CMR, Cardiovascular magnetic resonance.

---

lines are designed with extra length and are secured to the movable tabletop to ensure smooth patient transfer.

The electrocardiogram (ECG) and invasive pressure data are sent from the MR-compatible monitoring equipment via an optical network to a computer in the control room, where the cardiac technician is stationed. The appropriate measurement and recording of the data is made in the usual way. The technician has access to monitors that show the appropriate x-ray or CMR images of the procedure. The person carrying out the procedure in the room can view the CMR images and any monitoring data (e.g., ECG, invasive pressure data) with the addition of commercially available MR conditional LCD monitors or projectors available for use in the magnetic resonance imaging (MRI) room for display.

Blood samples taken during the procedure are labeled in the room and passed to the technician in the control room via a wave guide.

Reliable and accurate ECG synchronization is essential for CMR and in particular CMR-guided cardiac catheterization. When catheters are manipulated in the heart, there is the potential to cause arrhythmias (tachyarrhythmia or heart block). It is therefore important to perform accurate monitoring of the cardiac rhythm at all times during XMR catheterization. Obtaining a reliable ECG in the magnet, particularly during some CMR sequences, can be difficult. The magnetohydrodynamic effect and gradient noise can seriously disturb the ECG signal.[156,157] Vector electrocardiogram (VCG) is a QRS detection algorithm that automatically adjusts to the actual electrical axis of the patient's heart and the specific multidimensional QRS waveform. In our experience, this greatly improves the reliability of R-wave detection to nearly 100%. A reliable R-wave, with the P-waves and T-waves that are also always clearly seen with VCG, allows detection of nearly all arrhythmias. There are now MR-conditional hemodynamic monitoring systems available (such as Invivo, GE, Medrad) that are sufficient for basic monitoring, but there are still not commercial hemodynamic monitoring systems available specifically for use during MR guided cardiac catheterization.

Another complication of performing cardiac catheterization under CMR guidance is the noise generated during scanning. There is a headphone and microphone system in the room reducing the noise, allowing staff to communicate with each other in both the scanner and control rooms. There are techniques using infrared technology to allow full wireless coverage in the scanning and control rooms to allow use of multiple headsets (such as Optoacoustics, Clear-Com, Gaven).

Some CMR coils have x-ray–visible components and would need to be removed between CMR imaging and x-ray imaging of patients. It is therefore necessary to have specifically designed coils sufficiently radiotranslucent to be left in place during XRF without deterioration of image quality. We use these types of coils in our procedures so that patients do not have to be disturbed when moving from one imaging modality to the other.[158]

The XMR suite has positive-pressure air handling and filtration appropriate for a catheterization laboratory. There is a scrub room that is also RF and x-ray shielded and can be accessed both from the XMR suite and control room. This room acts as an RF lock, allowing access to the XMR suite during CMR scanning.

Performing X-Ray and Cardiovascular Magnetic Resonance Interventions

In a typical XMR interventional procedure, after the induction of anesthesia, the patient is transferred from an MR-compatible trolley to the CMR end of the XMR facility and positioned on the CMR scanner tabletop (Fig. 48.8A). The monitoring and anesthetic equipment are attached. A three-lead ECG, separate from the VCG, is used for cardiac monitoring during MR scanning. The VCG electrodes are placed on the subcostal margin, outside the x-ray field of view, and the VCG is used for triggering CMR scans. An MR-compatible pulse oximeter and noninvasive blood pressure monitoring equipment are also attached. The exhaled anesthetic gases are monitored for end-tidal carbon dioxide as well as the concentration of the volatile anesthetic agents. Flexible phase array RF coils are used. These coils are relatively x-ray lucent and thus do not need to be removed between MR and x-ray imaging.

The patient is then placed in the CMR scanner, and a multibreath-hold three-dimensional (3D) SSFP scan of the heart and great vessels (echo time 2, repetition time 4, flip angle 50 degrees, 80 to 120 slices reconstructed to 1 mm cubic voxels) is obtained.[8,159] Using an interactive SSFP sequence (8 to 10 frames per second), with real-time manipulation of scan parameters, the likely imaging planes needed for subsequent catheter tracking, ventricular function, and flow quantification are stored. The patient is then transferred to the x-ray end of the room. Draping and vascular access are carried out as for routine cardiac catheterization; in addition, a second large drape is placed over the patient (see Fig. 48.8B).

The patient is transferred back to the MR scanner after safety checks are performed, including an operating theater-style check of all metallic objects used under x-ray. The second drape is then lifted up and taped to the top of the magnet, which in effect provides sterile draping of the bore and sides of the magnet (see Fig. 48.8C). An end-hole or side-hole balloon angiographic catheter (4 to 7 Fr) is placed in the sheath, and with the balloon inflated with CO_2 (see Fig. 48.3), the catheter tip is passively visualized using the interactive sequences described earlier. The previously stored imaging planes are used, along with interactive slice selection, to track the catheter. Because only the tip of the catheter is visualized, care is taken not to push the catheter too fast and thus beyond the CMR imaging plane. This also ensures that the catheter does not accidentally form loops and possible knots.

A duplicate CMR control console is positioned next to the bore of the magnet so that the interactive window can be easily visualized while the catheter is being manipulated. Therefore this procedure requires two experienced operators, one to move the catheter and one to alter the CMR imaging planes to ensure that the catheter tip is tracked, using the real-time interactive sequence. Alternatively simple maneuvers such as moving the imaging plane or toggling between different views, as well as starting or stopping scanning can be done using pedals that are connected to the scanner host computer.

Once the catheter is positioned in the desired vessel or chamber, appropriate pressure data and saturation/blood gas samples are obtained,

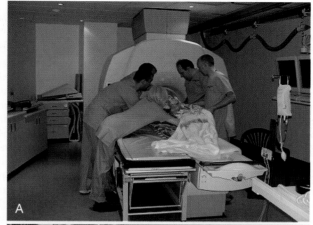
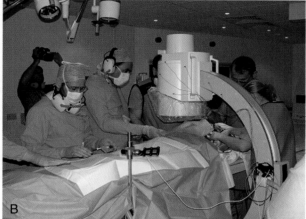
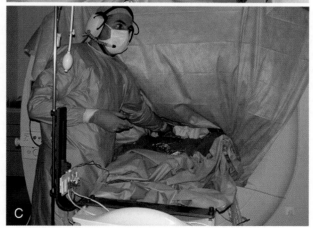

FIG. 48.8 X-ray and magnetic resonance intervention. (A) Patient is placed on the magnetic resonance tabletop. (B) Patient is slid across to the x-ray half of the room for sheath insertion. (C) Passive catheter manipulation is performed under magnetic resonance guidance.

as for routine cardiac catheterization. In addition, ventricular function (short-axis balanced SSFP) and flow (phase contrast) scans can be performed using the appropriate previously stored imaging planes. If catheter manipulation into a particular heart chamber or vessel using CMR guidance alone is difficult, the patient is transferred back to the x-ray end of the room, where catheterization can be continued under XRF (e.g., to use a guidewire or a braided catheter). The patient can be transferred back to the CMR scanner for further CMR measurements once the catheter is positioned satisfactorily.

Early Experience in Humans

In our institution we had the first clinical experience of CMR and combined CMR and x-ray (XMR) guided cardiac catheterizations,[5,67,93] which allowed for a significant reduction of overall x-ray dose. CMR/XMR catheterizations were initially employed and validated against standard cardiac catheterization for the assessment of pulmonary vascular resistance (PVR).[5,67] We used CMR to assess pulmonary vascular resistance in the patients because it allowed for simultaneous measurement of pulmonary arterial flow and invasive pressures. We found moderate-to-good agreement between the Fick method and the CMR method of deriving PVR at baseline conditions. However, in the presence of nitric oxide, which is used to assess pulmonary vasoreactivity, there was less agreement between the two methods. There was not only worsening in agreement but also a large bias when PVR was measured in the presence of 100% oxygen and nitric oxide. We believe this is the result of errors in the Fick method rather than the XMR method, which has important implications for patient management. This novel MR technique proved to be a more accurate method to quantify PVR in humans; it also offers reduced exposure to ionizing radiation.[6,67]

In the past few years the indications have widened to include assessment of anatomy and function, cardiac output, and hemodynamic measurements during pharmacological stress.[8,68,70,72,160] We have also described an initial clinical experience of CMR guided structural cardiac interventions using a CMR compatible guide wire.[90] CMR catheterization has been employed successfully into routine clinical practice at several centers with experience of over 100 cases.[7] At our own unit, we have performed over 214 MRI catheterizations in the first 10 years of the program[8] in a range of patient weights from 2.3 kg to 108 kg, with a good safety profile. This includes the CMR-guided interventions in humans, as described later. The majority of the assessments were for PVR evaluation. We found that PVR assessments in this way were a safe and accurate tool, which allowed for risk stratification of patients with congenital heart disease being considered for intervention.[68] We also identified discrete PVR thresholds below which good long-term outcomes could be achieved following surgical repair or intervention, with a successful biventricular repair at resting PVR values ≤ 6 WU/m^2 and Fontan completion at ≤ 4 WU/m^2. Additionally, we identified that a baseline Qp:Qs ≤ 2.75 in biventricular circulations with left-to-right shunts predicted a PVR ≥ 6 WU/m^2 with 100% sensitivity and 48% specificity as a possible noninvasive surrogate.

Pharmacological stress studies with dobutamine were employed to increase the heart rate and simulate physiological heart rate responses to exercise to assess the circulation at rest and under stress. These studies involved measurements of cardiac output and invasive pressures at baseline and were repeated with dobutamine infused at a rate of 10 µg/kg per minute for 10 minutes or once a stable heart rate or blood pressure rise had been observed and repeated at 20 µg/kg per minute. Thus far, these have been employed in the assessment of patients preliver transplant[8,73] and in patients with a functionally single ventricle.[72,74] Our experience is that titration in this manner has a very good safety profile.

Isoprenaline stress studies have been used to assess for latent coarctation.[76,161] This involved measurement of aortic blood flow and pressure gradients across the site of aortic coarctation at baseline and with isoprenaline (isoprenaline sulphate) at a dose of 0.02 µg/kg per minute increasing to a maximum of 0.7 µg/kg per minute. The dose was titrated upwards until the heart rate increased by $\geq 50\%$ from baseline and maintained once a stress steady state was achieved.

Interventional Cardiac Applications

Animal models have shown immense potential for interventional CMR. The interventions shown to be feasible with passive and active catheter techniques include balloon angioplasty of arterial stenoses,[162–167] stenting of vessels,[121,168–171] and atrial septal puncture/septostomy.[172,173] Device closure of atrial septal defects is another application that has been explored.[174–177] CMR-guided percutaneous pulmonary and aortic valve stent implantation have also been performed successfully (Fig. 48.11).[168,178] In addition, more complex interventions, such as percutaneous coronary catheterization and intervention, have been demonstrated in healthy animals using CMR[179–182] but limitations in spatial resolution are unlikely to result in coronary interventions being a key area for CMR guided interventions.

Further animal studies employing XFM also offer potential interventions in congenital heart disease such as percutaneous VSD closure[183] and successful transcatheter creation of bidirectional Glenn shunts in pigs.[184] The application of interventions has now been extended to humans.[90,167] This includes balloon dilation of aortic coarctation and pulmonary valvuloplasty in patients under CMR guidance alone. In our experience, the youngest patient where this has been achieved was 3.5 years.[8,90]

Novel catheters and guidewires have made possible targeted intramyocardial injection of progenitor stem cells in myocardial infarction in animal models.[39,109,185,186] Using real-time CMR and direct apical access in porcine hearts, prosthetic aortic valves were implanted in the beating heart.[187] This breakthrough application may allow CMR guidance of minimally invasive extraanatomic bypass and beating-heart valve repair. MR guidance of intramyocardial gene therapy is another exciting field.[188] The ability of CMR to detect myocardial fibrosis and scar tissue could also open up the utility for targeted myocardial biopsy, with researchers working on developing appropriate biotomes.[3] This may well improve the poor diagnostic yield of myocardial biopsy in the evaluation of cardiomyopathy.[189]

Electrophysiology and Radiofrequency Ablation

Electrophysiology studies and radiofrequency ablation have long been done under XRF and ultrasound guidance because of the lack of suitable CMR compatible hardware. However, CMR offers significant advantages over XRF with rapid 3D segmentation of the heart and myocardial tissue characterization, which allows for visualization of the arrhythmogenic substrate as a target for radiofrequency ablation of arrhythmias and assessment ablation induced cardiac lesions. Initial experience in the application of CMR required part of the procedure to be performed under x-ray fluoroscopy with CMR imaging performed at the beginning of the procedure for planning purposes, used in guiding the procedure with XFM, and performed again at the end of the procedure for evaluation. XRF guidance is conventionally used to guide such procedures because it offers excellent temporal resolution and good visualization of catheters. However, as a projection imaging modality, more than one view is necessary to gain an appreciation of the 3D location and path of catheters. This implies moving the x-ray c-arm to obtain different projections. A few centers use a biplane x-ray system for the same purpose. The anatomic context of the acquired images can be difficult to interpret because soft tissues, such as the heart and blood vessels, are not visible during x-ray exposure. Therefore we developed a real-time XMR guidance system for cardiovascular interventions that allows the use of both CMR and x-ray imaging for guidance, thereby overcoming some of the failings of exclusive XRF guidance.[190]

During intervention, the guidance system can provide a real-time MR anatomy overlay onto x-ray images. One monitor is used to display the control interface and the second monitor shows the image overlay. During fluoroscopy, the system acquires x-ray images and computes the registration matrix from the tracking data at 10 frames per second and updates the overlay display at 3 frames per second. Using this unique XMR technology, we have carried out RF ablation in pulmonary veins, atria, and ventricles to treat arrhythmias successfully in 30 patients (Fig. 48.9).[190] This CMR to x-ray registration method also allows us to relate the position of measured electrophysiology data to cardiac motion data from 3D CMR images. The XMR technology is also being used to perform stent implantation in patients with coarctation of the aorta (Figs. 48.10 and 48.11). Three-dimensional electromechanical models of the heart have been created that allow simulation of cardiovascular pathologies to test therapeutic strategies and plan interventions (Fig. 48.12).[191,192]

However, there are tools for real-time visualization and active tracking of cardiac catheters for diagnostic and ablation procedures.[193–197]

These have led to successful electrophysiological studies and RF ablation of right atrial flutter in humans.[198,199] Early clinical studies have proved safe, with reliable navigation and mapping for RF ablation. RF ablation of the cavo-tricuspid isthmus was performed under active MR guidance, with brief cine sequences for catheter position confirmation (Fig. 48.13). This is currently limited to adults and, to date, there are no reports of this approach in children. It is anticipated that further development of this technique would benefit adults and children with congenital heart disease with complex intracardiac anatomy and potential arrhythmic substrate from multiple scar sites.

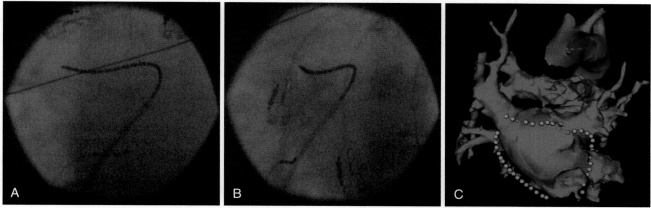

FIG. 48.9 (A, B) Biplane x-ray views of the linear ablating catheter in the left atrial roof position. (C) Posterior three-dimensional view of the left atrium derived from a gadolinium cardiovascular magnetic resonance angiography scan. The green dots show the mapped locations of the linear ablating catheter in three positions: (1) left atrial roof position; (2) left upper pulmonary vein to mitral valve annulus position; and (3) right upper pulmonary vein to mitral valve annulus position.

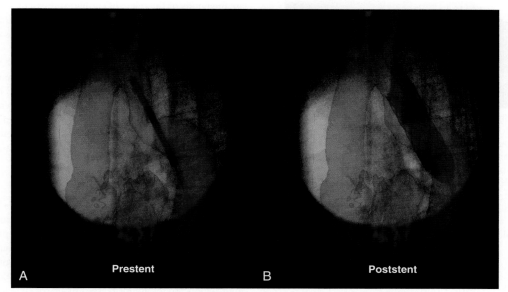

FIG. 48.10 Cardiovascular magnetic resonance angiography (MRA) image superimposed onto the x-ray cardiac catheter image during stent implantation. (A) Undilated stent and guidewire across the coarctation site. (B) The combined images show that the implanted open stent lies in a satisfactory position, distal to the origin of the left subclavian artery and across the coarctation narrowing. Stent implantation was performed in the x-ray half of the x-ray and magnetic resonance facility. Magnetic resonance imaging was used before stent insertion to acquire the three-dimensional cardiovascular MRA images and after the procedure (guidewires removed) to confirm satisfactory position of the stent and relief of aortic obstruction.

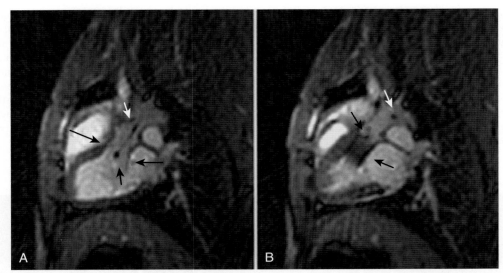

FIG. 48.11 Percutaneous aortic valve stent implantation in a swine before (A) and after (B) valve stent implantation under cardiovascular magnetic resonance. White arrow indicates guidewire, and black arrows note the position of the aortic valve annulus and subsequent stent. (Courtesy Dr. Titus Kuehne, German Heart Institute, Berlin, Germany.)

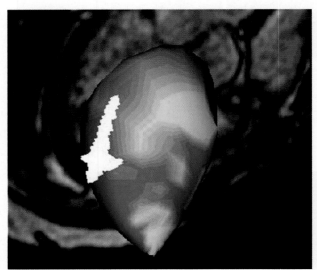

FIG. 48.12 Patient undergoing x-ray and cardiovascular magnetic resonance (CMR)-guided biventricular pacing. Composite image showing one slice of a CMR cardiac anatomic scan with a superimposed surface model of the left ventricle. Cardiac electrical modeling was used to estimate myocardial conductivity for the left ventricle. The conductivity is represented by the color coding, with blue showing areas of low conductivity and yellow showing areas of normal conductivity. The white region shows the area of scarring segmented from late enhancement magnetic resonance imaging. There is good correspondence with predicted low conductivity and the region of the scar.

Future Directions

CMR-guided catheterization is clearly feasible and safe in pediatric and adult practice for diagnostic purposes, particularly in the accurate assessment of PVR. The early experience in CMR guided interventions is also promising, with major advances being made in electrophysiological studies and RF ablation in adults. The main benefits include reduction of x-ray dose and better visualization of complex anatomy for both diagnostic and interventional cardiac catheterization. Developments in image registration and overlay techniques also allow for immediate use of 3D datasets for procedural guidance in the CMR scanner. Improvements in the accessibility of these imaging platforms will increase their application in the clinical arena. Meanwhile, there still needs to be improved spatial and temporal resolution of CMR, particularly to guide pediatric interventions.

There is a pressing need for industry participation in the development of CMR compatible cardiac catheters and devices specifically designed for CMR-guided cardiac catheterization. This is particularly relevant in congenital heart disease, where complex anatomy requires wires and end-hole catheters with good steerabilty and torque to negotiate the bends of the relevant cardiac and vascular structures. Development of such equipment needs to keep pace with the rigorous processes of regulatory approval involved in bringing devices and sequences from a prototype stage to clinical applications.

The cost associated with installing expensive XMR suites does also limit the widespread application of interventional CMR but costs will eventually come down. Over time, there will need to be some verification in terms of the cost effectiveness of these techniques and its role in improving patient outcomes. However, CMR-guided catheterization in children will continue to develop as a consequence of the continued strive for better anatomical and physiological data and avoidance of radiation.

CONCLUSION

CMR-guided catheterization is clearly feasible and safe in pediatric and adult practice for diagnostic purposes with promising early data on interventions, limited by the lack of available hardware. The potential benefits of 3D anatomic guidance for interventional cardiologists, radiologists, and surgeons, including the useful additional physiologic information and the ability to assess tissue response to therapy with CMR, makes this remarkable imaging modality unique and one that offers great promise for safe guidance of complex cardiovascular interventions.

ACKNOWLEDGMENTS

Some of the work described in this chapter was performed by a team of academic and clinical staff at the Evelina London Children's Hospital,

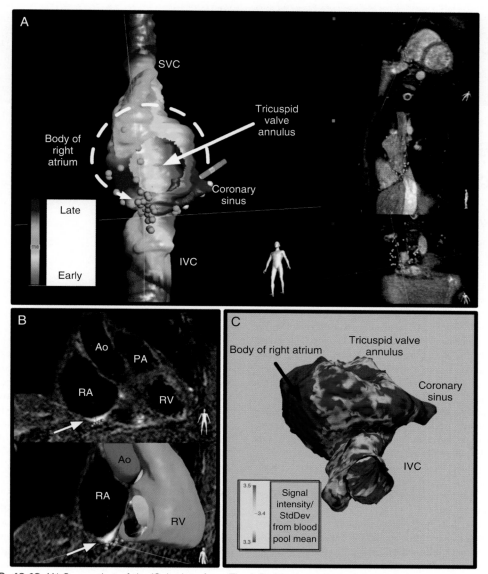

FIG. 48.13 (A) Screenshot of the iSuite interface. The left side demonstrates a magnetic resonance generated mesh of the right atrium *(RA)*. Local activation time is overlaid on the map, in a manner analogous to electroanatomical mapping systems such as Carto. The green catheter, in the coronary sinus, is used for pacing. A line of block is seen at the site of the red dots (ablation lesions), with superior to inferior activation of the lateral wall of the RA, confirming block. The dotted arrow indicates direction of electrical activation. On the right side are three orthogonal multiplanar reconstructions of the balanced steady-state free precession whole heart that is used as a map for navigation. The multiplanar reconstruction planes are automatically recalculated based upon the catheter position. (B) T2-weighted imaging immediately postablation. The white arrow indicates regions of increased enhancement at the cavotricuspid isthmus, at the site of the projected ablation points *(red dots)*. (C) Magnetic resonance imaging performed three months post ablation. A three-dimensional late gadolinium enhanced image has been reconstructed on a mesh of the RA, in the same patient as A and B. The enhancement is seen at the sites of prior ablation. *Ao,* Aorta; *IVC,* inferior vena cava; *PA,* pulmonary artery; *RV,* right ventricle; *SVC,* superior vena cava. (Courtesy Dr. Henry Chubb, King's College London.)

London, United Kingdom and the Division of Imaging Sciences and Biomedical Engineering at King's College London. The authors thank Sanjeet Hegde for his work on the previous edition of this chapter. In addition, we wish to acknowledge Tobias Schaeffter, Kawal Rhode, Aphrodite Tzifa, Stephen Keevil, Marc O'Neill, Henry Chubb, Israel Valverde, James Wong, Sujeev Mathur, Aaron Bell, Jas Gill, Shakeel Qureshi, Eric Rosenthal, Edward Baker and Derek Hill in the Departments of Imaging Sciences, Pediatric and Adult Cardiology. We would also like to acknowledge members of the Anesthetic Department; and staff from the Radiology Department who have provided considerable support.

REFERENCES

A full reference list is available online at ExpertConsult.com

49

Cost-Effectiveness Analysis for Cardiovascular Magnetic Resonance Imaging

Afshin Farzaneh-Far, Juerg Schwitter, and Raymond Y. Kwong

Explosive growth in medical imaging technology during the past few decades has provided physicians with an unparalleled ability to diagnose abnormalities of the cardiovascular system. However, in some cases, scientific enthusiasm and economic forces have helped diffuse new technologies widely without careful assessment of their costs and benefits to patient care. This growth in available imaging technologies has contributed to the continuous increase in health care spending seen since the 1970s. Despite a steady decline in deaths from coronary artery disease (CAD) in the United States, there has been an increase in health care expenditures attributable to heart disease, with an estimated cost of $316 billion dollars in 2010.[1] An analysis of Medicare claims between 1999 and 2008 revealed that 78% of this growth in cardiovascular services was attributed to noninvasive testing—primarily nuclear stress imaging and echocardiography.[2]

Given these rising costs, there is increasing pressure worldwide from government agencies, insurance companies and other stakeholders to demonstrate proof of value for all medical expenditures.

Cost-effectiveness analyses compare the costs and outcomes for a new intervention with an existing alternative treatment, strategy, or intervention. The questions such analyses aim to answer are: how much does the new intervention cost compared with current practice and is it more effective; and if so, how much more? Cost-effectiveness analyses aim to provide the same information commonly used for making decisions about purchasing decisions in everyday life (Fig. 49.1). If a new strategy or potential purchase is more effective and less costly than the currently available option, it is almost certainly worth doing, and in general such a strategy is called "dominant." Likewise, if the new strategy is less effective and more costly, no one is likely to use it. However, the more usual outcome of a cost-effectiveness analysis of a health technology is that the new technology may be more effective, but also more costly. A judgment then needs to be made as to whether the benefit obtained is worth the cost, and how certain we can be about that assessment. Cost-effectiveness analyses aim to provide a framework for making such decisions.

It is clear that cost-effectiveness analysis is critical for the future of cardiac imaging, given rising costs and increasing scrutiny from third-party payers. In this chapter we will provide a brief overview of the techniques of cost-effectiveness analysis, as applied to cardiovascular magnetic resonance (CMR) and review the current literature as it pertains to CMR in both US and European contexts.

BASIC TERMINOLOGY

A detailed review of the technical methods of cost-effectiveness analysis is beyond the scope of this chapter, and readers are referred elsewhere.[3–6] However, cardiovascular imaging physicians need to have a basic understanding of the terminology used in this field. Cost-effectiveness analysis tries to provide a framework to compare different management strategies or treatments within the constraint of limited resources.[4] It aims to maximize health for a given budget. Although often used interchangeably, the terms "cost-minimization," "cost-benefit," "cost-effectiveness," and "cost-utility" have distinct definitions (Fig. 49.2).

Cost-Minimization Analysis

When clinical equivalence is demonstrated through rigorous trial data then a cost-minimization analysis can be a useful economic tool. The rationale being that if two therapies (or management strategies) are equally effective, the cheaper one is favorable from an economic perspective. In reality it is often very difficult to determine clinical equivalence, so caution must be used when interpreting results from such analyses.

Cost-Benefit Analysis

In a cost-benefit analysis, both the cost and the benefit, which in this case is improved health, are measured in monetary terms. This requires placing a dollar value on grades of health and duration of life. Although this methodology is appropriate in the analysis of many economic systems, placing a direct monetary value on human health and life extension can be problematic.

Cost-Effectiveness Analysis

Due to the difficulty of assigning a dollar value on human health, many health economists prefer cost effectiveness, which describes the relationship between cost and a measure of health relevant to the intervention being analyzed—such as life-years gained, disease free survival in a cancer treatment study, or reductions in blood pressure in a trial of an antihypertensive. The central metric of cost effectiveness is the cost-effectiveness ratio with cost in the numerator (in dollars, euros, etc.) and effectiveness in the denominator.[7,8] In the context of a cost-effectiveness analysis, the cost of a particular therapy is the sum of all resources consumed. This may include the direct cost of care (i.e.,

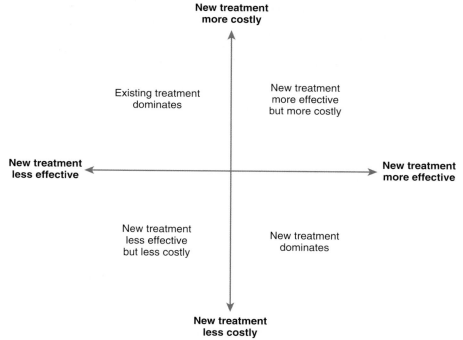

FIG. 49.1 Types of economic evaluations used in health care.

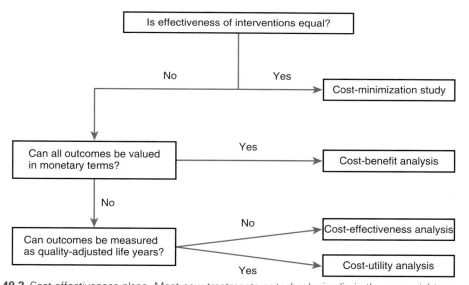

FIG. 49.2 Cost-effectiveness plane. Most new treatments or technologies lie in the upper right corner.

hospital, drugs, treatments, diagnostic tests, physician fees), indirect costs (i.e., lost productivity from work, travel, day care), as well as intangible costs (i.e., pain, suffering).

For a particular treatment or test, the cost-effectiveness ratio in isolation is of little value, unless compared with an alternative treatment/test (or no treatment/test). Cost-effectiveness analysis may therefore be better characterized as an incremental cost-effectiveness ("comparative effectiveness") ratio as detailed in the formula below:

$$\text{Incremental cost-effectiveness ratio}$$
$$= \frac{\text{Cost}_{\text{new strategy}} - \text{Cost}_{\text{current practice}}}{\text{Effect}_{\text{new strategy}} - \text{Effect}_{\text{current practice}}}$$

Quality-Adjusted Life Year

In its most basic form, the "effectiveness" of a treatment can be represented as the years of life gained. However, for most interventions improvements in quality of life are more prominent, giving rise to a quality-adjusted life year (QALY). The QALY applies a weighting factor to account for varying degrees of health for each year of life gained or lost. By convention, perfect health is assigned a value of 1, and death a value of 0. For all of the health states in between, there is a deduction in QALY.

Cost-Utility Analysis

A cost-utility analysis is a type of cost-effective analysis that uses QALY to measure treatment effect. It therefore allows for the comparison of different treatments across different diseases such as dialysis in end-stage kidney disease versus transcatheter aortic valve replacement for aortic stenosis. Cost-utility analyses are important from a public health policy and societal standpoint.

Societal Perspective

Depending on the specific health care system, there are many different stakeholders: governments, insurance companies, hospitals, physicians, employers, and patients. Each participant has a different perspective with regard to cost and effect. It is important to recognize that what may be cost-effective from a societal standpoint may not be from the perspective of an individual hospital or medical practice or institution. The societal perspective attempts to look at the aggregate costs and effects on all members and is the one most often employed in cost-effectiveness analysis.[9]

Time Horizon

The time horizon is the period of time for which the analysis is conducted. It has significant impact on both costs and effects, because over time the costs of an intervention may change (e.g., because of emergence of other competing techniques, drop in clinical demand, etc.) and effectiveness provided has a limited longevity. Short-term versus long-term costs/effects may be very different and thus can alter the cost-effectiveness ratio of a given therapy depending on the time horizon used in the analysis.

Cost-Effectiveness Thresholds

There are several commonly used thresholds seen in the literature, which are sometimes used to define the boundaries of a cost-effective therapy. For example, in the United States, $50K/QALY is a commonly cited threshold, as compared with £20K/QALY in the United Kingdom. Such thresholds are somewhat arbitrary and do not necessarily reflect a society's willingness to pay, leading some to suggest alternative methods to determine what is cost-effective—such as using annual average income.[10] These threshold values are therefore highly dependent on regional economic and cultural forces.

CHALLENGES IN CONDUCTING COST-EFFECTIVENESS ANALYSIS IN CARDIOVASCULAR IMAGING

Cost-effectiveness analyses for diagnostic technologies differ from the evaluation of therapeutic interventions in many respects.[11] One of the most important and challenging differences is the indirect relationship between results of a diagnostic test and health outcomes. Diagnostic tests only provide intermediate results, often a surrogate of a disease state, which may influence treatment decisions but not directly alter hard clinical health outcomes.

Many factors can alter the chain of events between diagnostic test performance and ultimate outcomes. For example, the diagnostic test may be technically inadequate, or it may be technically adequate, but the reader may fail to correctly interpret the images. The correct interpretation may not be accurately transmitted or received by the referring physician, or the referring physicians may vary in their treatment decisions based on their clinical discretion. In addition, the patient may choose not to comply with the recommended treatments. Perhaps most importantly, ultimate outcomes are usually driven by the effectiveness of the treatment(s) used. Therefore consideration needs to be given not only to the diagnostic imaging study, but also to the cost effectiveness of any subsequent therapies instituted as a result of imaging. This complicates study design because investigators must also account for the efficacy and cost of possible downstream therapies resulting from

diagnostic test results, as well as ensuring strict protocol adherence to management strategies with minimization of patient crossover.

Although imaging procedures share many of the features of other diagnostic tests, there are several issues that may be unique to imaging: (1) imaging results are often multidimensional (e.g., presence or absence, location, size, etc.) rather than one-dimensional (e.g., plasma creatinine level); (2) clear quantitative cut-off points are often not established (i.e., results are presented in terms such as "mild," "moderate," or "severe"); (3) images can incidentally reveal other diseases (e.g., an unsuspected lung mass); and/or (4) some imaging procedures may be associated with increased risk of harm (e.g., radiation exposure or renal dysfunction).

Historically, the performance of an imaging test has been evaluated simply in terms of diagnostic accuracy and prognostic utility. However, the downstream decision-making and resource utilization occurring after a diagnostic test are very complex and involve numerous factors that are difficult, if not impossible, to model or predict. For example, Shaw et al. showed significant variation in clinical decision-making after presentation of the same nuclear perfusion imaging results to clinicians.[12]

Finally, it should be noted that disease prevalence in the study population plays an important role in any assessment of cost effectiveness because it affects diagnostic performance through Bayesian principles. For example, cost-effectiveness analysis of CMR in symptomatic patients with CAD cannot be applied to a broad population of asymptomatic patients without known CAD.

COST-EFFECTIVE ANALYSES OF CARDIOVASCULAR MAGNETIC RESONANCE

Differences in health care systems across the world greatly impact cost-effectiveness analyses. To a large extent, the assumptions and conclusions of these studies are limited to the country or region in which they were performed. Therefore in the following sections of this chapter we will attempt to separately review studies performed in the United States and Europe.

US Perspective

Cost-effectiveness studies of CMR within the US health care system have been very limited to date (Table 49.1). This relates to significant difficulties in ascertaining costs, compared with many European countries, which have universal health care systems; as well as the relatively limited clinical adaptation of CMR in CAD, compared with other imaging modalities in the United States.

It is extremely difficult to accurately assess actual costs in the US health care system. In many instances, there is complex and opaque accounting—with varying cost-to-charge ratios resulting in differences between what is charged or billed and actual payments or costs received. The "charge" is the price the consumer is billed by the health care facility for the service. This charge is highly variable depending on the hospital and other local factors, which can be very unclear. The actual payment received may be a small fraction of the charge, and varies widely among hospitals, states, and third-party payers. Consequently, investigators frequently use cost estimates derived from the United States' Centers for Medicare and Medicaid Services (CMS) average payments. These cost estimates published by the CMS can serve as an averaged metric for a significant portion of the US population. They can be looked up online using the Healthcare Common Procedure Coding System (HCPCS) or Current Procedural Technology (CPT) codes of the procedures (http://www.cms.gov/apps/physician-fee-schedule/search/search-criteria.aspx).

Within the US system, direct CMR costs include the cost of using and maintaining the equipment (technical fee) and the cost of study interpretation (professional fee). The costs of the medications used in

TABLE 49.1 **Summary of Major Cost-Effectiveness Studies for Cardiovascular Magnetic Resonance Performed in the United States**

Author	N	Study Population	Study Conclusions
Miller et al.[13]	110	Patients presenting to ED with chest pain and negative ECG/biomarkers randomized to stress CMR in an observation unit vs. standard inpatient care	Patients randomized to stress CMR had a significantly reduced median hospitalization cost
Miller et al.[14]	109	Patients presenting to ED with chest pain and negative ECG/biomarkers randomized to stress CMR in an observation unit vs. standard inpatient care	Cardiac-related costs at 1 year after discharge were significantly lower for participants randomized to stress CMR than those receiving standard inpatient care ($3101 vs. $4742 [P = .004])

CMR, Cardiovascular magnetic resonance; *ECG*, electrocardiogram; *ED*, emergency department; *US*, United States.

stress imaging and any contrast agent also factor into the overall costs. There is huge variability in price between different hospitals, counties, and states, as well as the insurance reimbursement. This cost variability is a significant barrier to accurate and meaningful cost-effectiveness analysis. These problems are further compounded by the variable utilizations of downstream testing and procedures influenced by some regional or local factors.

Despite these challenges, reports of cost-effectiveness analysis of CMR in the United States are developing. Miller and colleagues investigated the cost effectiveness of CMR for patients presenting with acute chest pain to a US hospital.[13] They sought to determine whether stress CMR in an observation unit would reduce costs among patients with emergent non-low-risk chest pain who otherwise would be managed with an in-patient care strategy. Emergency department patients (N = 110) at intermediate or high probability for acute coronary syndrome without electrocardiographic or biomarker evidence of a myocardial infarction were randomized to stress CMR in an observation unit versus standard in-patient care. At 30 days, no subjects in either group experienced an acute coronary syndrome. The stress CMR patients had a reduced median hospitalization cost of $588, and 79% were managed without hospital admission. In a follow-up study, they sought to compare the direct cost of medical care and clinical events during the first year after discharge.[14] They used direct costs of cardiac-related care and clinical outcomes (myocardial infarction, revascularization, cardiovascular death). Cardiac-related costs at 1 year were significantly lower for participants randomized to stress CMR than those receiving conventional inpatient care ($3101 vs. $4742 [P = .004]). There was no significant difference in occurrence of major cardiac events between the two groups at 1 year (6% vs. 9%, respectively [P = .72]).

European Perspective

There are more published data regarding cost effectiveness of CMR in the European context—predominantly from Switzerland, Germany and the United Kingdom (Table 49.2). However, it is important to realize that there are significant differences between different European countries in terms of health care economics and delivery. Thus studies in one country cannot necessarily be extrapolated to other countries in Europe.

Boldt and colleagues used a mathematical model based on Bayes' theorem to compare cost effectiveness and utility of stress CMR and single-photon emission computed tomography (SPECT) versus invasive coronary angiography as the standard of reference in a German population with CAD prevalence rates ranging from 0% to 100%.[15] From a third-payer perspective, stress CMR was more cost-effective than SPECT for any CAD prevalence and this was true for costs per correct diagnosis of CAD as well as for costs per QALY gained. However, this rank order changed in favor of invasive coronary angiography when CAD prevalence was above 60%. The authors concluded that, from

an economic point of view, first-line invasive coronary angiography is a reasonable alternative to stress CMR for patients with a pretest likelihood greater than 60%. Similar results were obtained in a study by Moschetti et al., where diagnostic performance of perfusion CMR, as observed in the European CMR registry, was used for comparison with invasive coronary angiography.[16] In this registry population with a CAD prevalence of 21%, perfusion CMR yielded the correct diagnosis of CAD, at lower costs than invasive coronary angiography when calculated for the German health care system—which is consistent with the earlier findings of Boldt et al.[15] In the European CMR registry, costs were also calculated for the UK, Swiss, and US health care systems, with similar results demonstrating reduced costs by CMR in patient diagnosis and management.[16]

Moschetti et al. also compared ischemia detection by perfusion CMR with fractional flow reserve (FFR).[17] To provide all information necessary for a decision on revascularization, both strategies were coupled with invasive coronary angiography. Specifically, in the CMR+coronary angiography arm, all patients with ischemia on perfusion CMR were investigated by additional invasive coronary angiography, whereas in the hypothetical coronary angiography+FFR arm, all patients underwent first-line invasive coronary angiography and patients with >50% diameter stenosis were further studied by FFR. To calculate the fraction of patients with >50% diameter stenosis, the stenosis–FFR relationship reported in the literature was used.[18] Furthermore, it was assumed that the outcome would be the same for both strategies, given growing evidence demonstrating excellent prognosis in patients with either negative perfusion CMR or negative FFR.[19–21] These two strategies, that is CMR+coronary angiography and coronary angiography+FFR, were applied to a population with CAD prevalence rates ranging from 0% to 100%. The CMR+coronary angiography strategy was more cost-effective than the coronary angiography+FFR strategy below a CAD prevalence of 62%, 65%, 83%, and 82% for the Swiss, German, UK, and US health care systems, respectively. These numbers have important implications. If one collects the percentage of patients undergoing revascularizations after invasive coronary angiography, the pretest probability of CAD for patients undergoing coronary angiography can be estimated. Accordingly, for the Swiss, German, UK, and US health care systems, the literature reports a pretest probability of significant CAD of 34% to 45%, 43%, 42%, and ~38%, respectively, all considerably below the calculated thresholds needed for cost effectiveness of the angiography+FFR strategy.[16,17,20,22–24]

Walker and colleagues compared 8 different diagnostic pathways applying exercise treadmill testing, SPECT, or CMR in various combinations using patients from the UK CE-MARC study.[23] Patients were assigned to different states such as true positive for patients who were correctly identified and revascularized, true negative for those without significant stenosis, and false negative for patients who were misidentified

TABLE 49.2 **Summary of Major Cost-Effectiveness Studies for Cardiovascular Magnetic Resonance Performed in Europe**

Author	Design	Country	N	Study and Methods	Study Conclusions
Pilz et al.[27]	Cost minimization	Germany	250	Determination of costs between a strategy of CMR perfusion vs. coronary angiography using propensity matching	CMR perfusion resulted in cost savings for all patients with the exception of patients at the highest risk of CAD based on Morise scores. This cost saving was achieved mainly through reduction of invasive angiography.
Walker et al.[23]	Cost effectiveness, Markov-model	UK	752	Cost-effectiveness analysis using a decision analytic model to compare eight strategies for the diagnosis of CAD based on CE-MARC data	CMR perfusion is more cost-effective (lower cost/QALY) than SPECT
Boldt et al.[15]	Cost effectiveness	Germany	—	Based on Bayes' theorem, a mathematical model was developed to compare the cost effectiveness and utility of CMR vs. SPECT in patients with suspected CAD	In patients with low to intermediate CAD probabilities, CMR is more cost-effective (both lower cost/diagnosis and cost/QALY) than SPECT. Direct coronary angiography as first test is most cost-effective at CAD prevalence >60%.
Thom et al.[26]	Cost effectiveness	UK	898	Comparison of cost effectiveness and outcomes of various initial imaging strategies in the management of stable chest pain in a long-term prospective randomized trial	Noninvasive cardiac imaging can be used safely as the initial diagnostic test to diagnose CAD without adverse effects on patient outcomes or increased costs, relative to angiography. Noninvasive imaging avoided 20%–25% of invasive angiography.
Petrov et al.[28]	Cost minimization	Germany	1158	Determination of costs between a strategy of dobutamine CMR vs. coronary angiography. Propensity matched.	Initial stress CMR strategy saved €12,466 of hospital costs per life year
Moschetti et al.[20]	Cost minimization	Germany, Switzerland, UK, US	3647	Comparison of the costs of a CMR-guided strategy vs. two invasive strategies in the EuroCMR registry population	A CMR + CXA strategy for patients with suspected CAD provides cost reduction compared with a hypothetical CXA + FFR strategy in patients with low to intermediate disease prevalence in all four countries
Pletscher et al.[25]	Cost effectiveness, Markov-model	Switzerland	752	Cost-effectiveness analysis using a decision analytic model to compare eight strategies for the diagnosis of CAD based on CE-MARC data	CMR perfusion is more cost-effective (lower cost/QALY) than other strategies using SPECT or direct coronary angiography

CAD, Coronary artery disease; *CE-MARC*, Clinical Evaluation of MAgnetic Resonance imaging in Coronary heart disease; *CMR*, cardiovascular resonance imaging; *CXA*, coronary angiography; *FFR*, fractional flow reserve; *QALY*, quality-adjusted life years; *SPECT*, single proton emission computed tomography; *UK*, United Kingdom; *US*, United States.

and not revascularized or who died as a result of the mortality risks associated with CAD. The proportion of patients in each state was dependent on the sensitivities and specificities of the various tests in the diagnostic strategy, and each state was then linked to cardiovascular events. They found only two strategies as potentially cost-effective for the diagnosis of CAD, both of which included CMR. In one strategy CMR followed a positive or inconclusive stress test, followed by coronary angiography if CMR was positive or inconclusive (strategy 3). In the other strategy, coronary angiography followed a positive or inconclusive CMR (strategy 5). In this study, these two strategies appeared cost-effective at the lower and higher end of the threshold range used in the United Kingdom (i.e., at £20,000 and £30,000 per QALY gained), for a typical case patient (60-year-old male with a prior likelihood of significant stenosis of 39.5% based on CE-MARC data[21]). Similar modeling was applied to the Swiss health care system by Pletscher et al.[25] In their study, a CMR-based work-up of a typical patient (60-year-old

male with a prior likelihood of significant stenosis of 39.5% based on CE-MARC data[21]) was also the most cost-effective strategy. They concluded that the strategy of inconclusive stress testing followed by CMR followed by coronary angiography (if CMR is positive or inconclusive) with all positive stress tests followed by coronary angiography (without CMR testing) was the strategy with highest QALYs gained at lowest costs.[25] Similar to the UK study, the strategy of coronary angiography following a positive or inconclusive CMR was the strategy with the second highest QALYs gained.[25] Thus for both UK and Swiss health care systems, a CMR-based diagnostic strategy appears most cost-effective in comparison with other noninvasive testing algorithms. Boldt et al. found similar results in the German system with CMR being superior to SPECT.[15] However, another cost-effectiveness study performed in the United Kingdom found that cost effectiveness was similar between coronary angiography, CMR, SPECT, and stress echocardiography.[26] This study has been criticized for being underpowered and having a very low percentage of avoided coronary angiography procedures (ranging between 20% and 25%) when starting with a noninvasive test.[26]

CONCLUSION

The field of CMR has developed over recent years on the basis of a large and growing body of published evidence showing excellent diagnostic and prognostic performance across a wide range of cardiovascular conditions. However, given the rising costs of imaging, there is increasing pressure worldwide from government agencies, insurance companies, and other stakeholders to demonstrate proof of value for all medical expenditures. Therefore demonstrating the cost effectiveness of CMR across a spectrum of disease will be critical to ensure continued growth and appropriate utilization. These studies will need to include large randomized patient populations comparing CMR-guided treatment strategies with standard management, as well as registry data reflecting real-world clinical practice. As the health care environment continues to evolve it is clear that fiscal constraints on cardiac imaging will likely increase, as the current rate of growth is unsustainable in many parts of the world. Despite their limitations, cost-effectiveness analyses will be pivotal in demonstrating the value of CMR and its impact on patient outcomes.

REFERENCES

A full reference list is available online at ExpertConsult.com

50

Cardiac Positron Emission Tomography/ Magnetic Resonance

Felix Nensa and Thomas Schlosser

For decades, cardiovascular magnetic resonance imaging (CMR) and positron emission tomography (PET) have been clinically established imaging modalities in cardiovascular medicine. For several years, a new multimodality imaging system, PET/magnetic resonance (MR), using sequential or even integrated scanner platforms has been available. This hybrid imaging technique is gradually being implemented into the clinical setting for cardiac imaging.

Because of its unique capabilities, CMR has become a key imaging modality in clinical cardiology practice and a widely accepted standard of reference for the quantification of left and right ventricular function, the assessment of global and regional wall motion abnormalities and tissue characterization (scar, fibrosis, edema), as well as valve function. In contrast, PET is superb at quantification of myocardial perfusion and coronary flow reserve as well as visualization and quantification of particular metabolic processes at the molecular level.[1] Combining both methods there is a range of complementary information, suggesting the use of integrated cardiac PET/MR may be justified in routine setting for evaluation of different disease entities. However, the exact role and value of PET/MR for cardiovascular imaging has not yet been determined. Critical evaluation of cardiac PET/MR is needed regarding incremental value beyond diagnostic information provided by PET and CMR alone. Because cardiac PET/MR is still in its infancy, this chapter will be based on published studies and case reports, available evidence, and where not yet available, on personal experience and expert opinion.

TECHNICAL ASPECTS AND IMPLEMENTATION

Positron Emission Tomography/Magnetic Resonance Scanners and Instrumentation

To generate fused PET/MR images, several approaches exist. In the past the only practicable solution was to use software to register and fuse separately acquired PET and MR data. Although this method works relatively well for body areas with little deformability such as the head, imaging the heart poses problems with respect to coregistration as a result of patient breathing and cardiac motion, as well as patient positioning.[2] Therefore sequential PET/MR systems provide improvement of coregistration if the patient undergoes both scans in a row on a mobile table system without repositioning.[3] Compared with that, integrated PET/MR systems allow for a completely simultaneous data acquisition and in vivo observation of physiologic processes. Moreover, this technique minimizes the likelihood of movement-related misregistration and leads to a significant reduction of the scan time.

However, for PET/MR the technical problem of system integration is a major challenge attributed to the presence of magnetic fields. In PET/MR the real goal has been to fully integrate both systems without reducing the performance of the PET and the MR components. Uniform magnetic fields are of utmost importance in MR imaging. Thus any additional electronic circuits, which can distort the magnetic field, could potentially deteriorate the accuracy and quality of MR images. Besides the interference with the magnetic field, conventional PET photomultiplier tubes (PMT) were not designed to be used inside strong electromagnetic fields and do not function properly in or near these fields. Consequently, the main challenge in combining PET and MR into one integrated system has been the development of MR-compatible PET detector technology.[4] Current integrated PET/MR systems are either based on avalanche photodiodes[5] (APD; Siemens mMR Biograph) or silicon photon multipliers[6] (SiPM; GE Signa), where cross-interference with the MR is minimized.[7]

Attenuation Correction in Positron Emission Tomography/Magnetic Resonance

For the attenuation correction of acquired PET data, modern PET and PET/CT systems use attenuation maps (μ-maps) that contain the radiodensity of each body volume element for 511-keV photons. These are typically calculated using transmission scans with external radionuclide sources or coregistered computed tomography (CT) data, which needs an additional transformation to convert to the radiodensity for 511-keV photons. However, for integrated PET/MR systems without a CT or external radionuclide source, new techniques for the creation of attenuation maps are needed. One approach is based on tissue segmentation using specialized computer algorithms to segment MR data into a fixed number of tissue types with a priori assigned coefficients of radiodensity. The currently most common approach uses a multipoint Dixon sequence for the segmentation into lung, fat, soft tissue, and background.[8] However, one limitation of this method is that bones and calcifications are not assigned into a separate class but classified as soft tissue. Consequently, standardized uptake values of tissue close to bone might be significantly underestimated,[9] which could particularly apply to the retrosternal parts of the heart. However, underestimation seems to be rather small in cardiac imaging.[8,10]

To overcome this limitation, modified segmentation methods based on ultrashort echo time (UTE) sequences can be used, segmenting tissue with very short T2* (such as bone) into a separate class. However, due to a rather small field of view, this technique is not yet usable in cardiac PET/MR imaging.

Because of the fact that all objects between the patient and the PET detector can potentially attenuate and thus compromise the acquired PET data, all instrumentation used in the PET field of view during PET data acquisition has to be optimized for PET transparency.[11–13] This has particular significance for radiofrequency surface coils, due to their unfavorable attenuation profiles. However, dedicated PET/MR surface coils with minimal attenuation for gamma quanta are commercially available. Alternatively, technical methods exist which allow for integration of attenuation coefficients of standard coil systems into the attenuation map after these have been previously measured in a CT scanner; however, one limitation of this approach is that the expansion of the attenuation map presumes knowledge of the exact coil position in the acquired image area.[7]

Motion Correction
Electrocardiogram Gating
To assign image data to a specific cardiac phase, electrocardiogram (ECG)-based triggering is mandatory for MR and PET of the heart. However, during MR, and thus also during integrated PET/MR, ECG signals can be considerably distorted by the magnetic field and radiofrequency pulses. Therefore special care is needed when applying the electrodes and monitoring the signal. The comparably long cumulative acquisition times of most CMR protocols allow for an extensive parallel acquisition of PET signal, which typically compensates for the lost PET data because of ECG gating, resulting in reconstructed PET images of high quality.[14]

Magnetic Resonance-Based Motion Correction
One of the most promising, yet still experimental, technical new developments of combined PET/MR is the advantage of motion detection using ultrafast ("real-time") three-dimensional (3D) MR acquisition and tagging techniques. This allows for the MR-based estimation of motion-vector fields during PET acquisition, which can then be used to improve effective spatial resolution of PET and motion-induced inaccuracies in PET quantification. Recent advances in this area suggest a relevant utility of this technology for simultaneous PET/MR cardiac imaging.[15]

Image Postprocessing, Visualization, and Quantification
To achieve a wide acceptance of complex cardiac imaging scans in clinical practice, a semiautomated or even automated processing of cardiac imaging data is required. Meanwhile, several software products are available from commercial and academic sources. However, most of these software products focus on either CMR or PET, but a few software packages analyzing both cardiac PET and MR data are available as well (e.g., Munich Heart or syngo.via). For analysis of clinical cardiac PET/MR scans, the respective software solutions should include tools for the assessment of ventricular function, viability, fibrosis and scar, perfusion, flow quantification, and tissue composition (e.g., T1, T2, T2* mapping) as well as dedicated postprocessing of cardiac PET data, including creation of bull's eye plots and comparison of myocardial tracer uptake to normal databases.

Common Pitfalls
Despite its complexity, integrated cardiac PET/MR has been demonstrated to be a robust and reliable imaging modality. This is based on our own experience and hundreds of scans performed in several specialized cardiovascular imaging centers and research institutes around the world. Given a certain expertise and knowledge of common pitfalls, cardiac PET/MR has shown to be reliable and robust, and thus suitable for clinical routine imaging. Still, it is recommended that a team consisting of a radiologist and a nuclear medicine specialist with expertise in cardiac imaging should perform and interpret cardiac PET/MR, supervising technicians with cardiac imaging experience.

Segmentation and Misalignment Errors
The validity of attenuation-corrected PET data is directly dependent on the validity of the underlying MR tissue segmentation because the creation of μ-maps is based on the MR data segmentation. MR image artifacts or unexpected behavior of the segmentation algorithm can cause more or less severe tissue misclassification, compromising the validity of attenuation-corrected PET data caused by wrong attenuation-coefficients in the μ-map. Typical MR artifacts in cardiac imaging originate from foreign objects like implantable port systems, sternal wires, artificial heart valves, or artificial joint replacement of the humerus. Thus it is imperative that cardiac PET/MR reading should include visual inspection of the underlying μ-maps. If significant errors are evident, findings in attenuation-corrected PET data should be interpreted with caution and correlation with uncorrected PET data should be performed. If in doubt, an experienced reader should perform these tasks.

Another typical attenuation-correction (AC)–related issue results from patient motion. In a typical setting, the MR-based μ-maps are created in the beginning of the study and are later used for the AC of PET data that get continuously acquired over time in list mode. If the patient changes body position following μ-map creation, this results in misalignment between attenuation coefficients and PET data, which can cause severe PET image artifacts and quantification bias. As a simple workaround, it is recommended to perform repeated μ-map creation, interleaved between main MR acquisitions. If patient motion is retrospectively detected, PET list-mode data can be truncated to an interval before or after patient motion and an appropriate μ-map can be selected for attenuation correction.

Truncation of Field of View
Because of lack of space within the magnet and relatively long scan times, cardiac PET/MR is usually performed with the patient's arms aligned along the body axis. Depending on the patient's body habitus, this can result in parts of the arms being placed outside the MR field of view. This can cause so-called truncation artifacts at the edges of the attenuation maps, which can translate to errors in the attenuation-corrected PET data. These artifacts can at least partially be avoided by extension of the MR field of view by the use of optimized readout gradients[16] or by partial correction with PET emission data using maximum likelihood reconstruction of attenuation and activity (MLAA).[17] However, the MLAA algorithm is restricted to radiotracers that accumulate in the skin because it is based on contour detection in PET images.

Patient Preparation for Fludeoxyglucose Positron Emission Tomography/Magnetic Resonance Studies
Fludeoxyglucose (FDG) is still by far the most widely used tracer for cardiac PET. Normal myocardium is a very insulin-sensitive tissue that uses a variable mixture of glucose, lactate, ketone bodies, and free fatty acids under uncontrolled metabolic conditions, with a preference for fatty acids. Depending on the clinical question (inflammation/tumor vs. viability), myocardial metabolism needs to be shifted to either free fatty-acid or glucose utilization in cardiac PET with FDG. Therefore careful patient preparation is of utmost importance. It is strongly recommended to perform detailed patient interviews regarding the compliance to the preparation protocol. This is ideally performed by a nuclear medicine specialist before tracer injection. In cases of incompliance, the PET/MR scan can be postponed or certain countermeasures (e.g., insulin injection, unfractionated heparin injection, fatty-acid loading) can be taken. In addition to interviews, it is recommended to perform blood testing of glucose level and possibly insulin and free fatty-acid levels.

For cardiac FDG-PET of inflammation, infiltration, and tumors, suppress glucose uptake into normal cardiomyocytes by means of low insulin levels and high levels of fatty acids to differentiate between inflammatory infiltrates or tumor tissue and normal myocardium. This can be achieved using several techniques, including prolonged fasting, high-fat low-carbohydrate diet, fatty-acid loading, and additional injection of unfractionated heparin.[18–20] However, fasting has been observed to be a major reason for patient discomfort, potentially contributing to increased cancellation rates during cardiac PET/MR scans.[14] In a recent study, we have described a high-fat low-carbohydrate protein-permitted diet without fasting that yields an 84% success rate regarding suppression of normal myocardial glucose uptake. Cancellation rate was less than 3% and thus comparable with routine CMR scans.[21]

For FDG-PET of myocardial viability it is necessary to significantly raise insulin levels to favor the uptake of glucose by normal cardiomyocytes. In principle, several techniques including hyperglycemic clamping, administration of hypolipidemic agents (e.g., Acipimox), and oral glucose loading are available. In our department, the following protocol for oral glucose loading has proved to be reliable, simple to perform, and well received by patients: patients fast before the scan, which normally means skipping breakfast in the morning. The glucose level of diabetic patients should be below 150 mg/dL (8.3 mmol/L). Before the FDG injection, the patients orally receive 75 g glucose in a preparation that is commercially available for glucose tolerance tests.

RADIATION EXPOSURE

The effective radiation dose for patients undergoing cardiac FDG-PET usually ranges between 4 and 7 mSv.[22] Because the overall PET/MR study duration is determined by the comparably long CMR acquisition time, this allows for a significant prolongation of the PET acquisition interval, which might result in a significant reduction of the administered activity and therefore the effective dose. In our own institution the effective dose of cardiac FDG-PET/MR is approximately 2.5 ± 1.2 mSv, yielding still significantly better PET image quality than our standard cardiac FDG-PET/CT scans and leaving room for further reduction of the administered activity. Such radiation exposure goes significantly below that reported for 64-slice coronary CT angiography[23] and competes with what is possible with third-generation dual-source CT.[24]

CORONARY ARTERY DISEASE

Suspected and Known Coronary Artery Disease

Published data on simultaneous PET/MR in patients with suspected or known coronary artery disease (CAD) is still sparse. The available data from PET/CT and MR studies indicate that simultaneous PET/MR has the potential to be a powerful tool for the detection of CAD and the assessment of myocardial viability. In integrated imaging protocols with PET tracers for perfusion imaging, viability imaging could be performed using late gadolinium enhancement (LGE) CMR, which seems not only to be the most sensitive modality for the detection of myocardial scar, especially for small subendocardial scars, but would also allow the omission of FDG imaging. This could greatly simplify the PET scan because the complex task of a dual tracer study would become obsolete. Moreover, myocardial perfusion PET has been demonstrated to achieve the highest diagnostic accuracy in noninvasive assessment of significant coronary artery stenosis and, in addition, allows for the absolute quantification of myocardial blood flow.[25]

In side-by-side comparison using sequential FDG-PET/CT and LGE CMR in patients with known CAD, a close agreement between both modalities was found for the detection of transmural myocardial scars. However, a significant number of segments with subendocardial LGE showed normal FDG uptake by PET, thus indicating a higher sensitivity of LGE imaging for the detection of small myocardial scars.[26] These findings have not yet been confirmed using simultaneous FDG-PET/MR.

Preliminary data show the feasibility of simultaneous PET/MR perfusion imaging using ^{13}N-ammonia. In this context, a protocol for the parallel acquisition and comparison of simultaneous PET and MR measurements of myocardial perfusion at rest and during pharmacologic stress has been developed.[27] A more recent study compared ^{13}N-ammonia PET/MR with single-photon emission computed tomography (SPECT) perfusion imaging and reported superior specificity and diagnostic accuracy of PET/MR in patients with reversible ischemia.[28]

Acute Coronary Syndrome

Infarct size is a strong predictor of outcome in patients with acute myocardial infarction (AMI). Both FDG-PET and LGE-CMR are clinically established techniques for the assessment of infarct size in the chronic state. Initial PET/MR studies in the subacute phase after AMI have also demonstrated moderate-to-good agreement between myocardial segments showing LGE and reduced FDG uptake[14,29,30] (Figs. 50.1 and 50.2). Furthermore, CMR in the subacute phase of reperfused AMI can differentiate between myocardial edema, microvascular obstruction, and intramyocardial hemorrhage, which is a potential indicator for reperfusion injury with additional prognostic impact also for the right ventricle.[31–33]

Other studies have observed a certain mismatch between PET and CMR. In cases of underestimation of infarct size using PET, this could be explained by the higher spatial resolution of CMR and a higher sensitivity to detect subendocardial infarction. However, recently performed studies have identified patients with AMI where some myocardial segments demonstrated reduced FDG uptake but no LGE[14,34] (Fig. 50.3). These myocardial segments had wall motion abnormalities comparable with that of infarcted (in terms of LGE) segments and showed only partial functional recovery after 6 months.[30]

The discrimination between reversible and irreversible myocardial dysfunction in the subacute phase after AMI is of high clinical and scientific interest. From the clinical perspective, reversible dysfunction of myocardial segments will contribute to global left ventricular recovery. On the other hand, dysfunction of noninfarcted myocardial segments in periinfarct regions is associated with the salvage area, that is, the difference between the area at risk and the final infarct size. A PET/MR study in patients with reperfused AMI has found that the area of reduced FDG uptake correlates with the area at risk (as determined by the endocardial surface area) and, in the absence of necrosis, is localized in the perfusion territory of the culprit artery.[14] This has been further substantiated by another study comparing the area at risk by FDG-PET to the area at risk by T2-mapping using simultaneous PET/MR.[35]

If finally confirmed, infarct size, area at risk, and salvage area could be assessed with cardiac FDG-PET/MR and used as surrogate parameters for the evaluation of strategies to reduce infarct size, such as preconditioning and postconditioning or remote conditioning.

INFLAMMATORY HEART DISEASE

In recent years, FDG-PET/CT has attracted growing interest in the detection and monitoring of inflammatory diseases; however, until now, no widespread clinical use of FDG-PET/CT has been observed for the diagnosis of inflammatory heart disease.[36] In contrast to PET, CMR is an established imaging modality in the diagnostic workup and management of patients with cardiac inflammation.[37–39] It is well known that CMR can identify even small areas of myocardial damage using the LGE technique or T1-mapping. In addition, CMR is a robust tool to accurately detect and even quantify regional and global wall motion abnormalities, to assess myocardial edema and hyperemia, as well as pericardial effusion. Thus a combination of multiparametric CMR with the high sensitivity and outstanding quantification capabilities of FDG-PET could represent a very powerful imaging modality for cardiac

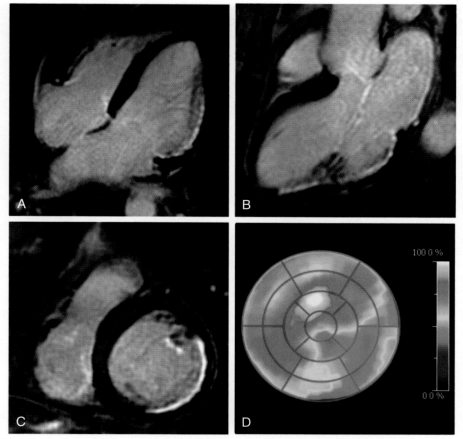

FIG. 50.1 Fludeoxyglucose-positron emission tomography (PET)/magnetic resonance scan in a 59-year-old male patient after reperfused acute occlusion of the left circumflex artery and a corresponding subendocardial infarction of the lateral and inferior myocardial wall. (A) Four-chamber, (B) three-chamber, and (C) short-axis views show the extent of the late gadolinium enhancement. (D) PET data mapped onto a polar plot and overlaid with the 17-segment model of the left ventricle. (From Nensa F, Poeppel TD, Beiderwellen K, et al. Hybrid PET/MR imaging of the heart: feasibility and initial results. *Radiology.* 2013;268:366–373.)

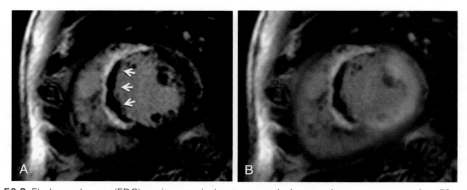

FIG. 50.2 Fludeoxyglucose (FDG)-positron emission tomography/ magnetic resonance scan in a 53-year-old male patient with reperfused acute occlusion of the proximal left anterior descending artery and consecutive acute myocardial infarction. The short-axis late gadolinium enhancement scan shows large transmural infarction of the septal and anteroseptal wall with a hypointense area of microvascular obstruction (A, *arrows*). No FDG uptake was observed in the infarct area (B). (From Nensa F, Poeppel TD, Beiderwellen K, et al. Hybrid PET/MR imaging of the heart: feasibility and initial results. *Radiology.* 2013;268:366–373.)

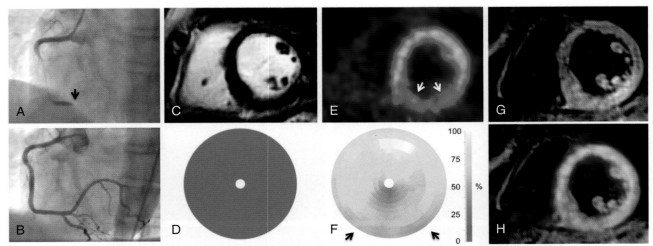

FIG. 50.3 Cardiac angiography and fludeoxyglucose positron emission tomography/magnetic resonance (FDG-PET/MR) in a 44-year-old woman with an acute occlusion in segment three of the right coronary artery. Cardiac angiograms show the culprit lesion before (A, *arrow*) and after (B) reperfusion (pain-to-balloon time <40 min). PET/MR was performed 3 days after the cardiac event. Late gadolinium enhancement (LGE) polar plot shows a complete absence of infarction (D), a finding that was also confirmed on the source LGE MR image (C). Source PET image (E) and polar plot (F) show substantially reduced FDG uptake in the perfusion territory of the right coronary artery (F, *arrows*). T2-weighted MR image shows myocardial edema in the inferior wall (G), a finding that was in good agreement with the reduced FDG uptake seen on the fused image (H). (From Nensa F, Poeppel T, Tezgah E, et al. Integrated FDG PET/MR imaging for the assessment of myocardial salvage in reperfused acute myocardial infarction. *Radiology.* 2015;276:400–407.)

inflammation. In the near future, a number of non-FDG tracers against inflammation biomarkers, as recently demonstrated for Ga-68 pentixafor,[40] could add significant clinical value to cardiac PET/MR.[41]

Myocarditis

To date, no published studies exist that evaluated PET/MR as a diagnostic tool in patients with suspected or known myocarditis. An initial case report has demonstrated the potential of FDG-PET/MR in a patient with myocarditis caused by parvovirus B19.[42] In this report, a typically focal subepicardial LGE was observed which was closely matched by intense FDG uptake in this area and accompanied by myocardial edema and hyperemia (Fig. 50.4). Although CMR would have been sufficient for the detection and diagnosis of myocarditis in this case, it highlights the ability of FDG-PET to quantify inflammatory activity, particularly suitable for the use in disease monitoring. A similar case report was published in a patient with myocarditis due to Epstein-Barr virus infection, with a more diffuse FDG uptake in the lateral wall that closely matched LGE and myocardial edema.[43]

Neutrophils and the monocyte/macrophage family express high levels of glucose transporters and hexokinase activity, which results in increased uptake and accumulation of FDG in inflammatory infiltrates. As such, FDG uptake is truly complementary to LGE (representing myocardial necrosis), T2-weighted CMR (representing myocardial edema) and early gadolinium enhancement (representing myocardial hyperemia) and could be useful to extend the so-called Lake Louise Criteria in the imaging assessment of suspected myocarditis.[44] In future, FDG-PET could not only complement CMR in the diagnosis of myocarditis, but could also allow for quantitative assessment of inflammation and monitoring of disease activity or improve differentiation between acute and chronic/persistent myocarditis. This is particularly relevant because more severe myocardial inflammation is thought to predict progression to dilated cardiomyopathy, increased risk of arrhythmias, and chronic heart failure. Nevertheless, further studies showing added diagnostic

value of FDG-PET/MR and, most importantly, improved patient outcome need to be performed.

Cardiac Sarcoidosis

In patients with sarcoidosis, cardiac involvement is a strong predictor of worse outcome, which often manifests in arrhythmia and heart failure. Thus early diagnosis and discrimination between active and chronic states are prerequisites for adequate treatment and can contribute to the reduction of overall morbidity and mortality. Commonly, treatment of cardiac sarcoidosis comprises both symptomatic management of cardiac dysfunction and immunosuppressive therapy. However, immunosuppression needs to be carefully balanced against harmful side effects. Hence, alongside early diagnosis, continuous monitoring of disease activity with the objective of guided dose adaptation is needed. Accurate detection and monitoring of cardiac sarcoidosis still remain challenging, especially as endomyocardial biopsy significantly suffers from sampling error and can cause severe complications such as myocardial perforation and pericardial tamponade. Therefore noninvasive techniques such as CMR and FDG-PET represent promising alternatives in the clinical workup of patients with cardiac sarcoidosis.[45] In fact, both CMR and FDG-PET are recommended for the assessment of cardiac sarcoidosis.[45] CMR has been demonstrated to predict death and other adverse events in suspected cardiac sarcoidosis[46] and a metaanalysis (7 studies, 164 patients) reported a pooled 89% sensitivity and 78% specificity for FDG-PET in the detection of cardiac involvement in sarcoidosis.[47] In a comparative study of CMR and FDG-PET, CMR provided a higher negative predictive value and thus might be superior for ruling out cardiac involvement.[48]

Also, there is some evidence that a combination of FDG-PET and CMR might provide added value.[49] In fact, both techniques visualize different pathologic correlates of cardiac sarcoidosis. Although the LGE technique can accurately detect myocardial necrosis, fibrosis, and scarring, FDG uptake is a quantitative surrogate parameter of increased

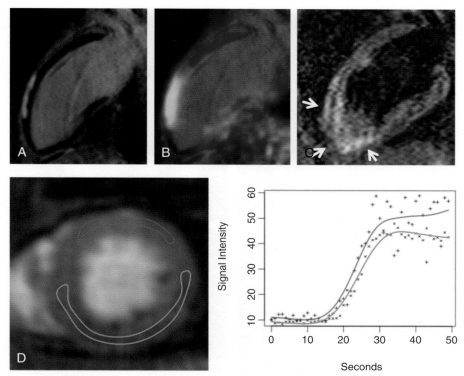

FIG. 50.4 Multiparametric fludeoxyglucose (FDG) positron emission tomography/magnetic resonance scan in a patient with acute viral myocarditis caused by parvovirus B19. Subepicardial late gadolinium enhancement (A) was found in the left ventricular (LV) anterior wall that was in excellent agreement with increased FDG uptake (B). T2-weighted images revealed an edema in the LV apex (C). Dynamic perfusion imaging revealed hyperemia in the LV anterior wall (D, *plot at bottom right*). (From Nensa F, Poeppel TD, Krings P, et al. Multiparametric assessment of myocarditis using simultaneous positron emission tomography/magnetic resonance imaging. *Eur Heart J.* 2014;35:2173.)

glucose metabolism, a hallmark of inflammation. Thus a combination of CMR and FDG-PET has the potential to provide both accurate detection and an assessment of disease activity. Several case reports have demonstrated the feasibility of integrated FDG-PET/MR in the detection[50,51] and therapy monitoring[52] of cardiac sarcoidosis (Fig. 50.5). One study in 51 consecutive patients with cardiac sarcoidosis has found improved diagnostic accuracy of combined FDG-PET/MR over FDG-PET and CMR alone.[53] Despite the sparseness of available studies, integrated FDG-PET/MR holds great potential in the imaging of cardiac sarcoidosis. However further evaluation, particularly with respect to clinical outcome of patients, is warranted.

Endocarditis

Infective endocarditis is a potentially lethal disease if not immediately treated with antibiotics. In patients with prosthetic valves, complications of inflammation include prosthetic-valve dehiscence, paravalvular leaks, and abscesses. CMR is a robust imaging modality that can visualize the infected valve, identify and quantify valve regurgitation, and may even detect dislocation of the prosthetic valve.[54] However, severe image artifacts frequently found in the vicinity of mechanical valves are a well-known limitation of CMR and can significantly compromise image quality and diagnostic accuracy. Review of nonattenuated PET images is always mandatory because extinction artifacts in MR images lead to erroneous μ-maps causing underestimation of tracer uptake in attenuation-corrected PET images. In addition to the morphologic imaging of CMR, FDG-PET allows for the assessment of inflammatory activity and may be well suited to monitor therapy

response, as already discussed in the context of myocardial inflammation. Until now, no studies on the use of FDG-PET/MR in infectious endocarditis have been published. However, one case report demonstrates the feasibility of FDG-PET/MR in a patient with Loeffler endocarditis.[55]

CARDIAC TUMORS

Given the role of CMR in the imaging of cardiac masses and the overall significance of FDG-PET in oncologic imaging, a combination of both seems to be a powerful combination for the diagnostic workup of cardiac tumors. Both modalities alone have already been demonstrated to yield high diagnostic accuracy in the differentiation of benign and malignant tumors, which is, in most cases, the crucial question before treatment. Nevertheless, in a small pilot study including 20 patients with cardiac masses, integrated assessment using PET/MR yielded improved diagnostic accuracy over PET or MR only assessment[56] (Fig. 50.6). Moreover, a *Journal of the American College of Cardiology* imaging vignette shows the potential of PET/MR in the diagnosis of cardiac and paracardiac masses with histopathologic correlation.[57] Considering the already strong diagnostic performance of PET/CT and CMR, high cost, and limited availability of PET/MR scanners, integrated PET/MR imaging might be reserved for selected cases of cardiac tumors where true benefit can be expected. Such cases could include the planning of surgery in patients with complex cardiac infiltration or the differentiation of scar tissue versus relapse in follow-up scans after surgery or radiation therapy of cardiac malignancies.[56]

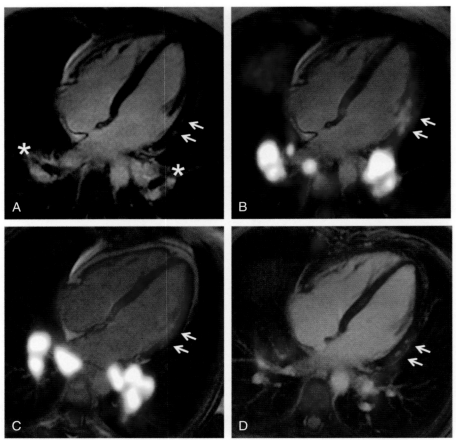

FIG. 50.5 Fludeoxyglucose positron emission tomography/magnetic resonance (FDG-PET/MR) scan in a patient with general malaise, acute retrosternal chest pain, and palpitations. Baseline scan (A, B) showed bilateral hilar lymphadenopathy (A, *asterisks*) and focal late gadolinium enhancement in the lateral left ventricular wall (A, *arrows*). Both lymph nodes and myocardial lesions showed intense FDG uptake (B, *arrows*) and sarcoidosis with myocardial involvement was diagnosed. After 4 weeks of treatment, PET still demonstrated increased lymphonodular and myocardial (C, *arrows*) FDG uptake, whereas FDG uptake was significantly reduced after 4 months of treatment (D, *arrows*). In contrast with FDG uptake, myocardial late gadolinium enhancement remained constant in all three scans, and thus was not an indicator of treatment response. (From Nensa F, Tezgah E, Poeppel T, et al. Diagnosis and treatment response evaluation of cardiac sarcoidosis using positron emission tomography/magnetic resonance imaging. *Eur Heart J.* 2014;36:550.)

REPORTING

The practical implementation as well as the interpretation of cardiac PET/MR scans should be performed with cooperation between the radiology and nuclear medicine departments by experts in cardiac imaging. The documentation of the procedure should comprise a joint consensus report by a radiologist and a nuclear medicine specialist.

All examination-related patient preparation should be carefully recorded (e.g., fasting or other dietary precautions, glucose loading). The name, dose, and route of administration of regulated nonradioactive drugs and contrast agents should also be stated. Blood glucose level and, if available, free-fatty acids level before FDG administration and heparin injection should be reported. Study-specific details should include the radiopharmaceutical, the amount of injected activity in megabecquerels (MBq), the route of administration (intravenous), and the date and time of administration. Furthermore, the used PET/MR system and instrumentation, such as coils, should be specified.

A description of the procedure should include the time interval between administration of the tracer and the start time of the acquisition, as well as a brief description of the CMR protocol. Also, the position of the patient's arms (elevated vs. aligned to the body axis) should be specified.

Depending on the CMR sequences used, the report should provide detailed information about the localization and extent of structural abnormalities of the myocardium including edema, perfusion deficits, infarcts, microvascular obstruction, hemorrhage, and fibrosis. Usually, the report should include data of left and/or right ventricular function analysis, analysis of regional wall motion, and myocardial mass. It also may include ventricular dimensions, which correlate to dimensions as measured in echocardiography to improve comparability.

For PET, the report should include a description of the location, the extent, and the intensity of pathologic tracer accumulation (specified as standardized uptake values) or reduction related to normal tissue. Extracardiac pathologies should be reported as well. If present, confounding factors that might influence the sensitivity or specificity of the study should be mentioned such as ubiquitous and undesired high or low tracer uptake in the myocardium (depending on the preparation and acquisition protocol).

In the conclusion, the study should be identified as normal or abnormal. The question asked in the study requisition should be directly

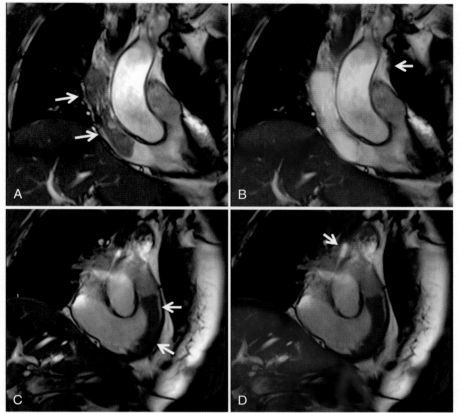

FIG. 50.6 Images of a patient with history of breast cancer (A, B). Images of a patient with anal cancer (C, D). In both patients, large intracavitary masses were initially found in echocardiography. Arrows in (A) and (C) show steady-state free precession (SSFP) images of large tubular masses in superior vena cava and right atrium (A) and in right ventricular outflow tract (C). (B, D) Fusion images of SSFP and positron emission tomography (PET) clearly demonstrating malignancy in the patient with breast cancer (B) and benign mass in the patient with anal cancer (D). However, closer inspection of PET images revealed mediastinal lymph node metastases in both patients (B, D; *arrows*). (From Nensa F, Tezgah E, Poeppel TD, et al. Integrated 18F-FDG-PET/MRI in the assessment of cardiac masses: a pilot study. *J Nucl Med.* 2014;56:255–260.)

addressed. If possible, a definite diagnosis should be stated. If necessary, recommendations for further imaging procedures should be given. Joint approval from a radiologist and a nuclear medicine specialist should be performed.

CONCLUSION

Integrated PET/MR has been clinically available for a few years and available studies and case reports have shown cardiac PET/MR to be reliable and suitable for clinical use. The MR system is not affected by the integrated PET, and MR-based AC provides sufficient accuracy for most clinical applications.

PET/MR has the potential to provide a more accurate and earlier diagnosis, as well as monitoring of cardiac diseases using the complementary strengths of both techniques. The prospects of multiparametric imaging need to be translated into diagnostic advantage. This requires dedicated multiparametric imaging protocols, specialized software for the integrated reading of multiparametric PET/MR studies, and the

definition of new compound biomarkers. Further technical improvements like MR-based PET motion correction will lead to higher spatial and temporal resolution, enabling advanced applications such as the imaging of valves and coronary arteries. Finally, the translation of innovative PET tracers from preclinical imaging into the clinical routine will open up exiting new possibilities. Promising fields of application include suspected CAD and AMI, inflammatory heart diseases such as myocarditis and cardiac sarcoidosis, and different cardiomyopathies, as well as cardiac tumors.

However, before the future clinical establishment of cardiac PET/MR, further studies need to demonstrate added value in comparison with current standard diagnostic procedures regarding diagnosis, monitoring, and, most importantly, patient outcome, to justify the investments in this rather complex and expensive technology.

REFERENCES

A full reference list is available online at ExpertConsult.com

51

Guidelines for Cardiovascular Magnetic Resonance

Christopher M. Kramer and Michael Salerno

Cardiovascular magnetic resonance (CMR) has become an increasingly important tool in the armamentarium of the cardiovascular imager. It has also had an increasingly prominent role in guidelines developed by various societies, including the Society for Cardiovascular Magnetic Resonance (SCMR), American College of Cardiology (ACC), American Heart Association (AHA), European Society of Cardiology (ESC), and other societies. The role of guidelines is to direct the field, reduce unwarranted variability, and improve the overall quality of the practice of cardiovascular imaging. Because it often takes years from concept to publication for societal guideline recommendations to be developed, they generally lag behind the state of the science and clinical trials and therefore must be taken into context. This chapter will review the state of CMR in recent guidelines.

The SCMR has put out several guideline documents. The first was the 2008 document that created standardized protocols for performance of CMR.[1] These protocols included most CMR procedures performed, from stress imaging to evaluation of cardiomyopathies, pericardial diseases, and so on. Some of the CMR manufacturers used these guidelines to create protocols on their scanners that could be used to follow these guidelines. These protocols were updated in 2013[2] and newer imaging pulse sequences, such as T1 and T2 mapping, were incorporated into the protocols.[2a] These will continue to be updated as the field evolves. Neither of these documents covered congenital heart disease protocols in sufficient depth and thus SCMR commissioned a separate protocol document to cover these diverse disease processes.[3]

Soon after the initial protocols document was published, the SCMR commissioned a document reviewing standardized reporting guidelines.[4] This document reviewed idealized reports for studies including how to report stress tests, volumetric studies, and so on. Many centers and report vendors have incorporated these guidelines into their reporting templates. Finally, the SCMR developed a document reviewing proper analysis techniques for various types of CMR images.[5] These included guidance for the quantification of left ventricular (LV) volumes from cine imaging and scar quantification from late gadolinium enhanced (LGE) images amongst others. This document set the standards for analysis that are being used in most CMR laboratories around the world.

In 2010, the ACC published a document that reviewed the state of the art in CMR including most of the standard clinical techniques and the evidence behind them.[6] This document was a consensus document with input from other societies including the AHA, SCMR, American College of Radiology (ACR), and North American Society of Cardiovascular Imaging (NASCI). The document was quite comprehensive and served as an up-to-date review of the field at that time. However, it did not serve as a guideline because no recommendations were made as to when a certain CMR procedure should or should not be used in a given clinical scenario. This document replaced an older consensus document regarding indications for CMR that was published in 2004 and developed through the ESC.[7]

CMR plays an important role in US multimodality guidelines with additional guidelines soon to be published. One crucial set of expert documents are the appropriate use criteria (AUC) developed by the ACC, in conjunction with many other societies that outline which imaging tests are (A) appropriate, may be (M) appropriate, or are rarely (R) appropriate, given a particular clinical scenario. The first set of AUC guidelines for CMR was published in conjunction with computed tomography (CT) in 2006[8] and evaluated each single imaging modality against appropriateness. This document evaluated only 33 clinical scenarios and identified 17 as appropriate for CMR, 7 as uncertain (now termed may be appropriate), 9 as inappropriate (now termed rarely appropriate). Appropriate indications for CMR included: (1) stress testing in patients who had intermediate pretest probability of coronary artery disease (CAD) and were unable to exercise or had an uninterpretable electrocardiogram (ECG); and (2) those with a stenosis identified by x-ray or CT angiography of unclear significance. Most of the appropriate indications were in the structure and function category, such as postmyocardial infarction, cardiomyopathies, myocarditis, complex congenital heart disease, cardiac masses, pericardial disease, and preatrial fibrillation ablation. Myocardial viability and valvular assessments were also deemed appropriate.

The initial AUC documents were single modality. Since that time, the field has evolved toward the development of multimodality imaging documents. The first of this type was the 2014 publication regarding the evaluation of patients with suspected or known ischemic heart disease.[9] In the ischemic heart disease document, CMR stress testing was rated appropriate in the same scenarios as listed previously for the single modality document, but also in symptomatic patients with high pretest probability of CAD. CMR was also deemed appropriate in patients with new systolic or diastolic heart failure and those with high-grade ventricular arrhythmias. Additional appropriate indications for CMR include patients with abnormal resting ECG and intermediate to high global CAD risk, and those with abnormal ECG stress studies or stenosis identified on prior x-ray or CT coronary angiography. Uncertain ECG stress findings or uncertain x-ray or CT coronary angiography results were also appropriate indications for CMR. Patients with new or worsening symptoms and prior ECG stress testing, nonobstructive CAD on x-ray angiography, obstructive CAD on CT coronary angiography, or coronary calcium score >100 were thought to be appropriate. Postrevascularization patients who were symptomatic with an ischemic equivalent were appropriate for CMR stress testing. Many other indications were considered as may be appropriate depending on the individual patient's clinical characteristics. AUC documents presently in preparation are in the structure and function category and will cover both myocardial and valvular diseases, which will likely include more of the key strengths of CMR.

Another set of guidelines for the management of patients with stable ischemic heart disease were published in 2012 by the ACC, in collaboration with multiple other organizations.[10] This document used slightly different gradings from the previously mentioned AUC documents. Recommendations are classified as class 1 (procedure should be performed), class IIa (it is reasonable to perform the procedure), class IIb (the procedure may be considered, or class III (procedure should not be performed). The level of evidence supporting the recommendations is also considered (A being the highest level with multiple randomized clinical trials or metaanalyses, B with a single randomized trial or nonrandomized studies, and C the lowest with only consensus opinions or case studies). Stress CMR received a class IIa recommendation (level of evidence B) for patients who are able to exercise with intermediate-to-high pretest probability of obstructive CAD and an uninterpretable ECG. This was lower than the class I recommendations for exercise stress echocardiography and stress single-photon emission computed tomography (SPECT) in the same setting. Similarly, stress CMR was classified as class IIa (level of evidence B) for patients in the same category but who are unable to exercise, which was again lower than the class I recommendation for pharmacologic stress echo and SPECT, likely because the latter techniques provide information about the patient's exercise capacity. For patients with known stable ischemic heart disease, CMR received a class IIa recommendation (level of evidence B) for patients who are able to exercise but have an uninterpretable ECG or for those who are unable to exercise regardless of ECG interpretability. CMR received a class I (level of evidence B) recommendation in patients with stable ischemic heart disease who are being considered for revascularization in the setting of known coronary stenosis with unclear physiologic significance. For patients with known stable ischemic heart disease and worsening symptoms who are incapable of exercise, again CMR was rated IIa (level of evidence B) whereas stress echo and SPECT were class I. In those with stable ischemic heart disease and silent ischemia who are unable to exercise, have an uninterpretable ECG, or were incompletely revascularized, all stress imaging modalities received a class IIa recommendation (level of evidence C). In summary, CMR was rated lower than stress ECG and SPECT in many of the clinical scenarios, but this document is several years old and it did state that more evidence would be generated in regards to the utility of CMR in these scenarios in the ensuing years.

In recent years, the ACC and ACR have partnered to develop two multimodality AUC documents that concern particular topics within cardiovascular medicine. The first such document covered imaging in heart failure and was published in 2013.[11] This document covered appropriateness of CMR, and all of the other major imaging modalities, in various clinical scenarios including new onset heart failure, ischemia, and viability evaluation, evaluation for implantable cardioverter-defibrillator (ICD) or biventricular pacemaker placement, and repeat evaluation of heart failure. CMR was rated as appropriate in many of these indications, with the exception of post-ICD or pacer placement because of the relative contraindication of CMR performance, as well as repeat evaluation of heart failure. The second ACC/ACR document covering AUC dealt with imaging in the emergency department and was published in 2015.[12] Clinical scenarios covered in this document included suspected ST elevation myocardial infarction (STEMI), chest pain and non-STEMI (NSTEMI), suspected pulmonary embolus, and suspected acute aortic syndrome. Appropriate roles for CMR in the emergency department were the use of stress CMR in the evaluation of the chest pain patient with myocardial infarction excluded, as well as in aortic syndromes. In many other scenarios, CMR was rated as may be or rarely appropriate.

ACC and ESC have led the way in the development of guidelines that cover specific disease processes and point out where CMR is of use in these diseases. The first such document was the 2008 ACC guideline for the management of patients with congenital heart disease.[13] CMR was recommended as an important modality to have available at a center that specializes in caring for the congenital heart disease patient. CMR was noted to be useful in many clinical conditions involving congenital heart disease, especially the postoperative patient, and was deemed complementary to ECG for many of these patients. In 2013, the ACC and AHA led the development of guidelines for the management of heart failure.[14] CMR received a class IIa level of evidence C recommendation for evaluation of LV volumes and function as well as for evaluation of myocardial scar and infiltrative diseases (class IIa, level of evidence B). By comparison, ECG received a Ia recommendation, level of evidence C, for initial evaluation of the heart failure patient. Any type of noninvasive evaluation (including CMR) was given a class IIa, level of evidence C, for evaluation of ischemia and/or viability in this setting, but with no discrimination between the various modalities. In the valvular disease management guidelines published in 2014,[15] CMR receives a class IA, level of evidence B, recommendation for evaluation of patients with moderate to severe aortic regurgitation or primary mitral regurgitation who have inadequate ECG windows and a class IA, level of evidence C, for evaluation of the aortic sinuses and ascending aorta for patients with bicuspid aortic valves and known aortic dilatation. CMR received a class IIb, level of evidence C, recommendation regarding its use in measuring right ventricular volumes in the setting of severe tricuspid regurgitation. With emerging literature regarding the utility of CMR in many more common conditions, its role in many of these guidelines will likely expand in the future.

CMR receives little mention in some of the ACC documents regarding common clinical conditions.[15a] For example, in the document regarding management of atrial fibrillation,[15] CMR was mentioned only in the data supplement as a potential method (with atrial LGE) to assess left atrial wall fibrosis. In the 2014 guideline covering management of the patient with NSTEMI, it is only recommended in the patient with stress (Takotsubo) cardiomyopathy.[16] In the 2015 supraventricular tachycardia guideline, CMR is only discussed as a method to assess the risk of arrhythmias in repaired tetralogy of Fallot patients.[17] In the 2013 AUC criteria regarding patient selection for ICD or cardiac resynchronization therapy (CRT), CMR is discussed as one of several imaging modalities to evaluate LV ejection fraction.[18] An exception to this lack of discussion of CMR in disease-specific guidelines is the 2014 Heart Rhythm Society document on patients with myocardial sarcoidosis,[19] which recommended CMR as a class IIA indication when a patient with extracardiac sarcoidosis has symptoms, ECG, or echocardiographic findings suggestive of possible cardiac involvement.

CMR indications are covered somewhat more frequently in current ESC documents than in ACC and AHA guideline documents but remains limited.[19a] In the 2016 ESC guidelines in regards to management of acute coronary syndromes,[20] CMR is discussed as an excellent method for the assessment of function, perfusion, and viability, but it does not have a particular recommendation for use in given clinical scenarios other than making the diagnosis of stress (Takotsubo) cardiomyopathy. CMR was given a more prominent role in the guideline document regarding the management of patients with sudden cardiac death.[21] For example, CMR or echocardiography was recommended as an evaluation for family members of patients with sudden cardiac death, and CMR is discussed as an alternative to echo for the evaluation of ventricular structure and function in patients with high-grade ventricular arrhythmias. CMR was recommended in pediatric patients with frequent premature ventricular contractions and it received a class IIB recommendation for the evaluation of patients with myocarditis.

In athletes with suspected structural heart disease, it was given a class 1C recommendation.

CMR was discussed quite extensively in the 2016 ESC heart failure guidelines.[22] It received a recommendation of class I, level of evidence C, for evaluation of LV structure and function in patients with poor echocardiographic windows and in patients with congenital heart disease. For discrimination of ischemic and dilated cardiomyopathy, CMR received a recommendation of class IIa, level of evidence C, and a class I, level of evidence C, for evaluation of infiltrative cardiomyopathies such as amyloidosis, Anderson–Fabry disease, sarcoidosis, noncompaction, Chagas disease, and hemochromatosis. CMR and other noninvasive stress modalities were given a class IIb, level of evidence B, recommendation in the evaluation of ischemia and viability in patients with ischemic cardiomyopathy before revascularization. In the 2014 Hypertrophic Cardiomyopathy guidelines,[23] CMR is discussed as a method to accurately measure increased wall thickness especially when some segment(s) are unable to be visualized by echocardiography (class IIa, level of evidence C). It also states that "CMR should be considered in patients with hypertrophic cardiomyopathy at their baseline assessment if local resources and expertise permit," class IIa, level of evidence B. CMR with LGE received a class IIa, level of evidence C, for evaluation of apical hypertrophic cardiomyopathy and for patients before septal myectomy or alcohol septal ablation. The document suggests repeating CMR every 5 years in stable disease or every 2 to 3 years in those with progressive disease (class IIb, level of evidence C).

In summary, CMR is slowly and steadily gaining traction in cardiovascular guideline documents. Overall, at the present time, ESC guidelines include a greater discussion of the role of CMR than ACC/AHA guidelines.[15a,19a] As more data become available from ongoing large multicenter clinical trials and registries, and with the ongoing expansion of CMR access, CMR will undoubtedly have an ever-increasing role in guidelines regarding the management of patients with cardiovascular disease.

REFERENCES

A full reference list is available online at ExpertConsult.com

52

Noncardiac Pathology

Muhammad Shahzeb Khan, Kiran Khurshid, and Faisal Khosa

Eyes do not see what the mind does not know (Anonymous).

Cardiovascular magnetic resonance (CMR) has been increasingly incorporated into clinical practice as a noninvasive method that offers superior structural and functional assessment of the heart, especially in patients presenting with complex cardiac pathology, congenital cardiac diseases and cardiomyopathies. Because CMR is a cross-sectional modality, it provides complementary information on noncardiac structures adjacent to the heart, including the mediastinum, lungs, chest wall, and upper abdomen. The acquisition of imaging field data outside the heart offers the opportunity for detection of these noncardiac findings.

Indications for CMR: The American College of Cardiology Foundation[1] has listed many conditions considered appropriate for CMR. The major indications include the following:
1. Assessment of right ventricular (RV) and left ventricular (LV) systolic function in cases of:
   - Cardiac failure
   - Arrhythmias
   - Pulmonary hypertension
   - Cardiomyopathy
2. Assessment of myocardial perfusion:
   - Ischemic heart diseases (angina)
3. Evaluation of cardiac blood flow in the following conditions:
   - Valvular heart diseases, for example, aortic regurgitation, mitral regurgitation, aortic stenosis, mitral and so on
   - Shunts: atrial septal defect, ventricular septal defect, patent ductus arteriosus and so on
4. Inflammatory/neoplastic conditions:
   - Pericarditis: constrictive, serous, inflammatory and so on
   - Cardiac tumors; myxoma, rhabdosarcoma, carcinoids and so on
   - Thrombus
5. Congenital cardiac diseases
6. Coronary artery imaging
7. Assessment of myocardial viability:
   - After myocardial infarction

The anatomic region, or more accurately, the field of view covered during a routine CMR extends beyond the conventional boundaries of the heart and associated major vessels to include all the thoracic viscera as well as the upper abdominal organs. Hence, it is not uncommon to encounter findings in the thoracic or upper abdominal viscera incidentally while conducting a routine CMR. In fact, studies have shown that the prevalence of the noncardiac findings on the routine CMR is quite high[2] and requires in certain cases prompt attention of not only the radiologist but also of the attending physician.

An in-depth knowledge of entities affecting different organs in the field of view and a keen eye to detect these noncardiac findings can lead to the reduction in morbidity, mortality in certain cases, and can also add up to screening value. In certain cases the detection and characterization of these noncardiac findings can pose a challenge to the interpreting medical personnel who are reviewing and reporting these studies.

WHAT IS AN INCIDENTAL NONCARDIAC FINDING?

Incidental findings are defined as the previously undiagnosed medical conditions that are discovered unintentionally and may be unrelated to the current medical condition which is being investigated or for which tests were being performed.

Location of the noncardiac incidental findings: in case of CMR, the organs or systems in which incidental findings may be identified include:
- Liver and gall bladder
- Kidneys and adrenal glands
- Spleen
- Peritoneum
- Lungs and pleura
- Breast
- Thyroid, esophagus, and vasculature
- Bones; involving ribs, vertebrae, and sternum

CLASSIFICATION OF INCIDENTAL NONCARDIAC FINDINGS BASED ON CLINICAL SIGNIFICANCE

The incidental findings encountered during CMR can be broadly divided into the following categories:
1. Clinically important incidental noncardiac findings: comprise findings that require further clinical or radiological workup and/or an intervention. Not effectively doing so in a timely manner can have negative consequences for the patient. Examples include:
   - Pulmonary nodules
   - Solid/complex lesions of solid abdominal viscera
   - Malignant breast lumps
   - Esophageal cancers
   - Thyroid masses
   - Aortic pathology including aneurysms or dissection, to name a few
2. Moderately important incidental findings: include the findings that may or may not have an effect on patient care depending on medical history or symptomology. In other words, mortality and morbidity is not directly related to the prompt diagnosis and addressing of these findings. Examples include, but are not limited to, the following:
   - Liver adenoma or focal nodular hyperplasia
   - Complex renal and adrenal lesions
   - Aortic plaques
3. Clinically unimportant incidental noncardiac findings: these are the findings that are benign and are inconsequential for the patient. Their presence however sometimes can point to disease

TABLE 52.3 Significant Findings That Changed Treatment

First Author	Field Strength Used (T)	Magnetic Resonance Image or Report Review	Interpreter	Significant Findings That Changed Treatment	Significant Findings That Required Further Invasive Testing
Dewey	1.5	Image	Radiologist	2	—
McKenna	1.5	Image	Radiologist	—	—
Chan	—	Report	Radiologist and/or cardiologist	6	3
Atalay	1.5	Image and report	Radiologist	9	6
Khosa	1.5	Image	Radiologist and/or cardiologist	7	—
May	1.5	Report	Radiologist and/or cardiologist	—	—
Wyttenbach	1.5	Image	Radiologist	—	—
Irwin	1.5	Report	Radiologist and/or cardiologist	8	—
Sohns	1.5	Image	Radiologist and/or cardiologist	13	8
Secchi	1.5	Image and report	Radiologist	—	—
Roller	1.5	Image	Cardiologist	—	—
Greulich	1.5	Report	Radiologist and/or cardiologist	8	—
Dunet	1.5 and 3	Image	Radiologist	11	—
Mahani	—	Report	Radiologist	—	—

findings. A recent metaanalysis[2] showed that the combined prevalence of major noncardiac pathology found on CMR that changed the patient management was only 1% (95% CI: 1%–2%). This value increased to 2% if anomalies of the great vessels were included. It is important to consider that none of the studies had a long-term (>3 years) follow-up of patients. Hence, it is difficult to comprehend how much these incidental findings can impact patient mortality.

IMPACT OF PATIENT'S GENDER ON INCIDENTAL FINDINGS

We found four studies[7,9,14,17] that investigated the relationship of patient's gender with the number of incidental findings. None of the studies reported any significant correlation between gender and noncardiac pathology except for Khosa et al.[14] This was primarily due to the benign finding of gynecomastia in men, which they had considered as an incidental finding, compared with other studies that had not taken gynecomastia into account. Once gynecomastia was excluded from the analysis, even Khosa et al. found no significant difference in frequency of noncardiac pathology among men and women (36% vs. 38%, respectively, $P = .85$). Moreover, Wyttenbach et al.[17] also explored the possible gender difference between those who had significant extracardiac findings versus those who did not. The analysis revealed no statistically significant difference ($P = .27$). Thus it can be implied that CMRs should be thoroughly studied for incidental findings in both the genders because they have similar odds of having an important or unimportant extracardiac pathology.

IMPACT OF PATIENT'S AGE ON INCIDENTAL FINDINGS

All the studies that investigated the link between patient's age and frequency of noncardiac pathology found statistically significant trends. Khosa et al.[14] showed that the age of those with noncardiac findings was more advanced than those without extracardiac findings (56 vs. 48 years, $P < .001$). Similar results were published by Chan et al.[7] (54 ± 16 years vs. 49 ± 16 years, $P < .001$) and Wyttenbach et al.[17] (58.3 ± 14 years vs. 49.1 ± 17 years; $P < .0001$). Atalay et al.[9] documented an interesting trend showing that no significant difference existed between middle age groups (40–59 years) and younger age groups (<40 years).

However, if the sample was categorized into <60 years and >60 years, a significant difference was noted not only in the prevalence of incidental findings (33% vs. 59%, respectively) but also in important noncardiac findings (1% vs. 12%). May et al.[16] also commented that the positive correlation of age and frequency of noncardiac pathology was mainly caused by increasing prevalence of incidental findings in people age older than 40 years. The literature suggests there is a sharp increase in prevalence of incidental findings from the age group 40 to 60 years. Thus it is vital that interpreting clinicians be on the lookout for noncardiac pathology, especially in the older population, considering it may have impact on clinical management.

CARDIOLOGY AND RADIOLOGY REVIEWING OF CARDIOVASCULAR MAGNETIC RESONANCE

Few studies have reported original data on the impact of a radiologist and cardiologist reading the CMR simultaneously. Khosa et al.[14] was one of the first to highlight this important issue. The results showed that a combined readout using a concomitant radiologist and cardiologist lead to a significantly increased reporting of all noncardiac findings ($P < .0001$). A combined readout was used in around 80% (384/495) of all CMR performed in the study. The serial readout (independent interpretation by a cardiologist and radiologist at separate reading sessions) resulted in only 15% of all noncardiac findings being reported, compared with 42% for combined readout. More importantly, this vast difference was also present when only the indeterminate and worrisome findings were considered (56% for combined readout vs. 33% for serial readout, $P = .03$). Hence the data showed that a concurrent readout may have an important impact on the detection of possible management-altering extracardiac findings.

Similar results were published by Greulich et al.[12] in 2014. Their data showed that a joint approach reported 200 previously unknown noncardiac findings in 138 patients versus 23 noncardiac findings in 23 patients when the report was read by a cardiologist alone ($P < .001$). The trend remained significant ($P < .0001$), even when only the major extracardiac findings were considered. In contrast with Khosa et al. and Greulich et al., Irwin et al.[13] found no significant association between detection of noncardiac pathologies and read-out by a cardiologist or a radiologist ($P = .38$). The reporting rates by a cardiologist and radiologist for noncardiac pathology were found to be 24.3% and 27.5%, respectively. Also, for major incidental findings, the reporting rates were found to be similar (12.5% for radiologist vs. 13.0% for cardiologist, $P = .84$).

IMPACT OF DIFFERENT CARDIOVASCULAR MAGNETIC RESONANCE SEQUENCES IN DETECTING INCIDENTAL PATHOLOGY

Many studies have investigated the association between different sequences of CMR and detection of incidental findings. McKenna et al.[8] found no significant difference ($P = .369$) between the coronal localizer, axial localizer, and short axis multislice sequences in detecting incidental noncardiac findings. The three sequences were able to visualize 47%, 46%, and 41% of all noncardiac pathologies, respectively. Review of these three sequences had significantly ($P = .013$) higher chance of detecting noncardiac findings compared with transmitral flow cine, aortic pulsatility cine, and the single slice vertical long axis cine. Their study established that localizer sequences, owing to their larger field of view, are critical in detecting noncardiac pathology on CMR.

Moreover, the study by Khosa et al.[14] showed that among the various CMR sequences, the following were most revealing of incidental findings:
- Thoracic single-shot fast balanced steady-state free precession (bSSFP) scout sequences in the sagittal, coronal, and axial planes (field of view 450×450)
- Axial T1 weighted fast spin echo (FSE) sequence

The authors postulated that 99% of the management-changing incidental noncardiac findings were detected on either one of these two sequences. Out of the total of 295 incidental noncardiac findings detected on the CMRs included in their study, 63% of the findings were picked up on the thoracic bSSFP scout sequence, whereas 60% of the noncardiac incidental findings were detected by the axial T1-weighted fast spin echo sequence. The other views highlighted in the study included assessment of LV and RV systolic functioning using bSSFP long axis, contiguous short axis, four-chamber, and LV outflow tract views and velocity encoded flow imaging of the proximal aorta and the proximal main pulmonary artery.

These sequences served as complimentary in some cases to the bSSFP and T1-weighted fast spin echo. In some instances, the other CMR sequences detected the incidental findings that were already known before the study. This study also reviewed the contrast enhanced CMR, which offered a very limited field of view, mainly of the heart and the major blood vessels, and hence did not play any meaningful role in displaying the noncardiac incidental findings.

Atalay and his colleagues[9] stated that out of the five principal pulse sequences in their study, axial stacked bright-blood and dark-blood sequences had the highest sensitivity for displaying incidental noncardiac findings (73% and 70%, respectively). The remaining imaging sequences yield was less than 25%. On subanalysis of their results, it was found that despite having lower overall detection rates for incidental findings, multiplanar viability imaging had the best sensitivity for visualizing abdominal noncardiac findings. Similarly, it was observed that bright-blood methods and axial dark-blood were the most revealing of incidental findings in the thorax.

As shown by other authors, Wyttenbach et al.[17] also demonstrated that coronal, axial, and sagittal scout sequences are the best to detect nonsignificant and also potentially management-changing extracardiac findings. Late gadolinium enhancement (LGE) and cine bSSFP images were the next best with a detection rate of 47% and 34%, respectively.

Because of difference in institutional policy, individual expertise, and preference, there is great heterogeneity between the type and number of different sequences used by each of the studies. This not only impacts the overall detection rate of noncardiac findings but also makes it challenging to pool the data regarding different CMR sequences and compare the available evidence.

COST EFFECTIVENESS OF REPORTING INCIDENTAL NONCARDIAC PATHOLOGIES

Although the cost effectiveness of CMR in the assessment of coronary artery disease (CAD) has been studied, to date there is no study that has investigated the economic impact associated with these findings. Roller et al.[18] briefly touched on this topic by suggesting that additional axial bSSFP chest sequences do not offer any benefit in the visualizing of additional incidental findings and concluded that, in a world of severe time constraints, reviewing these additional sequences for noncardiac findings is not cost effective when high quality survey images are already generated. However, they did not give any economic or cost analysis/evaluation. Furthermore, no data exists on the possible negative impact of reporting incidental findings on patient's anxiety and stress levels. Apart from patient anxiety, such incidental findings can culminate into potentially harmful interventions in the pursuit of a diagnosis that does not even exist. Hence, it is imperative that future research is geared toward characterizing the positive predictive value and specificity to avoid unnecessary financial and emotional implications in this cost-conscious era.

We also feel that increased communication between different physicians is vital to improve the relevance of noncardiac findings. The focus should not be on findings that can theoretically change management but on the findings that can practically change management in the specific subset of patient population. The true significance of each finding can only be gauged when it is put into each individual patient's clinical context. The interpreting clinician must be provided with important aspects of the patient's medical history to suspect a truly significant finding. However, this approach of suspecting extracardiac findings based on history removes the actual significance of incidental findings, which is to detect unsuspected findings. The real question remains how wide we should open our eyes to detect these findings and how long should we look for them on every image when a CMR study can have thousands of images.

Interphysician communication level can also reduce costs by comparing incidental noncardiac findings with previous reports and providing clear follow-up recommendations. Moreover, many authors who are in favor of reporting all incidental findings argue that physicians have an ethical obligation and a medicolegal duty to report all pathology in the field of view. We believe that until cost-benefit analysis studies come out, the most prudent way to approach the incidental findings will be to provide clear advice in the CMR report. The practice of writing detailed and specific reports can be the key tool in preventing health care dollars being spent on needless managements.

INCIDENTAL FINDINGS CLASSIFIED BY BODY SYSTEM

The thorax and upper abdomen are the primary regions that are included in the CMR field of view and hence where noncardiac pathology is observed. Most of the studies had the highest number of incidental findings in the thoracic region. Atalay's[9] study yielded a total of 114 noncardiac incidental findings limited to the chest territory out of the total of 240 findings. The other studies showing remarkable relevance of finding noncardiac incidental pathology limited to the chest included Khosa et al.,[14] with the study yielding 162 chest findings in a total of 495 cases. Other notable mentions include the studies conducted by Wyttenbach et al.,[17] Irwin et al.,[13] and Greulich et al.[12] as shown in Table 52.4.

TABLE 52.4   Incidental Findings Classified by Body System

First Author	Total Thorax Findings	Significant Thorax Findings	Total Abdomen Findings	Significant Abdomen Findings	Miscellaneous Findings	Significant Miscellaneous Findings
Dewey	3	2/3	6	0/6	0	0/0
McKenna	95	15/95	115	9/115	14	1/14
Chan	90	8/90	36	0/36	3	0/3
Atalay	114	12/114	46	3/46	2	1/2
Khosa	162	14/162	66	0/66	67	0/67
May	38	16/38	22	8/22	39	12/39
Wyttenbach	106	56/106	128	21/128	16	7/16
Irwin	110	7/110	38	1/38	32	0/32
Sohns	116	31/116	157	10/157	13	8/13
Secchi	—	—	—	—	—	—
Roller	—	21	—	3	—	1
Greulich	246	112/246	67	23/67	44	35/44
Dunet	—	—	—	—	—	—
Mahani	44	6/44	74	13/74	27	0/27

The metaanalysis by Dunet et al.[2] revealed that almost half of the minor extracardiac findings are observed in the thorax. The most common minor thorax findings were pleural effusion (15.7%) and parenchymal lung opacities or consolidation (11.8%). The abdomen, which constituted ~40% of minor incidental findings, was primarily affected by hepatic and renal cysts. Note that when considering only the major incidental findings, the thoracic region is by far the most common region where suspected lesions can be found (thoracic 72% vs. abdominal 20.2%). In terms of organs, lung parenchyma (15%), kidney (14.3%), and liver (16.4%) were the most commonly affected overall. These findings indicate that CMR practitioners should pay close attention especially to liver and lung parenchyma.

The most important incidental findings in the thorax region are briefly discussed here:

- Lung nodule: The close proximity of the lungs to the heart, and large field-of-view images on thoracic scout and axial T1-weighted spin echo images results in the inclusion of the lung fields in all CMR studies. A lung nodule is by far the most worrisome noncardiac incidental finding on CMR. Although the prevalence of lung nodules on routine CMR is quite low, ignoring or misinterpreting this finding can culminate in dire consequences. In the study by Atalay et al.,[9] 5 new cancers (including 2 that were pulmonary) were diagnosed on CMR. In many instances, the lung nodule may be benign requiring only periodic follow-up according to guidelines by the Fleischner Society; but in some instances, the lung nodule can show a more sinister pathology, morphing into lung cancer or metastasis (Fig. 52.1). Lung lesions are termed a lung nodule if the lesion is <3 cm or a lung mass if it is >3 cm. Because there is no effective universal screening available for lung tumors at present, early detection and management of lung lesions detected incidentally on chest imaging can have an important impact on the morbidity and mortality. Thus, it is vital that any lung nodule, diagnosed incidentally on CMR, be compared with prior imaging (i.e., CT) or followed-up to ensure stability. In addition, seemingly benign noncardiac lung findings such as atelectasis, pleural effusion, and air space disease can point to a graver pathology. It is therefore advisable to follow-up these noncardiac findings to resolution.
- Aortic dissection: This is another less prevalent but potentially lethal incidental finding requiring urgent diagnosis and treatment (Fig. 52.2). Moreover, the risk of aortic dissection is significantly

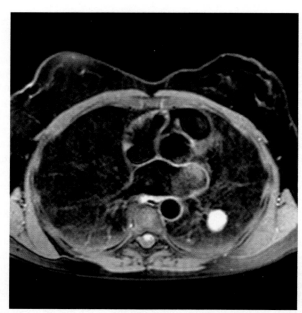

FIG. 52.1 Axial fat saturation T2-weighted axial spin echo demonstrating a bright lung nodule. Subsequent evaluation determined this to be pulmonary carcinoid.

higher in women, especially in the third trimester of pregnancy or postpartum.

- Thyroid nodules: The axial scouts and axial T1 spin echo thoracic stack often include images of the thyroid. Very few (4%–6%) of incidentally identified thyroid nodules are ultimately proven to represent thyroid malignancies. The vast majority are benign colloid nodules. The thyroid malignancy shows bimodal age distribution with the peaks occurring in the patients in their 20s and 70s. Thyroid cancers have an excellent prognosis if caught early, before the development of distant metastasis. Hence, their incidental finding necessitates follow-up. The studies conducted by May et al.,[16] Greulich et al.,[12] and a few others have laid special emphasis in observing the neck region while reporting CMR, to check for thyroid nodules.

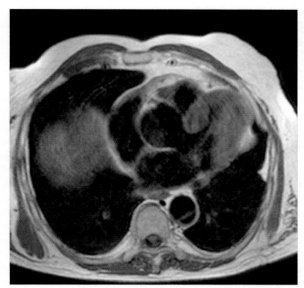

FIG. 52.2 Axial T1-weighted spin echo image demonstrating a descending thoracic aortic dissection.

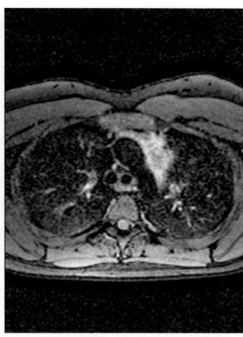

FIG. 52.3 Axial T1-weighted postcontrast image demonstrated an enhancing mediastinal mass representing lymphadenopathy in a patient with lymphoma.

- Lymphadenopathy: A relatively common noncardiac finding of the mediastinum and the neck region is enlarged lymph nodes. The study by Khosa et al.[14] showed lymphadenopathy in 4% of 495 overread CMRs, whereas Chan et al.[7] showed lymphadenopathy as an incidental noncardiac finding in <1% of 1534 of CMR reports. Greulich et al.[12] found 51 (5%) incidental lymph node findings in 1074 CMR studies. The reason why these studies identified nodal pathology in such large numbers may be because of the simultaneous or coreporting of a radiologist and a cardiologist. There is a multitude of causes of enlarged nodes, ranging from a reactive lymphadenopathy as a result of infection to a more gruesome malignant pathology. In cases of lymphoma, detecting lymphadenopathy incidentally on a routine CMR study can help establish early diagnosis and with proper referral may impact mortality. Fig. 52.3 shows an enhancing mediastinal mass in a patient with known lymphoma.
- Pulmonary embolism: Few studies have commented on the importance of pulmonary embolism as an incidental noncardiac CMR finding (Fig. 52.4). In the Dunet et al.[11] cohort, pulmonary embolism was the most frequent ($N = 15$, 3.1%) major extracardiac diagnosis. Eight of those patients were further tested, of which five were confirmed for pulmonary embolism. According to the literature[2] the pooled prevalence of pulmonary embolism as a major noncardiac finding is 1.2%.
- Breast lesions: The breasts are typically displayed in both scout images and thoracic T1-weighted spin echo images. Breast cancer is the most common cancer among women and if caught early can have excellent prognosis. Lesions of the breast, especially in women over the age of 40 years should always be reported, compared with mammography (if available) and followed-up closely for malignancy. In younger women, the CMR findings usually represent benign lesions such as a breast fibroadenoma or fibrocystic changes. In any case, it is best to further evaluate any breast pathology and to compare with prior imaging (e.g., mammography).
- Gynecomastia: The only study reporting gynecomastia as a noncardiac incidental finding was of Khosa et al.[14] who reported 41 cases of gynecomastia (Fig. 52.5). Gynecomastia is usually clinically unimportant. In some cases, it may indicate important undiagnosed

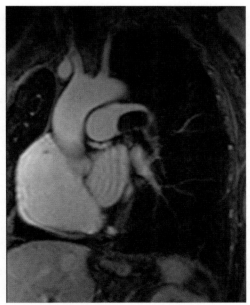

FIG. 52.4 Oblique coronary cardiovascular magnetic resonance angiogram demonstrating a pulmonary embolism in the left main pulmonary artery.

pathology, that is, pituitary tumor (prolactinoma), cirrhosis, or adrenal pathology.
- Skeletal lesions: Any incidental bone lesions should be thoroughly evaluated for metastasis. May et al.[16] in their research on pediatric population found cases of syringomyelia as a clinically significant incidental finding on CMRs performed on patients aged younger than 20 years. The other less prevalent vertebral lesions requiring

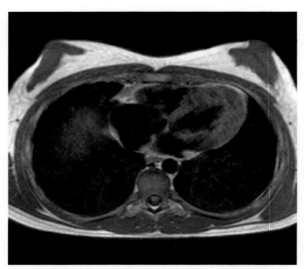

FIG. 52.5 T1-weighted axial image demonstrating bilateral gynecomastia.

attention and follow-up include indeterminate bone lesions, degenerative disc disease with herniation, and disc prolapse. Mild degrees of scoliosis usually do not require any follow-up. The study conducted by Khosa et al.[14] identified a few cases of scoliosis ranging from mild to severe degrees of deformity. Bony deformity of chest wall (pectus) and adjoining ribs may be congenital or indicative of nutritional deficiency.

- Soft tissue lesions: mostly lipomas, are seen as an insignificant incidental finding in the chest as well in the abdomen. Almost all CMR studies reported lipomas as an incidental pathology in various locations. In most cases, lipomas do not require follow-up.

Although the heart resides in the thorax, scout images and axial T1-weighted spin echo images frequently include the mid abdomen to upper-abdomen in the field of view. Frequently seen noncardiac findings in abdomen include:

- Renal cystic lesions: Most renal cysts are simple and prevalent among people of all ages, race, and gender. However, a minority of the cysts can be complicated representing a more serious underlying pathology, such as malignancy or polycystic kidney disease. Complicated cysts may show irregular margins, septations, calcification, or enhancement. Complicated cysts require further clinical follow-up, and in some cases removal. The frequency of renal cysts found in various studies is similar and constitutes 10% to 20% of all noncardiac findings. It has been shown that complex renal cysts represent 7% of all important noncardiac pathologies, whereas simple renal cysts contribute to 18% of all minor noncardiac pathology.[2] Only a few studies have commented on the presence of hydronephrosis as an incidental noncardiac finding. McKenna et al.[8] and Atalay et al.[9] all detected a couple of cases of hydronephrosis.

- Hepatic cystic lesions: These are mostly benign liver lesions showing predilection for the right lobe of the liver. In most cases, they do not require follow-up or monitoring. The simple cysts are benign developmental lesions that do not communicate with the biliary tree and originate from hamartomatous tissue. The cysts can be solitary or multiple, and seen in 2% to 7% of the population with no age or gender preference.[2] The studies conducted by Chan, Khosa, and Wyttenbach reported hepatic cysts as noncardiac findings (11.6%, 5.8%, and 14.8%, respectively). Pooled analysis reveals that hepatic cysts or hemangiomas are responsible for approximately 20% of all minor noncardiac pathology. In terms of clinically significant findings, hepatic masses and cirrhosis have frequency rates of 11.5%; other lesions encountered may be adenoma, focal nodular hyperplasia, and metastatic disease.[2]

- Gallstones: Widely prevalent in females 40 years of age and older, gallstones are normally considered clinically unimportant because they do not require any immediate medical attention. However, a stone in the gall bladder has the potential to dislodge into the common bile duct or pancreatic duct, causing choledocholithiasis or pancreatitis.

- Hiatal hernia: In most cases, a hiatal hernia is a clinically unimportant congenital or acquired anomaly discovered incidentally on CMR. In almost all cases, it does not require any further radiological or clinical follow-up. Hiatal hernia represents 5% of all minor noncardiac findings, whereas a diaphragmatic hernia constitutes only 0.6% of all noncardiac pathology.[2]

CONCLUSION: PROS AND CONS OF REPORTING INCIDENTAL FINDINGS

The documentation and reporting of noncardiac findings on CMR has been a matter of much debate. Those who are in favor of reviewing CMR images and reporting noncardiac findings claim that appropriate follow-up of these incidental findings in certain cases can serve as a screening tool for various diseases. Moreover, fatal diseases, such as lung and breast cancers, can be detected by keen observation of noncardiac pathology and patients may (although unproven) benefit from early interventions.

Those not in favor of reviewing CMRs for noncardiac pathology base their argument on the fact that most of the noncardiac findings are not clinically important or are benign and aggressive evaluation or pursuit of these usually yields futile results and potential morbidity. The follow-up can result in unnecessary financial strain on both the patient and the health care budget, resulting in a waste of resources. It also causes false alarm and undue worry among the patients. Finally, no prospective study has demonstrated any clinical benefit of early detection of noncardiac findings.

REFERENCES

A full reference list is available online at ExpertConsult.com

CMR Screening Form: Beth Israel Deaconess Medical Center (BIDMC)—CMR Center

Cardiac MR Center
East Campus/Gryzmish 4
Telephone – 617-667-8555
Fax – 617-975-5480

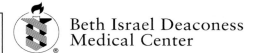
Beth Israel Deaconess Medical Center

Date of Birth ___/____/_____

Date __/___/20__ Name_____ Height___ in Weight_____ lbs

An MRI involves the use of a very strong magnet. For your safety, the presence of certain metallic objects must be determined _before_ you enter the exam room. Please place a check in the appropriate column for each item below.

	Yes	No		Yes	No
1. Have you had an MRI before?			17. Do you have a Port-a-cath or Hickman device?		
If yes, did you receive a contrast injection?			If yes, is it accessed?		
2. Pacemaker/Pacer wires/Implantable defibrillator			18. Are you on dialysis? If yes, how often:_____		
3. Metallic heart valve or any metallic stents			19. Please **list** all surgeries:		
4. Intracranial or brain aneurysm clip/brain surgery			_____		
5. Bio or neurostimulator, electronic device, or implant			_____		
6. Tattoo(s), Tattooed eyeliner If yes, location (s):_____			_____		
7. Body piercing If yes, location (s):_____			20. Please **circle** if you have any of the following medical conditions:		
8. Metal injury to the eye requiring medical attention			**Asthma/Hay fever Heart Disease Multiple Myeloma** **Thyroid Disease Pheochromocytoma Sickle Cell Disease**		

9. Shrapnel/gunshot (metal in body)			**FEMALES**	Y E S	N O	**MALES**	Y E S	N O
10. Eye prosthesis/surgery on eye								
11. Ear prosthesis/surgery on ear			21. Possibility of pregnancy?			24. Do you have a penile implant?		
12. Limb or joint replacement or pinning								
13. Tissue expander (e.g., breast implant)			22. IUD (intrauterine device) or diaphragm			If yes, make and model:		
14. Implanted pump (insulin, pain med, chemotherapy)						_____		
15. Are you wearing a patch that delivers medication?			23. Pessary (in pelvis)?			_____		
16. Do you have a history of difficult IV starts?								

Personal items such as these should be left in the lockers provided.

Cell phone/Electronic devices	Wallet/Keys	Watch/Jewelry	Credit and ATM cards	Hearing aids	Metal hair clips/pins/accessories

Cardiac MR Center
East Campus/Gryzmish 4
Telephone: 617-667-8555
Fax: 617-975-5480

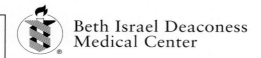

Beth Israel Deaconess
Medical Center

Date of Birth ____/____/_____

Ethnic Origin and Race: *We need this information to accurately calculate your kidney function.*

25. ETHNICITY: (Check one) ❑ Hispanic or Latino   ❑ Not Hispanic or Latino

RACE: (Check all that Apply)

❑ White   ❑ Black or African American

❑ Asian   ❑ Native Hawaiian or Other Pacific Islander

❑ American Indian or Alaska Native

Choyke questionnaire (Choyke PL, Tech Urol 1998;4:65–69)	Yes	No
26. Have you ever been told you have kidney problems?		
27. Have you ever been told you have protein in your urine?		
28. Have you ever had high blood pressure?		
29. Do you have diabetes?		
30. Have you ever had gout?		
31. Have you ever had kidney surgery?		

32. Please **list** below any allergies to medications, food, or latex: ❑ NONE	Reaction

33. Please **list** below all prescription and over-the-counter medications you take:	Last Dose Date & Time	
	/ /	:
	/ /	:
	/ /	:
	/ /	:
	/ /	:
	/ /	:
	/ /	:
	/ /	:
	/ /	:
	/ /	:
	/ /	:

34. Are you taking any of the following medications?   ❑ **NO**

❑ Revatia   ❑ Adcirca   ❑ Viagra   ❑ Levitra   ❑ Cialis   ❑ Sildenafil   ❑ Vardenafil   ❑ Tadalafil **Last Dose: __ am/pm __/__/20___**

These drugs can interfere with certain aspects of some cardiac MRI examinations. If you take <u>any</u> of these drugs for erectile dysfunction you should **refrain** from taking these medications for 48 hours (2 days) prior to your cardiac MRI. If you take any of these drugs for pulmonary hypertension you should **NOT** stop taking your medication, but MUST inform the Cardiac MR Center staff before your examination.

Patient Signature_____ Relationship (if not the patient)_____ Date __/__/20___

Signature of Nurse or Technologist_____ Date __/__/20___

CMR Sequence Protocols in Use (2018) at the Beth Israel Deaconess Medical Center (BIDMC)—CMR Center

Protocols

Protocol: [ ]   Resched/Prior Cancellation ☐   Prior CMR ☐

Protocol	Sequences
LV/RV function only	S1, F1, (F13 if AF or ectopy), P1, P2, S2, A1, S10, (S11 if Gd)
ARVC (+/− Gd)	S1, F1, F9, P1, P2, S2, S6, (G5Gd if abnl RV), S10 (S11Gd if Gd)
Mitral Valve (Prolapse)/AORTIC Valve	S1, F1, F6, P1, P2, S2, A1, S10, (S11Gd if Gd)
Pulmonic Valve/Pulmonary Artery	S1, F1, F9, P1, P2, S2, F8, A1, S10, (S11Gd if Gd)
Tricuspid Valve	S1, F1, F5, P1, P2, S2, A1, S10, (S11Gd if Gd)
Pericardial Constriction (Gd)	S1, F1, F13 (4Ch, MidSA), F11, P1, P2, S2, G5Gd, G6Gd, A1, S10, S11Gd
Pericarditis - Acute (Gd)	S1, F1, F11, P1, P2, S2, G5, G6, A1, S10, S11Gd
Cardiomyopathy (Gd)	S1, F1, P1, P2, S2, A1, G3Gd, G5Gd, (if +: G4Gd), S10, S11Gd
HCM/Amyloid add-on	F11, G1Gd, (Apical aneurysm: G7Gd)
Dilated (hemo, sarcoid, VT...) add-on	S7, S8, S9, G1Gd, G5Gd, (aneurysm: G7Gd), (first CMR: C2); (pre CRT/ICD: F11)
CAD Viability (Dobutamine - (fellow; Gd)	S1, F1, P1, P2, G3Gd, S2, A1, dobut 5mcg/kg/min x 5 min --> F1, S10, S11
PV Ablation (pre-ablation)	S1, F1, S2, (AF: BH-F12), (Sinus: P1, P2, S10, A5 (if Gd: S11, A3Gd, G5Gd, G8Gd), A1
PV Ablation: follow-up/?PV stenosis (Gd)	S1, F1, (AF: F13), (Sinus: P1, P2, S10, (S11Gd if Gd) (no P1, P2 if prior), A3Gd, G6Gd, A1
Coronary Arteries/Veins (+/− Gd)	S1, CAD-C3Gd (anomalous: TNG-A1); CABG grafts – C2), F1, S2, P1, P2, A1
Congenital (Fellow, Gd)[a]	S1, F1, (F3 if ASD), F5, P1, P2, S2 (P4-special views), A1, S10 (S11 if Gd)
Aorta (aneurysm, coarctation) (Gd)	S1, F1, P1, P2, S2, S4, A1 (A2Gd), (F10 if dissection)
Cardiac Mass/Tumor (Fellow, Gd)	S1, F1 (F13 if atrial), F5, P1, P2, S2, S6; special views, E1 (mass), A1, S10 (S11 if Gd)
Stress (exercise (fellow, Gd)	S1, F1, F12; out of magnet, exercise: F12, E2, rest E1, S2, P1, P2, G3Gd
Stress - vasodilator (fellow, Gd)	S1, F1; vasodilator: E2; rest: E1, S2, P1, P2, G3Gd

[a]Also see Chapters 40 and 41 for disease-specific congenital protocols as well as Fratz S, Chung T, Greil GF, et al. Guidelines and protocols for cardiovascular magnetic resonance in children and adults with congenital heart disease: SCMR expert consensus group on congenital heart disease. *J Cardiovasc Magn Reson*. 2013;15:51.

Also see Kramer CK, Barkhausen J, Flamm SD, et al. Standardized cardiovascular magnetic resonance (CMR) protocols 2013 update. *J Cardiovasc Magn Reson*. 2013;15:91.

Sequences – Structure/Function

⊙ Worksheet-test

Protocol Fellow [▼]

⟲ Scouts, LV/RV, AoV, PV, Ao/PA Flow   No Gd ☐

Structure (S)

(S1) Scouts – Sag/cor/axial	☐	Done	☐
(S2) T1w Bl blood (axial,5mm)	☐	Done	☐
(S3) T1w Bl blood w/fat sat (axial)	☐	Done	☐
(S4) T1w Bl blood (oblique/aorta)	☐	Done	☐
(S5Gd) Post Gd T1 axial	☐	Done	☐
(S6) DIXON axial stack	☐	Done	☐
(S7) T2 STIR (short axis stack)	☐	Done	☐
(S8) T2w Bl blood (axial)	☐	Done	☐
(S9) T2* (hemochromatosis)	☐	Done	☐
(S10) T1 & T2 mapping	☐	Done	☐
(S11Gd) ECV mapping	☐	Done	☐

Function: Breath-hold cine (F)

(F1) Short axis stack;2,3,4Ch;AoV	☐	Done	☐
(F2) Short axis LV stack (8/2)	☐	Done	☐
(F3) Left atrial short axis stack	☐	Done	☐
(F4) TFE cine left atrial stack	☐	Done	☐
(F5) 4 Ch (stack)	☐	Done	☐
(F6) LVOT/3 Ch stack	☐	Done	☐
(F7) 2 Ch (stack)	☐	Done	☐
(F8) Pulmonic valve (axial)	☐	Done	☐
(F9) RVOT/PA (stack)	☐	Done	☐
(F10) SSFP aorta candy cane	☐	Done	☐
(F11) CSPAMM (SAx3;2Ch;4Ch)	☐	Done	☐
(F12) Real-time 2/4/mid SA cine	☐	Done	☐

Function: Free-breathing cine (F)

(F13) Real-time 4Ch/midLVSAcine	☐	Done	☐

MRA/LGE/Flow/Stress/Coronaries

Early/Late Gadolinium enhancement (GE)

(G1Gd) Early GE – 3D PSIR	☐	Done	☐
(G2Gd) Early GE – 2D (2Ch, 4Ch)	☐	Done	☐
(G3Gd) LGE 3D PSIR LV SA	☐	Done	☐
(G4Gd) LGE 2D (2ch, 4ch)	☐	Done	☐
(G5Gd) High Res 3D LGE LV	☐	Done	☐
(G6Gd) High res 3D LGE LA	☐	Done	☐
(G7Gd) Long TI 3D LGE-LV Thromb	☐	Done	☐
(G8Gd) Long TI 3D LGE-LA Thromb	☐	Done	☐

MR Angiogram (A)

(A1) 3D Isotropic thoracic MRA	☐	Done	☐
(A2Gd) CE-MRA Aorta	☐	Done	☐
(A3Gd) CE MRA-pulmonary veins	☐	Done	☐
(A4) Non-contrast aorta MRA	☐	Done	☐
(A5) Non-con pulmonary vein MRA	☐	Done	☐

Flow/Phase velocity (P)

(P1) Ascending aorta-axial	☐	Done	☐
(P2) Pulmonary artery - coronal	☐	Done	☐
(P3) ASD - through plane	☐	Done	☐
(P4)Through plane of interest	☐	Done	☐

Stress/Exercise (E)

(E1) Rest perfusion (short axis)	☐	Done	☐
(E2) Vasodil stress perfusion (SA)	☐	Done	☐
(E3) Low dose dobutamine (SA)	☐	Done	☐
(E4) Physiologic stress-ergometry	☐	Done	☐

Coronary artery/graft imaging (C)

(C1) Targeted 3D cor MRA	☐	Done	☐
(C2) Whole heart cor 3D MRI	☐	Done	☐
(C3Gd) CE whole heart cor MRA	☐	Done	☐
(C4) Isotropic whole heart 3D MRI	☐	Done	☐
(C5) Whole heart cor vein MRI	☐	Done	☐

Analogous CMR Terminology Used by Various Vendors

Sequence Type	Philips	Siemens	GE	Hitachi	Canon (Toshiba)
Spin echo	SE	SE	SE	SE	SE
Multispin echo	Multi SE	Multi echo/MS	SE	SE	Multi echo
Fast spin echo	Turbo SE (TSE)	Turbo SE (TSE)	FSE (Fast SE)	FSE (Fast SE)	FSE (Fast SE)
Fast spin echo with 90-degree flip-back pulse	DRIVE	RESTORE	FRFSE	Driven Equilibrium FSE	T2 plus FSE
3D fast spin echo with variable flip angle	VISTA	SPACE	CUBE	isoFSE	3D MVOX
Ultrafast spin echo (echo planar fast spin echo)	Single shot TSE	HASTE	SS-FSE	Single shot FSE	FASE/SuperFASE
Chemical shift fat saturation		Fat-sat	CHESS		Fat-sat
Combined chemical shift and inversion recovery	SPIR		SPECIAL/SSRF		
Combined chemical shift and adiabatic inversion recovery	SPAIR	SPAIR			SPAIR
Dixon fat suppression	mDixon	Dixon	IDEAL/FLEX	fatSep	WFOP
Water excitation	ProSet	WE	SSRF		PASTA/WET
Inversion recovery	IR	IR/IRM	IR	IR	IR
Fast inversion recovery	IR TSE	Turbo IR/TIRM	FSE-IR	FIR	Fast IR
Short T1 inversion recovery	STIR	STIR	STIR	STIR	STIR
Long Tau inversion recovery	FLAIR/FLAIR TSE	FLAIR/Turbo FLAIR	FLAIR/Fast FLAIR	FLAIR/Fast FLAIR	FLAIR/Fast FLAIR
True inversion recovery (phase-sensitive inversion recovery)	Real IR/PSIR	Ture IR/PSIR	T1 FLAIR/PSIR	T1 FLAIR/PSIR	PSIR
Gradient recalled echo	FFE	GRE	GRE	GE	Field Echo (FE)
Spoiled gradient echo	T1-FFE	FLASH	SPGR	RSSG	T1-FFE/RF Spoiled FE
Ultrafast gradient echo	T1-TFE /T2-TFE THRIVE, eTHRIVE	TurboFLASH VIBE	Fast GRE/Fast SPGR VIBRANT/FAME/LAVA	RGE SARGE	Fast FE RADIANCE/QUICK 3D
Ultrafast 3D gradient echo	TFE/3D T1-TFE	MP-RAGE	3D FGRE, 3D fast SPGR	MP-RAGE	
Ultrafast gradient echo with magnetization preparation	IR TFE	T1/T2 TurboFLASH	IR-prepped, DE-SPGR, BRAVO		Fast FE
T1-weighted gradient echo with fat suppression	THRIVE, eTHRIVE	VIBE	LAVA, LAVA XV, LAVA FLEX, FAME	TIGRE	QUICK 3D

Sequence Type	Philips	Siemens	GE	Hitachi	Canon (Toshiba)
Coherent gradient echo	FFE	FISP	GRASS	Rephased SARGE	FE
Coherent gradient echo with echo refocusing	T2-FFE	PSIF	SSFP	Time-Reversed SARGE	SSFP
Balanced gradient echo	Balanced FFE (BFFE)/BTFE	TrueFISP	FIESTA	BASG	True SSFP
Coherent balanced gradient echo with dual excitation		CISS	FIESTA-C	PBSG	
Echo planar	EPI	EPI	EPI	EPI	EPI
Gradient recalled echo plus spin echo (hybrid echo)	GRASE	TGSE			Hybrid EPI
Spoiled gradient echo using combined multiple free induction decays	M-FFE	MEDIC	MERGE		
Spin echo black-blood (cardiac)	Black-blood prepulse	Dark-blood prepared TSE, HASTE	Double IR FSE w/ blood suppression		
Spin echo fat-suppressed black-blood (cardiac)	Black-blood prepulse with SPIR or SPAIR	TIRM	Double IR FSE with blood suppression		
Single shot black blood	Single shot TSE (SSH-TSE)/ Ultrafast spin echo (UFSE)	HASTE	Single shot-FSE (SS-FSE)	Single shot fast SE	Fast advanced SE (FASE)
Time-of-flight MR angiography	Inflow MRA	TOF	TOF		
Fluroscopic triggering sequence	Bolus TRAK	Care Bolus	Fluoro trigger	FLUTE	VISUAL PREP
Time-resolved contrast-enhanced MR angiography with k-space manipulation	4D-TRAK	TWIST	TRICKS		
Contrast-enhanced MR angiography	CE Angio	CE-MRA	CE-MRA	CE-MRA	CE-MRA
Noncontrast angiography (inflow balanced SSFP with inversion recovery saturation)	TRANCE/B-TRANCE	NATIVE TrueFISP	Inhance Inflow IR (IFIR)	VASC-ASL	Time-SLIP
Contrast-enhanced MR with moving table (bolus-chase)	MobiTrak, MobiFlex	TimCT	SmartStep		
Real-time interactive scan	Interactive	CARE	iDRIVE		
Susceptibility-weighted imaging	Venous BOLD	SWI	SWAN		
Parallel imaging technique	SENSE	iPAT	ASSET		RAPID
Parallel imaging	SENSE	mSENSE	SENSE	SENSE	SENSE
Parallel imaging with k space–based algorithm		GRAPPA	ARC		

3D, Three-dimensional; *MR,* magnetic resonance.
Prepared with the assistance of Patrick Pierce, RT(MR), and Tim Leiner, MD, PhD.

INDEX

Page number followed by *t*, *f*, or *b* indicates table, figure, or box, respectively.